OXFORD MED

Paedi
Neurology

Oxford Specialist Handbooks published and forthcoming

Oxford Specialist Handbooks in Paediatrics

Paediatric Neurology

Fourth Edition

Edited by

Rob Forsyth

Senior Lecturer in Child Neurology, Newcastle University;
and Honorary Consultant Paediatric Neurologist, Newcastle
Hospitals NHS Foundation Trust, Newcastle upon Tyne, UK

Daniel E Lumsden

Consultant Paediatric Neurologist Evelina London Children's
Hospital; and Adjunct Clinical Senior Lecturer, Biomedical
Engineering and Imaging Sciences, King's College London, UK

and

Filipa Rodrigues

Paediatric Neurologist, Local Health Unit of the Aveiro Region;
and Egas Moniz Health Alliance Clinical Academic Centre,
University of Aveiro, Portugal

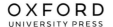

OXFORD
UNIVERSITY PRESS

OXFORD
UNIVERSITY PRESS

Great Clarendon Street, Oxford, OX2 6DP,
United Kingdom

Oxford University Press is a department of the University of Oxford.
It furthers the University's objective of excellence in research, scholarship,
and education by publishing worldwide. Oxford is a registered trade mark of
Oxford University Press in the UK and in certain other countries

First Edition published in 2007
Second Edition published in 2012
Third Edition published in 2018
Fourth Edition published in 2024

Published in the United States of America by Oxford University Press
198 Madison Avenue, New York, NY 10016, United States of America

British Library Cataloguing in Publication Data
Data available

Library of Congress Control Number: 2024940102

ISBN 978–0–19–889264–9

DOI: 10.1093/med/9780198892649.001.0001

Printed in the UK by
Bell & Bain Ltd., Glasgow

For our families:
Pip, Ellen and Beth for the journey and the joy;
Rebecca, Abby, and Jonathan for their love, support and tolerating the
time to write;
Mum and dad for their example. My brother for the unconditional love.
João and Luis for being there and all the laughs.
To those we meet through our work who support us and teach us
so much.

Preface

Preface to the Fourth Edition

In the years since the first edition of this book the science and practice of paediatric neurology have changed more than we could have possibly anticipated. Genetic advances continue to revolutionize investigation and have dramatically shortened the diagnostic journey travelled by families and clinicians alike; and with new treatments in many areas, most notably neuromuscular disease, and epilepsy, we are moving from 'describers of disorders' to 'deliverers of interventions'. New treatments have transformed the experience of neurological disease for many families, created new clinical phenotypes to study and understand, and create new challenges to meet ever growing expectations of what's becoming possible. In all this change, the core skills of attentive listening and careful examination, and the communication of understanding, reassurance, and hope become ever more relevant: reprieve from the diagnostic odysseys that perhaps preoccupied us in the past gives us more time to focus on the human.

This marks the first edition that has not benefited from Richard Newton's wisdom. We thank him for all that he brought to the project; and welcome Dan and Filipa to the editorial team bringing younger and, in Filipa's case, international perspectives from which this edition has greatly profited.

Preface to the Third Edition

In the few years since the second edition, the themes of our second edition preface seem to have become ever more relevant. The 'next generation' genetics revolution is indeed sweeping through paediatric neurology as we were predicting then. Gene panels bring 'one stop shops' for some of our common diagnostically challenging scenarios (such as early onset epileptic encephalopathies), but also new clinical challenges in the interpretation of findings of uncertain significance. In the last 30 years, we have developed the clinical skills to handle and interpret advanced neuroimaging: in the next decade or so we will need to develop analogous skills in the interpretation of genetic data.

It is an enormous privilege to be practicing in such a rapidly developing, fascinating speciality: but as ever it is the humanity we bring to the bedside that matters most.

Preface to the Second Edition

The very gratifying response to the first edition of this book has justified our belief in the value of a team approach: contributors with their fingers on the pulse of advances in our field, steadied at the helm by two editors with experience and perspective. It has, again, been a great privilege: never has Lord Acton's advice to 'learn as much from writing books as from reading them' been better heeded!

We have appreciated the very constructive suggestions for improvement of the first edition and followed them where we can. We have added respiratory consults to Chapter 6, and included more neuroradiology diagrams and images in situations where they offer clarity. A section on late-onset metabolic disease is added with an emphasis on how this group of disorders might catch us out.

With an ever-increasing list of genes and autoantibodies to think about it is important to remember those everyday skills we carry, honed as juniors in our specialty: listening to what is truly being said, careful clinical examination, focused investigation, and above all the communication of understanding, reassurance, and hope to families and young people facing challenges they never dreamed existed. You will find due emphasis on this in the text.

We trust this book will become a trusted companion. Please continue to tell us how it can be improved!

Preface to the First Edition

Medicine is a communal discipline, and this book has benefited greatly from being written in community by trainees (who remember the recent struggle to grasp a complex area) and older colleagues who can add particular emphases and perspective. We've striven to provide a combination of practical advice on clinical approach and 'at a glance' oversights and *aides-memoire* to topic areas. We also wanted to address a number of practical issues that occupy a lot of time in practice but that are rarely addressed in more conventional textbooks.

Acknowledgements

Stavros Stivaros, of Royal Manchester Children's Hospital provided some MR images. Hilary Reidpath, Senior Technician in the Neurophysiology Department at the Royal Hospital for Sick Children Glasgow and Dr Ming Lai, Consultant Neurophysiologist at the Royal Victoria Infirmary Newcastle upon Tyne kindly supplied EEG illustrations.

We are very grateful to Anna Basu, Tracy Briggs, Hilary Cass, Nuno Cordeiro, Christian de Goede, Pooja Harijan, Cheryl Hemingway, Imelda Hughes, Susan Kafka, Ram Kumar, Omar Kwaja, Andrew Lux, Chris O'Brien, Ki Pang, Kate Riney, Sophia Varadkar, Grace Vassallo, and John Walter who contributed so generously to previous editions.

We are grateful to Saboo Chowdhury and Pip Gaunt for proofreading, but any remaining errors are, of course, our responsibility.

Contents

Detailed contents

Contributors to the fourth edition

Omar Abdel-Mannan
Speciality Trainee in Paediatric Neurology, Great Ormond Street Hospital, London, UK

Simon Bailey
Honorary Professor of Paediatric Neuro-oncology, Newcastle University and Great North Children's Hospital, Newcastle upon Tyne, UK

Rob Forsyth
Senior Lecturer and Honorary Consultant Paediatric Neurologist, Newcastle University and Great North Children's Hospital, Newcastle upon Tyne, UK

Yael Hacohen
Consultant Paediatric Neurologist, Great Ormond Street Hospital, London, UK

Anthony Hart
Consultant Paediatric Neurologist, Kings College Hospital, London, UK

Rachel Kneen
Consultant Paediatric Neurologist, Alder Hey Children's Hospital, Liverpool, UK

Dan Lumsden
Consultant Paediatric Neurologist, Evelina Children's Hospital, London UK.

Robert McFarland
Professor and Honorary Consultant Paediatric Neurologist, Newcastle University and Great North Children's Hospital, Newcastle upon Tyne, UK

Sithara Ramdas
Consultant Paediatric Neurologist, Oxford University Hospitals NHS Trust and Oxford Children's Hospital, Oxford, UK

Filipa Rodrigues
Paediatric Neurologist, Centro Hospitalar Baixo Vouga, Aveiro, Portugal

Vicky Tsang
Clinical Pharmacist, Evelina Children's Hospital London, UK

Brian Wilson
Consultant Clinical Geneticist, Newcastle upon Tyne Hospitals NHS Foundation Trust, Newcastle, UK

Symbols and abbreviations

❶	Warning
►	Important
►►	Don't dawdle
♂	Male
♀	Female
ℬ	Online
➔	Book
3,4-DAP	3,4-diaminopyridine
5HIAA	5-hydroxyindoleacetic acid
5MTHF	5-methyl terahydrofolate
AAC	assistive/augmentative communication
AADC	Aromatic L-amino acid decarboxylase
AASA	L-alpha-aminoadipic semi-aldehyde
ABC	Airway, breathing, circulation
ABG	Arterial blood gases
ABI	Acquired brain injury
ACC	Agenesis of the corpus callosum
ACE	Angiotensin converting enzyme
AChR	Acetylcholine receptor
ACTH	Adrenocorticotrophic hormone
AD	Autosomal dominant
(AD)ANE	(Autosomal dominant) acute necrotizing encephalopathy
ADAR	Adenosine deaminase acting on RNA
ADC	Apparent diffusion coefficient (in MRI)
ADEM	Acute disseminated encephalomyelopathy
ADH	Antidiuretic hormone
ADHD	Attention deficit hyperactivity disorder
ADI/ADOS	Autism Diagnostic Inventory/ Observation Schedule
ADS	Acquired demyelinating syndrome
AFB	Acid fast bacilli
AFM	Acute flaccid myelitis
AFP	Alpha-feto protein

AGAT	Arginine-glycine amidinotransferase
AGS	Aicardi–Goutières syndrome
AIDP	Acute inflammatory demyelinating neuropathy
AIDS	Acquired immunodeficiency syndrome
AIS	Arterial ischaemic stroke
ALL	Acute lymphoblastic leukaemia
ALTE	Acute life-threatening event (see also BRUE)
AMAN	Acute motor axonal neuropathy
AMC	Arthrogryposis multiplex congenita
AMPA(-R)	α-amino-3-hydroxy-5-methyl-4-isoxazole proprionic acid (receptor)
AMRF	Action myoclonus renal failure syndrome
AMSAN	Acute motor and sensory axonal neuropathy
ANCA	Antineutrophil cytoplasmic antibodies
AOA	Ataxia oculomotor ataxia
APD	Afferent pupillary defect
AQP4	Aquaporin 4
ART	Anti-retroviral treatment
ASA	Arginosuccinic acid
ASL	Arterial spin labelling (MRI sequence)
ASM	Antiseizure medication (was 'antiepilepsy drug', AED)
ASOT	Anti-streptolysin 'O' titre
AT	Ataxia telangiectasia
ATPO	Antithyroid peroxidase antibody
AVED	Ataxia with vitamin E deficiency
AVM	Arteriovenous malformation
BAER/P	Brainstem auditory evoked response/potential
BBB	Blood brain barrier
BD	(Latin: bis in die) = twice daily
BFMDRS	Burke-Fahn-Marsden Dystonia Rating Scale

BH4	Tetrahydrobipterin (neurotransmitter synthesis cofactor)		CK(-MB)	Creatinine phosphokinase (MB = cardiac muscle related isoform)
BIND	Bilirubin-induced neurologic dysfunction (kernicterus)		CLIPPERS	Chronic lymphocytic inflammation with pontine perivascular enhancement responsive to steroids
BMD	Becker muscular dystrophy			
BNF-C	British National Formulary for Children		CLN	Neuronal ceroid lipofuscinosis subtypes (see also NCL)
BOLD	Blood oxygen level dependent (MRI brain activity signal)		CMAP	Compound muscle action potential
BPAN	Beta-propeller protein-associated neurodegeneration		CMD	Congenital muscular dystrophy
BRUE	Brief Resolved Unexplained Events		CMS	Congenital myaesthenic syndrome
BVVL	Brown-Vialetto-van Laere (syndrome)		CMT	Charcot-Marie tooth Disease
			CMV	Cytomegalovirus
CACH	Childhood ataxia with CNS hypomyelination (= Vanishing White Matter disease)		CNS	Central nervous system
			CNV	Copy number variant
CADASIL	Cerebral autosomal dominant arteriopathy with subcortical infarcts and leukoencephalopathy		COACH	cerebellar vermis hypo- or aplasia, oligophrenia, congenital ataxia, ocular coloboma, and hepatic fibrosis
CAE	Childhood absence epilepsy		COVE	Childhood onset visual epilepsy
CAMHS	Child and adolescent mental health services		COVID	Coronavirus (SARS-CoV2) disease
CAR-T	Chimeric antigen receptor (CAR) T-cell		COX	Cytochrome oxidase
CBF	Cerebral blood flow		CP	Cerebral palsy
CBT	Cognitive-behavioural therapy		CPEO	Chronic progressive external ophthalmoplegia
CBZ	Carbamazepine		CPH	Chronic paroxysmal hemicranias
CDD	Creatine deficiency disorder			
CDG	Congenital disorder of glycosylation (also known as carbohydrate deficient glycoprotein syndrome)		CPP	Cerebral perfusion pressure
			CPR	Cardiopulmonary resuscitation
			CRP	C-reactive protein
CFM	Cerebral function monitor		CRPS	Chronic regional pain syndrome
CGH	Comparative genome hybridization		CRTR	Creatine transporter
			CSE	Convulsive status epilepticus
CGRP	Calcitonin gene related peptide		CSF	Cerebrospinal fluid
			CSI	Craniospinal irradiation
CHARGE	Coloboma, heart defects, (choanal) atresia, (growth) retardation, genital/urinary and ear abnormalities (syndrome)		CSW	Cerebral salt wasting
			CSWS	Continuous spike-wave discharges during slow-wave sleep
CHM	Commission on Human Medicines		CTA	Computerized tomographic angiography
CIDP	Chronic inflammatory demyelinating neuropathy		CTG	Cardiotocograph
CINCA	Chronic infantile neurological cutaneous and articular (syndrome)		CVI	Cerebral (or cortical) visual impairment
			CVP	Central venous pressure
CIS	Clinically isolated syndrome		CVST	Cerebral venous sinus thrombosis

CVVH	Continuous veno-venous haemofiltration	EEM	Epilepsy with eyelid myoclonia
CXR	Chest X-ray	EIDEE	Early infantile developmental epileptic encephalopathy
DA	Dopamine		
DBS	Deep brain stimulation	EIMFS	Epilepsy of infancy with migrating focal seizures
DCD	Developmental coordination disorder		
		ELISA	Enzyme-linked immunosorbent assay
DEE	Developmental and epileptic encephalopathy		
		EMAtS	Epilepsy with myoclonic–atonic seizures
(D)EE-SWAS	(Developmental) epileptic encephalopathy with spike-and-wave activation in sleep		
		EMG	Electromyography
		EOG	Electrooculogram
DEXA	Dual-energy X-ray absorptiometry	EOS	Early onset sarcoid
		EPC	Epilepsia partialis continua
DHAP-AT	Dihydroxy acetone phosphate acyl transferase	ERG	Electroretinogram
		ESES	Electrical status during slow-wave sleep (synonymous with CSWS)
DI	Diabetes insipidus		
DIDMOAD	Diabetes insipidus, diabetes mellitus, optic atrophy, and deafness		
		EVD	Extra-ventricular drain
		EZ	Epileptogenic zone
DIS	Disseminated in space (MS criterion)	FCA	Focal cerebral arteriopathy
		FCD	Focal cortical dysplasia
DIT	Disseminated in time (MS criterion)	FFEVF	Familial focal epilepsy with variable foci
DKA	Diabetic ketoacidosis	FII	Factitious or induced illness
DM	Myotonic dystrophy	FIRES	Febrile infection-related epilepsy syndrome
DMD	Duchenne muscular dystrophy		
DMSA	Dimercapto succinic acid (kidney radioisotope scan)	FISH	Fluorescent in-situ hybridization
DNC	Death by neurological criteria	FLAIR	Fluid attenuated inversion recovery—MRI sequence
DNET	Dysembryoplastic neuroepithelial tumour		
		fMRI	Functional MRI
DRD	DOPA responsive dystonia	FMTLE	Familial mesial temporal lobe epilepsy
DRPLA	Dentato-rubral-pallido-luysian atrophy		
		FND	Functional neurological disorder
DSA	Digital subtraction angiography		
DSM(-IV)	Diagnostic and Statistical Manual of mental disorders (fourth edition)	FS+	Febrile seizures 'plus'
		FSH	Facio-scapulo-humeral muscular dystrophy
		FTT	Failure to thrive
DTI	Diffusion tensor imaging (MRI)	FVC	Forced vital capacity
DWI	Diffusion-weighted image (MRI)	GA	General anaesthetic
		GABA	Gamma amino-butyric acid
EAF	Epilepsy with auditory features	GAD	Glutamic acid decarboxylase
EBV	Ebstein–Barr virus	GAG	Glycosaminoglycans
ECG	Electrocardiogram	GAMT	Guanidinoacetate methyltransferase
ECMO	Extra-corporeal membrane oxygenation		
		GAS	Group A streptococcus
EDH	Extra-dural haemorrhage	GBS	Guillain-Barré syndrome
EDMD	Emery Dreifuss muscular dystrophy	GC-MS	Gas chromatography mass spectroscopy
EE	Epileptic encephalopathy		
EEG	Electroencephalogram	GCS	Glasgow coma score

GCT	Germ cell tumour
GEFS+	Generalized epilepsy with febrile seizures plus
GFAP	Glial fibrillary acidic protein
(e)GFR	(estimated) Glomerular filtration rate
GGE	Generalized genetic epilepsies
GHB	Gamma hydroxy-butyrate
GIT	Gastrointestinal tract
GLUT1(DS)	Glucose transporter enzyme 1 (deficiency syndrome)
GMFCS	Gross motor function classification syndrome
GMFM	Gross motor function measure
GMH	Germinal matrix haemorrhage
GORD	Gastroesophageal reflux disease
GSD	Glycogen storage disease
GTC	Generalized tonic–clonic seizure
GTCA	Epilepsy with generalized tonic–clonic seizures alone
HAART	Highly active anti-retroviral therapy
HCG	Human chorionic gonadotrophin
HELLP	Hemolysis, elevated liver enzymes with low platelet count
HHT	Hereditary haemorrhagic telangiectasia
HHV	Herpes hominis virus
HIE	Hypoxic-ischaemic encephalopathy
HIV	Human immunodeficiency virus
HLA	Human leucocyte antigen—the major human hostocompatability antigens
HLH	Haemophagocytic lymphohistiocytosis
HMN	Hereditary motor neuropathy
HMSN	Hereditary sensory motor neuropathy
HNPP	Hereditary neurolpathy with liability to pressure palsies
HOCUM	Hypertrophic obstructive cardiomyopathy
HPE	HIV-associated progressive encephalopathy
HPO	Human phenotype ontology
HSAN	Hereditary sensory and autonomic neuropathy

HSCT	Haematopoietic stem cell transplantation
HSV(E)	Herpes simplex virus (encephalitis)
HUS	Haemolytic uraemic syndrome
HVA	Homo-vanilic acid
IBD	Inflammatory bowel disease
ICD(-10)	International Classification of Diseases (version 10)
ICF	International Classification of Functioning, Disability, and Health
ICHD	International Classification of Headache Disorders
ICP	Intracranial pressure
IDDM	Insulin dependent diabetes mellitus
IEF	Iso-electric focussing
IEM	Inborn errors of metabolism
IESS	Infantile epileptic spasms syndrome
IGE	Idiopathic generalized epilepsy
IHS	International Headache Society
IIH	Idiopathic intracranial hypertension
IIM	Idiopathic inflammatory myopathy
ILAE	International League against epilepsy
IM	Intramuscular
INAD	Infantile neuraxonal dystrophy
IOP	Intraocular pressure
IPH	Intraparenchymal haemorrhage
ITB	Intrathecal baclofen
IU	International unit
IUD	Intrauterine device
IUGR	Intrauterine growth retardation
IV	Intravenous
IVA	Isovaleric acidaemia
IVH	Intraventricular haemorrhage
IVIG	Intravenous immunoglobulin
IVMP	Intravenous methylprednisolone
JAE	Juvenile absence epilepsy
JEV	Japanese encephalitis virus
JME	Juvenile myoclonic epilepsy
JRA	Juvenile rheumatoid arthritis
KF	Kaiser–Fleischer (ring)

KSS	Kearn Sayre syndrome		MNGIE	Myopathy and external ophthalmoplegia; Neuropathy; Gastrointestinal; Encephalopathy
LCHAD	Long-chain 3-hydroxyacyl-CoA dehydrogenase			
LCMV	Lymphocytic Choriomeningitis Virus		MOG(AD)	Myelin oligodendrocyte glycoprotein (antibody-mediated disease)
L-DOPA	L-3,4-dihydroxyphenylalanine (levodopa)		MPAN	Mitochondrial membrane protein-associated neurodegeneration
LETM	Longitudinally-extensive transverse myelitis			
LEV	Levetiracetam		MPS	Mucopolysaccharidosis
LGMD	Limb girdle muscular dystrophy		MRA	Magnetic resonance angiography
LGS	Lennox–Gastaut syndrome		MRC	Medical Research Council
LHON	Leber's hereditary optic neuropathy		MRI	Magnetic resonance imaging
			MRS	Magnetic resonance spectroscopy
LKS	Landau–Kleffner syndrome			
LMN	Lower motor neurone		MRV	Magnetic resonance venography
LMWH	Low molecular weight heparin		MS	Multiple sclerosis
MACS	Manual ability classification system		MSLT	Multiple sleep latency test
MAO(I)	Mono-amine oxidase (inhibitor)		MSUD	Maple syrup urine disease
			MTHFR	Methyltetrahydrofolate reductase
MAP	Mean arterial pressure			
MCAD	Medium chain acyl coenzyme A		MTLE-HS	Mesial temporal lobe epilepsy with hippocampal sclerosis
MCT	Medium chain triglyceride		MUP	Motor unit potential
MCV	Motor conduction velocity		NAA	N-acetyl aspartate
MDEM	Multiphasic disseminated encephalomyelitis		NAI	Non-accidental (head) injury
MECP2	Methyl-CpG-binding protein 2 gene—common Rett syndrome gene		NARP	Neuropathy, ataxia, and retinitis pigmentosa
			NBIA	Neurodegeneration with brain iron accumulation
MEGDEL	3 MEthylGlutaconic acid Deafness, Encephalopathy, and Leigh-like neuroimaging		NCL	Neuronal ceroidal lipofuscinosis (see also CLN)
MEI	Myoclonic epilepsy in infancy		NCSE	Non-convulsive status epilepticus
MELAS	Mitochondrial encephalomyopathy, lactic acidosis, and strokelike episodes		NCV	Nerve conduction velocity
			NEAD	Non-epileptic attack disorder
			NEC	Necrotizing enterocolitis
MERRF	Myoclonic epilepsy and ragged-red fibre		NEDA	No evidence of disease activity (demyelinating disease endpoint)
MERS	Mild encephalopathy with a reversible splenial lesion			
MG	Myaesthenia gravis		NF	Neurofibromatosis
MHRA	Medicines and Healthcare products Regulatory Agency		NGS	Next generation sequencing
			NGT	Naso-gastric tube
MIBG	Metaiodobenzyl guanidine (Iodine123)		NICE	National Institute of Clinical Excellence
MLD	Metachromatic leucodystrophy		NICU	Neonatal intensive care unit
MLF	Medial longitudinal fasciculus		NIH	National Institutes of Health
MMA	Methylmalonic acidaemia		NIHSS	NIH stroke severity (score)
MMSE	Mini-mental state examination			

NIPPV	Non-invasive positive pressure ventilation	
NIV	Non-invasive ventilation	
NKH	Nonketotic hyperglycinemia	
NMDA(-R)	N-methyl-D-aspartate (receptor)	
NMO(SD)	Neuromyelitis optica (spectrum disease)	
NPC	Niemann–Pick disease, type C	
NPV	Negative predictive value	
NSAID	Non-steroidal anti-inflammatory	
NTD	Neural tube defect	
OCD	Obsessive compulsive disorder	
OCP	Oral contraceptive pill	
OCT	Optical coherence tomography	
OD	Once daily	
OFC	Occipitofrontal (head) circumference	
OGB	Oligoclonal bands	
OGD	Oesophagogastroduodenoscopy	
OKN	Optokinetic nystagmus	
OMS	Opsoclonus-myoclonus syndrome (Kinsbourne)	
OSA	Obstructive sleep apnoea	
OT	Occupational therapist	
PANDAS	Paediatric autoimmune neuropsychiatric disorders associated with streptococcal infection	
PANS	Paediatric acute neuropsychiatric syndrome	
PCH	Pontocerebellar hypoplasia	
PCR	Polymerase chain reaction	
PCWP	Pulmonary capillary wedge pressure	
PDD	Pervasive developmental disorder	
PDE	Pyridoxine dependent epilepsy	
PDH	Pyruvate dehydrogenase	
PECS	Picture exchange communication system	
PED	Paroxysmal exertional dyskinesia	
PEDI	Pediatric Evaluation of Disability Inventory	
PEEP	Positive end-expiratory pressure	
PEG	Percutaneous endoscopic gastrostomy	

PEHO	Progressive encephalopathy with oedema, hypsarrhythmia, and optic atrophy
PEJ	Percutaneous endoscopic jejunostomy
PERM	Progressive encephalomyelitis with rigidity and myoclonus
PET	Positron-emission tomography
PHACES	Posterior fossa malformations–hemangiomas–arterial anomalies–cardiac defects–eye abnormalities–sternal cleft and supraumbilical raphe syndrome
PHT	Phenytoin
PKAN	Pantothenate kinase-associated neurodegeneration
PKD	Paroxysmal kinesigenic dyskinesia
PKU	Phenylketonuria
PLAN	PLA2G6-associated neurodegeneration
PLEDS	Periodic lateralized epileptiform discharges
PLEX	Plasma exchange (plasmapheresis)
PLP	pyridoxal 5 phosphate
PMD	Pelizaeus-Merzbacher disease
PME	Progressive myoclonus epilepsy
PML	Progressive multifocal leucoencephalopathy
PNDC	Progressive neuronal degeneration of childhood with liver disease (Alpers)
PNET	Primitive neuroectodermal tumour
PNKD	Paroxysmal non-kinesigenic dyskinesia
PNPO	Pyridoxine 5'-phosphate oxidase
PNS	Peripheral nervous system
PO	By mouth (Latin per os)
POLE	Photosensitive occipital lobe epilepsy
PPT	Palmitoyl-protein thioesterase
PPV	Positive predictive value
PR	Rectally (Latin per rectum)
PRES	Posterior reversible encephalopathy syndrome
PRN	As required: Latin pro re nata
PTA	Post-traumatic amnesia
PTH	Parathormone
PTSD	Post-traumatic stress disorder

PVL	Periventricular leucomalacia	SNAP	Sensory nerve action potential
QDS	Four times daily (Latin quater die sumendus)	SNP	Single nucleotide polymorphism
RAPD	Relative afferent pupillary defect	SPECT	Single photon emission computerized tomography
RAS	Reflex asystolic syncope/reflex anoxic seizure; also rapid antigen screen	SSADH	Succinic semi-aldehyde dehydrogenase
		SSEP	Somatosensory evoked potentials
RCDP	Rhizomelic chondrodysplasia punctata	SSPE	Subacute sclerosing panencephalitis
RCPCH	Royal College of Paediatrics and Child Health	SSRI	Selective serotonin reuptake inhibitor
RCT	Randomized controlled trial	STIR	Short tau inversion recovery (MRI sequence)
REM	Rapid eye movement		
ROM	Range of movement	SUDEP	Sudden unexpected death in epilepsy
RRMS	Relapsing-remitting multiple sclerosis	SUNCT	Short-lasting unilateral neuraligform headache with conjunctival injection and tearing
SAH	Sub-arachnoid haemorrhage		
SALT	Speech and language therapist		
SC	Subcutaneous	SWAS	Spike-and-wave activation in sleep
SCA	Spinocerebellar ataxia		
SCID	Subacute combined immunodeficiency	SWI	Susceptibility-weighted imaging (MRI sequence)
SCIWORA	Spinal cord injury without radiological abnormality	SWS	Sturge–Weber syndrome
		SXR	Skull X-ray
SD	Standard deviation	TBE(V)	Tick borne encephalitis (virus)
SDH	Subdural haemorrhage	TBI	Traumatic brain injury
SEGA	Sub-ependymal giant cell astrocytoma (in tuberous sclerosis)	TBM	Tuberculous meningitis
		TDS	Three times a day (Latin ter die sumendus)
SeLEAS	Self-limiting epilepsy with autonomic features	TIA	Transient ischaemic attack
		TM	Transverse myelitis
SeLECTS	Self-limiting epilepsy with centrotemporal spikes	TORCH	Toxoplasmosis, rubella, cytomegalovirus, herpes virus (congenital infection syndrome)
SeLFNIE	Self-limited familial neonatal-infantile epilepsy		
SeLIE	Self-limited (familial) infantile epilepsy	TPN	Total parenteral nutrition
		TPO	Thyroid peroxidase (antibody to)
SeLNE	Self-limited (familial) neonatal epilepsy	TPP	Tripetidyl amino peptidase
SFEMG	Single fibre electromyography	TS(C)	Tuberous sclerosis (complex)
SHE	Sleep-related hypermotor (hyperkinetic) epilepsy	TTH	Tension-type headache
		TTP	Thrombotic thrombocytopenic purpura
SHH	Sonic hedgehog (tumour subtype)		
		ULD	Unverricht–Lundborg disease
SIADH	Syndrome of inappropriate antidiuretic hormone secretion	ULN	Upper limit of normal
		UMN	Upper motor neurone
SLE	Systemic lupus erythamotosus	USS	Ultrasound scan
SMA	Spinal muscular atrophy	VATER	Vertebral defects, anal atresia, tracheoesophageal fistula, oesophageal atresia, radial, and renal anomalies
SMARD	Spinal muscular atrophy with respiratory distress		
SMEI	Severe myoclonic epilepsy of infancy		

vCJD	Variant Creutzfeldt–Jakob disease
VDRL	Venereal disease reference laboratory (syphillis test)
VEGF	Vascular endothelial growth factor
VEP/VER	Visual evoked potential/response
VI	Visual impairment
VLBW	Very low birth weight
VLCFA	Very long-chain fatty acid
VMA	Vanillylmandelic acid
VNS	Vagal nerve stimulator
VP	Ventriculo-peritoneal
VPA	Valproate
VUS	Variant of uncertain significance (genetics)

VWM	'Vanishing white matter' leukodystrophy (=CACH, q.v.)
VZV	Varicella zoster virus
WCE	White-cell enzymes
WES	Whole exome sequencing
WGS	Whole genome sequencing
WHO	World Health Organization
WISC	Wechsler Intelligence Scale for Children
WNV	West Nile virus
WPPSI	Wechsler Preschool and Primary Scale of Intelligence
WPW	Wolff–Parkinson–White
X-ALD	X-linked adrenoleucodystrophy

Chapter 1

Clinical approach

The consultation

'I've learned that people will forget what you said, people will forget what you did, but people will never forget how you made them feel.'

Maya Angelou

- For the family, an eagerly or apprehensively awaited time: to hear the worst, dispel fears, learn more, get tests, get help, and to find a cure.
- For doctors, often a severely time-limited interchange: to meet the family's agenda, diagnose, arrange a management plan, and form a relationship.

Setting the scene

Make people feel at ease: greet them at the door and welcome them in. Arrange furniture appropriately. In a ward setting, avoid talking across the bed. Use a setting conducive to communication.

Seeing a child for the first time

- Read the notes before seeing the child!
- Introduce yourself. Many doctors may be involved with this child's care: what's your role?
- Make sure you know who everyone is (is that mother or grandmother? Aunt or social worker? Father or boyfriend?)
- Establish what the child likes to be called (and if necessary, how to pronounce their name).
- Establish what the family is expecting to be discussing: this may not be your agenda or that of the referring clinician.
  - 'What have you been told about why I have been asked to see you?'
  - 'What do you want to get from this time together?' Confirming an esoteric diagnosis may be less important to the family than getting basic understanding and services.
- Encourage parents to ask questions.
  - Consider providing question prompt sheets before the appointment.
- Consider how life would be for you in similar circumstances: it will help you pinpoint solutions.
- Make sure the child understands what is to be discussed (occasionally families will not have divulged the purpose of the hospital visit).
- Explain how much time is available for the consultation: in complex situations, it may be helpful to be able to reassure everyone that this will be the first of several opportunities to talk together.
- Explain what will *not* be happening: children may be dreading blood tests that are not planned.
- The child is why you are all there: include him/her as much as possible.

Review appointments

▶ Again encourage questions from the family to establish the consultation agenda: what are their main concerns? Then:

- Is the diagnosis right?
- Is the medication list up to date?
- Update the problem list.
- Chase any results outstanding.

- Changes in family circumstances.
- Check for any investigations that ought to have been sent (e.g. in a 'legacy' case).
- Again, ensure addressing practical needs has not been lost in the hunt for a diagnosis.

Special circumstances

Giving bad news

Parents want significant news:
- Together.
- As soon as possible.
- Sympathetically and in private.
- With accuracy.

They also want:
- Help with how to pass on news to family and friends.
- To have the child present.

Language to use, language to avoid

Remember parents will hang on to every word. Do not be too negative. Compare: 'I am sorry, but I have some very bad news for you. Your child has cerebral palsy' with 'I have some news you may not have been expecting. Your child has cerebral palsy. This may be something you have heard of but know little about. I shall do my best to explain something about it to you and then explain how we can help'.

Present a balanced view on therapies. It is easy for parents to turn to remedies that promise 'cure'. Your understandable wish to spare them unnecessary pain is better achieved by protecting them from unscrupulous purveyors of miracles. Generally, we can promise maximization of developmental potential and prevention of secondary complications. Remember that parents will recall little of what you said at a first consultation and misunderstand half of that. Try always to see both parents together at important interviews. See if an advocate is available for them (health visitor, social worker, ward nurse, or a friend they know well).

❶ If you have been trying to give bad news, and the parents are not clearly upset, consider whether they really heard what you were trying to say.

The dying child
- Acknowledge that parents feel loss before death actually occurs.
- Address parents' feelings as well as, and separately from, day-to-day management issues.
- Respect parental wishes in difficult end-of-life decisions (see Withdrawal of care decisions in Chapter 5 **➲** p. 587).

Seeing parents after their child has died
- Discuss any post-mortem findings.
- Re-explain the cause of the illness in the light of the findings.
- Dispense with misconceptions about the illness, death, or care.
- Alleviate guilt.

- Involve bereavement support organizations and consider psychological referral.
- Arrange genetic counselling if appropriate.
- Give an update on the transplant recipient if relevant.
- Any unanswered questions?
- Accept thanks, donations, and offers to help with research.

What, where, and when

'Where's the lesion? What's the lesion?'

This is the catch-phrase of the classical (adult) neurological approach: its applicability to paediatric neurology is limited only by the greater frequency of global rather than focal neurological disease in children.

> ❶ Examination gives the 'where'; history gives the 'what'.

Examination findings, plus some neuroanatomical knowledge, locate the problem (the 'where?')

Clinical assessment of the likely site(s) of involvement is crucial to the planning of further investigation (including where to direct neuroimaging studies). It can also prevent the chance finding of an unexpected imaging abnormality (an 'incidentaloma', see Unexpected findings on MRI in Chapter 2 ➋ p. 74) distracting evaluation, if its location means that it cannot be relevant to the presenting symptoms or signs. The signs you elicit at examination, evaluated in light of neuroanatomical knowledge and pattern recognition, indicate the location(s) of the problem.

Some examples:

- The cause of a spastic hemiparesis will lie in the contralateral corticospinal tract. It may be possible to localize further:
  - If there is also an ipsilateral visual field defect the lesion probably involves the subcortical white matter (as that's where the visual pathways and corticospinal tracts intersect).
  - Associated seizures suggest cortical (grey matter) involvement.
- The co-occurrence of ipsilateral fourth, fifth, and sixth cranial nerve signs implies cavernous sinus pathology.
- Unilateral hypoglossal nerve involvement and ipsilateral ataxia are hallmarks of the lateral medullary syndrome: the lesion is localized as precisely as any MRI scan can!

Even in the more common situation of more widespread neurological involvement (e.g. a child with psychomotor regression) it is useful to try to define the system(s) involved based on examination. Seizures and cognitive impairments imply cortical grey matter involvement; movement disorders implicate basal ganglia and thalami; pyramidal motor signs implicate the central white matter.

The history tells you the pathology (the 'what?')

Recall the classic 'surgical sieve' of causes: infective, inflammatory, neoplastic, paraneoplastic, iatrogenic, toxic, metabolic, etc. The 'what?' of diagnosis comes from the history, particularly the time-course of the onset of symptoms and signs.

For *any* sign (e.g. hemiparesis) or *any* symptom (e.g. headache):

- Near-instantaneous onset (see Fig. 1.1A) suggests a vascular cause: haemorrhage or infarction.
- Development (B) over days might suggest inflammation. Evolution over weeks may be due to expansion of a space-occupying lesion.

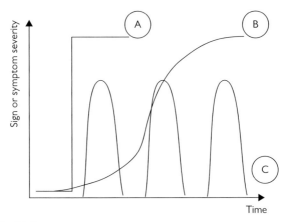

Fig. 1.1 Time-courses.

- Paroxysmal symptoms or signs occurring episodically with intervening spells of complete normality (C) are most commonly due either to epileptic or to migrainous processes (true transient ischaemic attacks are rare). Both are capable of a wide repertoire of episodic phenomena. Again, the time-course can be helpful: epileptic events tend to last seconds to a few minutes; migrainous events tend to evolve over tens of minutes and to last up to several hours.

'When' was the process?

The effects of lesions depend both on age at insult and time since insult in complex ways. Lesions acquired before the establishment of the normal function of the affected region can be relatively silent (e.g. neonatal infarction of dominant hemisphere 'language' cortex) if adjacent or homologous contralateral brain regions can take on that function. Conversely, the effects of a lesion acquired in early childhood to a region of the brain still developmentally 'silent' may remain latent until the region's function can be assessed clinically (see Age at injury and time since injury in Chapter 4 ➜ p. 220).

A less frequently considered aspect is the 'momentum' of a lesion. A very slowly developing lesion (such as a low-grade tumour) may be clinically very silent as the surrounding brain has time to 'accommodate' its presence. Conversely pronounced clinical manifestations imply a 'high momentum' lesion of recent onset and rapid evolution. This can be a useful consideration when, for example, considering an extensive infiltrative abnormality on MRI. If such an extensive lesion is relatively clinically silent, it has been there a long time and developed slowly.

History taking

'Listen to the patient, he is trying to tell you the diagnosis.'

William Osler

An accurate history often contributes far more to successful diagnosis and management than either examination or investigation.

Specific questions relevant to specific presentations are dealt with in Chapter 3.

Some general points:
- History taking should be *interactive*. 'Have I got this right? You're saying …'; 'No, that's not quite right: it's more like …'.
- History taking can be *iterative*. It may be important to revisit aspects of the history in the light of examination or investigation findings.
- The experience of *giving* a history (as a child or a parent) can itself be therapeutic if elicited carefully. Hearing your experiences retold as a coherent story can help make sense of the experience. Knowing that the story is familiar to the doctor and that he/she will be able to make additional 'sense' of it is a bonus.
- Children as young as 3 can give useful first-hand history, even if their language is limited. Young children can, however, be very influenced by perceptions of what they 'ought' or 'ought not' to be saying.
- School age children deserve an opportunity to speak to you alone although this must be balanced against the reassurance a child gains from observing a good rapport between physician and parent, and against the lost opportunity for indirect observation of the child that talking to the parent offers.
- A child's *inability* to give a history may itself be informative.

History of presenting complaint

Hear what *was* said, not what you thought was said! Patients do not complain of ataxia or dystonia. If the mother said 'he keeps falling over' but you heard 'ataxia' you have already closed your mind to a range of non-cerebellar causes of balance problems, weakness, and other causes of falls. Occasionally a well-intentioned parent will use quasi-medical language ('He's having absences: that's what you call them isn't it, doctor?'), which must be gently discouraged.
- The family will see the presenting complaint as the most important part of the history. If for some reason other aspects are important in your assessment you need to explain why.
- For acute presentations, it is usually possible to start at the beginning of the story ('Tell me when your child was last entirely well') and take the story forward. For very long-term pictures, it may be more useful to start with the present situation and fill in backwards.
- The time-course of symptom onset is crucial to determining pathology (see The history tells you the pathology (the 'what?') in this chapter ❥ p. 5).
- Evaluating whether very long-term/insidious onset symptoms were present from birth or appeared after a few months of normal development can be challenging. Likewise, it can be difficult to distinguish static from slowly progressive symptoms.

❶ Static ability is rarely normal. If ability is not demonstrably improving with time, consider whether it may be regressing.

Developmental history

Some less commonly emphasized, but useful, developmental milestones, particularly of early cognitive/linguistic development:

- *Hand regard* (prolonged periods of fascinated observation of hands) is an important prelude to establishment of hand use, seen at about 3–5 months, followed by foot regard (holding feet and bringing them into view) several weeks later.
- The distinguishing of familiar carers from strangers, from 9 months.
- *Object permanence*: the understanding that objects continue to exist even if they cannot currently be seen. Once established, 'peek-a-boo' becomes a game, and distraction hearing tests become impossible (as the child becomes aware of an examiner out of sight behind her). From 9–10 months.
- *Theory of mind*: the recognition that 'there is another 'I' in my mother who can be interested in things that interest me'. Typically established by 18 months and demonstrated by the set-up of opportunities for *shared attention*, e.g. bringing an interesting object to mother to look at, or by glancing at mother for a reaction to *my* actions (e.g. ones I know will meet disapproval) (see Pervasive developmental disorder in Chapter 3 ➋ p. 125). Shared attention is a vital prerequisite for language development: a child is only going to associate the 'C-A-T' sound his mother is making with the furry animal he is watching if he understands that she is thinking about it too.
- *Proto-linguistic behaviour*: pointing—again as a demonstration of shared attention—often with vocalizations meaning either 'get me that' (proto-imperative) or 'look at that interesting [aeroplane/bus/cat] mummy' (proto-declarative). From ~18 months.
- *Symbolic play*: using representational toys in imitative play (making meals for doll). From ~18 months.
- *Naming body parts* ('where's Amy's nose?') from ~18 months.
- *Cooperative play* including turn-taking, from ~3 yrs.

Piaget (1898–1980) created a very influential model of child cognitive development based on sequential stages:
- the Sensorimotor stage (0–2 yrs);
- the Pre-Operational stage (2–7 yrs);
- the Concrete Operational stage (7–11 yrs); and
- the Formal Operations stage (>11 yrs).

The model is undoubtedly over-simplistic, and more relevant to educational theory than clinical developmental assessment. However, some insights (such as the prevalence of 'magical thinking' and the imbuing of inanimate objects with personalities in the pre-operational phase) are clinically useful.

❶ A boy not walking independently by 18 months' age must have creatine kinase (CK) checked to exclude Duchenne muscular dystrophy.

▶ For early developmental milestones in the context of autism spectrum concerns, see Pervasive developmental disorder in Chapter 3 p. 125.
▶ For early visual developmental milestones, see Table 3.17 in Chapter 3 p. 209.
▶ For early hearing and language developmental milestones, see Specific language impairment in Chapter 3 p. 123.

Examination

General appearance

Table 1.1 lists helpful clinical features of some paediatric neurological disorders.

Table 1.1 General medical manifestations of some neurological diseases

Big head	Most commonly familial: for evaluation, see 'Large head: >2SD above mean for age' in Chapter 3 ◐ p. 162
Small head	Familial, or any cause of cerebral atrophy. For evaluation, see 'Small head: <2SD below mean for age' in Chapter 3 ◐ p. 164
Big fontanelle	Zellweger
Hair abnormalities	Stiff, wiry: trichopoliodystrophy (Menkes)
	Hirsutism: infantile GM gangliosidosis, Hurler, Hunter, Sanfilippo, I-cell disease
	Grey: ataxia telangiectasia, Cockayne, Chédiak–Higashi, progeria
Skin findings	Telangiectasia: ataxia telangiectasia, hereditary haemorrhagic telangiectasia
	Angiokeratoma: Fabry, juvenile fucosidosis, sialidosis with chondrodystrophy
	Icthyosis: Refsum, Sjögren–Larsson
	Hypopigmentation: trichopoliodystrophy (Menkes), Chédiak–Higashi, tuberous sclerosis (ash-leaf macules), hypomelanosis of Ito
	Hyperpigmentation: Niemann–Pick, adrenoleukodystrophy, Farber, neurofibromatosis 1 (café au lait), xeroderma pigmentosum
	Thin atrophic skin: ataxia telangiectasia, Cockayne disease, xeroderma pigmentosum, progeria
	Thick skin: I-cell disease, mucopolysaccharidoses I, II, III, infantile fucosidosis
	Subcutaneous nodules: Farber, neurofibromatosis 1, cerebrotendinous xanthomatosis
	Xanthomas: Niemann–Pick
	Blotching: dysautonomia
Enlarged nodes	Farber, Niemann–Pick, juvenile Gaucher, Chédiak–Higashi, ataxia telangiectasia (lymphoma)
Stridor, hoarseness	Infantile adrenoleukodystrophy, Farber, infantile Gaucher, Pelizaeus–Merzbacher, Chiari II malformation
Big (orange) tonsils	Tangier disease
Severe swallowing problems	(Any severe bulbar, pseudobulbar, cerebellar, basal ganglia pathology)
	Infantile Gaucher

Table 1.1 (Contd.)

Dysautonomia	Neurodegeneration with Brain Iron Accumulation, severe dystonia, infantile adrenoleukodystrophy, Zellweger
Heart abnormalities	Pompe, Hurler, and other mucopolysaccharidoses, Fabry, infantile fucosidosis, Refsum, Friedreich, abetalipoproteinaemia, tuberous sclerosis, progeria, Zellweger
Strokes	MELAS; Fabry, trichopoliodystrophy (Menkes), progeria
Organomegaly	Most mucopolysaccharidoses, infantile GM1 gangliosidosis, Niemann–Pick, Gaucher, Zellweger, galactosaemia, Pompe, mannosidosis
Gastrointestinal problems	Malabsorption: MNGIE syndrome (myopathy and external ophthalmoplegia; neuropathy; gastrointestinal; encephalopathy), Wolman disease, abetalipoproteinaemia Non-functioning gallbladder: metachromatic leukodystrophy, infantile fucosidosis Jaundice: Niemann–Pick types A and C, Zellweger, galactosaemia Vomiting: dysautonomia, urea-cycle defects Diarrhoea: Hunter syndrome
Kidney problems	Renal failure: Fabry, nephrosialidosis Cysts: Zellweger, von Hippel–Lindau, tuberous sclerosis Stones: Lesch–Nyhan Aminoaciduria: specific aminoacidurias, Lowe syndrome, Wilson
Bone and joint abnormalities	Stiff joints: mucopolysaccharidoses (all but type I-S), mucolipidoses (most), fucosidoses, Farber disease, sialidoses (some), Zellweger, Cockayne Scoliosis: Friedreich, Rett, ataxia telangiectasia, severe dystonia, all chronic illnesses with muscle weakness especially anterior horn cell involvement Kyphosis: mucopolysaccharidoses
Endocrine dysfunction	Adrenals: adrenoleukodystrophy, Wolman Hypogonadism: xeroderma pigmentosum, ataxia telangiectasia, some spinocerebellar degenerations Diabetes: ataxia telangiectasia; Friedreich
Short stature	Morquio, other mucopolysaccharidoses, Cockayne, progeria, diseases with severe malnutrition
Neoplasms	Ataxia telangiectasia, xeroderma pigmentosum, neurofibromatosis (1 and 2), von Hippel–Lindau, tuberous sclerosis, basal cell nevus syndrome (Gorlin)
Hearing loss	Hunter, other mucopolysaccharidoses, adrenoleukodystrophy, Cockayne disease, Kearns–Sayre, Leigh, and other mitochondrial diseases, other spinocerebellar degenerations, Usher syndrome

Source: data from Traeger EC and Rapin I. 'Differential Diagnosis'. In: Rowland LP (ed.). Merritts' Neurology, 10th edition. Philadelphia, PA, USA: Lippincott, Williams and Wilkins, Copyright © 2000 Lippincott, Williams and Wilkins.

Dysmorphic appearances

Dysmorphology is a demanding discipline. Beyond the easily recognized gestalts of Down, Angelman, and other syndromes, it is best to seek specialist opinions from clinical genetics colleagues. Computer databases of neurogenetic and dysmorphic syndromes can be useful but require care to ensure the most informative 'handles' have been identified. Deciding whether a child is 'subtly dysmorphic' is a dangerous business and cannot happen without having met both parents! Ask parents 'who in the family do you think he/she resembles?'

Hypertelorism is a particularly 'hard' and useful finding if present.

Head circumference measurement

See Head size abnormalities in Chapter 3 ➲ p. 162 for assessment of abnormal head size. Head circumference charts are provided in Figures 1.2. and 1.3.

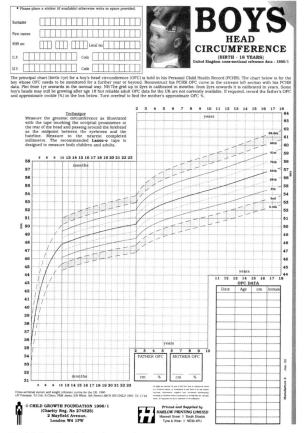

Fig. 1.2 Boys' head circumference charts.

Reproduced with the kind permission of the Child Growth Foundation. Copyright © 2016 Child Growth Foundation. Further information and supplies ✆ www.healthforallchildren.com

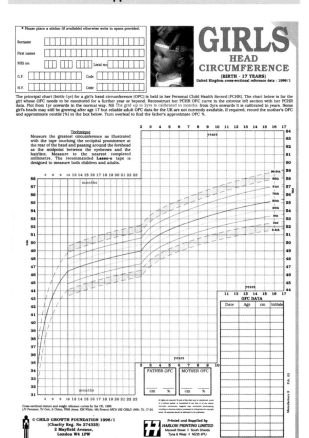

Fig. 1.3 Girls' head circumference chart.

Reproduced with the kind permission of the Child Growth Foundation. Copyright © 2016 Child Growth Foundation. Further information and supplies ℘ www.healthforallchildren.com

Higher cognitive function

A conceptual framework is very useful in interpreting and organizing in-formal impressions of higher cognitive function gained incidentally during examination.

Conscious level

Consciousness implies both *wakefulness* (eyes open, not asleep) and *aware-ness of external events*. These can be dissociated; see Recognition of 'low level' states in Chapter 4 ➔ p. 218.

Orientation

In time, place, and person. Orientation also implies the resumption of regis-tration and recall of events ('who came to visit you this morning?'). In the context of acquired brain injury, return of full orientation marks the end of post-traumatic amnesia (PTA), the length of which is a sensitive indicator of severity of injury, see Acquired brain injury, prognosis in Chapter 4 ➔ p. 222.

Attention and concentration

Two-, three-, and four-year olds should be able to recall immediately two, three, and four random digit sequences ('8, 1, 9') respectively. Between 5 and 10 yrs of age, 5–6 digits forward and 3–4 digits in reverse order are typical. Over 10 yrs of age, <5 digits forward or <3 digits reversed should be concerning. Serial 7s subtracted from 100 should be assessed.

Memory

Retrograde: recall of birthdays, ages, names of family members and pets, meanings of simple words. Anterograde (registration): recall three words after 3 min.

Frontal lobe function

Relatively selective impairment of executive function is common after traumatic brain injury. Decline of frontal lobe function may be an early in-dicator of cognitive regression. It is not normally fully established until mid-adolescence, however, so these tests are not useful in younger children.
- In what ways are these similar: an apple and a banana? A coat and a dress? Praise and punishment? A poem and a statue?
- Understanding of proverbs ('a rolling stone gathers no moss', 'too many cooks spoil the broth', 'still waters run deep', 'a bird in the hand is worth two in the bush') is reassuring although they are culturally dependent.
- Demonstrate the Luria 'fist-edge-hand' sequence. Put your dominant hand down on the table or your thigh repeatedly, firstly in a fist, then with the outstretched hand ulnar side down, then flat palm down. Demonstrate once and ask child to repeat five times.
- Cognitive estimates: 'What's the largest object normally found in a house?'

Praxis

- Constructional: 'Draw a clock face'.
- Ideomotor/ideational: 'Imitate brushing your teeth', 'wave bye-bye', copy the examiner's arbitrary gesture.

Communication

Verbal expression

Spontaneous speech. Immediate repetition of a simple sentence. Naming items. Dysphasia or dysarthria. Word generation ('name as many animals/words beginning with F as you can in 1 min').

Verbal comprehension

Understanding one-, two-, or three-stage requests.

Non-verbal

Use of gestures.

Cognitive 'syndromes'

Frontal lobe dysfunction

Deficits in attention, impulsivity, perseveration on a topic ('stuck in a groove'). Tendency to interpret sarcastic, ironic, or figurative language literally. Good superficial social 'chit-chat' (over-learned) but poor 'emotional intelligence'. Poor *executive function* (i.e. organizing and prioritizing, problem solving) in adolescents: can reflect frontal grey or subcortical white matter damage. In extreme situations (e.g. large frontal tumour), incontinence and inappropriate defecation/urination or sexualized behaviour may be seen.

Temporal lobe dysfunction

- Language dysfunction (receptive or expressive dysphasia) in dominant temporal lobe disease.
- Visual field defect (superior, contralateral quadrantanopia).
- Memory deficits: poor anterograde memory due to hippocampal injury typical of traumatic brain injury.

Parietal lobe dysfunction

Poor two-point discrimination, graphaesthesia (interpretation of letters drawn on the hand), or shape discrimination (identification of a coin or paper clip in the contralateral hand, particularly in non-dominant lobe disease). Apraxia. Inferior contralateral quadrantanopia.

Global dementia

There are very few causes of new-onset dementia in children old enough to perform the Mini-Mental State Examination (MMSE); however, such instruments may be a useful reassurance, where apparently deteriorating school performance is due to depression or other emotional factors. It is, however, very language-oriented, with relatively limited testing of memory, visuospatial function, or executive skills.

Cranial nerves

Olfactory nerve (I)

Not routinely examined. The most common cause of 'anosmia' is rhinitis! To assess this formally, first check nostril patency (sniff with the other nostril occluded) then use pleasant odours (chocolate, etc.). Very irritant odours can be detected somatically by the nasal mucosa (trigeminal nerve).

Optic nerve (II)

- See Table 1.2 for eye signs in neurological disease.
- For an approach to the evaluation of visual disturbances, see Visual disturbance in Chapter 3 ⟳ p. 209.

Acuity

Assess informally using books for the appropriate reading age. In preliterate children, note the ability to reach for small items (e.g. tiny 'hundreds and thousands' cake decorations, which are safe if ingested) Formal techniques such as preferential looking can assess visual acuity accurately even in infants.

Fields

For the interpretation of visual field defects, see Figure 3.7 in Chapter 3 ⟳ p. 211.

In older children, visual fields can be tested by confrontation with both eyes open. Isolated nasal visual field defects (without temporal field defects) are rare other than in relation to chronic vigabatrin use (see Vigabatrin in Chapter 7 ⟳ p. 707), thus a binocular approach is an effective screen. If deficits are identified, then test each eye separately. In infants, gross field preservation can be inferred by the re-fixation reflex: the child re-fixing on a target as it moves from central into peripheral vision in each direction.

Fundoscopy

'The eye is anatomically an extension of the brain; it is almost as if a portion of the brain were in plain sight.'

EH Hess

It follows that fundoscopy is an indispensable skill for the paediatrician!

In younger children (age 5–7), make a game of having them sit in your (swivelling!) clinic chair, put mummy behind you and ask them to 'tell mummy off if she makes funny faces' to help them fix on her and not your ophthalmoscope. Fundoscopy in toddlers requires an assistant to attempt to secure attention, and patience! In neonates get the mother to hold child against her with head on her shoulder looking to side whilst quietly awake.

Perform fundoscopy in the child's right eye with your right eye and vice versa so as not to block the view of the non-examined eye with your head and thus prevent their fixing on a distant target. Keep your glasses on if worn but remove the child's. Darkening the room (e.g. drawing curtains) helps pupillary dilatation, but a very dark room may cause distress and prevent the child fixing on the target.

▶ Optic neuritis (papillitis) and papilloedema have very similar fundoscopic appearances but distinguishing them in practice should not be difficult: visual loss is prominent in papillitis and is usually the presenting complaint (only in the mildest cases is it limited to loss of colour vision). Visual impairment is only ever a very late feature of papilloedema.

Red reflex

View from arm's length distance with the lens at zero. Observe the corneal light reflex at the same time. Normal red reflex appearances vary in different ethnic groups: if in doubt, check appearances in parents. An abnormal red reflex can be absent (dark pupil), partially obscured (by an opacity in lens or media), or of an abnormal colour or brightness (e.g. typically near-white in retinoblastoma).

Venous pulsation

- The retinal veins are the thicker of the two populations of retinal vessels visible.
- Pulsation, if seen, *confirms normal intracranial pressure*, which can be very useful reassurance (e.g. in the evaluation of headache) but is *absent in 10% of the normal population.*
- Rest your thumb on the eyebrow and stabilize the ophthalmoscope on your thumb: this minimizes distracting parallax effects due to movement of the ophthalmoscope relative to the eye.
- Pulsation is best seen at the 'knuckle' where the vessel turns perpendicular to view to enter the optic cup (Fig. 1.4 A), as a pulsation of the vein profile particularly at tortuosities (B), or as movement of the light reflex on the surface of the vein.

Pupil reactions

Anisocoria

Deciding which is the abnormal pupil can be difficult!

- A *dilated* pupil may be due to a partial third cranial nerve lesion: usually associated with eye deviation inferolaterally and/or eyelid ptosis.
- A *small* pupil again associated with ipsilateral ptosis is likely to represent a unilateral Horner syndrome. Asymmetry will be more marked in

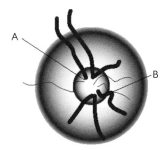

Fig. 1.4 Venous pulsation.

the dark. 0.5% apraclonidine eye drops will reverse the miosis (i.e. pupil dilates). Test for the ipsilateral anhidrosis by sliding a clean metal teaspoon lightly over the forehead and noting the slight drag on crossing to the stickier, sweatier normal side. For an approach to the evaluation of Horner syndrome, see Horner syndrome in Chapter 3 ➔ p. 135.

• Isolated anisocoria is usually benign, although often a cause of anxiety.
  • Tonic pupil is a common benign cause of anisocoria. The affected pupil is larger and reacts poorly to light (thus asymmetry may be more marked in, or on initially moving to, brighter conditions) but contracts briskly on accommodating to a near target.
  • Hyoscine patches (used to control drooling) can cause anisocoria if the child touches the patch and then rubs his/her eye!

Afferent pupillary defect (APD)

A non-reactive pupil can arise from a lesion either in the afferent (optic nerve) or the efferent (third nerve) limb of the pupillary light reflex. Due to the bilateral consensual nature of the pupillary light reflex, an eye with an interrupted optic nerve but intact third nerve will still constrict when the opposite eye is illuminated, but both pupils will dilate when the injured eye is illuminated.

Partial APDs can be subtle and hard to identify reliably. Key to accurate assessment is careful timing in the 'swinging penlight test'. Illuminate one pupil for a count of 5 then immediately swing over to the other pupil for another counted 5 then back, and continue repeatedly, keeping the time neither pupil is illuminated to an absolute minimum, until a consistent impression is gained of whether one pupil is dilating as the torch swings onto it.

❶ Head trauma is one context where recognition of an APD is crucial: the optic nerve can be involved in orbital fractures and the dilated pupil due to the APD might otherwise be interpreted as a third nerve lesion and a sign of ipsilateral uncal herniation (see Examine for signs of herniation in Chapter 6 ➔ p. 614). The difference will be that the consensual response will be present: in APD the pupil will constrict when the other eye is illuminated.

Oculomotor, trochlear, and abducens nerves (III, IV, and VI)

For an approach to the evaluation of abnormal eye movements, see Eye movement abnormalities in Chapter 3 ➔ p. 130.

▶ The 3rd, 4th, and 6th cranial nerve nuclei, and their interconnections span the pons: it is rare for any significant pontine pathology to spare eye movements.

Inspection

• Note that broad epicanthic folds or a broad nasal bridge can give the appearance of a pseudo-squint.
• Observe for ptosis.
• Note pupil size (small on the side of Horner); aniridia; colobomata.
• Note symmetry of position of the light reflex (the dot of light due to the reflection of the ophthalmoscope light on the iris when examining for red reflex). This is very useful in detecting subtle non-alignment of eyes in the neutral position.

Table 1.2 Eye findings in neurological disease

Telangiectasia	Ataxia telangiectasia, Fabry
Corneal opacity	Wilson (KF ring) Mucopolysaccharidoses I, III, IV, VI; Mucolipidoses III, IV; Zellweger (variable); Fabry; sialidosis with chondrodystrophy; Cockayne; xeroderma pigmentosum
Lens opacity	Wilson, galactosaemia, Marinesco–Sjögren Lowe, sialidosis (rarely significant clinically); mannosidosis; cerebrocutaneous xanthomatosis
Glaucoma	Mucopolysaccharidosis I, Zellweger (infrequent)
Cherry red spot	Tay–Sachs; sialidosis (usually); Niemann–Pick type A (50%); Infantile GM1 gangliosidosis (50%); Farber (variable); multiple sulphatase deficiency (metachromatic leukodystrophy variant)
Macular and retinal pigmentary degeneration	Most NCLs; mucopolysaccharidoses I-H and I-S, II, III; mucolipidoses I; abetalipoproteinaemia; Refsum; some spinocerebellar syndromes; Kearns–Sayre syndrome; Neurodegeneration with Brain Iron Accumulation (some); Cockayne; Sjögren–Larsson (some); Usher
Optic atrophy	Krabbe; metachromatic leukodystrophy; most sphingolipidoses (late); adrenoleukodystrophy; Alexander disease, Canavan disease, Pelizaeus–Merzbacher; neuraxonal dystrophy; Alper; Leber; some spinocerebellar degenerations
Nystagmus	Sensory nystagmus; Pelizaeus–Merzbacher; metachromatic leukodystrophy; Friedreich and spinocerebellar degenerations; neuraxonal dystrophy, ataxia telangiectasia; Leigh syndrome (inconstant); Marinesco–Sjögren syndrome; Chédiak–Higashi; opsoclonus-myoclonus (jerky eye movements may be mistaken for nystagmus), GLUT1DS (jerky eye movements may be mistaken for nystagmus)
Ophthalmoplegia	Kearns–Sayre and Leigh; Niemann–Pick with vertical ophthalmoplegia; abetalipoproteinaemia; ataxia telangiectasia; infantile Gaucher; Tangier

Abbreviations: KF, Kayser–Fleischer ring; NCL, neuronal ceroid lipofuscinosis.

Source: data from Traeger EC and Rapin I. 'Differential Diagnosis'. In: Rowland LP (ed.). *Merritts' Neurology*, 10th edition. Philadelphia, PA, USA: Lippincott, Williams and Wilkins, Copyright © 2000 Lippincott, Williams and Wilkins.

Eye movements

In an older child, test smooth pursuit of a slowly moving target and saccadic eye movements ('Look at mummy… now look at me') separately.

In a younger child, observe spontaneous eye movements.

In an infant, eye movements can be observed by inducing nystagmus. A rotating striped drum will induce optokinetic nystagmus (OKN) confirming the integrity of horizontal eye movements and indirectly indicating sufficient visual acuity to discern the stripes.

In the absence of an OKN drum, stand holding an infant close in front of your face and then turn slowly on the spot. This induces nystagmus (again confirming the integrity of horizontal eye movements). If the child's visual acuity is adequate to fix on your face, the motion-induced nystagmus will be rapidly suppressed despite continuing rotation.

▶ Distinguish a paralytic disorder of eye movement from non-paralytic squint (where each eye considered separately is capable of a full range of movement but binocular movement is dysconjugate).

Abnormal conjugate eye movements
- Down (sunsetting in ↑ intracranial pressure).
- To one side: 'away from' an irritative lesion (seizures, frontal lobe lesion); 'toward' an old lesion (stroke) in part due to associated visual field deficits or visual inattention in the contra-lesional visual field.
- Nystagmus (can also be dysconjugate).

Abnormal dysconjugate eye movements
- Squint.
- Cranial nerve palsies.
- Head tilt (to compensate for squint; posterior fossa tumour).

See Figures 1.5 and 1.6.

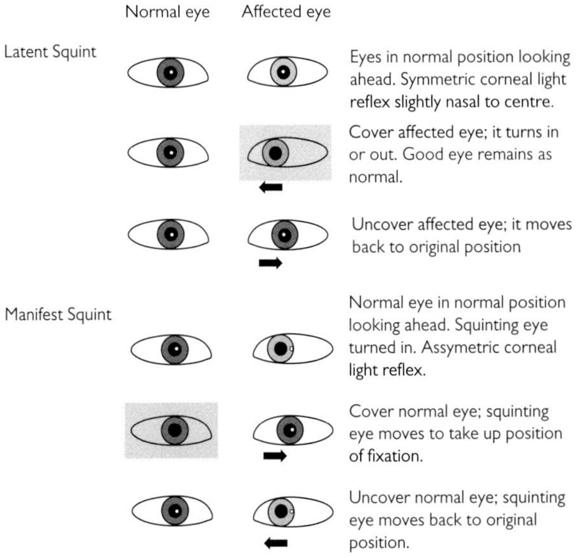

	Normal eye	Affected eye	
Latent Squint			Eyes in normal position looking ahead. Symmetric corneal light reflex slightly nasal to centre.
			Cover affected eye; it turns in or out. Good eye remains as normal.
			Uncover affected eye; it moves back to original position
Manifest Squint			Normal eye in normal position looking ahead. Squinting eye turned in. Assymetric corneal light reflex.
			Cover normal eye; squinting eye moves to take up position of fixation.
			Uncover normal eye; squinting eye moves back to original position.

Fig. 1.5 Cover test.

Cranial nerve	Ocular muscle	Function	Palsy		Aetiology
			Normal	Palsied	
III Oculomotor nerve	Medial rectus Superior rectus Inferior rectus Inferior oblique	Adduction, intorsion, adduction Elevation, intorsion, adduction Depression, extorsion, adduction Elevation, extorsion, abduction	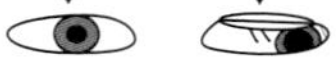	Looking straight ahead: ptosis, dilated pupil, eye 'down-and-out' (not myasthenia if pupil dilated)	**Congenital**: rare, 50% have associated neurological abnormalities **Acquired**: Trauma Tumour Raised intracranial pressure Vascular (migraine; posterior communicating artery aneurysms–pupil dilates first) Inflammation or infection ADEM, meningitis)
IV Trochlear nerve	Superior oblique	Depression, intorsion, adduction	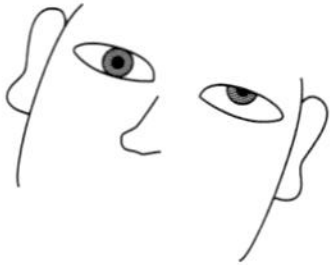	Head tilt-and-turn away from paralysed side. To test, tilt head toward affected side (shown here): see defect in depression	**Congenital**: commonest of ocular palsies, rarely due to birth trauma or perinatal events **Acquired**: Trauma (closed head injury) Tumour (brain-stem glioma) Myasthenia
VI Abducens nerve	Lateral rectus	Abduction	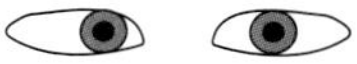	Looking left: left eye fails to abduct	**Congenital**: usually isolated, rare, spontaneous recovery **Acquired**: Trauma (commonest) Tumour (brain-stem glioma, histiocytosis) Raised intracranial pressure Vascular (AVM) Inflammation (ADEM)

Congenital cranial dysinnervation disorders

Moebius syndrome: congenital facial weakness accompanied by abduction deficit in one or both eyes. Other cranial nerve palsies also may occur.

Duane retraction syndrome: on attempted adduction, limitation or absence of abduction, variable limitation of adduction and palpebral fissure narrowing because of globe retraction.

Aplasia of one or both VI nuclei. Mostly sporadic. 50% have associated brain-stem deficits (e.g. crocodile tears, sensorineural deafness).

Fig. 1.6 Cranial nerve palsies affecting eye movements.

Diplopia

Paralytic eye movement abnormalities, particularly if of acute onset, will give rise to subjective diplopia. Diplopia will be worst (i.e. image separation greatest) when attempting to look in the direction of the affected eye movement.

The false image (the most lateral one) will be from the affected eye and will disappear when the affected eye is occluded, although younger children will struggle to report this reliably. Covering one eye with red glass and asking children to consider the red image can help.

Diplopia is often distressing, and children may cover or occlude one eye and dislike having it open.

▶ Reported double vision that persists with one eye covered is almost certainly functional: only a very unusual and readily confirmable ocular cause such as lens dislocation could otherwise give rise to this.

Trigeminal nerve (V)

For an approach to the evaluation of disturbances of facial sensation, see Facial sensation abnormalities in Chapter 3 ➋ p. 141.

Examine perception of light touch and temperature in the normal manner. Note whether boundaries of any reported area of altered perception correspond to the anatomical boundaries of the divisions of the trigeminal nerve (see Facial sensation abnormalities in Chapter 3 ➋ p. 141).

Corneal reflex

Approach with a wisp of cotton wool from the side to avoid a blink due to visual threat. Touch the cornea over the infero-lateral quadrant of the iris (i.e. the coloured part of the eye). Note whether a blink is elicited and ask whether the sensation felt similar on each side. Informally, observing the blink produced by brushing eyelashes elicits similar information.

Motor functions of trigeminal nerve

Test the ability to resist attempted jaw closure (lateral pterygoid).

Jaw jerk

Elicit by asking the child to let their mouth fall open, gently holding their chin and tapping your own thumb: explain what you are going to do before approaching the child's face with a tendon hammer! Not normally detectable. A readily elicited, exaggerated jaw jerk confirms that an upper motor neuron picture is of cerebral, rather than high cervical spine origin.

Facial nerve (VII)

For an approach to the evaluation of abnormal facial movement, see Facial movement abnormalities in Chapter 3 ➋ p. 137.

Ask the child to imitate facial expressions (grimace, frown, smile, forced eye closure). Examine the symmetry of movements. The child should normally be able to completely bury their eyelashes in forced eye closure which you should not be able to overcome. Distinguish upper motor neuron involvement of the seventh cranial nerve (minimal effect on eye closure or eyebrow elevation) from lower motor neuron cranial nerve lesions (eye closure typically marked affected).

❶ Do not mistake asymmetric crying facies of a newborn for a unilateral lower motor neuron facial nerve injury! See Asymmetric crying facies in Chapter 3 ➋ p. 137.

Auditory nerve (VIII)

For an approach to the evaluation of hearing loss, see Hearing loss in Chapter 3 ➜ p. 169.

Middle ear disease (chronic serous otitis media; 'glue ear') is a common cause of conductive hearing loss in younger children, also in children with Down syndrome and any disorder of palatal function (acquired palatal palsies as well as cleft palate).

Rinne tuning fork testing is reliable in children as young as 5 if performed carefully.

- 'This is behind [press base of fork against mastoid]; and this is in front [hold next to ear]. Which is louder? Behind? [Press fork against mastoid again] Or in front? [Fork next to ear]'.
- If in doubt, hold the fork against the mastoid until the child reports that they have just stopped being able to hear it and then check whether they can still hear it next to their ear (should be able to: air conduction should be better than bone conduction).
- The Weber tuning fork test (whether the tuning fork placed centrally on the forehead is louder in one or other ear) is less reliable in children.

Cranial nerves IX and X

Palatal and bulbar function

For an approach to the evaluation of poorly articulated speech, and swallowing difficulties, see Speech difficulties and Swallowing and feeding problems in Chapter 3 ➜ p. 197 and 201.

The gag reflex tests sensory and motor components of IX and X. In the conscious child, it is rarely necessary to elicit a gag reflex formally to assess palatal and bulbar function: this can be inferred from observation of feeding and swallowing behaviour. Symmetry of palatal movement can be assessed by observing whether the uvula is midline and moves vertically upward on saying 'aah'. Unilateral IX nerve injury causes the uvula to move to the side of the cerebral lesion. In practice, IX, X, and XI are very closely related, and isolated injury to one nerve is rare. Hoarseness or stridor implicates X nerve involvement.

In the disabled child, demonstration of the presence of a detectable gag reflex is not an adequate demonstration of the safety of oral feeding, and a formal feeding and swallowing assessment is required (see Feeding in Chapter 4 ➜ p. 253).

Cranial nerves XI and XII

Neck and tongue movements

Confusion sometimes arises as the action of the sternomastoid is to turn the head to the *contralateral* side (the distance from the mastoid process to the sternum, i.e. the length of the sternomastoid muscle, is less when it is turned away than when the head is midline). Assess power by asking the child to turn their head to the contralateral side and then prevent you pushing back. Also assess shoulder shrug power (spinal accessory nerve).

The integrity of 12th nerve function is assessed by observation of the tongue at rest in the open mouth (fasciculation?), the symmetry of tongue movement on attempted protrusion, and if required, by palpating from outside the pressure with which the tongue can be pressed against the inside of the cheek on each side (and its symmetry). Chronic 12th nerve lesions may result in ipsilateral tongue atrophy and wasting.

Peripheral nervous system

Examination of the peripheral nervous system comprises both the formal static assessment of appearance, tone, power, coordination, reflexes, and sensation adapted from the adult approach, and the sensitive, dynamic, integrated evaluation that comes from consideration of posture and gait. The latter forms a very sensitive screening test that will detect all but perhaps the mildest of pyramidal weaknesses, although formal neurological evaluation may be very helpful in identifying the cause of a puzzling gait or postural abnormality.

Formal peripheral neurological examination

Appearance
- Note symmetry of muscle bulk and limb length.
- Inspection of shoes can be helpful unless they're very new: uneven wear of the soles may reflect a tendency to weight-bear on one part of the foot. Mild pyramidal weakness (causing perhaps only a subtle tendency to toe-walk) may be reflected in greater wear at the toe.
- Fasciculation is rare outside the context of neonatal (type 1) SMA where it most prominently affects the tongue.

Tone
- Younger children can find it hard to 'just relax', which can cause misleading impressions of ↑ tone. Posture may be a more useful indicator of ↓ tone.
- ↑ tone may be due to muscles contracting involuntarily, or due to changes in the viscoelastic properties of soft tissues. The latter can be difficult to distinguish from spasticity but importantly won't respond to medication.
- Involuntary muscle contraction may give rise to spasticity, dystonia, and/or rigidity. These features may co-exist, particularly after acquired brain injury or in the context of cerebral palsy. It is important to recognize the underlying form of elevated tone, as failure to do so can result in ineffective therapies being applied, and effective therapies overlooked.
  - Pyramidal stiffness or *spasticity* is *velocity dependent* (the more rapidly a muscle is passively extended the tighter it will be; manifest as a catch when muscles are passively extended rapidly) and has a 'clasp-knife' quality to it (i.e. resistance to movement to a certain point beyond which it 'collapses').
  - The stiffness of *dystonia* is velocity *independent* and uniform through range of movement. It can sometimes be brought out by passively moving the arm whilst asking the child to perform repeated movements (e.g. clenching and opening the fist) in the contralateral limb.
  - The stiffness of *rigidity* does not vary with the velocity or direction of movement across the joint range, but unlike dystonia is not associated with the body part taking up an abnormal posture. Rigidity is much less common than spasticity and dystonia in children.

Power
See Table 1.3.
- Younger children may be confused by requests to 'pull against me' in formal power testing.

Table 1.3 Medical Research Council (MRC) muscle strength scale

0	Nil
1	Flicker of movement
2	Movement, gravity eliminated across the whole joint range
3	Sustained antigravity power across the whole joint range
3+	Momentarily against resistance
4/4+	Movement against resistance
5−	Unsure if weak
5	Normal

Source: data from Medical Research Council. *Aids to the examination of the peripheral nervous system (Memorandum No. 45)*, London: Her Majesty's Stationery Office, Copyright © 1981 Crown Copyright, https://www.mrc.ac.uk/documents/pdf/aids-to-the-examination-of-the-peripheral-nervous-system-mrc-memorandum-no-45-superseding-war-memorandum-no-7/, accessed 06 Aug 2023.

- The most effective approach to a formal examination of power in a child above about 4 yrs of age is usually: 'Let me show you how I want you to hold your arms [move arm passively to desired test position, e.g. symmetrical 'chicken wing' posture] ... OK, hold them there ... Now don't let me move them [examiner tries to move them]'.
- Examine shoulder abduction on each side simultaneously, then elbow flexion on each side before elbow extension, etc. Formal examination of power in the legs is best performed in supine lying, although seated assessment is possible.
- A useful technique to screen for subtle hemiparesis is to ask a child to stand still for 20s with arms outstretched, palms upward, and eyes closed. Mild pyramidal weakness results in pronator drift: a downward and internally rotating (pronating) drift of the affected arm.
- Dynamic assessment of power by examination of posture, gait, and movement may be more informative.

Proximal weakness of shoulder and hip girdle (associated with complaints of difficulty raising head from pillow, combing hair, raising arms above head, getting up from chair, climbing stairs) usually implies muscle disease, and distal weakness (difficulty opening bottles, turning keys, buttoning clothes, writing), generally neuropathic disease. There are, however, exceptions to these generalizations: see Peripheral weakness in Chapter 3 ➔ p. 180.

▶ Assessment of fatiguability is important if neuromuscular junction disease is suspected. This is most readily assessed in the limbs by assessing baseline shoulder abduction strength then fatiguing one arm (e.g. asking an older child repeatedly to lift a heavy book held in one hand above his head) and then reassessing shoulder abduction looking now for asymmetry. Fatiguability of eye movements is assessed by the ability to maintain upgaze.

Reflexes
- The successful elicitation of a deep tendon reflex requires the muscle belly to be relaxed yet moderately extended. Attention to optimal limb position is thus helpful. Young children may also be disconcerted by the idea of being hit! For both these reasons, examination of reflexes in the upper limb can be helped by your holding the arm, placing a finger or thumb over the tendon and striking your own finger or thumb (and making jokes about what a strange thing that is to do).
- With the child's hands on his/her lap, press firmly with your thumb over the biceps tendon just above the elbow and strike your thumb. Elicited jerks are often as much felt (through your thumb) as seen.
- Supinator reflexes can be elicited by striking your fingers placed just proximal to the wrist over the radial side of the partially supinated forearm as it rests in the child's lap.
- Triceps may require a slightly different approach: hold the arm abducted at the shoulder to 90° and with the forearm hanging down passively (you won't have a hand free, so strike the tendon directly).
- In younger children, adequate relaxation of quadriceps muscles for elicitation of knee jerks can be assured with both child and examiner being seated and facing each other. Put the child's feet either up on the front edge of your chair or (if clean!) on your knees.
- Plantar responses are elicited in the usual manner. Note the very first movement of the hallux. A +ve Babinski comprises upward initial movement of the hallux and/or spreading (fanning) of the toes but is normal below 18 months of age.
- Abdominal reflexes are elicited by scratching the skin along a dermatome towards the midline. They may be absent in 15% of the normal population and may be asymmetrical. They can help localize thoracic spinal cord lesions, though they are less reliable than a sensory level to pinprick (Table 1.4). In children with scoliosis, their absence may indicate a syrinx.

Sensation
- Examine spinothalamic (pain and temperature) and dorsal column (light touch, proprioception, and two-point discrimination) function separately in all areas pertinent to the clinical scenario (see Fig. 1.7). Loss of spinothalamic with preserved dorsal column sensation is an

Table 1.4 Reflex root levels

Reflex	Root level
Biceps	C5,6
Brachioradialis	C5,6
Triceps	C6,7
Knee	L3,4
Ankle	S1

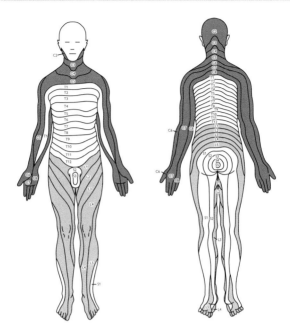

Fig. 1.7 Dermatomes.

important sign of syringomyelia; see Syringomyelia in Chapter 4 ➜
p. 226 and Figure 2.11b in Chapter 2 ➜ p. 70.
- Perception of the cold of a metallic object such as a tuning fork is a
  more acceptable means of assessing of spinothalamic function than
  pinprick!
- Subjective reporting of altered sensation should not be over-
  interpreted: if a child can discriminate hot and cold or sharp and blunt,
  and locate light touch accurately, then function is intact.
- In assessing light touch, hold cotton wool *still* against the skin without
  moving it. Tickle (which may be elicited by stroking) is a spinothalamic,
  not dorsal column, sensation.
- Joint position sense may be assessed at a single joint in the older
  child in the usual manner, but it is more useful to screen for impaired
  proprioception by performing the Romberg test (looking for ↑ body
  sway in standing with eyes closed).

Coordination

- Coordination of leg movements is assessed in walking: see Posture and gait in this Chapter ➲ p. 37.
- Ask the child to move his finger from tip of his nose to the tip of your finger: emphasize you're looking for accuracy, not speed.
  - Cerebellar or proprioceptive problems impair accuracy i.e. not landing precisely on the tip of the nose (dysmetria). Other movement disorders (such as tics or myoclonus) will interfere with the intended trajectory, but a child will usually slow down just before reaching the target to ensure an accurate landing (with the help of intact cerebellar function).
- Cerebellar dysfunction gives rise to patterns of ataxia that can be distinguished (Table 1.5).
  - Midline cerebellar (vermis) disease tends to affect midline (i.e. trunk) coordination, giving rise to wide-based gait.
  - Hemispheric cerebellar disease tends to cause limb ataxia (seen on finger–nose testing), which in uni-hemispheric disease will be asymmetric (ipsilateral to the affected cerebellar hemisphere).
- Ataxia can occasionally also be due to lack of proprioception (joint position awareness), so-called *sensory ataxia*. This failure of proprioception can be compensated to some extent by vision: these children's ability to stand still is much worse in the dark or with their eyes shut (positive Romberg sign).
- Developmental coordination disorder (dyspraxia) manifests as poor functional coordination in complex motor action sequences (e.g. shoe-tying; or the throw a ball–clap hands whilst it is in the air–catch it again manoeuvre), but there is *no abnormality* on formal testing of cerebellar function.

Innervation of the upper limbs

See Figures 1.8–1.12.

Table 1.5 Patterns of cerebellar dysfunction

Cerebellar lesion	Signs
Posterior (flocculo-nodular lobe; archi-cerebellum)	Eye movement disorders: nystagmus; vestibulo-ocular reflex; postural and gait dysfunction
Midline (vermis; paleo-cerebellum)	Truncal and gait ataxia
Hemisphere (neo-cerebellum)	Ipsilateral limb ataxia: dysmetria, dysdiadochokinesis, 'intention' tremor; dysarthria; hypotonia

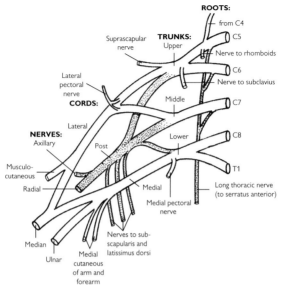

Fig. 1.8 Brachial plexus.

Reproduced with permission from MacKinnon P and Morris J. *Oxford Textbook of Functional Anatomy*, Volume 1, 2nd edition, Oxford: Oxford University Press, Copyright © 2005 Oxford University Press.

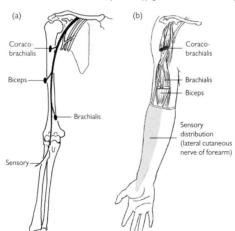

Fig. 1.9 Course of musculocutaneous nerve (a) supply to muscles (b) supply to skin.

Reproduced with permission from MacKinnon P and Morris J. *Oxford Textbook of Functional Anatomy*, Volume 1, 2nd edition, Oxford: Oxford University Press, Copyright © 2005 Oxford University Press.

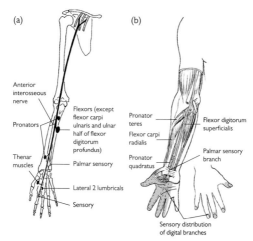

Fig. 1.10 Course of median nerve (a) supply to muscles (b) supply to skin.

Reproduced with permission from MacKinnon P and Morris J. *Oxford Textbook of Functional Anatomy*, Volume 1, 2nd edition, Oxford: Oxford University Press, Copyright © 2005 Oxford University Press.

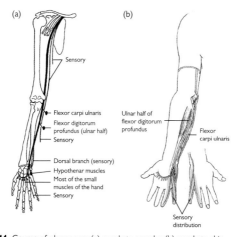

Fig. 1.11 Course of ulnar nerve (a) supply to muscles (b) supply to skin.

Reproduced with permission from MacKinnon P and Morris J. *Oxford Textbook of Functional Anatomy*, Volume 1, 2nd edition, Oxford: Oxford University Press, Copyright © 2005 Oxford University Press.

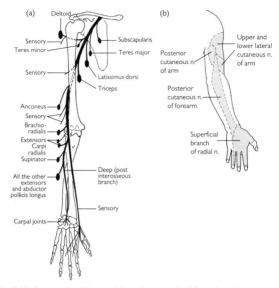

Fig. 1.12 Course of radial nerve (a) supply to muscles (b) supply to skin.

Innervation of lower limb

See Figures 1.13–1.17.

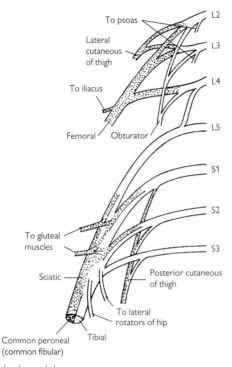

Fig. 1.13 Lumbosacral plexus.

Reproduced with permission from MacKinnon P and Morris J. *Oxford Textbook of Functional Anatomy*, Volume 1, 2nd edition, Oxford: Oxford University Press, Copyright © 2005 Oxford University Press.

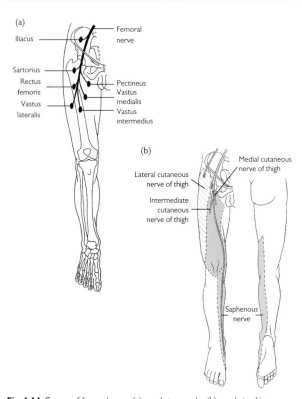

Fig. 1.14 Course of femoral nerve (a) supply to muscles (b) supply to skin.

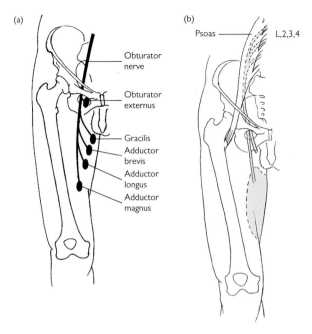

Fig. 1.15 Course of obturator nerve (a) supply to muscles (b) supply to skin.

Reproduced with permission from MacKinnon P and Morris J. *Oxford Textbook of Functional Anatomy*, Volume 1, 2nd edition, Oxford: Oxford University Press, Copyright © 2005 Oxford University Press.

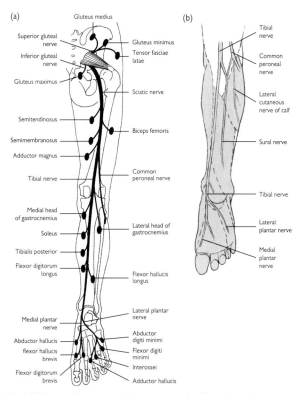

Fig. 1.16 Course of sciatic nerve (a) supply to muscles (b) supply to skin.

Reproduced with permission from MacKinnon P and Morris J. *Oxford Textbook of Functional Anatomy*, Volume 1, 2nd edition, Oxford: Oxford University Press, Copyright © 2005 Oxford University Press.

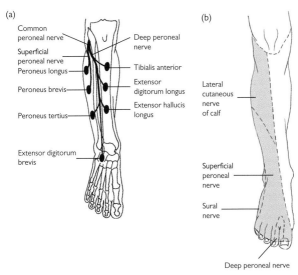

Fig. 1.17 Course of common peroneal nerve (a) supply to muscles (b) supply to skin.

Reproduced with permission from MacKinnon P and Morris J. *Oxford Textbook of Functional Anatomy*, Volume 1, 2nd edition, Oxford: Oxford University Press, Copyright © 2005 Oxford University Press.

Posture and gait

Posture

- Note extraneous movements (tics, chorea, etc.).
- Note whether stance is broad based.
- Ask the child to stand with their feet together, arms outstretched, and still with their eyes open. Is this difficult? Is it harder with their eyes closed? (Positive Romberg test sign implying poor proprioception.) A downward drift and pronation of one arm in this procedure implies mild pyramidal weakness.
- Is the child able to stand straight? Hip or knee flexion contractures may result in a 'crouch' stance.

Gait

Whilst it is usually fairly straightforward to recognize whether a gait is normal or not, putting your finger on exactly what is wrong in an abnormal gait can be challenging. For discussion of an approach to evaluation of abnormal gait, see Gait abnormalities in Chapter 3 ⊋ p. 157.

Neurological gait 'gestalts'

Neurological disease can cause one of several 'gestalt' gait appearances that allow pattern recognition.

- *Hemiparetic gait*. Equinus posture of the foot: tendency to catch a toe on the floor either resulting in the leg moving laterally during swing phase (circumduction), or compensatory hip flexion. Swing of the ipsilateral arm is impaired: may be held in a flexed posture. Greater wear on the sole of the shoe at the toe on the affected side can be seen.

- *Bilateral spastic gait*. Legs cross midline when viewed from in front with hips internally rotated ('scissor gait'): knees scraping together. Bilateral toe walking, and/or crouched stance due to bilateral flexion contractures at hips is seen. There is arm involvement in spastic bilateral CP.

- *Ataxic gait (cerebellar)*. Wide-based, staggering irregularly. Tandem gait (heel–toe walking along a line) is very difficult. Unilateral cerebellar disease gives ipsilateral ataxia (in tandem gait tends always to fall to same side; or compare the child's ability to walk round a chair clockwise and anticlockwise).

- *Sensory ataxia*. As cerebellar ataxia, but markedly worse with eyes closed. The child watches his feet intently as he walks.

- *Proximal weakness* (e.g. Duchenne dystrophy). Marked lumbar lordosis. A 'waddling' gait resulting from exaggerated rotation and 'throwing' of the hips to each side, accompanied by exaggerated alternating lateral flexion of the trunk (moving the body's centre of gravity as near to the hip joint as possible—to lessen the work the gluteal muscles have to do when the contralateral leg is off the floor). The ability to climb stairs is very limited.

- *Flaccid foot drop*. Weak foot dorsiflexion (tibialis anterior) results in the toe scraping the floor during the swing phase. 'Slapping' footfall sound. Tendency to step 'high' on the affected side flexing the hip to lift the foot clear of the floor.

- *Antalgic*. Due to pain: reluctance to weight-bear on the affected side: spending *less time on that leg*. Restricted range of movements, painful.

- *Functional*. Awkward posture, with tense, small, laboured shuffling steps, or exaggerated staggers or unsteadiness (astasia-abasia), which actually requires intact coordination to be able to reproduce: see Functional neurological symptoms in Chapter 4 p. 335.

- *Dystonic* and *athetotic* gaits can be variable and occasionally bizarre. They can be mistaken for functional gait disturbances (and vice versa). Dystonic gaits are typically accompanied by sustained posturing of the arms, trunk, head, and neck: involvement of one foot and ankle is a common presentation. Dystonia will also be demonstrable at rest. Dystonic gaits may show apparently bizarre variability, e.g. much less evident when running than walking, or when walking backward rather than forward.

When you don't recognize a pattern

See also Gait abnormalities in Chapter 3 → p. 157.

- Children with a cerebral palsy and other chronic neurodisability
  can have very idiosyncratic gaits due to the presence of additional
  biomechanical factors (contractures limiting the range of joint
  movement; limb length discrepancy, misalignment, or other orthopaedic
  factors). These will, however, be identifiable during static examination
  on the couch.
- Observe walking and running gaits over a significant distance and
  repeated requests. Do not try to take in all aspects of a child's gait
  simultaneously: there is too much to watch. In challenging situations,
  it can be helpful to video the gait to permit unhurried evaluation.
  Complex situations (certainly if surgery is being considered) may
  require formal gait analysis.

  To limit information overload in the clinic situation, consider:
- Just *listening* to the gait!
  - Is the child spending less time weight-bearing on one leg than the
    other? This implies *antalgia*: i.e. the child is avoiding weight-bearing
    because of unilateral (or at least asymmetric) *pain*.
  - Is the cadence irregular (ataxia)?
  - Is the sound of the foot fall normal (e.g. the split 'contact-slap' of a
    foot drop, or the single foot fall of a toe walker)?
- Base. Think about the track of footprints the child would leave in sand:
  - Wide- or narrow-based?
  - Watch where the feet fall and their distance from an imaginary centre
    line. Symmetrical? Consistent?
- Toe–heel or heel–toe?
- Hip internally rotated or externally rotated?
- Is it a weak gait? Waddle? Difficulty stepping up? Gowers?
- Starting at the feet and working up, consider the alignments of limb
  segments and the range of movement at each joint during the gait cycle
  and correlate with findings at rest on static examination.

Gowers' manoeuvre and sign

See Figure 1.18.

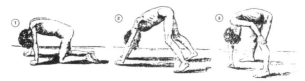

Fig. 1.18 Gowers' manoeuvre and sign.

Reprinted from *The Lancet*, Volume II, Gowers WR, Clinical lecture on pseudohypertrophic muscular paralysis, pp. 73–5, Copyright © 1879, with permission from Elsevier.

▶ Remember the key feature that defines a +ve Gowers' sign is not so much the 'walking up legs' which may be absent if the proximal weakness is mild, as the need to turn from supine lying to prone as a prelude to getting up.

Location of peripheral signs

Remember, the 'where' comes from signs (i.e. patterns of weakness, and/or distribution of sensory disturbances) interpreted in the light of neuroanatomical knowledge (see What, where, and when in this chapter ➋ p. 5).

Patterns of weakness
See Table 1.6. If the pattern suggests peripheral nerve involvement, this needs to be narrowed down further on the basis of Figures 1.7 and 1.8–1.17 as involving either a specified peripheral nerve, or a nerve root (radiculopathy). In the latter case, the pattern of weakness does not correspond to a particular peripheral nerve but to a *root level*. It will normally be associated with a corresponding dermatomal sensory loss although a very focal lesion can selectively involve the ventral or dorsal root only causing isolated weakness or dermatomal sensory loss respectively.

For example, weak ankle dorsiflexion could represent a common peroneal nerve injury (Fig. 1.17) or an L5 root injury (Fig. 1.13), but in the latter case sensory loss additionally includes the sole of the foot, lateral side of the knee, and the back of the thigh. Also, the L5 root pattern of motor weakness involves hip abductors and foot inverters.

Table 1.6 Patterns of weakness according to site of lesion

	Brain	Cord	Peripheral nerve	Neuro-muscular junction	Muscle
Pattern of weakness	Axial, truncal, or generalized hypotonia	Paraplegic or quadriplegic	Root or nerve distribution	Generalized	Variable distribution with individual conditions
Wasting	N	N	Y	N	Y
Fasciculation	N	N	Y	N	N
Tone	↑	↓	↓	Normal	Normal
Power	Normal or slight ↓	↓	↓	↓	↓
Reflexes	↑	↓ or absent*	↓	Normal	Normal
Plantar reflex	Upgoing	Initially downgoing; upgoing later*	Downgoing	Normal	Normal

* Note signs are initially of a LMN pattern in the acute phase of spinal shock.

Autonomic instability is seen in both peripheral nerve lesions (GBS) and acute spinal shock.

Neonatal neurological examination

Gestational age

Interpretation of clinical and investigation findings will crucially depend on an accurate knowledge of gestational age. If there are doubts about timing of maternal last menstrual period, then various assessment scales based on physical characteristics (development of cartilage in pinna; breast bud; external genitalia) are available.

▶ Assessments of gestational age based on tone and posture (e.g. the presence of 'scarf sign') should not be used for a neonate who has come to specialist neurological attention, whose tone is quite probably abnormal for age!

External appearance

- Note head size and shape and plot OFC.
- Palpate fontanelles (anterior and posterior).
- Observe for stigmata of neurocutaneous syndromes.
  - Cutaneous feature of neurofibromatosis are absent in neonates.
  - Of tuberous sclerosis (TS) features, only hypopigmented macules are present in the newborn. In Caucasian infants in whom TS is a consideration, Wood's (UV) light examination is mandatory.
  - A variety of inconsequential diffuse pigmentary changes may be seen under Wood's light. Pathognomonic lesions are 'ash leaf' (biconvex, 'lens-shaped') often with the long axis aligned along a dermatome.
- Note spontaneous limb posture (see below Tone and Power) and joint contractures.

Alertness

Level of alertness is a sensitive 'summary' indicator of central nervous system (CNS) function. Nursing staff and/or parents' assessments over several hours will be very informative. Avoid examining immediately after a feed (sleepy) or when very hungry and distressed.

Cranial nerves

Acuity and eye movements

- Tracking of a bright red ball or similar target should be elicitable in >90% of infants of >34 weeks' gestation.
- Dysconjugate eye movements are normal in the newborn if not visually attending, and roving eye movements are normal at <32 weeks.
- Oculokinetic nystagmus (OKN) (analogous to the repeated pursuit-re-fixation that occurs on looking at the passing scene from a train) simultaneously assesses acuity and eye movements. A rotating drum or tape with black and white stripes can be used.
  - It can also be conveniently examined by holding the child upright close to the examiner's face and then turning on the spot for several rotations first one way then the other. The rotation induces repeated nystagmus comprising a brief tonic eye deviation to one side (confirming intactness of horizontal eye movements in that direction as well as vestibular input) that is then overcome as the child's re-fixates on the examiner's face (i.e. demonstrating sufficient acuity to re-fixate).

- Note that visual tracking in its narrowest sense can probably be maintained by subcortical visual systems and may not exclude significant occipital cortex pathology. However, a responsive smile in a slightly older infant is necessarily cortical.

Pupils and fundoscopy

The physiological pupil reaction to light is consistently detectable at >32 weeks. More premature infants will blink to bright light.

Fundoscopy should include confirmation of a normal red reflex. Opacities in the cornea or media require a formal ophthalmological assessment to exclude cataract. A white retina is a potential sign of retinoblastoma and requires urgent referral.

Facial movement (VII)

- Any asymmetry of facial movement is typically very evident when crying. Lower motor neuron facial nerve injury can be seen after forceps delivery due to pressure over the zygoma. Bilateral facial palsy can be seen in Moebius syndrome.
- Asymmetric crying facies is an important benign differential of unilateral lower motor neuron facial nerve injury. This is caused by developmental hypoplasia of the depressor angularis oris muscle resulting in a failure of the lower lip on the affected side to grimace fully. The asymmetric crying facies may be mistaken for facial nerve injury but the face above the mouth (particularly the nasolabial folds) will be normal. An association with structural heart disease is reported but uncommon.

Hearing

'Alerting' responses to perceived auditory stimuli may be very subtle, and clinical assessment can be difficult. Universal neonatal hearing screening programmes are increasingly widespread.

Bulbar function

In practice, a history of efficient sucking and swallowing is the most useful indicator of bulbar function.

Sternocleidomastoid

Most readily examined in the supine position, lying with the head over the edge of the cot and supported by the examiner's hand. As this is slowly lowered, the sternocleidomastoid will become more apparent and palpable.

Peripheral neurological examination

Tone and power

- Distinguishing the hypotonic child from the child who is hypotonic *and peripherally weak* is key to the assessment of the 'floppy' neonate (see Floppy infants in Chapter 3 ➔ p. 143).
- For assessment of the abnormally *stiff* neonate, see The stiff, rigid infant in Chapter 3 ➔ p. 199).
- Interpretation of findings on assessment of tone must bear in mind gestational age: the pathological 'frog-leg' posture of a term infant with a neuromuscular disease would be normal at 26 weeks.
- Resting tone becomes increasingly flexor (i.e. limbs held spontaneously in a gently flexed position) with gestation, with flexor tone developing

in the legs before the arms (hips and knees held flexed by 32 weeks; elbows held flexed after 36 weeks).
- Observation of spontaneous limb movement is the best indication of power: particularly helpful is whether antigravity power is being seen, i.e. whether limbs are being lifted off the bed.
- Observation of the quality of spontaneous limb movement (its rhythmicity, jerkiness, amplitudes, etc.) is an extremely useful and sensitive indicator of neurological status and outlook, but again depends on gestation, and requires considerable experience and practice (the 'General Movements Assessment' approach pioneered by Heinz Prechtl). Jitteriness is usually a non-specific indicator of biochemical disturbances (e.g. hypoglycaemia) rather than intrinsic neurological disease.
- Before reporting asymmetry of tone, ensure the head is midline and that one is not simply detecting the physiological asymmetric tonic neck reflex.
- The Moro reflex is primarily useful as a means of inducing movements that can be assessed for symmetry and evidence of peripheral weakness (Table 1.7). It should not persist beyond 6 months.

The most common peripheral nerve injury in neonatal practice is a proximal cervical root injury at C5/6/7 (usually unilateral) due to shoulder dystocia and a difficult delivery.
- The classic Erb palsy comprises weakness of shoulder abduction, elbow flexion, and finger extension (see Entrapment neuropathies in Chapter 4 ⊃ p. 438). The arm is held extended, internally rotated with flexion at the wrist. No biceps reflex can be elicited although one may be present in the triceps. Sensation is diminished in the lateral aspect of the arm.

Deep tendon reflexes
Plantar reflexes are not informative in infancy. It can be hard to state confidently that deep tendon reflexes are pathologically exaggerated or depressed: alertness, sedative drugs, systemic illness, and many other factors can lead to temporary symmetric changes in reflexes. Asymmetry of reflexes is, however, very informative. Neither crossed adductor responses nor a few beats of unsustained clonus are pathological in the neonate.

Table 1.7 Normal age of disappearance of primitive reflexes

	Normal age at abolition
Babinski	12–18 months
Grasp	4–6 months; in toes 9–10 months
Moro	5–6 months
Rooting	3–4 months
Stepping	3–4 months
Sucking	3–4 months
Asymmetric tonic neck reflex	3–4 months

Sensory examination

In practice, the most common indication for sensory examination is in defining sensory levels in spina bifida. Although thankfully much rarer, be alert to trauma to the cervical spinal cord resulting in a flaccid tetraparesis with variable ventilatory function. To the novice, this picture may be mistaken for a globally suppressed, asphyxiated neonate. Pointers include the clinical context (breech extraction, no biochemical evidence of global hypoxic ischaemic insult) with a combination of preservation of facial alertness but lack of perception of painful stimuli. A limb may still withdraw from pain due to local spinal reflexes, but crying implies central perception of the stimulus.

Real-world examination sequences

Real-world neurological examination of the neonate

Care should be taken to avoid prolonged undressing that risks hypothermia, particularly in the sick neonate.

In supine lying (in cot)
- Note alertness.
- Note head shape, dysmorphic features, neurocutaneous stigmata.
- Palpate fontanelles.
- Examine range of doll's eye movements.
- Note visual interest in face. If there is particular concern/interest in visual acuity, consider OKN suppression assessment (see Acuity and eye movements in this chapter ➔ p. 41).
- Note symmetry of cry/smile.
- Note spontaneous antigravity limb movements.
- Deep tendon reflexes.
- Gentle arm traction to observe head lag.

In prone lying (in hand)
- Note tone (omit in sick neonate).

Return to cot
- Ophthalmoscopy: symmetry of light reflex; red reflex; fundoscopy.
- Moro reflex. Primarily indicates integrity of the peripheral nervous system.
- Head circumference.

Real-world neurological examination of the infant

Sitting on mother's knee
- Note alertness; visual interest in faces; spontaneous vocalization.
- Observe range and symmetry of eye movements tracking an interesting object. Re-fixation on objects moved peripherally from central vision implies intactness of the visual field in that direction.
- Note the level at which the mother has to support the trunk, e.g. under arms, around waist, at pelvis, etc.
- Opportunistically note upper limb and hand movements for symmetry and completeness; note hand regard, bringing of hands to the midline.
- Offer an object (e.g. a small ring) and note the symmetry of hand use, transfer of object between hands and/or to the mouth.

On the couch
- Lying supine, note attempts to sit up or roll over.
- From supine lying pull to sit and note head lag.
- In sitting, note the need for support. If not yet sitting unsupported, gently tip to each side to detect lateral righting reflexes and their symmetry.
- Lift an older infant (>6 months) onto their feet. Observe for scissoring. Optionally examine for forward and downward parachute reflexes.

Lying on mother's shoulder, head turned to side (looking outward)
- Ophthalmoscopy: light reflex; red reflex; fundoscopy.

Back on mother's knee
- Biceps, quadriceps deep tendon reflexes.
- Head circumference.

Real-world neurological examination of the toddler

This is the group par excellence where opportunistic observation forms the backbone of the examination. There is little to be gained from the attempted formal examination of a crying child.

Sitting (on mother's knee)
- Opportunistically note language, interaction with mother, family members, and strangers (i.e. you!)
- Opportunistically observe visual attention, range, and symmetry of eye movements.

Moving around the room
A playroom-type setting with equipment to climb in and onto is the most informative.
- Observe gait. Wide-based (allowing for age)? Symmetric?
- Observe climbing up step or stair. Observe picking an item off the floor from the standing position: squats down? Can rise from squat?
- Observe upper limb function ideally in the sitting position (e.g. colouring sat at desk) for handedness, dexterity, coordination in reaching.
- Encourage an independent walk or run (e.g. from one parent to other).

Back on mother's knee
- Biceps, quadriceps deep tendon reflexes.
- Ophthalmoscopy: light and red reflex (views of discs will require an assistant to secure the child's visual interest).
- Head circumference.

Real-world examination of a grossly normal older child

Higher mental function
- Informal impressions of language, understanding of, and participation in the consultation.
- Observation of 'restlessness': may indicate disorders of attention.

Cranial nerve function
- Pupil reactivity to light and accommodation.
- Fundoscopy.
- Pursuit eye movements.
- Binocular assessment of temporal visual fields to confrontation.
- Bite and waggle jaw from side to side (V); grimace and eye closure (VII).
- Symmetry of uvula movement on 'ahh' (IX); put out tongue (XII).
- Shrug shoulders (XI).

Peripheral nerve function
Isolated sensory losses without accompanying motor signs are very uncommon in paediatrics; ∴ motor examination suffices except in situations of specific concern.
- Stand with feet together, arms outstretched, palms upward, and eyes closed. This is a sensitive screen for even mild pyramidal weakness of

arms (causes slow pronation and downward drift of the affected arm) and incorporates the equivalent of a Romberg test.
• In the same position with eyes still closed, slowly bring one index finger up to touch the nose and repeat on the other side. Screens for cerebellar and/or proprioceptive loss.
• Walking and running gaits.
• Deep tendon reflexes.

Supplemental tasks if indicated
• Visual acuity/hearing when indicated by history.
• Gowers' manoeuvre.
• Assess for visceromegaly, heart murmurs, skeletal signs of storage disorders, skin changes.

Fog's test
Elicits associated movements in the upper limbs, when the child is asked to heel-walk, toe-walk, or walk on inverted or everted feet. In the 4-yr-old, the upper limbs normally mirror the pattern of movement in the lower limbs. This becomes much less marked or has disappeared entirely by 9–10 yrs of age. Asymmetries which are marked and reproducible point to a hemi-syndrome on the exaggerated side. The signs should not be over-read. The more demanding tasks, such as walking on the inner border of the feet, are more likely to reveal a mild, non-significant asymmetry with mildly excessive posturing in the non-dominant arm. Posturing which is bilaterally exaggerated for the child's age points to an underlying developmental dyspraxia or clumsiness, which is unlikely to be pathological.

Real-world examination of the unconscious child
For recognition of brainstem herniation syndromes and assessment of conscious level in emergency settings, see Examine for signs of herniation in Chapter 6 ➔ p. 614.

The examination of a stable unconscious child comprises assessments of brainstem function as manifest by cranial nerve signs; and hemispheric function as reflected by spontaneous or induced limb movement, although the latter are particularly sensitive to the effects of sedation and anaesthesia (or indeed paralysis!) and may not be assessable.

As well as observing, enquire of nursing staff as to what limb movements have been noted in recent hours occurring either spontaneously or induced by cares and other procedures.
• Document blood pressure, pulse, and respiratory rate.
• Localizing movements (e.g. reaching for nasogastric or endotracheal tube) implies largely intact cortical function.
• Abnormal flexion (decorticate posturing) implies loss of cortical function (but preserved subcortical function).
• Abnormal extension (decerebrate posturing) implies loss of hemispheric function on the contralateral side.
• Prognostically, the best motor performance is most relevant although asymmetry of motor performance is very informative.
• Tendon reflexes, and the presence of clonus and plantar responses can be examined in the usual manner. Reflexes can be suppressed by sedative agents, but asymmetry of reflexes is informative.

- Assess pupil size.
  - Pupillary abnormalities can reflect severe brainstem dysfunction or the effects of opiate sedation. Pupillary size and responses to light should be examined for evidence of either herniation (see Examine for signs of herniation in Chapter 6 ➔ p. 614) or afferent pupillary defect (see Afferent pupillary defect in this chapter ➔ p. 19), particularly in the context of orbital trauma.
- Demonstration of venous pulsation (see Venous pulsation in this chapter ➔ p. 18) or papilloedema on fundoscopy is informative in relation to intracranial pressure (ICP) although the absence of papilloedema cannot be taken as reassurance of normal ICP.
- Resting eye position is not very informative. Oculocephalic reflex eye movements are useful and can be elicited even in the intubated child with assistance to ensure the tube is not dislodged. The head is turned sharply to one side with eyes held open but the direction of gaze in space is preserved (i.e. the eyes move in the orbits to compensate for head turn, allowing evaluation of extraocular movement). These manoeuvres should not be performed in the context of traumatic injury unless and until the cervical spine has been 'cleared' as stable. As an alternative, consider the use of caloric testing (see Vestibulo-ocular reflexes in Chapter 5 ➔ p. 584).
- Elicit corneal reflexes.
- Note symmetry of nasolabial folds and any grimace or other induced facial expression.
- In an intubated child, assessment of gag is most usefully assessed by enquiring after the response nurses are noting to oropharyngeal suction (rather than suction of the endotracheal tube itself).

Synthesis

Synthesizing historical and clinical findings into a differential diagnosis and investigation plan is the essence of the clinical process.

❶ Neurologists' diagnostic pronouncements are sometimes and unwisely regarded as infallible by other paediatricians. Be aware of some causes of downfall!

Some general points

- Remember the examination findings locate the site of the problem, the history suggests its nature.
- Try to define the system(s) involved (i.e. the 'where?') in broad terms: central or peripheral nervous system? Cerebellum? Basal ganglia? Cerebral hemispheres? Bilaterally or unilaterally?
- Ultimately the history is the richer source of information and is more likely to lead you to the diagnosis.
- It is vitally important to be aware of the prior likelihood of particular conditions. Some conditions in paediatric neurology are orders of magnitude more likely than others. Familiarity with ethnic or other factors that cause local 'pockets' of particular conditions is important.
- Unusual presentations of common conditions are still probably more likely than common presentations of uncommon conditions.
- Humans have an inherent tendency to see the evidence that supports their working hypothesis, and not look for the evidence that might disprove it (so-called confirmation bias, see Box 1.1).

Box 1.1 Card sorting

In a classic psychological experiment subjects were shown four playing cards (Fig. 1.19):

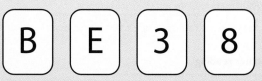

Fig. 1.19 Sorting cards.

Which two cards have to be turned over in order to check the validity of the hypothesis that 'every consonant has an even number on the other side of the card'? People tend to assume that the B and 8 cards must be turned over whereas B and 3 are correct. Whatever is on the reverse of the 8 card remains consistent with the hypothesis; it would be finding a consonant on the back of the 3 card that would disprove it.

- Actively try to disprove your diagnostic hypotheses!
- When all you have is a hammer, everything looks like a nail. Just because the child has been referred to a neurologist does not ensure this is a problem of neurological origin.
- Beware 'search bias', settling on the first plausible explanation you can think of for the picture: try to generate five! Consider each diagnosis in turn: what would the signs and symptoms be if the child had that diagnosis? This may prevent you dismissing uncommon but treatable conditions at an early stage because of a cognitive error that there is insufficient information yet to act.
- Beware 'availability bias'. People overestimate the likelihood of aeroplane crashes as a cause of death because, as newsworthy events, they can readily recall an example. Similarly just because you remember that disease X turned out to be the cause of sign Y last time, don't overestimate the likelihood of its being responsible again at the expense of other possibilities.
- Beware Kouska's fallacy. It can be hard to evaluate the significance of combinations of findings that you can't immediately connect and would normally be individually thought of as uncommon. It is more likely that the events are causally linked, either directly or indirectly (even if you can't see the link) than that they are really occurring coincidentally completely by chance. The assumption that the findings are independent is sometimes called Kouska's fallacy, after a fictional character who used this technique to disprove the existence of life!

▶ Remember:
- What else could it be?
- Is there anything that doesn't fit?
- Is it possible there's more than one problem?
- What is the family most worried about?
- Ask them to retell the story from the beginning.
- Details that were omitted first time, different wordings, or emphases may be seen to have significance in light of other data.

Further reading

Groopman JE (2008) *How Doctors Think*. Mariner Books

Neurodiagnostic tools

Principles of investigation

Sensitivity, specificity, and all that jazz ...

This subject tends to bring some people out in a rash. Unfortunately it is of fundamental importance to paediatric neurology, so bear with us! Refer to Table 2.1.

Table 2.1 Sensitivity and specificity

	Disease truly present	Disease truly absent
Test result +ve (abnormal)	A (true +ves)	B (false +ves)
Test result –ve (normal)	C (false –ves)	D (true –ves)

Sensitivity
The probability that the test will identify a case when the disease is present, given by the fraction $A/(A+C)$. Answers the question: if the test is administered to a group of people *all of whom actually have the disease*, in what proportion will it be (correctly) +ve?

Specificity
The probability that the test will be –ve when the disease is not present, given by the fraction $D/(D+B)$. Answers the question: if the test is administered to a group of people *none of whom* actually have the disease, in what proportion will it correctly give a normal, –ve result?

Positive predictive value (PPV)
The probability of the disease truly being present if the test is +ve, given by the fraction $A/(A+B)$.

Negative predictive value (NPV)
The probability of the disease being absent if the test is –ve, given by fraction $D/(C+D)$.
   PPV and NPV answer the question 'just how informative *is* a +ve (or, for NPV, –ve) test result?'
- While PPV may sound like sensitivity it is not: it has been 'turned round'. The probability, given that an animal is a cat, of it having four legs (the sensitivity of the four-leg test in identifying cats) will generally be greater than the probability, given that an animal has four legs, of it being a cat (the PPV of the four-leg test).
- PPV and NPV *depend on the prevalence of the condition in the population you are studying*, i.e. how likely it was that the disease was present *before* you applied the test. Relying on the four-leg test to identify cats in Battersea Dogs' Home is unwise *because the prior likelihood of finding cats in a dog pound is very low*. If you apply a test to look for a condition that under the circumstances is improbable, false +ves are quite likely and can even outnumber true +ves.

Utility indices
The positive and negative utility indices (UI) are numbers that quantify the ultimate value of a test in ruling in (positive UI) or ruling out (negative UI) a diagnosis. A test may have a high PPV but ultimately be of little use as it's

rarely +ve in the population you're testing. The positive UI is defined as sensitivity × PPV, and the negative UI as specificity × NPV.

An extreme example of looking for a disease in a situation where it is unlikely

- Suppose we're searching for a disease with a prevalence in our population (the prior probability) of 1 in 100 000 (there are considerably rarer conditions in paediatric neurology).
- We have a test with 99% specificity and sensitivity (much better than many tests in paediatric neurology).
- We test 1 million people, and given the prevalence expect there are 10 true cases in this population. The test has 99% sensitivity, so assume it picks up all 10 (it only misses 1 case in 100).
- However, it also has 99% specificity, meaning that 1 time in 100 it will say the disease is present when it is not. Unfortunately therefore, in testing the 999 990 people who don't have the disease, it will *falsely* state the condition is present when it isn't 1% of the time (i.e. on *just under 10 000 occasions!*)
- So how useful was a +ve test result here? (i.e. what is the PPV?) Unfortunately, not very much. We will get a total of 10 010 +ve test results, of which only 10 are truly +ve, a PPV of ~0.1%.
- What difference has applying the test made to the odds that the condition is present in a given individual? Beforehand, (the 'prior likelihood') it was 1 in 100 000. Now, having applied the test, and assuming the individual is among those with a +ve test result, the so-called posterior likelihood is 1 in 10 010—only nine times higher.
- *Applying the test has done little to increase the certainty with which we can say the individual is affected by the disease.* This is all because the disease was so improbable in the population to start with.
- In this example the prior likelihood has to get above 1% (by careful clinical evaluation and selection of a population in which the condition is reasonably likely in which to apply the test) before the true +ve test results outnumber the false +ves!

❶ This sort of situation is potentially common in paediatric neurology, where individually rare disorders are sought with imperfect tests. This is why it is dangerous blindly to apply batteries of tests looking on the off chance for diseases that are improbable in the clinical context.

The nose-picking principle of paediatric neurology

'Performing an investigation in paediatric neurology is like picking your nose: you don't want to find a result and *then* have to figure out what to do with it!'

In other words, perform investigations:

- Only when you have reasonable clinical grounds to suspect the condition being sought (to avoid generating potentially false +ve results whose significance you are uncertain of).
- Only when the test result will influence a management decision.
  - This may include establishing a diagnosis for purposes of genetic counselling, prognostication, or parental peace of mind, even if no specific treatments exist.

Principles of neuroradiology

See Table 2.2 for a comparison of the radiological characteristics of common neurological pathologies.

Computerized tomography

- X-ray-based technique delivering a radiation dose 10–100 times that of a standard chest X-ray. This is a significant disadvantage in children, particularly if multiple studies are anticipated.
  - It's estimated one excess case of leukaemia and one excess brain tumour are caused per 10 000 head CT scans performed in children under 10.
- Main advantages are speed (important if a child is critically ill) and its adequacy for many neurosurgical management decisions. CT thus retains a major role in the early management of neurotrauma.
- As an X-ray technique, it is better suited than MRI to study of the bony skull and to the detection of intracranial calcification.
- In the assessment of fractures (e.g. of the orbital roof) and craniosynostosis, 'bone windows' will be used: adjusting the 'brightness' and 'contrast' of the image to increase sensitivity at the white end of the grey scale. This is at the expense of detail in the intracranial cavity that appears as an 'underexposed' void.
- Spiral CT (Fig. 2.1) is particularly useful for the imaging of the skull itself but involves an even higher radiation dose.

White (or light grey) on CT is an X-ray absorbing substances and in practice will be either:
- Blood.
- Bone (or calcification).
- Contrast.
  - Intravenously injected contrast media enhance highly vascular structures such as arteriovenous malformations, some tumours, and abscesses.

Distinguishing these is generally straightforward: blood is not as white as calcium/bone (i.e. it appears light grey rather than white), and you will know if contrast has been given!

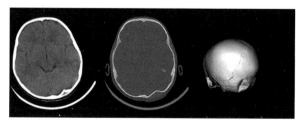

Fig. 2.1 CT imaging of a left occipital depressed skull fracture using conventional windowing (left). The fracture is more obvious on the bone window image (centre). Spiral CT reconstructs a 3D image of the skull as if viewed from behind and to the left of the head. The fracture is clearly visible (right). Note that axial CT (and MR) images are conventionally oriented 'as if looking up from the feet' and thus a left-sided fracture appears on the right side of the image.

Areas of *reduced* X-ray absorption in brain tissue (appearing darker grey) are typically due to *oedema*. Air appears black.

Metallic implants (such as clips or intracranial pressure monitoring devices) tend to cause 'sunburst'-like beam hardening artefacts although this does not affect their functioning.

CT angiography
CT angiography studies are performed following injection of intravenous contrast by a high-velocity injector to achieve temporarily high concentrations. As with MRA (below), 3D reconstruction techniques are available. CTA is superior to MRA for evaluation of some forms of large vessel (particularly carotid) disease and vasculitis and can be useful in the early evaluation of cerebral haemorrhage.

CT venography may be helpful in confirming venous sinus patency in acute cases where MR venography is not readily available.

MRI
In a very strong magnetic field, protons (hydrogen nuclei) emit a weak radio signal that can be detected in an overlying coil. The signal is modified by the physico-chemical environment of the protons (e.g. the local water content) and it this information that is represented in the scan image. MRI does not involve ionizing radiation and is superior to CT in all situations other than imaging bone or detection of calcification. Image acquisition is, however, prolonged (typically 20–30 min or more for a full study) and a claustrophobic and noisy experience for young children.

- Neonates and infants can typically be scanned in spontaneous sleep after a feed.
- Oral sedation is widely used in toddlers because of limited anaesthetic resources but is less effective and arguably less safe than general anaesthesia. Sedation is increasingly ineffective over 5 yrs of age.
- General anaesthetic is safe and guarantees images unaffected by movement artefact, the child waking in the scanner, etc., but requires specialist (non-metallic) equipment and clinician time.
- The very strong magnetic fields of MR scanners can be a consideration. The function of cardiac pacemakers, intrathecal baclofen pumps, vagus nerve stimulators, and other devices can be affected. Smaller objects, such as arterial clips, may move, and larger metal implants such as spinal rods can create signal voids obscuring the normal anatomy. Metallic objects can also heat up and cause local tissue damage.

Gadolinium contrast medium (injected intravenously) highlights vascular structures and can be useful in the evaluation of inflammatory lesions but its use is intentionally restricted.

- Hypersensitivity to gadolinium is well recognized (0.1% population).
- An extremely rare progressive systemic disease (nephrogenic systemic fibrosis) has been linked to gadolinium exposure in individuals with impaired renal function.
- There is some evidence that gadolinium accumulates in the brain. The long-term significance of this is unclear.

MRI scanners are defined by the *field strength* of their main magnet, measured in Tesla (T).

- 3T machines are increasingly standard with 7T machines becoming available.

- Stronger magnets allow greater spatial resolution (ability to see more detail) and/or shorter image acquisition times.
- *Open scanners* are less claustrophobic and may allow a child to cooperate without anaesthesia; however, the open design results in a lower magnet field strength.

MRI sequences

Many different MRI sequences are possible, each reflecting different physio-chemical properties of brain tissue, and in turn suited to the detection of different brain pathologies.

T1

Tends to reflect visible appearances better than other sequences: lesions visible on T1 are likely to be visually identifiable at surgery. Grey matter looks grey and white matter lighter grey. Cerebrospinal fluid (CSF) looks black (Fig. 2.2).

T2

T2 weighting is particularly sensitive to the presence of *water*. Pathologically, areas of high T2 signal intensity reflect oedema, e.g. due to inflammation or tumour. Not surprisingly CSF is bright white (Fig. 2.3).

FLAIR (fluid-attenuated inversion recovery)

Can be thought of as T2 with the CSF signal specifically suppressed. This makes it particularly suitable for the detection of pathology immediately

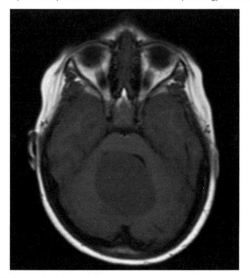

Fig. 2.2 T1 MRI. Typical T1-weighted image showing a large posterior fossa tumour (medulloblastoma). T1 appearances tend to reflect macroscopic appearances at surgery and suggest this tumour will be identifiable and potentially resectable.

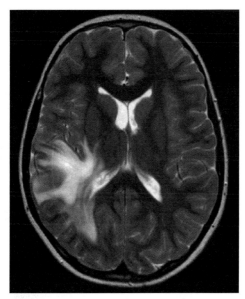

Fig. 2.3 T2 MRI. Typical T2-weighted image showing white CSF in lateral ventricles; grey matter is lighter grey than white matter. The large area of high T2 signal in the right parieto-occipital white matter reflects water, i.e. oedema, representing inflammation. This child presented almost asymptomatically with a quadrantanopic visual field defect (c.f. lesion 'momentum'; see 'When' was the process? in Chapter 1 ➲ p. 6) thus clinically a slow-growing tumour was suspected but, surprisingly, biopsy showed demyelination.

adjacent to the ventricles that can otherwise be 'swamped' by the CSF signal (e.g. subependymal nodules in tuberous sclerosis and white matter changes in multiple sclerosis).

MR angiography/venography

This is an important and widely utilized means of non-invasive imaging of large arteries and veins. Requires skilled interpretation, as artefactual flow voids giving the appearance of apparent vessel narrowing are quite common. It is significantly less reliable in evaluation of the posterior circulation. Useful for excluding venous sinus thrombosis (Fig. 2.4).

Diffusion-weighted imaging (DWI)

Quantifies the extent to which water is free to diffuse within tissues, which can be particularly affected by *cytotoxic oedema* (↑intracellular volume restricts diffusion through the extracellular space). Its main clinical application is acute stroke medicine where ischaemic tissue shows *restricted diffusion* before changes develop in other sequences, enabling consideration of

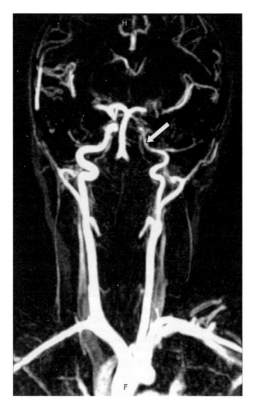

Fig. 2.4 MRA. Typical MRA image showing narrowing of left internal carotid proximal to the circle of Willis (white arrow) due to dissection.

emergency treatments such as thrombolysis. Areas of restricted diffusion have the opposite appearance to the ventricles (where water diffusion is entirely unrestricted). Under certain circumstances, *increased* diffusion can reflect ↑ extracellular space for diffusion (e.g. tissue loss or vasogenic oedema).

Diffusion-weighted imaging also forms the basis of diffusion tensor imaging (DTI) or 'tractography', a technique aimed at inferring white matter tract alignments (on the basis that water will diffuse more readily along a white matter tract than perpendicular to it; Fig. 2.5).

Fat-saturation sequences

A technique that selectively suppresses the signal from fat. Particularly useful for examination of the carotids in axial views of the neck in suspected

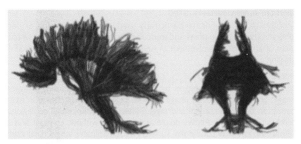

Fig. 2.5 Sagittal (left) and coronal (right) diffusion tensor images (tractography) of white matter fibres passing through corpus callosum in a healthy adult. False colour is typically added in these studies to aid visualization.

carotid artery dissection (see Investigation in Chapter 4 ⮎ p. 505) and can be at least as sensitive as MRA in this context.

Susceptibility weighted imaging (SWI)

A sequence sensitive to the presence of paramagnetic material, including intracranial calcification, but particularly *iron*. This includes iron deposition due to micro-haemorrhage and conditions such as the NBIAs (see Neurodegeneration with brain iron accumulation in Chapter 4 ⮎ p. 232). These areas appear black. It is particularly useful for the quantification of micro-haemorrhage that occurs in diffuse axonal injury after traumatic brain injury (allowing prognostication) and confirmation of suspected cavernomas (see Cavernous haemangiomas ('Cavernomas') in Chapter 4 ⮎ p. 512). It also shows blood vessels well (Fig. 2.6).

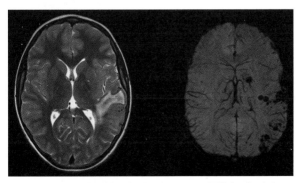

Fig. 2.6 Conventional T2w imaging (left) in this child with CNS scleroderma shows an area of left parietal oedema and hints at adjacent areas of micro-haemorrhage; these and many others are much more evident on the SWI imaging (right).

Short tau inversion recovery (STIR)

Sensitive to tissue oedema: particularly used in MRI examination of peripheral muscles. Myopathies and muscular dystrophies have distinctive patterns of anatomical involvement of muscles that can be delineated by STIR imaging.

Arterial spin labelling (ASL)

Involves tagging arterial blood by magnetic inversion, acquiring a tagged image, and then a second image without tagging. The difference in magnetization between control and tagged images is proportional to regional cerebral blood flow. Allows quantitative imaging without contrast and is sensitive in low flow conditions, such as AVMs. Facilitates longitudinal study of flow conditions, e.g. following revascularization surgery for moyamoya disease (see Moyamoya disease in Chapter 4 🠖 p. 507).

Functional MRI (fMRI)

Plays an important clinical role in the evaluation of epilepsy surgery candidates particularly if the seizure focus is near an area of potentially 'eloquent' cortex (see Surgical treatment of epilepsy in Chapter 4 🠖 p. 312).

Blood Oxygen Level Dependent (BOLD) imaging uses signals dependent on the ratio of oxy- to deoxy-haemoglobin in a region to infer local ↑ in blood flow, which in turn is taken as an indication of ↑ local neuronal activity.

• In *task-dependent* fMRI the BOLD signal is used to identify areas of brain activation associated with the performance of specific tasks (such as a movement or cognitive task) which together with carefully designed control tasks can be used to infer localization of that function.

• *Resting state* fMRI identifies patterns of inter-regional *functional connectivity*. Areas whose 'spontaneous' fluctuations in BOLD signal show temporal correlation are assumed to be functionally connected.

Magnetic resonance spectroscopy (MRS)

Chemicals have specific magnetic resonance signatures, which can be used to quantify their levels in a user-defined 'volume of interest', the minimum size of which is determined by scanner magnet strength but is typically ~ 1 cm^3. Substances assayed by MRS include lactate, choline, and creatine. ↑ lactate levels may indicate failure of aerobic metabolism (e.g. mitochondrial disease or in the centres of hypoxic tumours). Choline is found in cell membranes and levels are typically elevated in tumours. An absent creatine peak is the hallmark of the rare but treatable creatine deficiency disorders (see Creatine deficiency disorders in Chapter 4 🠖 p. 300).

Other imaging modalities

Cranial ultrasound

A non-invasive imaging modality particularly important in neonatal neurology. As in other forms of ultrasonography (e.g. echocardiography) ultra-high frequency sound waves are emitted from a probe that also detects returning echoes off underlying tissues. The distance of the reflecting structure from the probe can be inferred from the echo latency, and converted into a real-time image of the structures underlying the probe.

Its use in brain imaging is limited to the period before closure of the anterior fontanelle. It is particularly useful for assessment of ventricular size, and for the detection of intra- and peri-ventricular haemorrhage (blood is echogenic) and its non-invasive and portable nature makes it particularly suitable for use in sick neonates in intensive care settings. Because of the very narrow viewing window it is poor at imaging the cerebral cortex, sub-cortical structures away from the midline, and the posterior fossa.

Transcranial Doppler ultrasound
Increasingly used in neurocritical care as a quick and non-invasive evaluation of cerebral haemodynamics. An ultrasound probe is applied to thin areas of cranial bone (transtemporal, transorbital, submandibular and suboccipital acoustic windows) to measure blood flow velocity in major cerebral arteries. Used to assess perfusion in traumatic, hypoxic–ischaemic, and metabolic encephalopathy. Also used to predict stroke risk in sickle cell disease.

Cerebral angiography (digital subtraction angiography)
The 'gold standard' form of angiography for the evaluation and treatment of cerebrovascular disease. It requires invasive arterial (or venous) catheterization (typically percutaneously via femoral artery) and injection of radio-opaque contrast to visualize the arterial tree. In the newer digital subtraction angiography (DSA), a 'before-contrast' X-ray image is digitally subtracted from the image after injection, offering greater detail of fine-calibre vessels.

Very importantly, angiography also permits endovascular *treatment* of suitable arteriovenous malformations, aneurysms, or other vascular malformations (through the placement of endovascular coils or the use of glue embolization).

Positron emission tomography (PET)
A functional imaging technique using gamma cameras to localize the uptake in different brain regions of positron-emitting isotopes (which indirectly cause gamma emission). In principle positron-emitting isotopes can be incorporated into a wide variety of molecules and used to reflect and map a wide variety of brain processes. These include mapping of blood flow (oxygen-15), glucose metabolism (fluoro-deoxyglucose), and the presence of particular neurotransmitter receptors (e.g. labelled flumazenil binding to benzodiazepine receptors). The need for an on-site cyclotron for the manufacture of the short-lived isotopes is a major limitation but it has a role in localizing seizure foci in evaluation of candidates for epilepsy surgery.

Single photon emission computed tomography (SPECT)
'Poor man's PET'. Directly gamma-emitting isotopes can be injected, and conventional gamma camera imaging used, to map cerebral blood flow semi-quantitatively at the time of injection. Used in the evaluation of candidates for epilepsy surgery (by comparing ictal and inter-ictal patterns of blood flow) and in planning cerebral revascularization surgery.

Table 2.2 Radiological characteristics of neurological pathologies

Pathology	Ultrasound	CT	MRI-T1	MRI-T2/FLAIR	DWI	MRS	Other sequences
Oedema	Diffuse echogenicity	Hypodense. Reduced grey-white matter differentiation; sulcal pattern flattened	Hypointense	Hyperintense	Hyperintense. 'Cytotoxic': ↓ ADC (restricted diffusion) 'Vasogenic': ↑ ADC (↑ diffusion)		
Mitochondrial cytopathy		Focal hypodensities	Hypointense	Hyperintense	Vasogenic pattern (see above) in MELAS	Lactate doublet peak in mitochondrial disorders; NAA/Cr reduced	Perfusion imaging: ↑ perfusion indices
Infarction	↓ echogenicity	Hypodense	Hypointense	Hyperintense in chronic lesions (lags DWI changes)	Hyperintense with ↓ ADC (cytotoxic pattern) in recent lesions. Normal/↑ADC in older lesions	Lactate ↑, NAA/Cr reduced	Perfusion imaging: ↑mean transit time, reduced CBF (reduced perfusion)
Haemorrhage	↑echogenicity	Hyperdense	Hypointense, then hyperintense after a few days. Hypointense in chronic lesions	Hypointense early. Hyperintense cavity in later lesions	Hyperintense/low ADC (restricted diffusion)		
Abscess		Hypodense Contrast-enhancing	Hypointense	Hyperintense. Surrounding oedema hyperintensity typical	Hyperintense/low ADC (restricted diffusion)		Perfusion imaging: ↓ perfusion indices

Pathology	Ultrasound	CT	MRI-T1	MRI-T2/FLAIR	DWI	MRS	Other sequences
Demyelination		Hypodense/normal	Hypointense. Contrast enhancement in acute lesions	Hyperintense. Focal lesions with surrounding oedema (hypointense rim) in 'tumefactive' lesions	Variable ADC	↑Choline/Cr; myo-inositol and lactate peak. ↓ NAA/Cr	
Tumour (glioma)		Hypodense. Peri-lesional oedema and contrast enhancement in high-grade lesion	Hypointense. Contrast enhancement in high-grade lesion	Hyperintense High-grade lesions have oedema	Hypointense/ high ADC (more restricted diffusion in high-grade)	↑Choline/Cr ratio; ↓ NAA/Cr	Perfusion imaging: ↑perfusion indices in high-grade lesion
Fat/lipoma	↑echogenicity	Hypodense	Hyperintense, No contrast enhancement	Hyperintense			
Calcification	↑echogenicity	Hyperdensities	Variable (subtle)	Hypointense (subtle)			

Differential of ring-enhancing lesions:

Infective: toxoplasmosis, cysticercosis, TB, miliary bacterial abscesses.

Haemorrhage.

Lymphoma, high-grade glioma.

Demyelination.

Tumour.

Neuroradiological anatomy

See Figures 2.7–2.9.

1 Amygdala
2 Anterior commissure
3 Aqueduct
4 Caudate nucleus (head)
5 Caudate nucleus (tail)
6 Central sulcus
7 Cerebellum
8 Cerebral peduncles
9 Corpus callosum
10 Fornix
11 Fourth cranial (trochlear)
   nerve nucleus
12 Globus pallidus
13 Hippocampus
14 Hypophysis
15 Inferior colliculus
16 Infundibulum
17 Insula
18 Internal capsule
19 Internal capsule (anterior limb)
20 Internal capsule (genu)
21 Internal capsule (posterior limb)
22 Lateral ventricle
23 Mamillary bodies
24 Medulla (oblongata)
25 Motor strip
26 Optic chiasm
27 Optic tract
28 Pineal gland
29 Pons
30 Putamen
31 Red nucleus
32 Sensory strip
33 Septum pellucidum
34 Splenium of corpus callosum
35 Substantia nigra
36 Subthalamic nucleus
37 Superior colliculus
38 Tectum
39 Thalamus
40 Third cranial nerve
41 Third ventricle
42 Trigone
43 Visual cortex

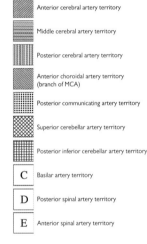

Anterior cerebral artery territory

Middle cerebral artery territory

Posterior cerebral artery territory

Anterior choroidal artery territory
(branch of MCA)

Posterior communicating artery territory

Superior cerebellar artery territory

Posterior inferior cerebellar artery territory

C Basilar artery territory

D Posterior spinal artery territory

E Anterior spinal artery territory

Fig. 2.7 Key to neuroanatomical sections in Figure 2.8.

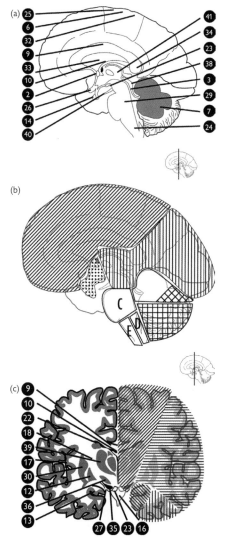

Fig. 2.8 Neuroanatomical sections.

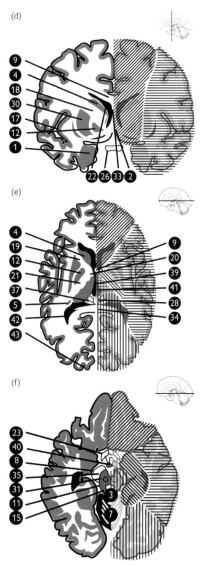

Fig. 2.8 (contd.)

(a)

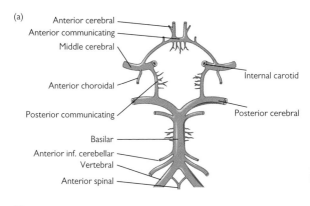

Anterior cerebral
Anterior communicating
Middle cerebral
Anterior choroidal
Posterior communicating
Basilar
Anterior inf. cerebellar
Vertebral
Anterior spinal
Internal carotid
Posterior cerebral

(b)

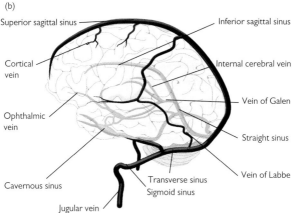

Superior sagittal sinus
Cortical vein
Ophthalmic vein
Cavernous sinus
Jugular vein
Inferior sagittal sinus
Internal cerebral vein
Vein of Galen
Straight sinus
Vein of Labbe
Transverse sinus
Sigmoid sinus

Fig. 2.9 Vascular anatomy. A (Top) Circle of Willis B (bottom) cerebral venous sinuses.
Adapted from Stroke Guidelines Adults & Children, Stroke Center Bern, Switzerland.

Anatomical terms in radiology reports

A number of potentially unfamiliar descriptor phrases are commonly used in neuroradiology reports:

Centrum semiovale

Refers to the subcortical white matter of the frontal and parietal lobes. This is essentially all the white matter superior to the lateral ventricles, extending fully anteriorly and posteriorly (area A in Fig. 2.10). The name comes from the approximately semi-circular outline (in each hemisphere) of this area in axial views.

Corona radiata

Effectively the 'transitional zone' of white matter (B) between the centrum semiovale and the internal capsule containing afferent and efferent fibres funnelling into the latter.

Corpus striatum

The internal capsule, basal ganglia, and the intervening white matter (C).

Trigone

The triangular junction of the temporal and occipital horns of the lateral ventricle and the main body (see location 42 in Fig. 2.8e).

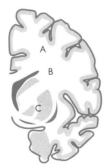

Fig. 2.10 Centrum semiovale and related structures.

Brainstem anatomy

See Figure 2.11.

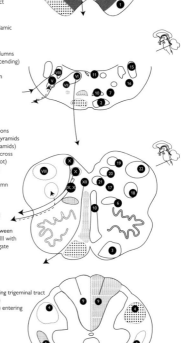

Note that some simplifications have been made:
The CN III and IV nuclei are shown in the same cut
although in fact they are at slightly different levels
(with CN IV more caudal). Similarly the origins of
CN IX, X, XII have been somewhat simplified.

Hatching patterns have been used to help "connect"
tracts at different levels.

Corticospinal/corticobulbar tract
(descending)

Pain and temperature (spinothalamic
tract) (ascending)

Vibration/light touch (dorsal columns
becoming medial lemniscus) (ascending)

Spinothalamic and dorsal column
modalities combine in medial
lemniscus at midbrain level

1 Descending corticospinal tract fibres in
   cerebral peduncles
2 Descending corticospinal tract fibres in pons
3 Descending corticospinal tract fibres in pyramids
4 Lateral corticospinal tract (crosses in pyramids)
5 Spinothalamic tract in spinal cord (fibres cross
   immediately from contralateral dorsal root)
6 Ascending spinothalamic tract in medulla
7 Ascending spinothalamic tract in pons
8 Spinothalamic fibres join with dorsal column
   fibres in medial lemniscus in midbrain
   (from here project to thalamus)
9 Ascending dorsal column fibres
10 Ascending dorsal column fibres in medial
   lemniscus
11 Medial longitudinal fasciculus running between
   midbrain and pons only, connecting CN III with
   IV and VI on each side to facilitate conjugate
   horizontal eye movement
12 Periaqueductal grey matter
13 Red nucleus
14 Substantia nigra
15 Cerebellar peduncle (middle)
16 Sensory fibres from CN VII (taste) entering trigeminal tract
17 Nucleus ambiguus (CN IX motor and X)
18 Sensory fibres from CN IX (oropharynx) entering
   trigeminal tract
19 Tractus and nucleus solitarius
20 Dorsal motor nucleus of CN X
21 Hypoglossal nucleus (CN XII)
22 Vestibular nuclei (CN VIII)

Fig. 2.11A Brainstem anatomy. Note that the neuroanatomical convention with
ventral at the bottom is the inverse of clinical axial neuroimaging.

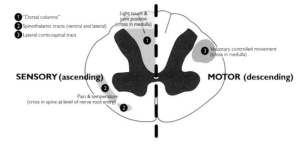

1 "Dorsal columns"
2 Spinothalamic tracts (ventral and lateral)
3 Lateral corticospinal tract

Light touch & joint position (cross in medulla)

Voluntary controlled movement (cross in medulla)

SENSORY (ascending)

MOTOR (descending)

Pain & temperature (cross in spine at level of nerve root entry)

NB: Neuroanatomical convention (with dorsal column to the top) is the inverse of radiological convention (ventral cord uppermost)

Anterior spinal artery syndrome
The blood supply to the cord is from the ventral side. Infarction results in a lower motor neuron weakness at the level of the infarct with upper motor neuron signs below, and a sensory level with loss of pain and temperature below this but with *relative preservation of dorsal column sensation*

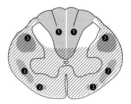

Syringomyelia or syringobulbia
The structures first involved in an expanding central cord cavity are pain and temperature sensing fibres as they cross immediately on entering from the dorsal roots to the contralateral ascending spinothalamic tract (dashed lines) resulting in pain and temperature (but not light touch) sensory loss in the affected dermatomes. If this happens in the pons or medulla (syringobulbia) then facial sensation is affected

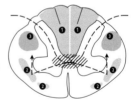

Hemicord syndrome (Brown-Séquard)
Initially described after sword fights (thankfully now rare!) asymmetric cord syndromes can result from vascular or demyelinating insults. Results in loss of ipsilateral dorsal column (light touch) and corticospinal tract (movement) function with contralateral loss of spinothalamic (pain and temperature) function below the level of injury. At T1 or above there will be an ipsilateral Horner syndrome..

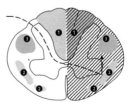

Fig. 2.11B Spinal cord anatomy.

MRI and brain development

Myelination changes with development

Normal MRI appearances of white and grey matter on T1 and T2 change markedly in the first two years of life, reflecting progression of myelination (Fig. 2.12).

Radiology of brain development

Radiological evidence of disordered brain development is a relatively common finding in MRI studies of children being investigated for developmental impairment or 'cerebral palsy', particularly if seizures are also present.

Brain development occurs in defined phases

- Neurons arise from proliferating cells adjacent to the ventricular system.
- Primitive nerve cells (neuroblasts) migrate centrifugally from the centre to the periphery, using radial glial cells as a guiding scaffold, creating the multi-layered cortex.
- An 'inside-out' sequence of development occurs: deepest layers are formed first, each successive migration passing *through* earlier, older layers to form more superficial layers, so that the youngest neurons are closest to the surface.
- Once neurons have reached their final location further differentiation occurs, dendrites form, and synaptic connections are made when growth cones contact their post-synaptic targets.
- Some neurons act as temporary targets for incoming fibres and form transient connections before being eliminated by apoptosis when a more appropriate and permanent set of target cells are in place.
- Synaptic formation starts in the second trimester and continues during post-natal life.
- Oligodendrocytes begin to lay down myelin sheaths from 26 weeks' gestation. Myelination occurs sequentially into the second decade. Fibres serving primary sensory and motor areas are myelinated shortly after birth while those associated with more complex cognitive functions are myelinated later (see Fig. 2.12).

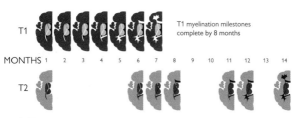

Fig. 2.12 Normal maturational changes in T1 and T2 imaging.

Adapted with permission from Staudt M, Krägeloh-Mann I, and Grodd W. [Normal myelination in childhood brains using MRI—a meta-analysis]. *RöFo*, Volume 172, Issue 10, pp. 802–11, Copyright © 2000 Georg Thieme Verlag Stuttgart.

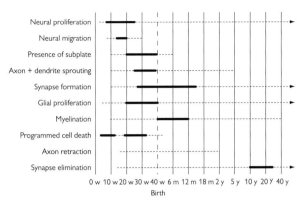

Fig. 2.13 Stages of brain development.

Reprinted from *Early Human Development*, Volume 82, Issue 4, de Graaf-Peters VB and Hadders-Algra M, Ontogeny of the human central nervous system: What is happening when?, pp. 257–266, Copyright © 2006, with permission from Elsevier.

- Myelination is radiologically complete by age 2. Before this age it can be difficult to distinguish terminal zones of myelination around the posterior horns of the lateral ventricles from small areas of periventricular leukomalacia or gliosis. Terminal zones of myelination should *not* be visible on T1.

Radiological patterns of disordered development reflect the stage at which developmental progress was disrupted (Fig. 2.13). This can either reflect a genetic (programming) error of brain development, or disruption by external injury or other noxious influences in what was an otherwise normally developing brain.

Evidence of bilateral, largely symmetrical changes indicate a likely genetic origin (with potential recurrence risk implications). Unilateral or strongly asymmetric patterns of involvement *generally* suggest acquired injury (with potentially lower recurrence risk implications); however, there are exceptions to this rule. Some radiological features may strongly implicate acquired pathogenesis (Fig. 2.14 A5–8; B4, 5).

Recognizable genetic brain malformation syndromes

Once a probable genetically determined brain malformation syndrome has been identified genetic evaluation is required because of different recurrence risk implications (the mother or sister of a boy with a *DCX* mutation may be asymptomatic but male offspring will be severely affected). An increasing number of genes have been identified as causing brain malformation syndromes comprising combinations of lissencephaly (smooth non-sulcated cortex), pachygyria (abnormally thick gyri) and/or grey matter heterotopia (islands or thin 'ribbons' of grey matter in subcortical white matter underlying apparently relatively normal cortex, reflecting the failure of a 'wave' of neuronal migration from the ependymal zone to the cortex to complete).

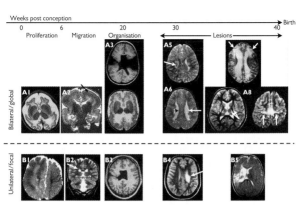

Fig. 2.14 Radiological appearances of developmental brain abnormalities.

Global patterns on top row (A1–8); focal or unilateral patterns on bottom row (B1–5)

1. Disorders of proliferation. A1. Extreme microcephaly with simplified gyral pattern; B1 hemimegalencephaly.

2. Disorders of migration. A2 lissencephaly with thick cortex and typical cell sparse layer (arrow); B2 focal periventricular heterotopia (arrow).

3. Disorders of organization. A3 polymicrogyria-schizencephaly with polymicrogyric cortex lining the bilateral clefts; A4 generalized polymicrogyria; B3 unilateral schizencephaly.

4. Lesion pattern early third trimester. A5 mild periventricular leukomalacia (PVL) with periventricular gliosis (arrow) but no white matter reduction; A6 severe PVL with irregular ventricular enlargement due to white matter loss (arrowhead) and periventricular gliosis (arrow); B4 unilateral periventricular lesion with white matter reduction and gliosis due to haemorrhagic infarction (arrow).

5. Lesion pattern late third trimester. A7 parasagittal hypoperfusion injury with cortical and subcortical damage in the parasagittal area (arrows); A8 acute severe term asphyxial insult of basal ganglia and thalamus lesions (left) with typical involvement of thalamus, globus pallidus, and putamen (arrows), and lesions of the central region (arrows, right).; B5 middle cerebral artery infarction with cortical, subcortical, and thalamic involvement.

Some of these genes have relatively characteristic appearances in terms of the distribution of changes although increasingly genetic investigation of brain malformation appearances is by gene panel.

- *DCX*. X-linked recessive with severely affected boys. The lissencephaly and/or subcortical band heterotopia is predominantly frontal.
- *LIS1*. Autosomal recessive. The lissencephaly and/or subcortical band heterotopia is predominantly posterior.
- *TUBA1A*. Autosomal recessive. More widespread lissencephaly and/ or subcortical band heterotopia (as *LIS1*) plus cerebellar hypoplasia ± agenesis of the corpus callosum.
- *ARX*. X-linked recessive. Temporal and/or posterior lissencephaly.

Unexpected findings on MRI

With widespread availability of MRI, it is common for radiological studies to identify unexpected findings of uncertain relevance, sometimes somewhat frivolously referred to as 'incidentalomas'. These can cause anxiety to in-experienced clinicians, radiologists, and, of course, families. Assessing their significance can occasionally be challenging.

- Remember the 'nose-picking principle' (see The nose-picking principle in this Chapter ➔ p. 53). Minimize the risk of unearthing incidentalomas by resisting the temptation to perform non-indicated examinations!
- Remember the 'what and where' approach (see What, where, and when in Chapter 1 ➔ p. 5) and particularly the 'where'. If the site of the incidentaloma is distant from the likely site of pathology, given the examination findings, then it is easier to be reassuring about its non-significance.

Recognized 'normal variants'

Refer to Figure 2.15 A–J.

Cavum septum pellucidum

The septum pellucidum is the membrane separating the anterior horns of the two lateral ventricles. In foetuses the two layers of the septum are separated around a central cavity containing CSF. The large majority of these spontaneously close in early infancy but may persist into adulthood. Note the MRI signal characteristics of the contents are those of CSF on all sequences (Fig. 2.15 A and B).

Prominent perivascular spaces

There is a potential, CSF-containing space around all cerebral arteries and arterioles as they enter the brain, formed by elongations along the vessel of the pia mater. These are also known as Virchow–Robin spaces. Prominence of these spaces is associated with some neurological diseases (such as mucopolysaccharidoses) but is more commonly a normal variant (Fig. 2.15 C).

Arachnoid cysts

Cysts can form in the arachnoid mater due to its filmy, self-adherent, nature (the name 'arachnoid', i.e. spider-like, is a reference to spiders' webs). Small cysts, such as that shown, are commonly asymptomatic (the location at the anterior pole of the temporal lobe is typical). They can, however, spon-taneously enlarge and very large cysts may rarely cause space-occupation symptoms either directly or indirectly via obstruction of CSF flow and re-quire neurosurgical treatment. Haemorrhage into very large cysts is also recognized; however, a cyst as small as that illustrated is very benign and should be ignored.

The evaluation of their relevance in some other situations can be more com-plex. They can give rise to seizures and in children with epilepsy with congruent EEG data consideration should be given to surgical treatment (Fig. 2.15 D).

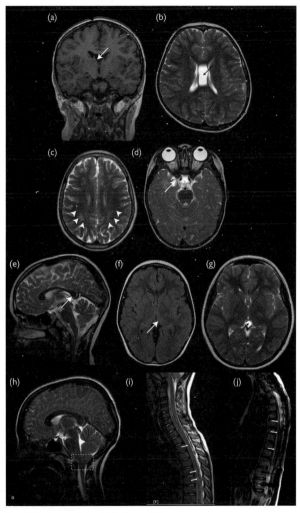

Fig. 2.15 Common incidental findings on MRI.

Pineal cyst
Cysts arising from the pineal gland are generally benign, however larger cysts can again cause obstruction of CSF flow and pressure effects which may require neurosurgical intervention. Follow-up imaging once, after 12 months, may be recommended for larger cysts (>10 mm diameter). Note that the signal characteristics of the contents of a pineal cyst match those of CSF on T1 and T2 but not FLAIR (Fig. 2.15 E–G).

Descent of cerebellar tonsils
Minor degrees of tonsillar descent are a common finding, particularly in younger children with relatively small posterior fossae. If the degree of descent is <5 mm it is very probably benign and incidental. In situations of greater tonsillar descent, radiological evidence of foramen magnum crowding and symptoms of occipital headache that worsen with cough, laugh, or sneezing, the findings may be significant (Fig. 2.15 H) (see Chiari malformations in Chapter 4 ➔ p. 359).

Prominent central canal of spinal cord
A prominent central canal of the spinal cord is a common finding and almost always incidental (Fig. 2.15 I). The concern is usually that the appearance may represent a *syrinx*. In practice, isolated syrinxes are very rare: nearly all are associated with other pathology affecting CSF flow such as a Chiari II malformation (see Chiari malformations in Chapter 4 ➔ p. 359) or previous meningitis/arachnoiditis. In the example of a syrinx shown in Figure 2.15 J for comparison, the radiological evidence of associated scoliosis (reflected in the fact that the whole length of the spine cannot be imaged in a single plane) is further indication of the pathological nature of this case.

In unclear situations, a follow-up study after an interval of 12 months may clarify its non-progressive nature. Recall that testing spinothalamic sensation in relevant dermatomes is the most sensitive clinical indicator of a syrinx (see Syringomyelia in Chapter 4 ➔ p. 226 and Fig. 2.11 B in this chapter ➔ p. 70).

'Mild cortical atrophy', 'Prominent subarachnoid spaces'
In comparison to adult brains, the subarachnoid space around the cerebral hemispheres in pre-adolescent children tends to be somewhat larger, particularly frontally (this relates to the fact that maturation of frontal lobe function—which is accompanied by demonstrable enlargement—is an adolescent phenomenon). This can lead to normal appearances being reported by adult neuroradiologists with less paediatric experience as 'mild cortical atrophy' or similar phrases.

If appearances are striking, and head circumference is large, consider benign external hydrocephalus or, far more commonly, benign familial macrocephaly (measure parental head size!) (see Head size abnormalities Figure 3.3 in Chapter 3 ➔ p. 162).

White matter abnormalities on MRI

Definitions
- *Leukoencephalopathy*: any disorder of white matter, whether genetic or acquired (includes leukodystrophies).
- *Leukodystrophy*: genetically determined white matter diseases.

Approach

The first step is to distinguish *hypomyelination* or delayed myelination from *dysmyelination* (i.e. a leukoencephalopathy). This is done by comparison of the T1 and T2 characteristics of the white matter in relation to the appearance of grey matter structures.

Because of physiological changes in white matter signal appearance in the first two years of life reflecting myelination (Fig. 2.16), this distinction can be difficult before the age of 18–24 months. After this time, white matter should normally be dark (reflecting completed myelination) on T2.

Further characterization is based on a combination of radiological features (particularly the anatomical location of abnormal white matter) and associated clinical features. Although diagnostic algorithms have been proposed (Schiffmann *et al.* (2009) Neurology 72: 750) variant and atypical forms complicate assessment; and this is another area where the development of large 'inherited white matter' gene panels has revolutionized the diagnostic approach.

The commonest leukodystrophies in UK practice are metachromatic leukodystrophy (MLD), X-linked adrenoleukodystrophy (X-ALD), and Krabbe disease; followed by Canavan, Alexander, CACH/VWM, and Pelizaeus–Merzbacher disease (see Fig. 2.17) however even with modern genetic testing a significant proportion of leukodystrophies remain undiagnosed.

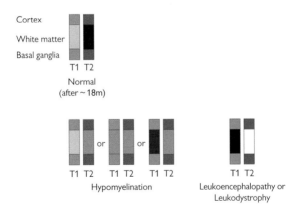

Fig. 2.16 Maturational changes of appearances of white and grey matter on T1 and T2.

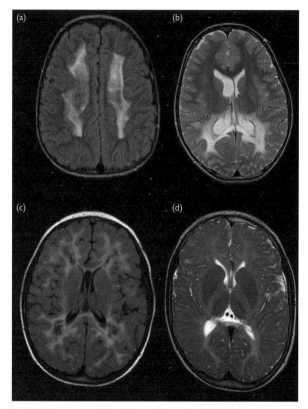

Fig. 2.17 Appearances of four leukoencephalopathies A: Typical deep, periventricular distribution of clearly leukodystrophic change with sparing of U fibres in metachromatic leukodystrophy. B: Posterior predominant confluent changes of X-linked adrenoleukodystrophy. C: FLAIR image showing diffuse white matter involvement (involving U fibres) with emerging cavitation in Vanishing White Matter disease. D: Global hypomyelination in Pelizaeus–Merzbacher disease.

An increasing number of leukodystrophies (notably at present X-ALD and some forms of MLD) have treatments available to children diagnosed sufficiently early in their disease course, making prompt diagnosis important (and screening of at risk younger siblings once a proband is identified) (see Late presentations of metabolic disease in Chapter 4 ➲ p. 484).

Principles of neurogenetics

The ultimate goal of diagnostic genetic testing is to establish the molecular basis of disease in order to optimize patient care, where possible permitting 'personalized medicine', in which therapy is tailored to the underlying molecular cause. Identifying the genetic cause of a disease can also help manage wider family concerns, by clarifying prognosis and reproductive risk in subsequent pregnancies.

- An extraordinarily rapidly moving field with advances in both what's technologically possible and aetiological understanding of a growing proportion of neurological conditions.
- The new 'massively parallel' sequencing technologies resemble screening tests (testing without strong prior hypotheses of what results are expected) and raise some of the same challenges: frequent identification of genetic data of uncertain clinical significance, i.e. data that is difficult to interpret based on current knowledge; and results with potentially unanticipated implications for the health of the child when older, or for the wider family.
- All involved need to understand these issues and formally consent to testing.

Much as with principles of neuroradiology, today's paediatric neurologist needs a pragmatic understanding of the capabilities and limitations of different types of genetic test so that they not only know which test to request but are also aware of possible test outcomes. The 'next-generation' techniques create major new challenges in the evaluation of findings: good clinical 'phenotyping' becomes more, not less important in the new genetic era.

- The boundary between cytogenetics (analysis of chromosome structure) and molecular genetics (analysis of gene sequence) has become blurred with the introduction of newer technologies, e.g. smaller structural variants within genes may be detected by both molecular and cytogenetic analyses.
- Clinically, it is more appropriate to differentiate between sequence or structural variation affecting a single gene (monogenic disorders) and larger chromosomal changes involving contiguous genes.

Cytogenetic testing

G-banded karyotyping

- Recognizable human genetic disorders can result from loss or gain of material in any one of the 22 autosomes or the two sex chromosomes. Until recently such imbalances were detected by direct visualization of Giemsa-stained condensed chromosomes under the microscope ('karyotyping') to report chromosome count, size, and staining patterns.
- Now almost completely superseded by array CGH but see Limitations of array-based analyses in this Chapter p. 81).
- Typical findings include:
  - differences in chromosome number (aneuploidies), such as trisomy 13, 18, or 21.
  - detection of large balanced and unbalanced structural rearrangements, e.g. chromosome translocations.
  - identification of mosaic abnormalities where not all cells express the same chromosomal complement.

Microarray-based comparative genomic hybridization ('array CGH', aCGH)

- A development of now largely superseded Fluorescence In Situ Hybridization (FISH) techniques that uses probes (tailored sequences of DNA with a fluorescent tag) that hybridize to and 'flag' the presence of DNA sequences identifying specific chromosomal loci. In contrast to FISH, aCGH employs tens of thousands of probes spread across all chromosomes to interrogate chromosome copy number at many loci in parallel.
- Detects copy number deficiencies or excesses (due to deletion or duplication) relative to a control sample known as *copy number variants* (CNVs).
- With multiple data points on the aCGH in some regions, resolution can be down to single gene level and can sometimes identify single gene causes of disease.

Single nucleotide polymorphism (SNP) arrays

- SNP ('snip') arrays exploit common (population-level) single nucleotide variants across the genome.
- Probing for these single nucleotide polymorphisms (SNPs) can provide copy number information in a similar way to aCGH.
- Additional information is available in terms of the nucleotide identity at each site. Individuals will be heterozygous (AB/BA) or homozygous (AA/BB) at each site randomly throughout the genome. A chromosomal deletion will result in both copy number loss and loss of heterozygosity, whereas a duplication will result in copy number gain and a 2:1 imbalance between SNPs.
- If copy number appears normal, but the expected variation in SNPs is lost in a chromosomal region, this is described as copy number neutral loss of heterozygosity; this implies both copies of this region are derived from the same parent (e.g. in uniparental disomy).
- SNPs represent common genetic variation and are not evenly distributed throughout the genome. This can be limiting factor in the application of this technology and may be overcome by combining with aCGH.

Interpreting aCGH and SNP array findings

- Assessing the clinical significance of CNVs (whether identified by aCGH or SNP) can be challenging. Individuals typically carry several tens of CNVs, most of which are not clinically important.
- Where a CNV has a clear disease association, specific clinical information is often available.
- Unique (rarechromo.org) provides helpful information leaflets for affected families, and there are GeneReviews articles for the commoner CNVs.
- There are many low penetrance neurosusceptibility loci CNVs; these represent risk factors for developmental delay, learning difficulties, and behavioural issues, but only a proportion of those sharing the CNV will be clinically affected (i.e. penetrance is reduced).
  - Many CNVs have been associated with several broad neurological phenotypes (e.g. autism, epilepsy) however many of these are also

seen (at lower frequency) in unaffected individuals i.e. appear to be predisposing, rather than directly causal (e.g. neurexin 1 (*NRXN1*) 'susceptibility' locus at 2p16).
- Where a CNV is not known to be a population variant (i.e. benign) or associated with disease, this is described as a variant of unknown significance (VUS). The first step typically is to check whether this is shared with an unaffected first degree relative, ideally the parents (in which case the CNV is unlikely to be clinically relevant).
- Database information on genes known to be in a deleted/duplicated area can aid interpretation.

Limitations of array-based analyses
- SNP and CGH arrays both provide a high resolution 'digital karyotype' with approximately 100-fold greater resolution than traditional 'analogue' karyotyping and have largely replaced the latter e.g. in the workup of children with congenital abnormality and/or developmental impairment.
- However as 'digital' methods sensitive only to copy *number* they have some important 'blind spots':
  - cannot detect inversions or balanced rearrangements that don't alter total copy number;
  - can't report location or orientation (e.g. inversions) of imbalances;
  - won't identify single nucleotide variants;
  - they are limited in their ability to detect low levels of *mosaicism* (situations where some but not all cells carry a CNV): the threshold is currently around 10%;
  - ring chromosome 20 mosaicism is a rare cause of severe epilepsy and learning difficulties with challenging behaviour (see Ring chromosome 20 in Chapter 4 ➲ p. 296). Ring chromosome 20 mosaicism should be specified if this is a consideration as traditional visual karyotyping of multiple cells will be required: examination of 50 cells will identify 6% mosaicism with 95% confidence.

Molecular genetics
- There are an estimated 20 000 to 25 000 protein-coding genes. Pathogenic variants in many of these have been associated with neurological disease.
- Conventional Sanger sequencing of individual candidate genes, dependent on suspected clinical diagnosis, has been the traditional approach to genetic testing. However, this approach is less effective when pathogenic variants in many genes can present in a similar way (e.g. the many genes capable of causing early infantile epileptic encephalopathies).
- In such cases next-generation or 'massively parallel' sequencing has revolutionized testing. Next-generation sequencing (NGS) technologies allow simultaneous assessment of a predetermined set of genes (a gene panel), all protein-coding genes (whole exome) or indeed all of a person's genetic material (whole genome) in a single assay.
- Several different techniques and sequencing platforms are used in a diagnostic setting. Short read approaches, sequencing fragments of a

few hundred base pairs, are more commonly used, but are less able to provide information on structural variation than long read technologies, which routinely sequence more than 10 kbp.

- The major challenge when using NGS approaches is the bioinformatic analysis of the data generated. The larger the panel of genes, the more variants will be found. For this reason, many laboratories prefer to sequence trios (an affected child and their parents) for very large panel, WES, and WGS analysis.
  - Data from a trio provides important information that can help determine the significance of a variant, e.g. whether a variant is *de novo* (present in the child but in neither parent) or has been inherited from an affected or unaffected parent. In the case of autosomal recessive disorders, trio data also provides the phase of variants (two variants in the same gene that occur on the same allele are in *cis*, two variants on different alleles are in *trans*).

Gene panels

Gene panel testing involves analysis of selected genes known to cause broad categories of neurological presentations, including early infantile-onset epilepsies, neuropathies, cerebral malformation disorders, and congenital myopathies. In practice panels are often 'virtual': the patient's whole exome or genome is sequenced, but only genes included in the panel are analysed.

- Panel testing is more time and cost effective than sequential testing of single genes and has largely replaced this (even in situations highly suggestive of a particular single gene such as a Dravet syndrome presentation, stand-alone *SCN1A* testing may no longer be available).
- Diagnostic success will depend on both the appropriate panel(s) being requested and, more importantly, the relevant gene being on that panel. Don't assume the panel is comprehensive.
- Panels need to be continuously revised and extended in light of further research, and reanalysis may be appropriate.

Gene-agnostic approaches

Whole Exome Sequencing (WES) involves sequencing the protein-coding regions of the genome only. *Whole Genome Sequencing* (WGS) data includes the non-protein-coding regions of the genome. Although the exome only comprises about 1.5% of the whole genome, it is thought that most disease-causing variants lie within protein-coding genes, whether in exons (which act as templates for translation after transcription and RNA splicing) introns (non-coding regions within genes that can influence e.g. RNA splicing) or regulatory elements (which can influence gene expression). In practice, gene-agnostic approaches using trios will identify variants in many different genes, which must then be filtered using the patient's phenotype, either through bioinformatics approaches using Human Phenotype Ontology (HPO) terms, or manual review.

Molecular genetic analysis and reporting

There are several considerations in the analysis and reporting of genetic variants identified on testing of large panels of genes, WES, and WGS.

- Initial screening may exclude common population variants if these have not been taken into account when population frequency thresholds have been set for bioinformatic filtering of the data. Conversely, variants that are frequent in one population may be rare in another population; it is therefore important to ensure that the correct reference populations have been used.

- Highly repetitive regions of the genome are difficult to assess, particularly with short read NGS methods. This is especially important when considering triplet repeat expansion disorders, e.g. some spinocerebellar ataxias, Friedreich ataxia, and myotonic dystrophy. Specialized testing may be required.

- Small structural variants below the threshold for detection on array may be missed.

- Detection of disorders relating to the *mitochondrial* genome may not be detected; specialized testing will be required.

- Detection of mosaicism is dependent on read depth; the greater the depth of sequencing, the greater the ability to detect low level mosaicism. When considering mosaicism, it is important to ensure that a relevant tissue is tested. For neurocutaneous disorders, DNA should be extracted directly from skin biopsies when these are available but note that culture may favour growth of cells that do not contain the pathogenic variant.

- Changes in methylation leading to imprinting disorders (e.g. Prader Willi syndrome and most Angelman syndrome cases) will not be detected by most NGS approaches. Specialized testing is likely to be required.

- Analysis is more complex in consanguineous families: homozygosity for a number of rare variants may be seen, and it may be challenging to determine which, if any, are causative.

- An apparently *de novo* variant in an affected child (i.e. not shared with either parent) does not rule out recurrence in future pregnancies. The pathogenic variant may be present at low level in ovary/testis (gonadal mosaicism); recurrence risk in this situation is thought to be around 1%.

Variants of uncertain significance (VUSs) are increasingly identified. They are typically described on a metaphorical 'temperature' scale from 'cold' (very unlikely to be relevant) to 'hot' (highly suspicious) based on information available at the time of reporting, with respect to the biological effect of the variant, the presenting phenotype, and the family history. Further information may alter variant classification, including evolution of the phenotype or additional family history.

Ethical issues and consenting for WES/WGS

Using trios for NGS testing is extremely valuable, but the relationship between samples is checked to ensure that the bioinformatics approach is appropriate; parents should be made aware when consenting that use of donor eggs and non-paternity will be apparent. When testing very large panels of genes, or using WES/WGS, it is possible that genes not directly related to the clinical question in hand will be analysed. Variants in genes that predispose to cancer or cardiac abnormalities, and for which surveillance or management is possible, will usually be reported, as determined by international consensus. It is important that families are aware of the possibility of such incidental findings, for both an affected individual and their parents independently, when providing consent for testing; individuals may choose to opt out of receiving incidental findings.

The role of the clinical paediatric neurologist

These newer genetic technologies create major challenges in the evaluation of the relevance if any of identified mutations (Table 2.3). Good clinical skills and phenotyping become more, not less important. When variants of uncertain significance, or when a number of possibly pathogenic variants are identified, accurate result interpretation relies upon clinical skills which synthesize serological, imaging, genetic, and clinical data to determine which variants may contribute to the disease phenotype and which do not. Neurologists, geneticists, and laboratory scientists increasingly need to work together as a multidisciplinary team.

Table 2.3 Uses of different genetic tests

Genetic test	Uses/examples
Karyotype	Aneuploidy, balanced and unbalanced structural rearrangements (>5 Mb) and mosaic abnormalities
aCGH/SNP array	CNVs, including <5 Mb and mosaic variations (>10% mosaicism) e.g. 16p13.11
Gene panels	Analysis of a predetermined group of genes causative of a certain neurological presentation, e.g. cerebral malformation disorders
Whole exome sequencing (WES)	Analysis of coding genes
Whole genome sequencing (WGS)	Coding gene and non-coding analysis
Methylation studies	Uniparental disomy, e.g. UPD 14 Imprinting defects, e.g. Angelman syndrome
Triplet repeat single gene analysis	Myotonic dystrophy and fragile X

Principles of neurophysiology

Electroencephalography (EEG)

- An aid to diagnosis, which must be interpreted in the context of the clinical history.
- EEG records the difference in electrical potentials generated by neurons in two locations over time.
- Potentials recorded are mainly post-synaptic membrane potentials generated from superficial cortical layers.
- Electrical potentials generated are attenuated by up to 90% by the CSF, skull, and scalp. They are of low amplitude (10–200μV) and must be amplified and filtered before they can be interpreted.

Best quality recording obtained by:
- Cleaning and preparing the scalp prior to electrode placement minimizing resistance and artefact.
- Activation procedures including hyperventilation and photic stimulation.

A 20 min recording is typical but this may be extended if there is a good chance that doing so will lead to events being captured.

Electrode placement

- Standard positions designated using the international '10–20 System', at 10% or 20% intervals of the distance between standard anatomical landmarks.
- Even numbers refer to right-sided electrodes, odd numbers to left-sided electrodes.
- F, frontal; Fp, fronto-polar; P, parietal; C, central; T, temporal; O, occipital; Z, midline; A, auricular (Fig. 2.18).
- Typically up to 16 pairs of electrodes (or individual electrodes versus a reference) are displayed in a montage suitable for the particular clinical question at hand.

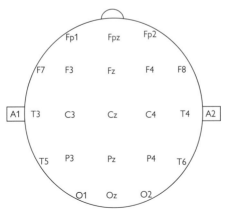

Fig. 2.18 EEG montage.

Indications for EEG

In the management of epilepsy

Do use the EEG:

- To help determine seizure type and epilepsy syndrome in individuals in whom epilepsy is *already* suspected or to reconsider a previous diagnosis of epilepsy (see The role of EEG in Chapter 3 ⊃ p. 154).
- To assess the risk of seizure recurrence in individuals presenting with a first unprovoked seizure.
- To re-evaluate a patient with a recent change in seizure semiology or prior to weaning ASM in seizure-free patients.

Do not use the EEG:

- To 'exclude epilepsy' when the clinical assessment suggests another cause (because of the danger of a false +ve result).
- Repeatedly if a clinical diagnosis has already been reached (consider sleep studies or other special procedures, see below).

An EEG should be performed only to *support* a diagnosis of epilepsy. Generally, an EEG would only be considered after more than one epileptic seizure but may in certain circumstances (e.g. at a 'one-stop' first seizure clinic) be ordered after a first seizure where the history is strongly suggestive of epilepsy.

In general acute neurology

One often-overlooked role of the EEG in general acute neurology is as an 'ESR of the brain'—or more accurately—of the cerebral cortex. The presence of normal age-appropriate background rhythms is a strong indicator of intact cortical function suggesting cortical sparing in any process under evaluation.

Special procedures

- Photic stimulation and hyperventilation are part of standard EEG assessment.
  - The individual and family need to know such activation procedures may induce a seizure and they have a right to refuse as a seizure may for example have driving licence implications.
- *Contraindications* to hyperventilation include:
  - Known large vessel cerebrovascular disease including moya-moya and sickle cell disease;
  - Severe cardiac or pulmonary disorders;
  - Pregnancy (also considered a contraindication for photic stimulaton).
- When a standard EEG has not contributed to diagnosis or classification, a sleep EEG should be considered. A 30-min minimum recording is advisable. In children, a sleep EEG is best achieved through sleep deprivation or the use of melatonin, and performed in the postprandial period.
- Prolonged video or ambulatory EEG (the latter typically for 48 h) may be used in special circumstances. Usually only helpful when the events are reported to be occurring at least daily.

- Video EEG (typically over several days) has an important place in the assessment of children for epilepsy surgery. Ictal records help define site(s) of seizure origin.

Basic EEG characteristics and reading reports

Separate consideration is given to the *background* (a general indicator of cortical function) and *paroxysmal activity* (related to epilepsy).

Background rhythms

Alter both with age (Fig. 2.19) and the child's arousal level. Normal background rhythm frequencies ↑ and amplitudes decrease with age. An alpha rhythm on eye closure (Fig. 2.20) should be present by age 8 ('8 Hz by 8 yrs'). During sleep the EEG slows.

The basic rhythms are

- Delta: <4 Hz.
- Theta: 4 to <8 Hz.
- Alpha: 8–13 Hz.
- Beta: >13 Hz.

A technical report will follow each record along with an opinion on the relevance of the findings to the clinical situation. Comment should be made on whether the background rhythms are appropriate for the child's age and on any asymmetries.

Paroxysmal activity

Many EEGs show non-specific abnormalities, such as an excess of dysrhythmic or slow wave activity in posterior areas. These findings are so common in the general population that they offer little or no support for a diagnosis of epilepsy: beware of over-interpreting them. More supportive of epilepsy would be persistent sharp, spike, or spike–wave complexes (Fig. 2.22). An ictal record, capturing a seizure, and demonstrating spike–wave discharge during the seizure is the only truly diagnostic finding. A persistent slow wave focus may indicate an underlying structural lesion.

Potential pitfalls of using an EEG

- Interictal EEGs are often normal in individuals with epilepsy.
- Individuals who have never had any seizures may have epileptiform abnormalities on EEG.
- Epileptiform spikes are common in conditions such as a cerebral palsy even when there is no history of seizures.
- Range of normal appearances are very age dependent: in particular, clinicians without experience of neonatal EEG may report normal neonatal EEG appearances as pathological.
- Some specific patterns, such as the eponymous spikes seen in self-limited epilepsy with centrotemporal spikes (SeLECTS), can also been seen in relatives without seizures and reflect a genetic tendency.

Cerebral function monitoring

Cerebral Function Monitors (CFMs) are devices used in intensive care and particularly neonatal intensive care settings to provide a form of continuous EEG monitoring.

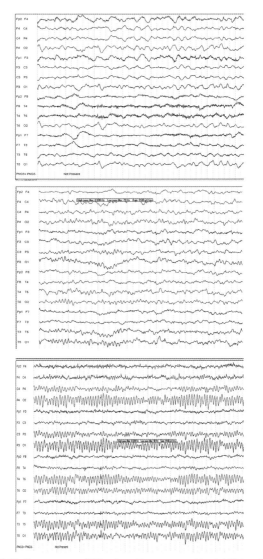

Fig. 2.19 Changes in normal EEG with age. From top, normal (awake) 10-day-old infant. Centre, normal 5-yr old: theta rhythms posteriorly with emerging alpha. Bottom, normal 12-yr old with well-developed alpha rhythm.

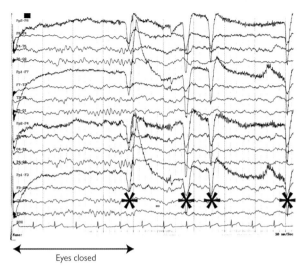

← Eyes closed →

Fig. 2.20 Normal alpha rhythm appearing particularly in occipital leads during eye closure, abolished when eyes open (also implied by the appearance of eye-blink artefacts caused by movement of the eyeball, asterisks).

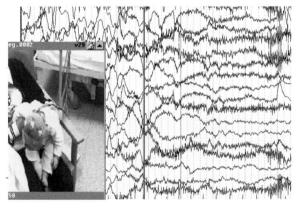

Fig. 2.21 Hypsarrhythmia. The high voltage, chaotic EEG associated with infantile spasms. At the instant of the flexion spasm shown in the video window (left) and marked by the central vertical line, the EEG loses amplitude, a so-called electro-decremental event, and becomes contaminated by movement artefact.

(a)

(b)

(c)

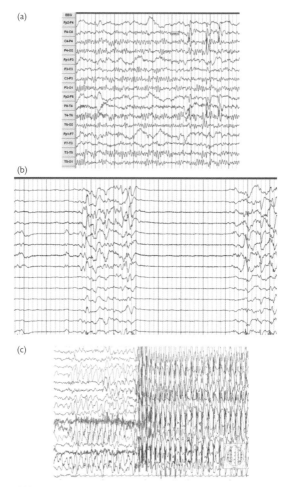

Fig. 2.22 Further EEG examples.

Top (A): Repeated single spikes in centro-temporal leads—in this example predominantly on right (even numbered leads). Appearance supports a diagnosis of Self-limited epilepsy with centrotemporal spikes (SeLECTS) in the appropriate clinical context (see Self-limited epilepsy with centrotemporal spikes in Chapter 4 ➲ p. 282). Centre (B) Burst suppression EEG—periods of abnormal slow high voltage synchronous 'burst' activity separated by periods of relative electrical silence. A non-specific indicator of major suppression of cortical function seen (for example) in deep barbiturate anaesthesia, and profound encephalopathy of any cause. Bottom (C) Generalized 3 Hz spike–wave activity typical of Childhood absence epilepsy (see Childhood absence epilepsy in Chapter 4 ➲ p. 288). The slow activity prior to the onset of the 3 Hz activity reflects hyperventilation-related changes.

CFMs display a simplified, compressed EEG signal known as the amplitude-integrated EEG (aEEG: the terms CFM and aEEG are often used interchangeably). The aEEG signal is derived from just one or two electrode pairs placed symmetrically on each side of the head, typically frontally. Time is shown on the x-axis with EEG amplitude shown on a semi-logarithmic scale on the y-axis. Raw EEG from the electrode pairs is typically displayed alongside together with electrode impedance information that verifies electrodes have good contact with skin.

- aEEG is primarily used to grade severity of encephalopathy (and particularly trends over time) as a prognostic tool in neonatal hypoxic–ischaemic encephalopathy and therapeutic hypothermia.
- Seizure activity is typically reflected by a sudden change, often into a narrower range, of amplitudes. Because of its very limited electrode coverage, sensitivity for the detection of subclinical seizure activity is low.
- Both excessively high and low amplitudes are abnormal: normal ranges depend on gestational age and whether the infant is awake or asleep.

Neurophysiological testing of central sensory pathways

Many central sensory neurophysiological techniques use repeated averaging of EEG recordings time-locked to a repeating visual or auditory stimulus to extract EEG features that consistently appear following the stimulus. They are *passive* responses that can be elicited in the uncooperative (ill or young) child.

Visual evoked potentials (VEPs)

- Uses a reversing checkerboard (or, if no response, strobe flash) typically 128 stimuli at 3 Hz with scalp electrodes placed 2 cm above the inion and 4 cm to the left and right of this point.
- The large volume of macular fibres means that this is essentially a test of retino-cortical conduction of the central retina.
- A five-component waveform is seen.
- The amplitude is typically variable and affected by visual acuity, the integrity of the visual pathway and stimulus type.
- The latency of the VEP (reflecting conduction velocity of fastest fibres) is much more repeatable. As with peripheral nerves, slowed conduction reflects *demyelination*.

Clinical application
- Detection of optic nerve pathology:
  - Demyelination (e.g. optic neuritis) results in an abnormal and markedly delayed wave form. As visual acuity returns, amplitude will improve but delayed latency is typically permanent.
  - Compression (e.g. craniopharyngioma or optic nerve glioma in neurofibromatosis). Amplitude of the waveform decreases. Can also aid monitoring of condition in idiopathic intracranial hypertension.
- Visual field abnormalities and acuity (specialist centres only):
  - Partial-field stimulation can provide basic indication of visual field integrity in uncooperative children (e.g. monitoring use of vigabatrin).
  - Reducing checkerboard square size until VEP is abolished gives an indication of visual acuity.
- Macular disease:
  - Ischaemic and toxic lesions result in disturbance of waveform and delayed conduction. Aids monitoring of progression.

Limitations
- Relatively insensitive to partial disruption of visual pathways.
- Gives no indication of actual visual processing, just arrival of data at occipital cortex.

Electroretinogram (ERG) and electrooculogram (EOG)

- Recorded by measuring the potential difference between electrodes from a contact lens electrode or a skin electrode applied close to the eye and a reference electrode on the forehead. A strobe flash is the stimulus. As the rapidity of flashes increases, a flicker ERG is obtained.

- ERG is a combination of rod- and cone-system responses. In light-adapted retina, the response is dominated by the cone system. In the dark-adapted state, there will be a pure rod response.
- The EOG detects the mass-change in ocular resting potential as the retina passes from the light-adapted to the dark-adapted state.
- Need sedation/anaesthesia for very young children.

Clinical application
- To determine the function of rods and cones, the function of the outer retinal layers and to determine the retinal level of a pathological insult.
- Rod function typically is lost early in retinitis pigmentosa.
- In early detection of retinopathy associated with neurodegenerative conditions.
- Ophthalmic artery occlusion.

Brainstem auditory evoked responses
- The short-latency responses measured in routine clinical practice reflect the function of the auditory nerve and pathways in the brainstem.
- Longer latency responses are used in research contexts to evaluate early steps of auditory processing (e.g. pitch perception).
- Short-latency tests are unaffected by sedation or general anaesthetic.
- Stimulus is a loud click at 10 Hz with contralateral ear masking.
- Five waveforms are evoked. Currently it is thought they are related to the following anatomical structures.
  - Wave I action potential of cranial nerve VIII.
  - Wave II cochlear nucleus (with VIII cranial nerve).
  - Wave III ipsilateral superior olivary nucleus.
  - Wave IV nucleus or axons of lateral lemniscus.
  - Wave V inferior colliculus.
- Peak latencies influenced by age, sex, auditory acuity, stimulus repetition rate, intensity, and polarity.

Clinical application
- Determining hearing threshold in an uncooperative child (e.g. neonate) although newborn population screening uses a different technology (oto-acoustic emissions).
- Identifying those who would benefit from a hearing aid.
- Defining the site of disruption of auditory pathways relative to the structures listed above.
- Intra-operative monitoring during cerebello-pontine angle tumour surgery to help preserve auditory nerve function.
- Longitudinal monitoring of ototoxic chelating agents in thalassaemia treatment.

Somatosensory evoked potentials (SSEP)
- Typically elicited by stimulation of the median nerve at the wrist, the common peroneal nerve at the knee, and/or the posterior tibial nerve at the ankle with recording from electrodes placed over the scalp, spine, and peripheral nerves.
- Depend on the integrity of fast conducting large diameter fibres travelling in the posterior columns of the spinal cord.

- Integrity at the level of the peripheral nerve, plexus, spinal root, spinal cord, brainstem, thalamo-cortical projections, or primary somatosensory cortex can be inferred.
- Less used clinically since the advent of MRI but remains useful for intra-operative monitoring in scoliosis or other spinal cord surgery.
- Persistently absent cortical SSEPs in the context of acquired brain injury is a very poor prognostic sign (see Prognostication after acquired brain injury in Chapter 5 p. 222).

Peripheral neurophysiological tests

These are becoming less important to routine practice, with the advent of gene panels for hereditary sensory motor neuropathies.

Nerve conduction studies

- Can be distressingly uncomfortable: have a low threshold for premedication (e.g. with oral morphine analgesia plus anxiolytic doses of diazepam). Some neurophysiologists prefer to study children under general anaesthesia although this precludes studying EMG changes associated with voluntary effort.
- A pick up surface electrode is placed to record the compound muscle action potential (CMAP) over the appropriate muscle group. A stimulating electrode is placed at two defined points along a given nerve pathway a known distance apart. Supramaximal stimulation is used to ensure the fastest fibres are being stimulated.

Nerve conduction studies

Measure amplitude, latency, configuration, and conduction velocities of motor, sensory, or mixed nerves. Conduction velocity is dependent on the diameter and degree of myelination of axons: in mixed-fibre nerves it is the conduction velocity of the *fastest* axons that will be reflected (so for example a selective neuropathy of slowly conducting small fibres would be undetected). In the newborn infant, the velocity is about half the adult level and does not reach adult values until 3–5 yrs of age or later.

Repetitive nerve stimulation

CMAPs are recorded following a volley of 6–10 supramaximal stimulations of a nerve, e.g. at 3 Hz. Changes in CMAP amplitude (e.g. sequential decrements) may indicate a disorder ('fatigue') of neuromuscular transmission. Some neuromuscular transmission disorders (Lambert–Eaton, botulism) can cause paradoxical sequential increments in CMAP amplitude.

- Demyelination is predominantly reflected in reduced conduction velocities (since fast conduction depends on myelin).
- Axonal neuropathies often show maintained conduction velocity but the amplitude of the action potential is reduced.
- Conduction block is a feature of acute and chronic inflammatory demyelinating polyneuropathies (i.e. Guillain–Barré, CIDP) and is demonstrated in *motor* nerve studies only. Patchy demyelination causes attenuation of the compound muscle action stimulated proximally but stimulation nearer the muscle (distal to the patchy demyelination) gives normal results.
- In practice, overlapping forms of these pictures are often seen

The late responses

These studies may be abnormal even when distal motor responses are normal as they test proximal function: they are useful in assessing radiculopathies, plexopathies, polyneuropathies, and proximal mononeuropathies.

H-reflex
The H-reflex is in effect a standardized, quantifiable electrical version of the clinical tendon reflex, and is typically studied in the posterior tibial nerve (soleus, assessing S1 integrity) or median nerve (flexor carpi radialis, C7). Asymmetry of response is key to determining abnormalities: under normal circumstances, latencies should not differ between sides by >1 ms.

F-wave
F-wave studies are used to assess the function of proximal segments of the motor nerve. They are long latency 'echo' muscle action potential seen after supramaximal stimulation of a nerve: the stimulus travels antidromically along the motor fibre and reaches the anterior horn cell at a critical time to depolarize it. It is best obtained in the small foot and hand muscles.

Electromyography

This is uncomfortable but best done on someone able to cooperate by voluntarily contracting individual muscle groups. These are studied by the insertion of a needle electrode. Sedation compromises the ability to co-operate but ensure analgesia!

• Muscle tissue is normally electrically silent at rest. Action potentials appear with voluntary contraction. Each potential is produced by groups of fibres responding to a single motor neuron. As voluntary effort increases, individual action potentials summate and become confluent to form a 'complete interference pattern', and the baseline disappears.
• Occasional small potentials ('spikes') are seen if the needle is near the motor end plate.
• A loudspeaker system is used to allow electrical activity to be heard: aural impressions can be informative.

> ❶ The main role of EMG is to help differentiate neuropathies and myopathies. Appearances can be ambiguous, however, and it is important to interpret the findings in the light of other aspects of the clinical picture, the technical adequacy of the study and the experience of the neurophysiologist. As with any other ancillary medical test, clinical correlation is crucial.

Neurogenic change (denervation)
• The interference pattern is reduced so that the EMG baseline becomes partially visible.
• Spontaneous fibrillation potentials occur at rest (resting muscle normally silent). These are sharp, bi-phasic and of short duration with low amplitude potentials of about 100 µV.
• High amplitude polyphasic fasciculation potentials of long duration also occurring at rest indicate anterior horn cell disease (notably spinal muscle atrophy).
• Individual motor unit potentials are either normal or of large amplitude, long duration, and polyphasic. They indicate collateral re-innervation by surviving neurons with ↑territory.

Myopathic changes
• Random loss of muscle fibres results in low amplitude EMG with polyphasic short duration potentials. Sound like 'crackles' on a loudspeaker.

Myotonia
- Spontaneous bursts of potentials in rapid succession (up to 100 per second or more) with waxing and gradually waning.
- The sound is characteristic, described as resembling a 'dive bomber' or accelerating motorcycle: tapping the muscle adjacent to the needle may provoke a burst.

Myasthenia
- Decay of the interference pattern with sustained effort.

Specialized EMG

Single fibre EMG
Single fibre electromyography (SFEMG) selectively records muscle fibre action potential from a single motor unit: its main uses are in the determination of jitter (a measure of neuromuscular junction transmission) and fibre density (muscle spatial organization).

There are age-dependent normal values for jitter, measurement of which is expressed as mean consecutive difference or mean sorted difference between the trigger potential and an adjacent muscle fibre potential.
- Neuromuscular junction disease is associated with ↑ jitter.
- Fibre density is the mean number of muscle fibre potentials on 20 separate insertions and increases with age. It is significantly ↑ in neuropathy.

Macro-electromyography
This is modified SFEMG using the distal 15 mm of the needle cannula. The large recording surface picks up electrical activity from all muscle fibres from a single motor unit. In general, macro-EMG motor unit potential amplitude and area correlate with motor unit muscle fibre number. They are therefore low in myopathy and high in neuropathy.

Quantitative electromyography
Motor unit morphology can be quantified by analysing the duration, amplitude, phases, turns, area or area/amplitude ratio for 20 or more randomly selected simple motor units from a given muscle.

Results may be compared with age-matched normative data. The most sensitive parameters for myopathy seem to be motor unit potential duration and area/amplitude ratio.

Exercise testing: short and long exercise test
Exercise may produce characteristic changes in CMAP amplitude in children with myotonic myopathies and periodic paralysis.
- In myotonic dystrophy and (particularly) myotonia congenita, exercise will produce an immediate fall in the amplitude of the CMAP followed by a prompt recovery within minutes.
- A long exercise test of 2–5 min with periodic breaks to prevent ischaemia is useful in the diagnosis of periodic paralysis. After an initial increment in amplitude, a progressive long-lasting fall in CMAP amplitude is seen (~50%, 20–40 min after exercise) with recovery in 1 h. This may also be seen in paramyotonia congenita.

Specialist investigations

Paediatric neurology involves a number of potentially unfamiliar investigations on blood, CSF, urine, and skin. A basic understanding of these tests, their uses, and limitations can aid their organization!

Cerebrospinal fluid

CSF glucose

Low CSF glucose can result from infection. In the absence of infection, a CSF glucose <2.5 mM raises the possibility of glucose transporter 1 deficiency syndrome (GLUT1DS), a *treatable* cause of infantile seizures, acquired microcephaly, ataxia, and developmental impairment (see Glucose transporter 1 deficiency syndrome in Chapter 4 ⧉ p. 301). Diagnosis rests on *paired* measurement of blood (taken first to avoid spurious elevation of plasma glucose from stress of LP!) and CSF glucose after a 4–6 h fast and demonstration of a ratio <0.5 (range 0.19–0.49).

Increasingly *SLC2A1* gene testing (as part of a panel) is supplementing or replacing biochemical testing for suspected GLUT1DS.

CSF protein studies

High CSF protein reflects either entry of plasma proteins (albumin) into the CSF (i.e. breakdown of the blood–brain barrier; BBB) due to inflammation; or intracerebral demyelination or tissue destruction (e.g. in some neurodegenerative diseases). Further studies can help clarify this.

Albumin ratio (useful ≤10 days of onset)

Albumin can cross the BBB but is not synthesized intrathecally, hence a ↑ CSF to serum albumin ratio indicates BBB breakdown. Normal value <0.0043 (CSF and serum albumin converted to same units).

IgG index (time independent)

Distinguishes local production of IgG (e.g. multiple sclerosis, viral encephalitis, SSPE) from leakage across BBB from serum. CSF and serum levels of IgG can be compared using albumin as a reference protein: a ↑ level indicates intrathecal IgG synthesis (normal value <0.6).

$$\frac{IgG_{CSF}}{IgG_{serum}} \times \frac{albumin_{serum}}{albumin_{CSF}}$$

IgG oligoclonal bands (useful ≥10 days of onset)

Indicated by the presence of two or more discrete bands in the G region on isoelectric focusing. Requires a paired serum sample: detection of oligoclonal bands in CSF absent in serum suggests the local production of IgG of restricted specificity, due to an intracerebral inflammatory response.
- Present in up to 95% of children with multiple sclerosis (tends to persist).
- Present transiently in Guillain–Barré, bacterial meningitis, and viral encephalitis. Significant false +ve rate in ~4% of non-inflammatory conditions. See Table 2.4.

Table 2.4 Interpretation of oligoclonal band findings Abbreviations: ALD, adrenoleukodystrophy; AT, ataxia telangectasia; OGB, oligoclonal band(s); SLE, systemic lupus erythematosus; SSPE, subacute sclerosing panencephalitis

Pattern	Description	Interpretation	Conditions
1	Negative, no OGBs in CSF or serum	Normal	Non-inflammatory
2	CSF OGBs with none in serum ('unmatched')	Isolated intrathecal IgG synthesis	CNS infection (encephalitis, meningitis, HIV, SSPE, borrelia); CNS inflammation (including demyelination); AT, ALD
3	CSF OGBs not present in serum with *additional* matched bands (i.e. combination of patterns 2 and 4)	Intrathecal IgG synthesis *and* (potentially independent) systemic inflammation	CNS infection; CNS inflammation (including demyelination); (para) neoplastic
4	Identical OGBs in CSF and plasma ('matched')	Systemic inflammation with CNS involvement	Infection; inflammation; autoimmune (SLE, vasculitis); (para)neoplastic; inflammatory neuropathy; neurodegenerative
5	Large *mono*clonal bands in serum and CSF	Clones of abnormal B cells	Lymphoma, myeloma

CSF neurotransmitters and folate metabolites

A number of rare disorders of neurotransmitter metabolism involving serotonin, catecholamines, tetrahydrobiopterin, and folate biochemistry, can result in movement disorders (see Neurotransmitter disorders in Chapter 4 ➡ p. 488). CSF neopterin levels are also elevated non-specifically in CNS inflammatory states.

Measurement of CSF levels of their metabolites is technically challenging.

- There is a rostro-caudal gradient of neurotransmitter metabolites: hence tubes provided by the laboratory are numbered to collect specimens in a specific order.
- If the CSF is blood stained it will either need to be centrifuged immediately and the supernatant transferred to a fresh tube, or the procedure should be abandoned until a later date.
- Samples must be frozen immediately into liquid nitrogen.

CSF lactate and pyruvate

Spurious elevation of lactate in CSF is less problematic than in blood and elevated CSF lactate is strong circumstantial evidence of a disorder of oxidative metabolism (including mitochondrial disorders). CSF lactate elevation also occurs in meningitis. Temporary elevations may occur immediately after seizures but these tend to be modest. CSF lactate tends to be low-normal or low in GLUT1 deficiency syndrome. Contamination of CSF with blood will falsely elevate CSF lactate (see CSF proline, below).

CSF lactate:pyruvate ratio is rarely more informative than CSF lactate alone; however, in the context of elevated CSF lactate and a suspected disorder of oxidative metabolism a low L:P ratio (<20) would support a diagnosis of pyruvate dehydrogenase deficiency (PDH). The ratio tends to be high (>25) in other respiratory chain disorders.

CSF amino acids
- Paired blood and CSF amino acid estimation is required for the diagnosis of non-ketotic hyperglycinaemia (normal CSF: plasma glycine ratio <0.025; ratio >0.1 often found in NKH).
- CSF proline levels should be extremely low (<5°µM): higher levels indicate contamination of CSF with blood, and provide useful 'quality assurance' when interpreting CSF:plasma ratios of other compounds (e.g. preventing a false +ve conclusion that CSF:plasma glycine ratio is elevated).
- Elevated CSF threonine may occur in pyridoxine-dependent seizures (threonine dehydratase is pyridoxine dependent); however, normal levels do not exclude this diagnosis.
- Low CSF serine may indicate a serine synthesis defect (may also have secondarily low 5MTHF levels): interpretation of CSF:plasma ratios requires fasting as plasma serine levels rise markedly after meals.

CSF interferon alpha
Interferon alpha (IFNα) is a cytokine produced in the early stages of viral infections such as HSV. It does not cross the BBB so elevated CSF levels indicate intrathecal synthesis. Normal <2 IU/mL; ↑ in neuro-lupus and Aicardi–Goutières syndrome. A paired blood sample may be helpful but CSF should be immediately frozen and sent to the appropriate laboratory.

Urine

Urine microscopy
Metachromatic granules in epithelial cells in early morning second sample of urine stained with toluidine blue are indicative of metachromatic leukodystrophy.

Urine catecholamine metabolites
Catecholamines are dopamine, noradrenaline, and adrenaline: their metabolites are the metadrenalines VMA and HVA. Elevated levels are useful in the diagnosis of neuroblastoma. There is a high false –ve rate for this test, which may be supplemented with an MIBG test (see Opsoclonus-myoclonus syndrome in Chapter 4 ➋ p. 395).

Urine organic acids
Abnormal profiles may be present all the time or only during metabolic decompensation. Many substances may create artefactual changes including concomitant valproate administration. Urine will keep in the fridge at 4°C overnight without the need for preservative but then should be stored

at −20°C. Capillary gas chromatography–mass spectrometry (GC-MS) is the preferred method of analysis.

There is a risk of false −ves if urine is too dilute or the child has recovered from metabolic decompensation. Results may be available within hours in emergency situations.

Urine amino acids

Analysis may be used to diagnose a metabolic defect or to monitor treatment of aminoacidurias. Secondary abnormalities are very common.

Urinary mucopoly and oligosaccharide screen

Urine mucopolysaccharide screening tests uses 2-D electrophoresis to detect greatly elevated levels of glycosaminoglycans (GAG) in mucopolysaccharidoses. There are three patterns of GAG excretion: ↑ dermatan sulphate and heparan sulphate (types I/II/VI and VII), ↑ heparan sulphate in type III, and ↑ keratan sulphate in type IV. Additionally, thin-layer chromatography is performed to identify the oligosaccharidoses (including mannosidosis and fucosidosis).

Urine alpha-aminoadipic semialdehyde (AASA)

α-aminoadipic semialdehyde dehydrogenase deficiency causes pyridoxine-dependent seizures. A ↑ serum/CSF pipecolic acid level is a non-specific marker (↑ in peroxisomal disorders, ↓ with long-term treatment) but urine AASA is specific for the condition and remains high even on supplementation, so diagnosis need not delay onset of empiric treatment.

Urine creatinine, creatine, and guanidinoacetate (GAA)

Disorders of creatine metabolism may be suspected from a low serum creatinine concentration. 24 h urinary creatinine, creatine, and GAA levels will help to differentiate between the deficiencies (see Creatine deficiency disorders in Chapter 4 ➜ p. 300).

Urine uric acid

Urinary uric acid/creatinine ratio is a simple but useful method of screening for disorders of purine metabolism.

Blood

For sample requirements see Table 2.5.

pH and base excess

This is usually assayed on arterial blood in the ICU setting but a well-perfused capillary sample is adequate for routine testing. Acidosis may accompany many metabolic conditions, notably mitochondrial cytopathies, organic acidopathies, and catabolic states. Alkalosis may accompany hyperammonaemia.

Free and acylcarnitine

Carnitine is required for the transport of long chain fatty acids (FAs) as acyl coenzyme A-esters across the mitochondrial membrane for FA oxidation. Low levels occur with primary defects or secondary to other causes. Acyl carnitines are toxic esters of carnitine produced in the transport and metabolism of FAs: ↑ levels occur in FA oxidation defects and organic acidaemias. The gold standard for analysis is now tandem mass spectrometry (MS/MS)

Table 2.5 Sample requirements for specialist investigations

Test	Sample
Amino and organic acids	3 mL of urine
Free and acylcarnitine	1 mL of LiHep or a dry blood spot
Transferrin isoelectric focusing	1 mL of clotted blood
Lysosomal storage disorders	
White cell enzymes	5 mL of EDTA
Mucopoly- and oligosaccharide screen	3 mL of fresh urine
Carbohydrate disorders	
Sugar chromatography	5 mL of urine
Peroxisomal disorders	Together 5 mL of EDTA
VLCFA	
Pipecolic acid	
Phytanic acid	
Plasmalogens	
Biotinidase	2–3 mL of LiHep
DNA mutations	5 mL of EDTA

EDTA = EDTA blood; LiHep = heparinized blood; VLCFA = very long chain fatty acids.

Note: most specific enzyme assays can be carried out on cultured skin fibroblasts, cultured amniotic fluid cells, or chorionic villus samples. Check with the laboratory.

because of small sample requirements, automation, and processing speed. A dried blood spot on a filter paper ('Guthrie card') will suffice, and a result is typically possible within 24 h in emergency situations.

Note that plasma acylcarnitine analysis may give false −ves in screening for MCAD deficiency as individuals with secondary carnitine deficiency may not show a significant elevation of C6–C10 acylcarnitines. Either urine organic acids (in acute episodes) or acylglycines should be analysed.

Ammonia

Hyperammonaemia is an important indication of urea cycle disorders and/ or liver dysfunction; however, artefactually ↑ ammonia levels due to improper sample collection are common. Blood obtained should be free flowing, and the laboratory forewarned to accept and promptly handle the sample, which should be transported on ice as red cells and glutamine in the serum can otherwise both also release ammonia.

Lysosomal ('white cell') enzymes

Measurement of enzyme activities in lysosomes can be used to identify children affected by lysosomal storage disease or heterozygote carriers, as well as to monitor the response to bone marrow transplant or enzyme replacement therapy. Many laboratories screen for a panel of enzymes; however, this may not include the enzyme you are specifically interested in! It is important that the laboratory has appropriate quality assurance procedures in place. (See Neurodegenerative conditions in Chapter 4 → p. 472.)

Buffy coat histology

When blood is centrifuged, the 'buffy coat' is the enriched white cell fraction, visible as a white layer between the red cells (bottom) and the plasma (top). This sample can be fixed and prepared for electron microscopy for inclusion bodies, which can be useful in the diagnosis of lysosomal disease and neuronal ceroid lipofuscinosis.

Peripheral blood film

Examination of a peripheral blood film by an experienced haematologist can be useful in a number of situations:

Vacuolated lymphocytes

Indicative of a lysosomal disorder (requiring further characterization).

Alder–Reilly granules

Dense metachromatic granules resembling toxic granulations seen in leucocytes in mucopolysaccharidoses.

Acanthocytes

Red blood cells with multiple, irregularly spaced thorn-like projections or spicules of variable size, associated with abetalipoproteinaemia, some cerebellar ataxias, some progressive neurodegenerative diseases such as NBIA/PKAN (see Neurodegeneration with brain iron accumulation in Chapter 4 → p. 478), DRPLA, end-stage liver disease, and hepatorenal failure. A small number of acanthocytes may be seen in other forms of severe haemolytic anaemia, particularly after splenectomy.

Basophilic stippling

Represents ribosomal RNA precipitated during staining• seen in heavy metal poisoning as well as thalassaemias, haemoglobinopathies, sideroblastic anaemias, and pyrimidine-5'-nucleotidase deficiency.

Lactate

Free flowing blood is typically collected immediately into perchloric acid to deproteinize it. For the laboratory to interpret the level the volume of added blood must be accurately known: this is usually done by pre-weighing the tube. Check local arrangements. Spurious elevations of plasma lactate levels are common (e.g. systemic hypoperfusion; restriction of blood flow locally with a tourniquet).

Transferrin isoforms

These should be examined to diagnose congenital disorders of glycosylation (CDGs; previously known as carbohydrate-deficient glycoprotein syndromes) arising from defects in genes coding for enzymes involved in the glycosylation of proteins. Transferrin is a sensitive and convenient marker, secreted by the liver and normally present in different isoforms due to differences in glycosylation. These can be separated by isoelectric focusing (IEF) due to differences in their charge, immunofixed and visualized with anti-transferrin antibody. The presence of abnormal isoforms indicates the possibility of a CDG. IEF only identifies abnormal glycosylation but not the cause of the abnormality: further analysis requires enzyme studies on fibroblasts.

- *False +ves*: uncontrolled fructosaemia, galactosaemia, liver disease.
- *False –ves*: have been described, particularly with samples taken in the first few weeks of life.

Very long chain fatty acids (VLCFAs)
- Most peroxisomal disorders can be detected by an accumulation of VLCFAs. Elevated VLCFAs, often with ↑ pipecolic and phytanic acid levels, imply either peroxisomal biogenesis or oxidation disorders. Decreased red blood cell (RBC) plasmalogens imply biogenesis defects; normal plasmalogens imply oxidation or mild biosynthesis defects.
- Normal VLCFA with ↓ RBC plasmalogens is seen in the peroxisomal form of rhizomelic chondrodysplasia punctata (RCDP); where the activity of dihydroxyacetonephosphate acyltransferase (DHAP-AT) may also be reduced.

Biotinidase
- The phenotypic range of this treatable deficiency state is broad (see Biotinidase deficiency in Chapter 4 🠖 p. 525). Consider testing especially where there is hypotonia, severe infantile epilepsy, alopecia, rashes, and hearing loss.

Bone marrow aspirate

Bone marrow aspirate histology may be informative in Gaucher and Niemann–Pick disease type C or in diagnosing CNS lymphoma.

Muscle biopsy

Histology

Dystrophic change
- Necrosis of fibres with phagocytosis, etc.
- Regeneration: splitting of fibres, hyalinized fibres.
- Atrophic/hypertrophic fibres, random.
- Excess collagen and fat.

Myopathic change
- ↑ fibrous septae.
- Muscle fibre variation in size.
- ↑ fat.
- Fibre type predominance.
- ↑ internal nuclei.

Neuropathic changes
- Fibre type grouping.

Histochemistry
- Abnormal fat, glycogen, or amyloid deposition.
- 'Ragged-red fibres' due to accumulation of abnormally proliferating mitochondria.

Immunohistochemistry
- Dystrophin (absent or deficient in Duchenne and Becker dystrophies).
- Sarcoglycans (deficient in limb girdle muscular dystrophy (LGMD) types 2C, D, E, F).
- Calpain (deficient in LGMD2A).
- Laminin A2 (deficient in some congenital muscular dystrophies).
- Merosin (deficient in merosin-deficient congenital muscular dystrophy).
- Emerin (deficient in Emery–Dreifuss dystrophy).
- Oxidative enzyme staining: Gomori, COX, SDH, NADH.

Chemistry
- Enzyme analysis (e.g. phosphorylase deficiency in McArdle disease, acid maltase deficiency in type II Pompe disease)
- Assay of enzymes of the respiratory chain (complexes I to IV) in mitochondrial disease.

Electron microscopy
- Ultrastructural change, e.g. nemaline rods, inclusion bodies.

Nerve biopsy
- Segmental demyelination and remyelination cause layers of myelin giving an onion bulb appearance to the myelin sheath, indicative of demyelinating disease.
- Axonal degeneration, loss of axons.

Skin biopsy
Electron microscopy
- Presence of inclusion bodies in apocrine sweat gland-containing skin are indicative of some neuronal ceroid lipofuscinoses.
- Abnormal glycogen-containing inclusions in Lafora body disease.
- Chromosome abnormalities, particularly in mosaicism or some neurocutaneous syndromes.

Fibroblast culture
Can be used for biochemical studies when:
- Genetic testing is not available/cannot exclude a diagnosis, e.g. cholesterol esterification studies and filipin staining for Niemann–Pick disease type C.
- When conventional tests are –ve but there is still a strong clinical suspicion, e.g. glutaric aciduria type 1.

Practical procedures

Skin biopsy

Skin is taken for histology and/or establishment of fibroblast cultures. While not specific, the diagnosis of a number of neurological conditions may be assisted by the demonstration at electron microscopy of inclusion bodies in apocrine sweat gland-containing skin (i.e. axilla). Fibroblast cultures can be established from skin taken immediately post-mortem.

Take the sample aseptically and include the full thickness of the dermis. Establishment of fibroblast culture may be indicated for enzyme analysis to investigate inborn errors of metabolism or chromosome analysis to look for tissue specific mosaicism (e.g. hypomelanosis of Ito). Skin for fibroblast culture must be scrupulously sterile or contaminants will prevent the culture establishing. Take a small sample (a few mm in diameter) to prevent necrosis of the centre of a larger sample.

Equipment needed
- Punch biopsy needle size 3 or 4 mm.
- Fine forceps (not essential).
- Scalpel and dressing pack.
- 0.5% lidocaine.
- 2 mL syringe.

Procedure
- Liaise with the laboratory for transport medium—ideally a technician should be present if fixation is required.
- If for histology, skin can be collected into 0.9% saline in a sterile universal container. For fibroblast culture, collection into tissue culture medium is strongly preferred (use saline only exceptionally).
- Decide on the site—liaise with the laboratory as this could depend on the reason for the biopsy, e.g. from pigmented and unpigmented skin in hypomelanosis of Ito looking for fibroblast mosaicism, axilla for apocrine sweat glands in Lafora body disease, or forearm for general eccrine glands.
- Prepare skin with alcohol, chlorhexidine, or Hibitane®—avoid iodine-containing compounds such as Betadine® as these interfere with cell growth in culture.
- Infiltrate around site with 0.2–0.5 mL 0.5% lidocaine if necessary.
- Push the punch biopsy into the skin to the hilt.
- Lift up with fine forceps or an orange needle.
- Cut away the tethered portion with a scalpel.
- If a punch biopsy is not available, then a tent of skin can be lifted with a green needle and cut across with a scalpel, but this leaves a ragged cut edge.
- Apply pressure to bleeding with a gauze swab.
- Divide into required portions according to the number of bottles.
- Apply Steristrips® to oppose the skin.
- Cover with dressing and a bandage.
- Samples destined for fibroblast culture can be stored for 24 h at 4°C in sterile saline or 3–5 days at 4°C in culture medium.

Lumbar puncture and manometry

Equipment needed
- Assorted LP needles sized according to the size of the child.
- Dressing pack or dedicated LP pack.
- Clorhexidine.
- Gloves.
- Manometer—have two available in case the pressure exceeds the upper limit of one.
- Universal bottles, a fluoride oxalate bottle for CSF glucose.
- Bottles for neurotransmitter studies (if relevant) should be provided by the laboratory along with instructions for order, volume to collect, and transport (dry ice or liquid nitrogen).
- Topical anaesthetic cream over the site if desired.
- 1% lidocaine.
- 2 mL syringe.
- Orange needle.
- Collodion.
- Sticking plaster.
- Experienced nurse and or play therapist to hold the child.
- Assistant to hold the bottles.

Procedure
- Lateral decubitus position with the child held tightly curled: your assistant needs to be confident!
- Take time to ensure the pelvis and back are in the vertical plane and not tilting away from you.
- Identify the L3–4 intervertebral space, located along a line joining the iliac crests.
- Prep the area.
- In a larger child infiltrate lidocaine subcutaneously and in the intended direction of the spinal needle.
- Insert the needle horizontally with bevel up and perpendicular to the skin, aiming towards the umbilicus (in infants and young toddlers keep nearer to 45°).
- Little or no resistance should be felt except for a 'pop' as the dura is penetrated.
- Remove the stylet, attach the manometer, straighten the legs, and measure the pressure when the CSF stops rising and swings with respiration.
  - Be aware that CSF pressure may be artificially elevated due to hypercarbia, use of certain general anaesthetic agents, PEEP from ventilation, or undue neck flexion constricting the jugular veins.
- Turn the tap to drip the CSF into bottles.
- Remove the needle.
- Apply pressure, collodion, and sticking plaster.
- Post-LP headaches is less frequent with 25 G pencil point (blunt) needles instead of the usual bevelled tip. However, the flow rate using this is very slow and may be a limiting factor.

Shunt tap

This should ideally only be performed by a neurosurgeon as different shunt designs have different access points, and some are not suitable for tapping. However, if this is not possible:

Equipment needed
- Povidone iodine.
- Dressing pack with gauze swabs, tweezers, gloves.
- Sticking plaster.
- 23 G butterfly needle.
- Manometer if needed to measure pressure.
- Sterile universal bottles.
- Glucose bottle (fluoride oxalate).
- Local anaesthetic cream may be applied before the procedure if desired.

Procedure
- Prep the site.
- Insert the butterfly into the tapping chamber.
- Connect to the manometer if desired while occluding the outlet valve.
- High opening pressure suggests distal obstruction.
- Absence of spontaneous flow or a poor drip rate suggest proximal obstruction.
- Obtain CSF for investigations.
- Remove the butterfly.
- Apply pressure then the sticking plaster.

Neuropsychological testing

The use of standardized neuropsychological tests can support both diagnosis and rehabilitation planning. Neuropsychological testing complements and supplements assessment by an educational psychologist.

Domains and modules

Development is considered to be 'domain specific'. A *domain* is a set of representations sustaining a particular area of knowledge (e.g. language). A *module* is a more specific term to describe an information-processing unit (e.g. phonological module within a language domain). Modules may be differentially vulnerable at different developmental stages.

Indications for neuropsychological testing

- Evaluation of developmental disorders.
- Detection of conditions not demonstrated on standard neurodiagnostic testing (e.g. subtle sequelae of traumatic brain injury).
- Monitoring the neuropsychological status of children (e.g. monitoring changes following surgery for a brain tumour or epilepsy surgery).
- Characterization of cognitive capacities in planning rehabilitation programmes.
- Research.

Assessment strategies

- Fixed test battery.
- Flexible—hypothesis driven—tests chosen on the basis of the referral question.
- Combination of the above.

Psychological capacities tested

Intelligence
- The Wechsler Intelligence Scale for Children (WISC), currently at version five (WISC-V), provides a robust verbal/non-verbal assessment for children aged 6–16 yrs. Four domain scores and an overall IQ score are provided:
  - Verbal Comprehension Index (similarities, vocabulary: information, comprehension)
  - Visual spatial perception (block design, visual puzzles)
  - Fluid reasoning (matrix reasoning, figure weights)
  - Working memory (digit span, picture span)
  - Processing Speed Index (reflecting performance in *timed* tasks including coding, symbol search)
- An equivalent instrument for younger children (>30 months) is the Wechsler Preschool and Primary Scale of Intelligence (WPPSI-IV).
- In younger children, a diagnosis of learning disability may be withheld until the child is older, with a temporary label of developmental delay.
- Instruments designed for infants below 18 months test sensorimotor function primarily.
- There is limited correspondence between test results in infancy and those in school age children in longitudinal studies.

Adaptive function
- A more pragmatic assessment of social function including temperament, sociability, affective status, and motivation to cooperate, that relates to the ICF concept of *Participation* (see Models of disability in Chapter 4 ➔ p. 243).
- Typical measures include the Vineland Adaptive Behaviour Scales.

Mental status evaluation
- The WISC provides verbal and performance scores, which may indicate differential hemisphere dysfunction. The overall IQ score is a summary of several aspects of cognitive function.
- Scatter in the subtest scores may suggest more detailed testing.

Further testing may include:
- Attention/inhibition.
- Mood and motivation.
- Orientation and memory.
- Speech and linguistic function.

Specific instruments exist for all these domains.

Visuospatial
Visuospatial tests assess right hemisphere function predominantly, although a left hemisphere influence may be present if verbal mediation occurs.

Visuomotor functioning
Closely related to visual item perception and visuospatial processing, visuo-motor functioning adds a manipulation or graphomotor component to the perceptual tasks.

Social-emotional functions
These are particularly important in children with non-verbal learning disabilities.

Executive functions
Capacities that include:
- Attending in a selective and focused manner.
- Inhibition of off-task responding.
- Self-monitoring.
- Flexible concept formation.
- Planning.
- Judgement.
- Decision making.

Observation of spontaneous behaviour is also necessary to assess executive function, as the 'structured' nature of formal assessment compensates for the deficits being sought. Qualitative data (the types of errors produced) may be useful in determining context-related processing difficulties from executive function problems. No single test of executive function can test all of the 'executive functions'.

What do the results mean?
This involves three stages:
- Assessing the age appropriateness of behavioural function.

- Evaluating the skills necessary to the function.
- Neuropsychological evaluation and interpretation of results in light of the function, and assessment as to whether the results constitute a distinct neuropsychological profile.

Tests in common use
- Bayley Scales of Infant Development.
- Griffiths Mental Development Scale.
- British Ability Scales (primarily used within education: essentially measures of progress in literacy and numeracy against National Curriculum standards).
- WISC versions.
- Vineland Adaptive Behaviour Scales.

Specialized tests exist for specific situations (e.g. development scales for children with visual impairment). Discuss with your clinical psychology service.

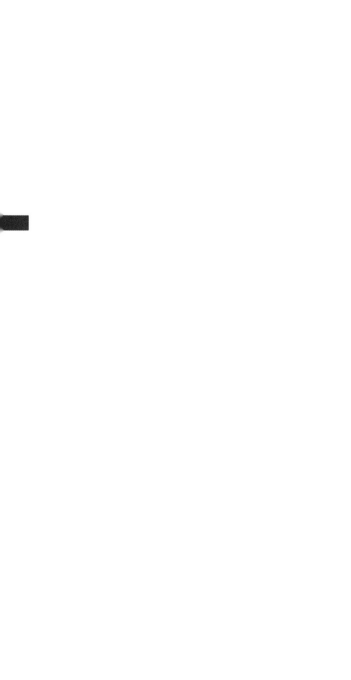

Chapter 3

Signs and symptoms

Agitation and confusion

Differential diagnosis

- Straightforward—if extreme—emotional reactions (panic, anger) to stress (e.g. prolonged hospitalization or chronic illness).
- Reactions to pain, particularly in children with severe learning disability who cannot report its location.
- Acute confusional state or delirium.
- Psychosis (schizophrenia, manic depression).
- Dementia: very rare in paediatric practice but will occur in later-onset neurodegenerative diseases.
- For differential diagnosis see Table 3.1.

Table 3.1 Differential diagnosis of agitation and confusion

	Delirium (acute confusional state)	Emotional reactions	Psychosis	Dementia
Prevalence	Common	Common	Rare as a new presentation in an acute hospital setting	Extremely rare
Onset	Acute or subacute	Acute or acute-on-chronic	Variable	Insidious
Course	Fluctuating, usually resolves over days to weeks	Usually days to weeks	Variable	Progressive
Conscious level	Often impaired, can fluctuate rapidly	Intact	Normal usually	Normal until late stages
Cognitive defects	Poor short-term memory, poor attention span	Absent	Absent	Poor short-term memory, attention less affected until severe
Hallucinations	Common, especially visual	None	Auditory; third person	Often absent
Delusions	Fleeting, non-systematized	None	Fixed and systematized	Often absent
Psychomotor activity	Unpredictable	Typically ↑	Variable (↑, ↓, catatonia)	Can be normal

Assessment

The key question is whether there is any *disorientation*: the hallmark of an acute confusional state. Subtle degrees of confusion are confirmed by specific testing of *orientation*. This has two components.

Awareness of time, place, and other people

- What is your name?
- How old are you?
- When is your birthday?
- Where do you live?
- Names of family members.
- Where are you now? (Are you at home?)
- Is it daytime or nighttime? Morning or afternoon?
- What time, day, month, year is it?

Orientation cannot be assessed in very young children. Formal tests of orientation (e.g. Children's Orientation and Amnesia Test) exist but are time-consuming and norms are age-dependent. A minor degree of disorientation in time (e.g. day of the week) can be normal in hospital!

Formation of new memories

- Who came to see you today?
- What was the score in your favourite football team's match/what happened in your favourite reality TV show last night?

Other features of acute confusional state

- Overactive and agitated, underactive and drowsy, or mixed.
- Fluctuates: worse at night.
- Anxious/irritable/depressed/perplexed.
- Thought abnormalities.
  - Reduced speed.
  - Muddled content.
  - Ideas of reference, delusions.
- Speech mumbling and incoherent.
- Visual illusions and misinterpretations:
  - Visual hallucinations are a marker of confusion until proven otherwise.
  - Typically of small, moving, fear inducing things such as insects or snakes.
  - May co-exist with visual misinterpretations as part of the clouded sensorium.

Acute management

One of many important reasons for correctly distinguishing an acute confusional state from emotional reaction is the very different approach to management. Emotional reactions will be managed by verbal de-escalation. However, attempts to argue, persuade, or cajole a child with an acute confusional state will be counter-productive: the mainstay of management is environmental modification. For investigation and management, see Acute behavioural disturbance in Chapter 6 ➔ p. 610.

Back pain

Always a cause of concern in childhood and adolescence. Consider the following:

Infection

Discitis in toddlers
- The child will often refuse to stand or will walk with a very straight back, 'guarding' the spine.
- May be febrile.
- Check FBC, ESR, blood cultures.
- Plain spine X-ray may show a narrow disc space.
- Have a low threshold for an MRI spine +/- bone scan.
- Treat for *Staphylococcus aureus* (usually for 6 weeks). If there is no response to IV antibiotics, consider needle aspiration. Seek microbiology advice.

Osteomyelitis
- Managed similarly. Always consider TB.

Skeletal causes
- *Disc herniation*. Uncommon in childhood. The pain is worse on raising the leg.
- *Spondylolysis*. Defect of the pars interarticularis: may have a fracture. Seen in gymnasts and rugby players.
- *Spondylolisthesis*. Slippage of a vertebra anteriorly. The significant cause of back pain in adolescents due to hyperextension from gymnastics, ballet, skating, etc. Treatment—symptomatic but if there is no improvement, may need surgery.
- *Osteochondritis*. Scheuermann disease, often seen with a kyphosis.
- *Rheumatic disease*: JRA, ankylosing spondylitis.
- *Scoliosis*: usually not painful, particularly in early stages.

Tumours
- *Malignant*: Neuroblastoma, lymphoma, leukaemia.
- *Metastatic:* Neuroblastoma, rhabdomyosarcoma, Wilms tumour, retinoblastoma, teratoma.
- Osteoma, osteoblastoma.

Intra-abdominal causes
- Pyelonephritis, retrocaecal appendicitis, pancreatitis.

Others
- Back pain can be the initial presentation of Guillain–Barré syndrome in toddlers, causing diagnostic confusion, although the fuller picture develops quickly.
- May be the presenting feature of transverse myelitis particularly if associated with paraesthesiae in the lower trunk or legs.
- Spinal cord infarction may present with sudden onset back pain (rare complication of trauma due to fat embolism; or as a complication of sickle cell disease).

- Functional disorder.
- Plexiform neurofibromas can cause pain without being externally visible.
- (Extremely rarely) as part of a generalized pain syndrome in acute attacks of porphyria (see Acute porphyria in Chapter 4 p. 487).
- Risk factors for benign causes: obesity, heavy school backpacks, joint laxity.

Behaviour disorders

A common situation where parents, teachers, and/or other carers are experiencing (perceived) difficulty managing a child. The general approach is to decide whether behaviour is a response to environmental factors, biologically mediated, or (often) a combination of both.

History

- What is the nature of the concern around behaviour?
- When was it first noticed? Recent onset after period of normality?
- Recent major life events?
- Where is it seen? Just at home or at school? In company of particular individuals?
- Are nursery/pre-school reports available?
- Are there concerns about developmental impairment?
- Is unrealistic parental expectation an issue?
- Any suggestion of poor parental child-management skills?
- Are there comorbidities?

Formulation

A response to environment?

Causes often difficult to define without detailed family assessment. Family factors include:

- Deprivation and neglect.
- Inconsistent or unskilled parenting.
- Unstable families.
- Violence in the home.
- Parents with anti-social personalities.

A child under pressure?

- Struggling at school with:
  - Specific learning difficulties.
  - Developmental coordination disorder.
  - Associated poor self-esteem.
  - (see School failure in this chapter ⊃ p. 191).
- Struggling with friendships:
  - Learnt (anti-) social behaviour.
  - Problems with inter-personal skills (autism)?

Biologically mediated?

- Any cause of developmental impairment (is the behavioural pattern more appropriate for the child's developmental than chronological age?) (see Developmental impairment in this chapter ⊃ p. 120).
- Autistic spectrum disorder (see Pervasive developmental disorder in this chapter ⊃ p. 125).
- Specific learning difficulties (e.g. dyslexia)—often reflecting in part poor self-esteem and a child under stress at school.
- Epilepsy (see Epilepsy and daily life in Chapter 4 ⊃ p. 317).
- Late-onset metabolic disease particularly when deterioration follows a period of normality (see Late presentation metabolic disease in Chapter 4 ⊃ p. 484).

A mixture of environment and biologically mediated disorders?
For example, the child with genetically determined learning difficulties under pressure at school adopting strategies for task avoidance or attention seeking. Each dimension needs assessment and appropriate intervention.

Specific patterns

Oppositional defiant disorder
The child is often negative and defiant with frequent loss of temper; arguing or non-compliant with adults. The child may be angry and resentful, irritable and easily annoyed, and deliberately provoking other people. Psychosocial interventions are the first-line treatment and should involve the child, family, and school focusing on psychotherapy, parent management training, and school-based interventions.

Conduct disorder
The child shows a persistent tendency to transgress normally accepted rules or the rights of others. This is often seen as bullying or threatening; initiating fights, and harming others; cruelty to people or animals; destroying property, fire-setting, theft, running away from home; truancy from school. Early intervention is crucial. Treatment options may include cognitive-behavioural therapy, family and peer group therapy, treatment of comorbidities (e.g. depression, ADHD).

Attention deficit disorder
A developmental disorder resulting in difficulty directing attention to tasks, listening to or following instructions, or organizing activities. Children exhibit distractibility, varying degrees of fidgetiness and impulsivity (e.g. interrupting and intruding on others).

Treatment (e.g. with methylphenidate, atomoxetine) may be indicated; a behavioural approach with firm, consistent handling with the definition of boundaries of acceptable behaviour usually used first, particularly for the under 5s.

Developmental impairment

When there is a suspicion of a developmental impairment, evaluate whether the delay is:
- Recent onset or longstanding.
- Static or progressive (regression).
- Global or specific (e.g. cognitive only).

Each area of development should be carefully assessed in turn. It is easy for one area of more obvious delay, such as gross motor, to 'mask' more subtle deficits in others, such as language.

An attempt should be made to quantify the degree of delay for all areas. This gives a profile of skills that can be reviewed over time to see if development is static, progressing, or regressing.

History
- What is the nature of the delay?
- When was it noticed?
- Are nursery/pre-school reports available?
- Are there concerns about other areas—motor, communication, social interaction, vision, hearing, general health?
- If there is a strong suggestion of developmental *regression* (i.e. the clear loss of previously established skills), see Psychomotor regression in this chapter ➋ p. 183.

Global developmental impairment

Causes
A genetic or syndromic cause is typically identified in ~20% of children investigated for isolated global developmental impairment, i.e. without neurological (particularly motor) signs, regression, dysmorphism, family history, or other evidence of genetic causes. The presence of any of these additional features greatly increases the chance of making a diagnosis. Metabolic testing contributes in ~1% of cases. Causes that are sometimes overlooked include:
- 'Mild' CP and dyspraxia: motor difficulty can disadvantage development in general: co-existent ADHD is common. Some authorities denote this combination DAMP: disorders of attention, motor processing, and perception.
- Less obvious genetic causes including Fragile X, 22q11 deletion syndrome, Sotos (not always obvious), Angelman (not always obvious in early stages), Rett (before stereotypies and regression become evident), maternal phenylketonuria (associated with microcephaly), some of the less dysmorphic mucopolysaccharidoses (type III), Duchenne muscular dystrophy, myotonic dystrophy, tuberous sclerosis, neurofibromatosis type 1, malformations of cortical development, especially subtle ones.
- Infection including HIV and CMV. Note that HIV encephalopathy can be the sole presenting feature of AIDS in children and is very treatable (see HIV and HIV-associated progressive encephalopathy in Chapter 4 ➋ p. 367).
- Antenatal exposure to toxins including alcohol.
- Postnatal exposure to toxins, e.g. lead (still important in some geographic areas).

History
- Birth history: maternal alcohol, medication, or recreational drug use; infection; movements *in utero*; oligo- or polyhydramnios; pre-, peri-, or postnatal risk factors for CP.
- Family history.
  - Ideally including grandparental generation;
  - Consanguinity;
  - Ethnicity;
  - Medical diagnoses? Early death?
  - Recurrent miscarriages;
  - Developmental delay/intellectual disability;
  - Seizures.
- Evidence of general clumsiness? Early oro-motor problems.
- Recurrent or persistent infections. Repeated hospital admissions.
- Risk factors for HIV infection.
- Is there a behavioural phenotype?

General examination
In order of diagnostic yield, examine head circumference, height, weight, face, then hands, then skin. See also Examination Table 1.1 in Chapter 1 ➔ p. 10 and see Psychomotor regression in this chapter ➔ p. 183.
- 'Gestalts' include 22q11, Cornelia de Lange, Kabuki (everted outer third of eyelid, 'thumb print' appearance to centre of bottom lip), 1p36 deletion (linear eyebrows, deaf, aggressive seizures).
- Skin abnormalities including signs of neurocutaneous syndromes.
- Microcephaly? Macrocephaly?
- Organomegaly?
- Neurological abnormalities particularly pyramidal or extrapyramidal motor signs.
- Eye signs: nystagmus, cataract, abnormalities on fundoscopy.
- Visual or hearing impairment?

Investigations
If no specific clues are found in the history, then the chances of finding a diagnosis are small, particularly in the absence of focal neurological signs and/or seizures.

However, a general screen is often taken with variations on the following:
- Blood: U&E, calcium, LFT, FBC, amino acids, (venous) blood gas, ammonia, lactate, thyroid function, CK.
- Urine: organic acids, amino acids, MPS/GAG, oligosaccharides.
- MRI of the head particularly in the presence of motor signs. Otherwise depending on severity of the delay, though subtle abnormalities are increasingly recognized with high resolution scans. MRI with spectroscopy should be considered in cases associated with development regression or refractory epilepsy.

The following may be considered if specific features in history or examination are suggestive.
- Maternal PKU status.
- EEG.

- Specific PCRs on stored Guthrie card blood spots (CMV, rubella) for suspected congenital infection.
- Plasma homocysteine.
- Plasma and urine creatine and guanidinoacetate for cerebral creatine deficiency syndromes (especially in boys). Rare but treatable with dietary modification. Freshly frozen urine is required. X-linked creatine transporter deficiency reported in 1% ♂'s with intellectual disability of unknown aetiology. See Creatine deficiency syndromes in Chapter 4 → p. 300.

Genetics review
An area of rapid technological change with important implications for clinical practice (see Principles of neurogenetics in Chapter 2 → p. 79).
- All children with isolated developmental impairment should have an aCGH and Fragile X testing.
- Consider an intellectual disability gene panel or equivalent.
  - The Deciphering Developmental Delay study (Wright CF *et al. Lancet*. 2015;385: 1305–14) reported a diagnostic yield of a further 27% from additional 'next-generation' techniques including whole-exome sequencing but this was in a selected population with strong prior suspicion of a genetic aetiology and samples available from parents as well as proband.
  - The yield in less selected cases of isolated early developmental impairment is less clear.
  - It is important to remain mindful of the 'blind spots' of gene panels and WES/WGS including insensitivity to triplet-repeat disorders (see Principles of neurogenetics in Chapter 2 → p. 79).
- In the absence of identified single-gene disorder, empirical (average) recurrence risks are approximately 1 in 7.5 for a brother and 1 in 20 for a sister of an index ♂; 1 in 12 for a brother and 1 in 15 for a sister of an index ♀.
- X-linked learning difficulties probably important in non-dysmorphic, otherwise healthy ♂ (accounts for ~ 10% all LD; at least 130 different genes).

Specific motor impairment/late walking

This often presents as a child with delayed sitting or walking. As the child will usually be young, the motor problem usually predominates and delay in other areas (language, etc.) may go unnoticed. For children who have achieved motor milestones but remain awkward or clumsy, see Gait abnormalities in this chapter → p. 157.

Causes
'Physiological' causes include:
- Familial delay.
- Variations on normal developmental patterns, e.g. 'bottom shuffling'.
- Ligamentous laxity.
- Prematurity with development not corrected for gestational age.

Common pathological causes include:
- Undiagnosed 'mild' CP.
- Developmental coordination disorder (dyspraxia).

- Duchenne muscular dystrophy in boys (vital to diagnose early for genetic counselling and family planning purposes).

Less common causes include hypothyroidism, Prader–Willi syndrome, cord lesions, and neuromuscular conditions, such as SMA, congenital muscular dystrophy, and hereditary sensorimotor neuropathies.

History
- Detailed developmental history to see if other skills are also delayed.
- Early hand preference?
- Early visual preference for one side?
- Floppiness?
- Weakness/stiffness (resistance when changing nappies, clothes).
- Disparity of skills of the upper limbs compared with the lower limbs.
- Oromotor difficulties.
- Bladder/bowel control (dribbling urine/constipation).
- Family history.

Examination
- Observation of level of alertness and of interest in the environment and social interaction can give an idea of whether there is cognitive impairment implying a more generalized 'central' cause.
- In toddlers, opportunistic observation of quality of movement in free play will often be more informative than attempted formal motor examination. Observe for asymmetry or stiffness and identify the limbs affected (see Real world examination of the toddler in Chapter 1 ➔ p. 46).
- Tone: ↑ or ↓? Central or peripheral lesion pattern?
- Long tract signs, contractures, scoliosis, persistence of immature reflexes, reflex level (check abdominal reflexes).

Investigation

▶▶ Creatine kinase (CK) **must** be checked in all boys not walking by 18 months.

- MRI of the brain if corticospinal, extrapyramidal, or cerebellar signs are present.
- If MRI of the brain is normal and signs are consistent consider MRI of the spine (given the need for sedation/GA to facilitate in younger children, it may be pragmatic to order these together at the outset).
- Consider investigations for neuromuscular disease (see Peripheral weakness in this chapter ➔ p. 180).

Specific language impairment

Assessment of language delay is complex!

Some concepts
- *Language*: a learned system of arbitrary symbols with socially shared meaning (this would include, e.g. the gestural symbols of sign languages).
- *Theory of mind*: a child's understanding there are other 'I's', other individuals with ideas, motives, etc. 'like me' in other people.

- *Shared attention*: the situation of child and adult (typically mother) simultaneously attending to the same external object (and the recognition by the child that this is occurring, which requires a theory of mind). Only in this situation might a child relate the 'c-a-t' sound he can hear his mother making to the furry animal he realizes they are both looking at and thinking about.
- *Speech*: the production and perception of oral symbols used for language.
- *Voice*: the acoustic characteristics of speech and non-speech sound.
- *Phonology*: the production of individual speech sounds.
- *Syntax*: the grammar of a language.
- *Pragmatics*: the social use of words.
- *Semantics*: the meaning of words.
- *Receptive function*: comprehension of speech or other communication.
- *Expressive function*: generation of speech or non-verbal communication.

Causes
Presentation of language delay can be conceptualized as being due to problems with:
- Developmental dysphasia.
  - Mixed receptive–expressive (e.g. verbal auditory agnosia).
  - Expressive (e.g. developmental verbal dyspraxia, dysarthria).
  - Higher order processing (e.g. semantic pragmatic disorder).
- Pervasive developmental disorders (PDD) including autism with weaknesses of theory of mind (see Pervasive developmental disorder in this chapter ➜ p. 125).
- Reading disorders (dyslexia).
  - Selective comprehension deficit.
  - Speech sound discrimination.
  - Dysnomia (inability to retrieve word from memory when needed).
- Emotional reactions as seen after major trauma or abuse, and selective mutism.

A neurologist can seek associated neurological conditions. These include:
- Epilepsy: non-convulsive status and Landau–Kleffner syndrome (see Epilepsy in Chapter 4 ➜ p. 273); other rare syndromes.
- Worster–Drought and bilateral perisylvian syndrome.
- Duchenne dystrophy.
- Cerebellar mutism after posterior fossa surgery (see Cerebellar mutism in Chapter 4 ➜ p. 520).
- Occasionally adrenoleukodystrophy can present with a receptive language problem.

History
- Current problem as seen by carers.
  - Supplemented by screening questionnaires or Speech and Language Therapist (SALT) reports to pinpoint areas of concern.
- How does the problem manifest in different situations: home vs school; with adults, peers, older, or younger children?
- How does the child communicate his needs?
- Dribbling/drooling, swallowing difficulties, aspiration, reflux?
- Deterioration over weeks or months after early normality?

- Epilepsy?
- Behavioural problems including ADHD and mood problems?
- Auditory agnosia?
- A detailed developmental history as relevant to PDD (see Pervasive developmental disorder in this chapter ➲ p. 125).

▶ Parents should understand about half of a child's speech at 2 yrs and three-quarters at 3 yrs.

Examination
- Oral cavity inspection: tongue, palate, dentition, tongue, and frenulum.
- Oral-motor examination to evaluate the strength of the muscles of the lips, jaw, and tongue (e.g. move the tongue from side to side, smile, frown, puff out the cheeks, etc.).
- Drooling?
- Coordination and sequencing of speech musculature. Ask the child to repeat strings of sounds (e.g. puh–tuh–kuh) as quickly as possible and perform actions such as licking a lollipop.
- Associated dyspraxia?
- Reading ability.
- Oral-sensory perception (identifying an object in the mouth through the sense of touch).

Assessment by other professionals
Evaluation cannot be made by a neurologist alone and should include SALT, psychologist, OT, and/or physiotherapist assessments.
- Cognitive ability.
- Irrespective of the nature of the problem, a cognitive assessment will inform prospects of a child communicating verbally or with an assistive device.
- Hearing assessment.
- Overall quality of verbal and non-verbal social communication skills (observation of the child in play: gesture, pointing, imitation).
- Quality of voice.
- Comprehension of language (evaluated using standardized tests).
- Expressive ability (word knowledge, use of grammar, ability to sequence a set of ideas, communication of needs).
- Observation of articulation: vowel and consonant sounds and combined sounds (syllables, etc.). Estimate of overall intelligibility of speech.

Investigations
- Limited role for formal neurological investigations.
- Consider:
  - MRI in selected cases where there is strong evidence of a motor disorder.
  - Sleep and waking EEG in suspected Landau–Kleffner and related disorders.

Pervasive developmental disorder

The now-superseded DSM-IV distinguished autism, Asperger syndrome, and 'pervasive developmental disorder not otherwise specified' (PDD-NOS, synonymous with ICD-10 term 'atypical autism'). The subsequent DSM-V (2013) subsumes all these terms under a single 'Autism Spectrum Disorder' rubric although the nosological validity of this remains controversial.

Several 'screening' tools (e.g. Checklist for Autism in Toddlers, CHAT) have been developed to help identify children with the disorders. They vary in quality and complexity and should only be used by those familiar with their usage and limitations.

> **!** Diagnosis of autism requires the assessment of more than one professional and observation of the child in more than one setting.

The condition is characterized by the triad of impairments in:
- Communication.
- Social interaction.
- Interests/imagination.

Many researchers regard weakness in theory of mind (see Some concepts in this chapter **◑** p. 123) as a key component.

Assessment requires standardized assessment instruments such as the ADI/ADOS (formal training in their use is required).

Early history
0–6 months
- Smiled back, responsive?
- Reciprocal vocalizations?
- Able to make him laugh, how?
- What sort of baby was he?

6–12 months
- Motor milestones.
- Cuddles?
- Peep-bo?
- Pleased to see you in the morning?
- Raised arms to be picked up?
- Wave bye-bye, clap?
- Turned to name?
- Musical, communicative babble?
- Cause and effect play?

12–18 months
- When did he walk?
- What was he like once on his feet? Did he explore?
- Did he bring toys for joint play?
- First words—when, what, to request, to name, or just copied and not for communication?
- Pointing—for need or to show?
- Referential eye contact?
- Looking at books together—joint attention?
- Imitative?
- Play—symbolic, repetitive, spontaneous, needed direction?
- Other behaviours—rigidity, routine?

18–24 months
- Self-help skills?
- Response to parents arriving/leaving?
- Response to familiar adults?
- Interaction with other children?
- Copy housework?
- Language development—if poor then how does he communicate needs?
- Response to nursery rhymes?

Current situation
Social interaction
- How does he show affection?
- Eye contact?
- Gesture/facial expression?
- Peer relationships—interested, inappropriate, passive?
- Sensitivity to feelings and expressions of others?
- Behaviour in public, appropriate social inhibitions?

Verbal and non-verbal communication
- How are needs communicated?
- Speech—echolalia, repetitive, stereotyped, idiosyncratic, appropriate?
- Does he ask questions appropriate to the occasion, listen, and understand answers?
- Is it possible to have a two-way conversation or does he direct topics?
- Does he expect you to know things you don't, go off on tangent?
- Literal interpretation?
- Appreciation of subtleties of humour—understand jokes or slapstick humour?
- What does he play with—truly imaginative, role-play?

Patterns of behaviour
- Preferred activities—obsessions, stereotyped, restricted?
- Range of things he plays with—fascination with non-functional/toy parts?
- Flexible with day-to-day activities or resistance to change?
- Motor mannerisms—hand flapping, spinning, rocking.

Other information
- Evidence of regression?
- Sleep pattern?
- Epilepsy.

Examination
- Neurocutaneous stigmata.
- Hearing and vision.
- Specific phenotypes of Rett syndrome, Fragile X, TS.

Investigations
- The following should be *considered*: plasma and urine creatine and guanidinoacetate, aCGH, *FMR1* (Fragile X), *MECP2*, EEG, MRI.

Exercise limitation and muscle pain

Relatively common complaints, but actual pathology is uncommon.
- Distinguish tiring and wanting to stop after a short distance, common in many neuromuscular (and other) conditions, from true *fatigue*: development of or increase in weakness with exercise. See Neuromuscular section: introduction in Chapter 4 ⊃ p. 429 for more details.

Causes

Non-neuromuscular causes such as post-viral illness are common. Also consider non-neurological causes such as arthropathy. Neuromuscular causes in children include the following:

Exercise limitation
- Myasthenia.
- Any significant neuromuscular condition.

Stiffness
- Myotonic dystrophy.
- Myotonia congenita.
- Paramyotonia.
- Periodic paralyses.
- Hypothyroidism.

Pain or cramps
- Poorly localized deep ache or discomfort: dystrophies or inflammatory myopathy.
- Localized, excruciating: viral myositis, muscle abscess, trauma, compartment syndrome.
- Cramps (painful contractions relieved by stretching): neuropathies, metabolic myopathy, e.g. McArdle disease (with second wind phenomenon) or carnitine palmitoyl transferase deficiency (fatigue with prolonged exercise, no second wind).

History

Exercise limitation
- Understand why this is happening: are there non-specific reasons or is the child actually weak?

Weakness
- Static or progressive.
- Fluctuating (myasthenia) or intermittent (periodic paralysis, myotonia congenita).
- Exercise-related (metabolic myopathy, especially with 'second wind' phenomenon).
- Pattern of weakness:
  - Proximal (reaching up, brushing hair, getting out of chair, or up off the ground). Typically *myopathy*.
  - Distal (gripping things). Often *neuropathy* although there are distal myopathies!
  - Both (myotonic dystrophy).

Stiffness
- Myotonia:
  - Difficulty with hand release.
  - 'Freezing' after a period of rest, or on standing from sitting, improves with gentle exercise (warming up phenomenon): myotonia congenita.
  - Freezing with on-going activity, exacerbated by cold: paramyotonia, periodic paralysis.

Pain
- Localized (infection, peripheral nerve lesion, metabolic myopathy) or generalized (dermatomyositis, viral, drugs, metabolic myopathy).
- At rest or during exercise (metabolic myopathy).

Family history
- Cataract (myotonic dystrophy).
- Diabetes, deafness (mitochondrial).

Myoglobinuria
- Urine 'like Coca-Cola'.
- 'Haematuria' on urine test strip but no red cells on microscopy.
- Metabolic myopathies but can also occur in dystrophies including Becker and Duchenne following strenuous activity.

Anaesthetic history
- Adverse reactions to previous anaesthetics.
- Family history of such reactions.

Involvement of other systems
- Cardiomyopathy.

Drugs
- Lipid lowering agents.
- Antipsychotics.

Examination
- See Neuromuscular section: introduction in Chapter 4 p. 429 for more details.

Eye movement abnormalities

Disorders of ocular movement disturb the conjugate eye movements that maintain binocular vision.

The key question to ask is whether this is a paralytic or non-paralytic squint, which is the same as asking:

▶ Is each eye—*considered alone*—capable of a full range of movement?

- If the answer to this question is yes, this is non-paralytic squint: a failure of *coordination* of the movements of each eye and by far the most common cause of non-conjugate eye movements.
- If no, then this reflects a 'lower motor neuron' lesion of eye movement pathways, i.e. a *paralytic* squint.

Non-paralytic squint

Affects 5% of pre-school children.

- Ocular alignment is poor in newborns. Constant alignment begins around 3 months of age and a 'nasal-ward' gaze bias persists until 6 months.
- Predisposing factors include very low birth weight, intraventricular or occipital-parietal haemorrhage, hydrocephalus, and trisomy 21.
- In neurologically normal children, squint can be caused by genetic factors, intraocular anatomy, or extraocular muscle conditions.
- A common cause is a very asymmetric refractive error (commonly long-sightedness) affecting one eye very much more than the other.
- Failure to correct such factors early, leading to dominance of the influence of the 'good' eye during a *critical window* between birth and about 2 yrs of age results in permanent and irreversible imbalance in the representation of inputs from each eye in the *ocular dominance columns* of the visual cortex, and permanent *amblyopia*, suppression of the visual input from the 'weak' eye (even if the ocular cause of the imbalance is subsequently corrected).
- Prevention is by correction of the primary ocular deficit, and *patching* of the good eye to 'force' use of the weak eye.

Squint types and ophthalmological jargon!

Latent strabismus (heterophoria)

- Intermittent.
- Brought on by stress/fatigue.
- Reveal with cover/uncover test (see Fig. 1.5 in Chapter 1 ⊃ p. 21).

Manifest strabismus (heterotropia)

- Constantly evident.

Convergent strabismus

- Eso*tropia* if manifest; eso*phoria* if latent.
- Inward deviation.
- Need to rule out long-sightedness, i.e. accommodative squint attempting to overcome hyperopia.

Divergent strabismus

- Exo*tropia* if manifest; exo*phoria* if latent.
- Outward deviation.
- Need to rule out intraocular disease.

Concomitant
- Latin: *concomito*, 'I accompany'.
- The misalignment, or relative angle, between the two eyes *remains constant* as the eyes look around.

Incomitant
- The relative angle between the eyes (the extent to which misalignment is evident) varies as the eyes move.

Pseudo-squint
- Pseudo-esotropia due to prominent epicanthic folds and a broad nasal bridge accounts for 50% of suspected squints. The cover test will be normal and light reflex central.

> ❶ Any *new* 'squint' (i.e. appearing *after* a period of established normal eye movement) warrants urgent neurological consideration including MRI; it may represent a cranial nerve palsy.

Paralytic squint
See Table 3.2.

Cranial nerve disorder
Lesion of cranial nerves III, IV, VI alone or in combination (see Fig. 1.6 in Chapter 1 ❸ p. 22).
- Trauma is commonest cause, followed by tumour.

Table 3.2 Causes of paralytic squint

Cranial nerves	Always consider ↑ intracranial pressure
	Idiopathic
	Trauma
	Vascular—cavernous sinus thrombosis* (usually spread of ear or sinus infection)
	Infection—meningitis, orbital cellulitis, diphtheria*, Gradenigo syndrome (middle ear infection)
	Inflammation—Miller–Fisher*
Ocular muscles	Mitochondrial myopathies (usually chronic and progressive external ophthalmoplegia; see Kearns-Sayre syndrome and chronic progressive external ophthalmoplegia in Chapter 4 ❸ p. 409)
	Thyroid disease
Neuromuscular transmission	Myasthenia gravis
	Botulism
	Tick paralysis

(Continued)

Table 3.2   *(Contd.)*

Cranial nerves	Always consider ↑ intracranial pressure
Brainstem	Tumour
	Vascular—AVM, haemorrhage, infarct, migraine, vasculitis
	Demyelination—ADEM, MS
	Toxic—tricyclics, ASMs
	Infection—basilar meningitis*

* Often bilateral involvement.

Ocular muscle disorders
- Congenital shortening of the superior oblique muscle or tendon (Brown syndrome).
- Congenital fibrosis of extraocular muscles (CFEOM): bilateral ptosis and restricted up-gaze, autosomal dominant.

Duane syndrome
- Rare congenital non-progressive disorder of horizontal eye movement.
- Congenital absence of VI nerve nucleus (cause uncertain), with associated aberrant innervation of lateral rectus by the III nerve.
- Clinically, results in limited horizontal eye movement, and often globe retraction and narrowing of palpebral fissure on attempted eye adduction.

Neuromuscular transmission
- Congenital and ocular autoimmune myasthenias (see Myasthenic syndromes in Chapter 4 ➋ p. 545).

Other eye movement disorder patterns

Vertical gaze palsy (supranuclear gaze palsy)
- Child cannot look up or down fully.
- Failure of upward gaze: dorsal midbrain damage (pineal region); Niemann–Pick; vCJD.
- Failure of downward gaze: rare; bilateral tectal/midbrain reticular formation lesions.

Horizontal gaze palsy
Apparent inability/unwillingness to look to one side; however, horizontal movements to doll's eye manoeuvre are present (i.e. this is a 'failure to generate the command' to look to one side: the mechanism to move the eyes is intact).
- Typically due to disease in cerebral hemispheres.
  - Lesion in the frontal eye fields in contralateral frontal lobe results in tonic deviation (usually toward side of the lesion) ± contralateral hemiplegia.
  - Parieto-occipital lesions giving rise to a hemianopia or hemi-inattention (i.e. unaware of visual targets on one side).
  - Gaucher disease.

Oculomotor apraxia (saccade initiation failure)
- Impairment of saccadic eye movements that redirect the eye to a new visual target.
- Child uses head thrusting with overshoot or blinking to move their eyes instead.
- Usually associated with neurological problems.
  - Congenital malformations—agenesis of corpus callosum or cerebellar vermis.
  - Neurodegenerative conditions—lysosomal storage diseases (Fabry, Gaucher), ataxia telangiectasia.

Internuclear ophthalmoplegia
- Normal horizontal eye movement requires connection between cranial nerve VI *ab*ducting one eye and cranial nerves III and IV *ad*ducting the opposite eye.
- Cranial nerves III and IV are higher in the brainstem (more rostral) than VI, so a connection passing vertically through the pons is required: the medial longitudinal fasciculus (MLF) (see Fig. 2.11a in Chapter 2 ➡ p. 69).
- MLF may be affected by demyelination, inflammation, infarction, intoxication, or traumatic axonal injury.
- The child is asymptomatic at rest but complains of diplopia on lateral gaze.
- Lesion of the right MLF causes failure of adduction of the right eye on attempted left gaze: left eye abducts normally.
- Both eyes may show nystagmus (more marked in the abducting eye).
- Can be bilateral resulting in intact abduction but impaired adduction of each eye.
- A combination of a lesion to MLF plus the ipsilateral VI nucleus or parapontine reticular formation) results in 'one-and-a-half' syndrome: loss of all horizontal eye movement *except* abduction of the contralateral eye.

Ptosis
- Drooping of one or both eyelids from birth is common. It is essential to distinguish congenital from acquired: *look at baby photographs*.

Congenital
- Horner syndrome (see Horner syndrome in this chapter ➡ p. 135).
- Myasthenia gravis.
- III nerve palsy.
- Syndromes associated with ptosis, e.g. Noonan, Saethre–Chotzen.

Congenital idiopathic
- Most common 'cause'.
- 70% unilateral.
- Eye movements normal.
- May have Marcus–Gunn phenomenon (synkinesis between III and V) resulting in winking when chewing.

▶ If examination findings suggest Horner or III lesion, MRI (including of the thoracic inlet) is required to exclude structural causes.

Acquired
- Horner syndrome (see Horner syndrome in this chapter ⊃ p. 135).
- Myasthenia gravis.
- III nerve palsy.
- Migraine.
- Trauma.
- Infection/inflammation of lid or orbit.
- Mitochondrial myopathies.

Ice pack test of ptosis for evaluation of possible myasthenia
If neuromuscular junction dysfunction is being considered in a child with ptosis, hold an ice pack firmly over one eye for 2 min. Improvement in the ptosis (i.e. better elevation of the eyelid) relative to the opposite (control) eye strongly suggests myasthenia as the cause of the ptosis (only reliable if baseline ptosis is bilateral and relatively symmetrical).

Nystagmus
Involuntary, rhythmic oscillation of the eyes, in which at least one phase is slow.
- *Pendular*: slow in each direction.
  - Assess visual acuity: can reflect difficulty fixing on target ('sensory nystagmus').
  - Optic atrophy (need to rule out optic glioma).
  - Demyelinating disease.
- *Jerky*: slower in one direction; named for the direction of the fast jerk return component. Always consider toxicity.

Horizontal
- Drug-induced (ASMs, psychoactive drugs, alcohol).
- Ictal.
- Vestibular (labyrinthine disease; usually with vertigo, nausea, vomiting, deafness, or tinnitus).

Vertical
- Downbeat (phenytoin, carbamazepine; cerebellar degeneration; heat stroke).
- Distinguished from nystagmus occurring only on looking down: sign of cervico-medullary junction or cerebellar lesion.
- Upbeat (medullary lesions).

Dissociated
- Monocular (spasmus nutans; chiasmatic tumour, amblyopia).
- See-saw (sellar and para-sellar tumour, retinitis pigmentosa).

Congenital onset nystagmus
A diagnosis of exclusion: all children with nystagmus require MR imaging.
- Relatively common.
- Present from birth but may not be identified until several months of age.
- Familial, idiopathic, or associated with visual impairment.
- Usually conjugate and horizontal.
- ↑ by fixation, visual interest, and arousal.

- ↓ by convergence and eyelid closure.
- Idiopathic (benign) congenital nystagmus typically has a 'null' direction of gaze in which the amplitude of the nystagmus is minimized: this may be eccentric, resulting in a head turn.

ⓘ Rotatory nystagmus in particular is a common presentation of pineal region tumours in infants but delayed presentation due to inappropriate reassurance by professionals is frequent.

Physiological
- High frequency (1–3 Hz), low amplitude, at extremes of lateral gaze (i.e. emerging during clinical examination of eye movements), especially with fatigue.

Horner syndrome

- The combination of ipsilateral mild ptosis, miosis (small pupil), variable anhidrosis, and enophthalmos.
- Pharmacological testing provides useful confirmation. 0.5% apraclonidine (α agonist) eye drops will reverse miosis. Demonstration of marked mydriasis (dilatation) with paredrine eye drops confirms normal function of the final, third-order neuron in the sympathetic pathway (i.e. if paredrine effect absent, this is the site of the lesion).
- The presence of iris *heterochromia*, where the ipsilateral iris is more blue or green and less brown than the normal contralateral iris (due to the absence of melanin) indicates the Horner syndrome is of congenital origin (there are additional causes of *isolated* iris heterochromia).
- Family photographs can be very helpful in establishing whether the Horner syndrome is congenital or acquired.
- Horner syndrome reflects disruption of the ipsilateral sympathetic pathway anywhere along its course. Important causes of acquired lesions include:
  - lateral medullary syndrome (occlusion of the posterior inferior cerebellar artery causing ipsilateral ataxia, XII lesion, and contralateral disruption of spinothalamic function, see Fig. 2.12).
  - syringomyelia.
  - brachial plexus injuries (Klumpke).
  - cervical ribs.
  - abnormalities of the aorta or carotid artery (e.g. dissection, aneurysm).
  - lesions in the upper thorax.
  - goitre.
  - middle ear disease.
  - cavernous sinus thrombosis.

▶▶ All cases of Horner syndrome require MRI: this must include the entire course of the sympathetic tract from medulla to upper thorax. Normal findings (i.e. 'idiopathic') are common in congenital onset situations.

Spasmus nutans
- Onset 6–12 months.
- Otherwise healthy child.
- Idiopathic, rarely associated with optic glioma.
- Triad of binocular nystagmus, titubation, and head tilt.
- High frequency, low amplitude, dysconjugate.
- Resolves spontaneously after 1–2 yrs.

▶▶ Diagnosis of exclusion: all children should be imaged.

Opsoclonus

Also known as the 'dancing eyes' phenomenon or saccadomania. A pattern of uncontrolled saccades, i.e. rapid, chaotic, multidirectional, but *conjugate* eye movements.

Associated with:
- *Neuroblastoma:* particularly as part of the 'dancing eyes, dancing feet', opsoclonus–myoclonus syndrome (see Opsoclonus–myoclonus in Chapter 4 ➋ p. 395).
- *Drugs:* amitriptyline, diazepam, phenytoin.
- (Probably) infections (Coxsackie B, para-influenza, Epstein-Barr) although some authorities suggest even supposed post-infectious cases are in fact due to occult neuroblastoma.
- GLUT1 deficiency see Glucose transporter-1 deficiency (see GLUT1DS in Chapter 4 ➋ p. 301) can present with eye movement abnormalities in infancy that can resemble opsoclonus.

Ocular flutter

Brief horizontal oscillatory eye movements occurring with fixation. A feature of eye movement disorders of cerebellar origin.

Proptosis

Any space-occupying mass behind the eye. Consider:
- Thyroid eye disease.
- Carotid-cavernous fistula or other vascular malformation (bruit?).

▶▶ All children presenting with proptosis will require imaging.

Facial movement abnormalities

Unusual movements

Tics
- Very common, particularly in boys.
- Peak ages at 5 yrs and then again around 10 yrs: majority largely or fully remit in adolescence.
- Worse with tiredness, stress, or boredom. Often disappear in sleep. Usually have family history.
- If accompanied by vocal tics consider Tourette syndrome (see Tic disorders and Tourette syndrome in Chapter 4 ⊃ p. 421).

Seizures
- Simple (clonic) partial motor seizures typically unilateral and due to structural lesions in contralateral primary motor cortex. If continuous, represents a form of *epilepsia partialis continua*, a feature of Rasmussen syndrome (see Rasmussen syndrome in Chapter 4 ⊃ p. 400) and Alpers disease (see Alpers-Huttenlocher syndrome in Chapter 4 ⊃ p. 409).
- Perioral seizures are a cardinal feature of SeLECTS (see Self-limiting epilepsy with centro-temporal spikes in Chapter 4 ⊃ p. 282) but are often nocturnal and thus may not be noted.

Myokymia
- Involuntary rippling movements often in the cheeks due to intrinsic pontine lesions (usually demyelination) or paraneoplastic. Very rare.

Hemifacial spasm:
- Intermittent twitching of facial muscles. Elevation of the ipsilateral eyebrow is seen with eye closure, as the internal part of frontalis contracts along with orbicularis oculi (described as 'Babinski's other sign'). Exclude structural lesions of the cerebello-pontine angle. Also a feature of gelastic seizures due to hypothalamic hamartoma. Very rare in children.

Facial weakness

See Table 3.3.
   Generalized, symmetrical facial weakness (tent-shaped, open mouth ± ptosis) may reflect a myopathic or neuromuscular junction pathology (see Neuromuscular conditions in Chapter 4 ⊃ p. 429).

Asymmetric crying facies
Frequently mistaken for facial nerve palsy in newborns and may result in a call from an anxious obstetrician after a forceps delivery!
- Due to unilateral congenital hypoplasia of the *depressor angularis oris* muscle (cause unknown).
- Results in an inability to pull down that corner of the mouth (and hence an asymmetric face particularly when crying).
- Facial nerve function (reflected in, for example, symmetry of the nasolabial folds) is in fact however, *normal*.
- Usually noticed within hours of birth.

Table 3.3 Causes of facial weakness

Congenital	
Developmental	Moebius syndrome (aplasia of facial nerve nuclei/muscles* often multiple cranial nerves)
	Goldenhaar syndrome, Poland anomaly, DiGeorge syndrome, osteopetrosis, trisomy 13/18
	Bilateral congenital perisylvian syndrome*
Trauma	Facial nerve compression against sacrum, forceps delivery
Muscle disorders	Congenital muscular dystrophy, congenital myasthenic syndromes, congenital myopathies, myotonic dystrophy
Acquired	
Idiopathic (fairly common)	Bell palsy (may also have pain/numbness around ear and impairment of taste)
Infective	Viral—herpes zoster oticus (Ramsay–Hunt syndrome, vesicles seen in ear canal), herpes simplex, mumps, EBV
	Borrelia (Lyme disease), TB, *Listeria*, diphtheritic neuropathy*, botulism (with ophthalmoplegia and dry mouth)
Vascular (rare in childhood)	Hypertension, diabetes, vasculitis
Inflammatory/autoimmune	Miller–Fisher syndrome*, otitis media, multiple sclerosis (rare), myasthenia gravis*
Tumour	Pontine glioma, cerebellopontine angle tumour, leukaemia, meningeal carcinoma, parotid tumour
Trauma	Temporal or basal skull fractures
Granuloma	Sarcoidosis* (very rare in childhood)
Metabolic	Hypothyroidism, hyperparathyroidism
Genetic	Melkersson syndrome—recurrent facial nerve weakness with fissured tongue and facial/lip oedema
	Fazio–Londe disease—progressive bulbar palsy (see Vitamin B2 in Chapter 4 ➲ p. 523)

* Often bilateral.

- A small number are associated with cardiac abnormalities but most commonly it is a benign incidental condition that is less obvious in older childhood (less time crying!) requiring reassurance only.

Decide if the involvement is an upper or lower motor neuron pattern
- Classically upper motor neuron (UMN) facial weakness results in preserved forehead power and eye closure (the mechanism is

controversial) but be aware that injury to *selected* lower branches of the facial nerve as they cross the cheek (e.g. by a parotid lesion) could result in the same pattern.

- UMN facial nerve weakness is unlikely to be isolated (e.g. likely to be accompanied by hemiplegia).

▶ Always assess for concurrent involvement of V, VI, VIII and lower cranial nerves: very helpful in localizing the lesion.

Supranuclear facial weakness
Voluntary facial movement (e.g. smiling for a photograph) originates in the face area of the motor cortex. Spontaneous (involuntary) facial expression of emotion has different, subcortical origins and can be selectively preserved.

Pontine lesion
- *Pseudobulbar palsy* due to high pontine lesions is a combination of (bilateral) upper motor neuron facial weakness with other lower cranial nerve defects, a hyperactive gag reflex, and typical emotional lability (weeping, laughing).
- Lateral pontine lesions result in facial analgesia and Horner syndrome ipsilateral to facial weakness.
- Lesions of the facial nerve nucleus itself inevitably result in ipsilateral sixth nerve weakness (due to a very close anatomical relationship) and usually contralateral hemiparesis.

Unilateral weakness of facial movement including forehead muscles (Bell palsy)
The facial nerve has a long course, during various stages of which it is closely related to other cranial nerves. Its long course through a very narrow canal in the temporal bone is also unique and probably underlies the vulnerability to traumatic or inflammatory injury.

Cerebellopontine angle lesion
- Facial nerve closely related to V, VI, and VIII nerves.

Intratemporal segment lesion
- In the proximal segment the facial nerve lies alongside the nervus intermedius: involvement of hearing (either loss or hyperacusis due to involvement of the nerve to stapedius) is unavoidable.
- At the geniculate ganglion, secretomotor fibres leave to travel forward in the greater petrosal nerve to the lacrimal gland. Loss of tearing from the ipsilateral eye implies lesion is proximal to this.
- In principle examination of taste in the anterior tongue should also have localizing value (chorda tympani), but in practice this is difficult as saliva carries material to other side of tongue too.

Evaluation of 'Bell palsy'
'Idiopathic' unilateral lower motor neuron facial nerve weakness (Bell palsy) is relatively common. Most cases probably due to post-viral infectious oedema, the selective vulnerability of the facial nerve being due to its long,

narrow intraosseous course. All cases require careful evaluation and consideration of the following possible causes:

- Hypertension.
- *Infection*: EBV, mumps, herpes zoster of the geniculate ganglion (Ramsay–Hunt syndrome), Lyme disease, otitis media, mastoiditis.
- *Trauma*: forceps delivery, maxillofacial fractures.
- *Infiltration*: brainstem tumour, Schwannoma, TB, leukaemia (expect other cranial nerve signs), lymphoma.
- In contrast to adult practice, sarcoid is a very rare cause.
- If bilateral or recurrent, consider evolving Melkersson–Rosenthal syndrome: recurrent paralysis with facial/lip swelling and fissured/furrowed tongue (rare) or any of the infective or infiltrative causes.

History
- Ask about noise intolerance (lesion in the proximal portion of the facial canal).
- Dry eyes/loss of tears.
- Tick bites (neuroborreliosis is an important cause of Bell palsy in Lyme-endemic areas), other infection.

Examination
- BP.
- Assess the degree of impairment of eyelid closure and risk to the cornea (Bell phenomenon of eyes rolling upward on attempted closure seen if lids are not fully closed).
- Parotid swelling.
- Otoscopy for otitis media, cholesteatoma, herpetic lesions.
- Mouth for herpetic lesion of hard palate.
- Testing taste in anterior two-thirds for chorda tympani involvement (difficult in practice).
- Exclude involvement of other cranial nerves (especially V: corneal reflex), presence of cerebellar and long tract signs: cerebellopontine lesion.

Management of Bell palsy
Good eye care with artificial tears and taping of the eyelid at night. If presentation is less than 7 days since onset, give prednisolone 1 mg/kg/day for 7 days and taper over 7 days. Some authorities additionally recommend empiric use of aciclovir (e.g. for 5 days) although this is controversial. It is of course clearly indicated in situations where a herpetic aetiology seems probable. Usually self-limiting with significant spontaneous recovery but if need be a physiotherapist should carry out facial rehabilitation.

Facial sensation abnormalities

Numbness, pain, or a combination of both. All very rare as isolated symptoms in children. See Table 3.4.

Table 3.4 Facial sensation abnormalities

Pain	Referred from eye (iritis/glaucoma), sinuses, teeth, jaw
	Post-herpetic neuralgia
	Migraine
	Cluster headache (usually retro-orbital)
	Multiple sclerosis (esp., paroxysmal)
	Trigeminal neuralgia
	Functional*
Numbness	Simple partial sensory seizures
	Migraine
	Shingles
	Multiple sclerosis
	Connective tissue diseases
	Sarcoidosis
	Dissociated sensory loss in syringobulbia (loss of pain sensation with preservation of light touch) tends to start peripherally on the face and spread to centre (sparing nose area until late)
	Functional*
Both pain and numbness	Preceding weakness in Bell palsy
	Tumour invading cranial nerve V —posterior fossa, base of skull, sinuses, salivary glands

*In the context of possible functional symptoms, it is important to remember the trigeminal nerve territory in some detail (see Fig. 3.1 in this chapter ⊃ p. 142): sensory disturbances that stop at the hairline (rather than the vertex), that extend down onto the neck, or that do not spare the angle of the jaw are not congruent with trigeminal nerve boundaries.

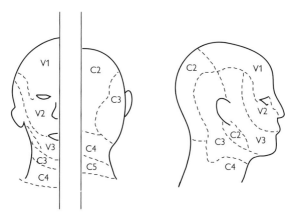

Fig. 3.1 Dermatomal boundaries on the head and neck.

Floppy infants

Floppy infants usually have poor head control, head lag, and truncal instability. When held in the air under the arms, infants will tend to 'slip through your hands'. This section discusses chronic floppiness in infants, which may have been present in the perinatal period or developed later. Acute floppiness can occur with any severe acute systemic illness and is not discussed in this chapter.

> ▶ Key question: is the child 'just' floppy, or floppy *and weak* (e.g. in supine lying does the child have enough antigravity power to lift and hold the limbs in the air?)
> **The presence of weakness implies a peripheral cause.**
> Beware of *mixed* pictures: for example an infant with peripheral hypotonia may be more at risk of hypoxic–ischaemic encephalopathy due to aspiration, causing an *additional*, central problem.

The approach to investigation depends on whether the floppiness is thought to be central (hypotonic but preserved power) or peripheral in origin (hypotonic and weak).

In most infants, the cause is central.

History

- *Maternal history*: systemic diseases, drug history, unrecognized myotonic dystrophy?
- *Family history*: consanguinity, sudden infant deaths.
- *Pregnancy*: foetal movement, drug exposure (e.g. ASMs), polyhydramnios/oligohydramnios, abnormal obstetric presentation.
- *Delivery*: Apgar score (muscle tone?), resuscitation, cord gases.
- *Postnatal*: feeding, alertness, response to stimuli, spontaneous activity, respiratory effort, seizures.
- *Time-course*: deterioration over time?

Examination

Typical findings in hypotonia of central origin
- Muscle strength usually normal.
- Reflexes normal or ↑ (may rarely be absent, especially in the first days of life).
- *Axial* tone often particularly affected with relatively preservation of limb tone.
- May have dysmorphic features, microcephaly, seizures, ↓ alertness, and poor visual tracking.

Typical findings in floppiness of peripheral origin
- Reduced axial *and* limb tone.
- *Anterior horn cell disease (e.g. SMA)*: generalized weakness, ↓ or absent reflexes, fasciculation, often described as very facially expressive and alert.
- *Peripheral nerve disease*: weakness more distal than proximal, ↓ or absent reflexes ± fasciculation.

- *Neuromuscular junction disease:* weakness particularly affecting eyelids, eye movements, or bulbar function. Reflexes normal.
- *Muscle disease:* weakness more proximal than distal, reduced reflexes.

▶ NB: examination of the mother is also important to exclude myotonic dystrophy and myasthenia gravis.
- Arthrogryposis is often due to peripheral or systemic conditions, but 50% ventilator-dependent children with arthrogryposis have a cerebral dysgenesis.

Causes of peripheral weakness

Neonate
- Neonatal myotonic dystrophy (see Myotonic dystrophy in Chapter 4 ⮞ p. 442).
- Transient neonatal myasthenia (see Transient neonatal myasthenia in Chapter 4 ⮞ p. 455).
  - affects around 12% of infants born to mothers with autoimmune (AChR antibody +ve) myasthenia gravis.
  - occurs via placental transfer of autoantibody.
  - transient feeding problems, poor suck, respiratory distress.
  - congenital myasthenic syndromes (inherited) tend to present a little later.
- Neonatal severe forms of inherited myopathies, e.g. central core disease, nemaline myopathy (see Congenital myopathies in Chapter 4 ⮞ p. 448).
- Trauma, including birth-related *spinal cord trauma.*
  - can be mistaken for birth asphyxia but alert, and no objective evidence of asphyxia insult (e.g. normal cord gases).
- 'Type 0' spinal muscular atrophy (see Spinal muscular atrophy in Chapter 4 ⮞ p. 452).
  - visually alert.
  - areflexic.
  - may have contractures.

Infant
- Spinal muscular atrophy type 1 (see Spinal muscular atrophy in Chapter 4 ⮞ p. 452).
  - visually alert infant.
  - may have bell-shaped chest from paradoxical breathing (diaphragm relatively spared, weak intercostal muscles).
  - may have visible tongue fasciculations.
- Hereditary sensorimotor neuropathies (see Hereditary motor neuropathies in Chapter 4 ⮞ p. 433).
- Infantile botulism: absolute constipation typically for a few days prior to presentation; weakness *descends* (cf. Guillain–Barré) with loss of head control early.
- Congenital myasthenic syndromes (see Congenital myasthenic syndromes in Chapter 4 ⮞ p. 455).
  - also important causes of apnoea and brief resolved unexplained events (BRUEs) in infants.

- Congenital muscular dystrophies (see Congenital muscular dystrophies in Chapter 4 ➲ p. 442) e.g. Fukuyama muscular dystrophy.
- Type II glycogen storage disease (Pompe disease) typically has modestly elevated CK (e.g. 2000–5000 IU/L).

Central causes

Neonate
- Trisomy 21.
- Prader–Willi syndrome (deletion 15q11): extreme floppiness with marked problems feeding and swallowing; mild dysmorphic features, hypopigmentation, undescended testes.
- Zellweger syndrome: peroxisomal disorder with dysmorphic features (high, prominent forehead), extreme floppiness, hepatosplenomegaly, seizures, and renal cysts.

Older infant
- Many infants with a cerebral palsy are floppy for some months before the onset of spasticity. Consider hypoxic–ischaemic insult, intraventricular haemorrhage, periventricular leukomalacia, developmental brain malformations, congenital infection (check for hepatosplenomegaly).
- Neurodegenerative diseases:
  - Tay–Sachs disease (visual impairment, cherry red spot).
  - metachromatic leukodystrophy (upper and lower motor neuron signs, high CSF protein).
  - Canavan disease: macrocephaly, leukodystrophy.
- Systemic disease:
  - hypothyroidism.
  - metabolic disorders, e.g. aminoaciduria.
  - electrolyte or glucose disturbance.
  - iatrogenic (drug toxicity, e.g. phenobarbital loading).
  - poisoning.
- Chronic disease of any nature.

Investigation

Suspected peripheral cause

▶ The availability now of treatments for SMA and Pompe where outcomes (particularly for SMA) depend crucially on early recognition; and the need to identify genetically determined muscular dystrophies etc before the birth of further siblings make the assessment of a peripherally weak young infant something of an emergency.

- Creatine kinase (markedly elevated in congenital muscular dystrophies; modestly elevated in Pompe).
- Low threshold for urgent '5q' SMA molecular genetics (typically still offered as a stand-alone test, not part of a panel).
  - Being incorporated into the national newborn screening programmes of an increasing number of countries.
- Nerve conduction studies, EMG.
- Consider muscle biopsy, gene panels.

Suspected central cause

As appropriate:
- Electrolytes including magnesium, calcium. Check glucose.
- Thyroid function (treatable!)
- Brain MRI (ultrasound may be appropriate in the first instance in neonates).
- EEG (may give prognostic information and help exclude seizures).
- aCGH or other selected genetic tests (e.g. trisomy 21, Prader–Willi syndrome).
- TORCH screen.
- Metabolic work-up.

Foot deformities

Causes

Numerous foot deformities are described: some have no neurological basis and can be idiopathic or familial.

- Metatarsus adductus (in-turned forefoot).
- Idiopathic congenital talipes equinovarus (club foot).
- Idiopathic toe-walking (see Toe-walking in this chapter ➲ p. 203).

Some *are* more commonly associated with neurological or other disease.

- *Pes planus ('flat feet')*: connective tissue disorders (Marfan); hereditary motor and sensory neuropathy (HMSN).
- *Pes cavus*: (plantar arch does not flatten on weight-bearing): cord lesion, HMSN, Friedreich ataxia, any neuromuscular condition.
- *Equinus deformity*: cerebral palsy, cord lesion, early Duchenne dystrophy, HMSN, dystonia.
- *Rocker bottom feet* (congenital vertical talus): chromosomal disorders (trisomy 18).

However, almost any neuromuscular condition can be associated with any foot deformity and a thorough neurological examination should be performed for all cases.

History

- New onset?
- Progressive symptoms?
- Ataxia?
- Dysarthria?
- Bladder or bowel involvement?
- Family history?
- Sensory symptoms?
- Functional limitations?

Examination

- Is it correctible?
- Does it fit into a particular type of foot deformity?
  - pes cavus;
  - pes planus;
  - metatarsus adductus;
  - varus or valgus deformity.
- Evidence of weakness?
- Reflexes.
- Spine.
- Wasting or (pseudo-) hypertrophy.
- Nerve hypertrophy.
- Reflexes.
- Weak dorsiflexion and eversion.
- Sensory impairment including saddle area:
  - Joint position and vibration; pain and temperature sensation.

Funny turns (paroxysmal episodes)

Paroxysmal events ('fits, faints, and funny turns') pose a diagnostic challenge as typically you will not witness the episodes, and diagnosis is dependent upon two descriptions: what the event felt like (from an older child, if awareness preserved) and what it looked like to an eyewitness observer. Medical attention is often not sought until the episodes have been independently witnessed, typically by a parent or teacher.

Although epilepsy is often uppermost in the minds of parents and referring physicians, a wide variety of other causes of 'funny turns' are recognized: some are unique to children and infants. False +ve diagnosis of epilepsy remains too common, and once a label is applied it can be difficult to remove.

> **!** Never make a firm diagnosis on the nature of paroxysmal episodes (and specifically never make a diagnosis of epilepsy) before taking a detailed history from an eyewitness. Never rely on 'what the mother says the teacher said she saw'.

Seizures

Epileptic
- An epileptic seizure is a clinical phenomenon associated with an abnormally excessive, synchronous discharge from a group of neurons.
- Clinical manifestations may include paroxysmal changes in motor, sensory, or cognitive function.
- The clinical component depends on the seizure's:
  - location;
  - extent of *generalization* (spread) over the cortex;
  - duration.

In principle, there are very few clinical signs and symptoms that cannot ever result from epileptic seizures, which complicates assessment. Seizures are, however, usually:
- *Stereotyped*: episodes resemble each other. Although a child can have >1 seizure type they are typically a small repertoire, each of which will be consistent.
- *Randomly distributed in time* (i.e. not usually confined to particular situations or contexts). Reflex epilepsies are the one exception to this.

Some movements are more likely to be seizures than others:
- Postures sustained for up to several seconds.
- Sustained head turns to one side, particularly if eyes are turned in the same direction.
- Subtle flickering of perioral and periorbital muscles.
- Shock-like jerks of the limbs, particularly if affecting both sides synchronously.

Conversely some movements are very *atypical* of seizures: this can be particularly relevant in the assessment of non-epileptic attack disorder:
- *Reciprocating* movements (e.g. back-and-forth, to-and-fro movements including side-to-side head movements and *alternating* kicking

movements of the limbs) except in the context of nocturnal frontal lobe epilepsy.
• Prolonged limp unresponsiveness.
• Pelvic thrusting.

The possibility of *sensory* seizures poses particular problems in relation to 'soft' phenomena such as episodic behaviour changes, outbursts of aggression, or reports of fluctuating awareness or concentration. Children with behavioural or developmental concerns are commonly referred with the question 'is any of it epilepsy?' Often the referrer of such children will have ignored the 'nose-picking principle' (see The nose-picking principle in Chapter 2 p. 53) and ordered an EEG showing non-specific abnormalities which have heightened anxiety.

Either of the following make a seizure disorder *less* likely:
• *Context-specificity*
  • For example events occur at home but not at school or *vice versa*, or only in the presence of certain individuals.
• *Content-specificity*
  • There is significant variability in the content of episodes (i.e. they're not stereotyped).
  • The occurrence of the event at that time makes sense: e.g. as an albeit disproportionate reaction to an immediately preceding frustration or irritation.
  • The content of the phenomena reflects context: e.g. the aggressive behaviour being seen relates in some way to what has immediately preceded it.

Event duration can be a helpful consideration. Seizures are typically brief—seconds to a minute or so. Phenomena extending or evolving over tens of minutes are less likely to be ictal: depending on the phenomenology, it may be worth considering a process with a migrainous basis, e.g. a 'migraine equivalent' (see Migraine in Chapter 4 p. 340).

History

How many different types of events are being seen? Give each episode type a 'nickname' (e.g. 'the big shaking ones') and for each:
• *Clarify frequency*. 'How unusual would it be to go a day/week/month without one?'
• Any patterns in terms of characteristic time of day or behavioural states?
• Any relationship to sleep?
• *Triggers*: sleep deprivation, travel, excitement, photic stimuli, exercise.
• Is there any warning? How long?
  • Warnings can be very brief and sometimes inferred, e.g. the child clings to a parent immediately prior to event onset.
  • 'Do you think your child knows one is coming?'
• How long does it last?
• How does it end, and how long does it take for the child to recover fully?
  • People's estimates of time are often inaccurate. Point out how slowly the second hand on the clinic clock actually moves to help them with estimates of duration.

- Is there any colour change? *Pallor at onset* suggests a primary cardiac mechanism due to structural or rhythm problems in an infant or, more commonly, neurocardiogenic syncope or reflex anoxic seizures (see Episodes with altered awareness in Chapter 4 ➋ p. 327).
  - Cyanosis is non-specific as a late feature, but *early cyanosis* suggests a primarily apnoeic mechanism such as occurs in cyanotic breath-holding episodes or gastro-oesophageal reflux.
- What motor phenomena occur? Explore what the words used mean to the witness (see Table 3.7).
  - 'Can you imitate for me now what he does?'
  - Determine any lateralization: which hand shows automatisms, which arm initially extends, which way do the head or eyes turn?
- Is the child's awareness affected by the episode? Older children can usually report whether they retain awareness (e.g. of what others are saying to them) during the episode.
- *Post-ictal symptoms*, behaviour, and impairment. Tiredness and sleep. Confusion, aphasia, or slurred speech. Lateralized or focal weakness. Headache may be associated with epilepsy, sometimes making it hard to distinguish migraine.
- Children are often referred with apparent 'lapses of awareness' for consideration of possible absence epilepsy. The typical scenario—'I have to call his name five times' before a child absorbed in his own thoughts (or computer game) responds—is distinguishable from a spell that actively interrupts a child mid-conversation or mid-mouthful.

▶ Video footage of phenomena can be immensely helpful.

Assessment

Identifying that events tend to occur in specific contexts can be very helpful in the recognition of a wide range of non-epileptic childhood paroxysmal events, many of which are benign normal variants. See Tables 3.5 and 3.6 for detailed descriptions.

Table 5.5 Situational clues to paroxysmal events at different ages

	Infant	Toddler	Child	Adolescent
In sleep	Benign neonatal sleep myoclonus	Night terrors	Parasomnias Confusional arousals	Parasomnias REM sleep disorders (e.g. sleep paralysis) Sleep walking
On feeding	GORD, Sandifer syndrome, shuddering spells	GORD, Sandifer syndrome		
Fever, intercurrent illness	Febrile seizures	Febrile seizures	Syncope	Syncope
Movement		(Kinesigenic) paroxysmal dystonias, dyskinesias	(Kinesigenic) paroxysmal dystonias, dyskinesias	(Kinesigenic) paroxysmal dystonias, dyskinesias
Pain, shock	Structural cardiac or dysrhythmia Reflex anoxic seizure	Structural cardiac or dysrhythmia Cyanotic breath-holding Reflex anoxic seizure	Structural cardiac or dysrhythmia Syncope	Structural cardiac or dysrhythmia Syncope
Hot weather, prolonged standing				Syncope
Tired, bored, meal-times, bed-time	Self-gratification events	Self-gratification events	Daydreaming	Daydreaming
Tired, bored, stressed			Tics	Tics
Excitement, emotion	Shuddering spells			Cataplexy
Boredom		Self-gratification	Stereotypies* Ritualistic behaviour*	Stereotypies* Ritualistic behaviour*
Absorbed in TV, computer game			Distracted	Distracted

*Particularly in children with learning difficulties or autism.

GORD, gastro-oesophageal reflux disease.

Source: data from National Institute for Health and Care Excellence. *The Epilepsies: clinical practice guideline*, 'Appendix A Differential diagnosis of epilepsy in adults and children', https://www.nice.org.uk/guidance/cg137/evidence/appendix-a-18513486, accessed 01 Oct. 2016. Copyright © 2004 NICE.

Table 3.6 Phenotypic clues to non-epileptic and epileptic attacks

	Infant	Toddler	Child	Adolescent
Rapidly repeating spasms	Infantile spasms Benign myoclonus of infancy Clonic seizure	Clonic seizure Focal seizure	Tics Behavioural stereotypy* Clonic seizure	Focal seizure tics Behavioural stereotypy* Clonic seizure
Stiffness	Tonic seizure¶ Coning† Hyperekplexia	Tonic seizure¶ Coning† Hyperekplexia	Tonic seizure¶ Coning† Hyperekplexia	Tonic seizure¶ Coning† Hyperekplexia
Loss of tone	Cardiac dysrhythmia	Reflex anoxic seizure Atonic seizures§	Syncope Atonic seizures§	Syncope Cataplexy
Sustained distorted posture	Benign paroxysmal torticollis	(Kinesigenic) paroxysmal dystonias, dyskinesias Drug reactions ICP elevations	(Kinesigenic) paroxysmal dystonias, dyskinesias Drug reactions ICP elevations	(Kinesigenic) paroxysmal dystonias, dyskinesias Drug reactions ICP elevations
Unsteadiness		Benign paroxysmal vertigo	Episodic ataxia Intoxication	Episodic ataxia Intoxication

* Particularly in children with learning difficulties.

¶ Tonic seizures can arise from acute cerebral hypoxia (e.g. reflex anoxic seizures, syncope).

† See Examine for signs of herniation in Chapter 6 ⊙ p. 614

§ Rarely the only seizure type present: typically in combination with other seizure types in Lennox–Gastaut syndrome or myoclonic-atonic epilepsy

Source: data from National Institute for Health and Care Excellence. The Epilepsies: clinical practice guideline, 'Appendix A Differential diagnosis of epilepsy in adults and children', https://www.nice.org.uk/guidance/cg137/evidence/appendix-a-185134863, accessed 01 Oct. 2016, Copyright © 2004 NICE.

Funny turns: likely epilepsy?

Consequences of both false-*positive* (regarding a non-epileptic phenomenon as epilepsy) and false-*negative* (failing to recognize epilepsy) diagnoses can be serious. However, the risks of false +ve diagnosis are almost certainly higher.

- In cases of genuine uncertainty, it is important to be comfortable regarding a diagnosis of epilepsy as 'unestablished'. Families must be helped to understand the importance of avoiding premature conclusions.
- Diagnosing epilepsy is hard! Even in specialist centres false +ve diagnosis rates have been estimated at 10 15%.
- It is a question that must be answered clinically, with recourse to EEG only for supportive evidence (see Potential pitfalls of using an EEG in Chapter 2 🠒 p. 87).

▶ Epilepsy is a tendency to recurrent, *unprovoked* (spontaneous) seizures, so even if you are sure the events are seizures, this may well still not be epilepsy.

- Deciding whether events are *recurrent* is usually fairly straightforward, although it is important to be sure that all 'recurrences' are of the same nature, i.e. the events are stereotyped.
- Deciding whether seizures are *unprovoked* is a vital consideration.

Epilepsy versus acute symptomatic seizures

- Acute symptomatic seizures arise as the immediate result of a variety of acute insults: hypoxia–ischaemia, hypoglycaemia, hypocalcaemia, metabolic derangements, infection, trauma, etc.
- Acute symptomatic seizures can also be recurrent, the most common example being recurrent febrile seizures. The diagnosis then is recurrent acute symptomatic seizures (of a cause to be identified), but not epilepsy.

Common non-epilepsy scenarios
- The toddler experiencing reflex anoxic seizures (see Reflex anoxic seizures in Chapter 4 🠒 p. 330) having caught a finger in a slamming door.
- The adolescent girl brought into the Emergency Room having passed out on a hot day at school.
- If there is a clear history of a trigger, *do not* get distracted into diagnosing epilepsy by the history of jerky limb movements and urinary incontinence at the *end* of the event.

▶ The details of the earliest stages of the episode—its context, premonitory symptoms, presence of pallor, etc.—are much more useful than late characteristics. It is much more useful to know how the event started than how it ended. (Unfortunately, the onset of the episode is also the phase least likely to have been observed.)

Although the generally unprovoked, spontaneous nature of epileptic seizures is emphasized to distinguish them from recurrent acute symptomatic seizures, there *are* of course well-described examples of true *reflex epilepsies*: photosensitivity to rapidly flickering light is the most common but rare reading epilepsies, epilepsies triggered by particular pieces of music or on immersion in water, etc., are recognized.

These latter are extraordinarily uncommon and in practice pose little diagnostic difficulty as one can arrange to perform EEG while exposing the child to the stimulus (seizures typically occur immediately). Photosensitivity is usually routinely sought in EEG studies.

▶ Of children with paroxysmal events in whom the initial diagnosis of epilepsy is tentative, fewer than 10% will ultimately prove to have epilepsy.
▶ The co-existence of multiple types of paroxysmal event (e.g. epilepsy and syncope; epilepsy and non-epileptic attacks) in one child is relatively common.

There is no such thing as epilepsy ...

... There are epilep*ses*.

Adopt a level approach to the diagnosis of epilepsy:
- *Disease* (*is* this epilepsy?)
- What *seizure types* are occurring?
- What is the *epilepsy type*?
- What is the epilepsy *syndrome*?

These questions correspond to the multilevel approach of the current ILAE epilepsy classification scheme. This enables rational decisions about the need for further investigation (e.g. imaging), guides therapy choices, and informs prognosis. The importance of searching for aetiology is emphasized at each step. Comorbidities, such as adverse social and educational effects should be monitored and appropriately managed (see Epilepsy and daily life in Chapter 4 ⊃ p. 317).

Aetiology and syndrome are discussed further in Chapter 4 (see Epilepsy ⊃ p. 273), but both require the identification of the seizure types present.

The role of EEG

Epilepsy novices overuse EEG in addressing the first question ('is this epilepsy?'), and underuse it in the remaining challenges of identifying seizure type(s), aetiology, and syndrome. Routine EEGs are of limited value in deciding whether an individual has epilepsy, with significant false –ve (sensitivity of first routine EEG ~60%) and more problematically false +ve rates (paroxysmal activity seen in >30%, and frankly epileptiform in ~5% of normal children). False +ve rates are even higher in children with a cerebral palsy, etc.

What seizure types are occurring?

As with deciding if events are indeed seizures, defining what seizure type(s) is/are occurring can be challenging. Family usage of terms such as 'jerk', 'shake', and 'fall' need to be understood fully, before they can be accurately 'mapped' onto conventional seizure descriptors (Table 3.7).

Table 3.7 Types of seizures

Jerk, shake	*Clonic* (rhythmic contractions followed by slightly slower relaxation) typically occurring immediately after a tonic phase as part of a tonic–clonic seizure, or confined to a body part as a focal seizure.
	Myoclonic seizures are isolated lightning-fast, brief contractions (positive myoclonus) or relaxations (negative myoclonus) of a muscle or a muscle group, occurring singly or in short runs, with full muscle relaxation between.
	Epileptic spasms have a slightly longer phase of sustained contraction than a myoclonic jerk and typically occur in runs. They occur as part of the infantile epileptic spasms syndrome but also in older children.
	Distinguishing these seizure types may be challenging clinically, and is a particularly important role for EEG.
Stiff	Usually a *tonic* seizure (sustained contraction for several seconds). There may be a low amplitude 'vibratory' (not tremulous) element to the contraction that is different from a clonic movement.
Fall	The term 'drop attack' is ambiguous.
	Atonic seizures result in a slump to the ground 'like a puppet having had its strings cut'.
	A *tonic* seizure resulting in rigidity can cause a child to fall 'like a felled tree'.
	Finally a child can be thrown to the ground by a large *myoclonic* seizure.
	In some seizures these are combined, as in myoclonic-atonic (previously known as myoclonic-astatic) seizures.
	Many centres now use surface EMG alongside EEG in order to determine whether, and for how long, there is muscle contraction associated with a seizure. This helps to distinguish tonic, atonic, and myoclonic events.
Vacancy	The word 'absence' creates a lot of confusion and diagnostic imprecision. An absence is a type of seizure *defined by its EEG features* that can cause loss of awareness, but loss of awareness can occur with *focal seizures with impaired awareness*.
	Most absence seizures are brief, lasting only a few seconds, but they may occur many times per day. They are often associated with subtle motor automatisms: lip smacking, chewing, or fiddling with the hands. Eyelid flickering may occur.
	Focal seizures with impaired awareness (e.g. originating from the temporal lobe) may be associated with loss of awareness and responsiveness to surroundings. They would typically be longer (30 seconds or more) and less frequent than absences and with more marked confusion or agitation. Again EEG can make a valuable contribution to distinguishing these two seizure types.

The child 'with generalized tonic–clonic seizures'

'GTC' tends to be used as a lazy shorthand in clinical records. It is important to define precisely what seizure types are occurring and detailed eyewitness accounts of the earliest phases of a seizure are invaluable if available.

It is *relatively rare* for a child to have an epilepsy defined by true GTCs alone.

- *Either*, they have GTCs together with other (possibly as yet unrecognized) seizures, e.g. in juvenile myoclonic epilepsy (see Chapter 4 ⊃ p. 288).
- *Or* they are experiencing focal to bilateral tonic–clonic seizures (e.g. in self-limited epilepsy with centrotemporal spikes; see Chapter 4 ⊃ p. 282).

Gait abnormalities

For acute presentations see The child who suddenly stops walking in Chapter 6 ⊃ p. 636.

History

- Nature of the problem?
- Onset?
- Static or progressive?
- Isolated or associated with other symptoms of delay?
- Constant or intermittent?
- Degree of functional impairment—what does it stop him doing?
- Exercise intolerance, stiffness, or pain?
- Vestibular symptoms?
- Involvement of bladder or spine?
- Family history of any form of abnormal walk or use of assistive devices?
- *Symptoms suggestive of proximal weakness*: difficulties raising head from pillow, combing hair, brushing teeth, shaving, raising arms above head, getting up from chair, stairs, and use of banisters, running, hopping, jumping.
- *Symptoms suggestive of peripheral weakness*: difficulties opening bottle caps or doorknob, turning key, buttoning clothes, writing, falling on uneven ground, tripping, hitting kerb.

Examination

- Give the child space to move.
- Observe posture and quality of movement of the upper limbs while the child is playing as well as during formal examination of the lower limbs.
- Look for asymmetry—mild hemiplegia?
- Perform a detailed neurological examination with movement to bring out the abnormality. These include walking forwards and backwards, running, jumping, hopping, timed stand on one leg, tandem walking, Fog's test (see Fog's test in Chapter 1 ⊃ p. 47).
- Gowers' manoeuvre (see Gowers' manoeuvre and sign in Chapter 1 ⊃ p. 39).
- Range of movement of hips, knees, and ankles.
- Tone, power, coordination, reflexes (including abdominal, sacral), sensory, joint position, touch, pain, and temperature, Rombergism.
- Check the spine.
- If foot deformity is present, examine the parents' feet.
- See later sections for more specific testing in different conditions.

Assessment

Consider the walking pattern in light of findings identified on static examination (e.g. that there is limited range of movement around a particular joint, or that a particular muscle group is weak) (see also Posture and gait in Chapter 1 ⊃ p. 37).

Is the gait antalgic?

The defining feature of an antalgic gait is that one foot spends less time on the ground than the other (i.e. the child is trying to limit weight-bearing on that leg because it is painful). An antalgic gait reflects painful orthopaedic or rheumatological disease: discuss with appropriate colleagues for further assessment.

Does the gait reflect other non-neurological pathology?
Other patterns of abnormal walking that can indicate non-neurological, bio-mechanical processes include:
- Circumducting gait:
  - typically reflects leg-length discrepancy (the circumducting leg is the longer one, although not necessarily the abnormal limb—it could be that the other is pathologically short);
  - can arise as a result of asymmetric pyramidal signs due to a foot held in plantarflexion.
- Steppage gait:
  - high-stepping gait;
  - can reflect difficulties achieving foot clearance on 'swing through' (c.f. circumducting gait);
  - high-stepping 'stamping' gait can reflect impaired proprioception;
  - can be symmetrical or asymmetrical.
- Trendelenburg gait:
  - The pelvis drops as the child enters 'stance phase', taking full body weight on one leg, because hip abductors on that side are unable to support the off-axis weight of the body.
  - Reflects hip abductor weakness either due to muscle disease (in which case usually bilateral and fairly symmetrical) or biomechanical factors.
- Equinus gait:
  - similar to steppage gait.

Further considerations
Consider the pattern of foot placement (i.e. the footprints the child would be leaving if walking on sand). Consider also wear patterns on the sole of the shoes.
- Abnormally wide-based? Consider ataxia.
- Abnormally narrowly-based? Consider spastic diplegia.
- Asymmetry of stride length? Interpret in light of static neurological findings, e.g. of limited joint range of movement.

Does the gait fit into a classic pattern?
See Posture and gait in Chapter 1 p. 37.
- *Long tract signs*: CP, leukodystrophy (X-ALD, MLD), tethered cord, hereditary spastic paraparesis.
- *Long tract signs and a root level*: occult spinal dysraphism or other pathology, transverse myelitis.
- *Cerebellar signs*: posterior fossa tumour, ataxia telangiectasia (AT), Friedreich ataxia.
- *Vestibular symptoms*: vestibulitis, benign paroxysmal vertigo.
- *Clumsiness also affecting other areas of motor coordination* (but without ataxia): dyspraxia.
- *Intercurrent illness or acute onset*: Guillain–Barré, CIDP.

- *Toe-walking alone*: idiopathic toe walker (see Toe-walking in this chapter ➲ p. 203).
  - toe-walking and other symptoms and signs: DMD, cord lesion.
- *Family history*, delayed motor development, proximal weakness: DMD, SMA.
- *Foot deformity*: club feet, CP, Friedreich.
- *Abnormal foot posture*: dystonia (e.g. DYT1-TOR1A).
- Family history (variable severity), symmetrical distal involvement, weak dorsiflexion and eversion, pes cavus, absent reflexes, nerve hypertrophy: HMSN.

A non-specific unusual gait is sometimes seen in children with a significant learning disability but without a specific diagnosis.

▶ Consider a functional gait disturbance when the features do not fit a recognized anatomical distribution but beware that functional and non-functional disorders may co-exist (e.g. astasia-abasia; see Gait and stance in Chapter 4 ➲ p. 336).

Investigate as indicated by differential diagnosis.

Head shape abnormalities

This is a common clinical scenario. The vast majority can be reassured. Head shape is determined by forces from within and outside the skull and by the timing of closure of cranial sutures (Fig. 3.2 and Table 3.8).

Intracranial forces affecting head shape

- Cerebellar agenesis causes a small posterior fossa.
- Large lateral ventricles cause bowing of the forehead.
- Dandy–Walker malformation causes bowing of the occiput.

Extracranial forces affecting head shape

- Constriction due to multiple pregnancy or bicornuate uterus.
- Scaphocephaly in premature babies; brachy- or plagiocephaly in hypotonic infants (effect of relative immobility).

▶ Benign positional posterior plagiocephaly is much more common following widespread introduction of supine sleeping for children to reduce risks of sudden infant death.

Craniosynostosis

- Results from premature closure of one or more cranial sutures.
- Isolated, or associated with other disorders, e.g ataxia telangiectasia, hyperthyroidism, mucopolysaccharidoses, rickets, sickle cell disease, thalassaemia major.
- Two-suture craniosynostosis is common (usually sagittal plus one other).

The hallmark clinically is *progressive* skull deformity. Plain SXR with Waters projection is a useful screening test but is unreliable particularly for lambdoid sutures. Spiral 3D CT is the definitive investigation but involves a high radiation dose. If confirmed, refer to specialist neurosurgical unit.

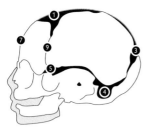 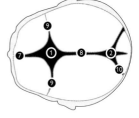

❶ Anterior fontanelle	❼ Metopic suture
❷ Posterior fontanelle	❽ Sagittal suture
❸ Occipital fontanelle	❾ Coronal suture
❹ Mastoid fontanelle	❿ Lambdoid suture
❺ Sphenoid fontanelle	

Fig. 3.2 Sutures and fontanelles.

Table 3.8 Description of head shape (sutures which may cause the shape with early fusion shown in parentheses)

Brachycephaly (both coronal)	Head abnormally wide and flat over occiput
Scaphocephaly/dolichocephaly (sagittal)	Abnormally long, narrow head
Plagiocephaly (one coronal or lambdoid)	Flattening on one side of head
Oxycephaly (all)	Pointed head
Turricephaly (also known as acrocephaly: coronal + others)	High, tower-like head with vertical forehead
Trigonocephaly (metopic)	Triangular head with prominent vertical ridge in mid-forehead

Specific syndromes with craniosynostosis as a feature
- *Crouzon syndrome*: autosomal dominant. Premature closure of any or all sutures plus maldevelopment of facial bones. Characteristic facies. Prominent eyes, beak nose, large tongue. May have intellectual disability.
- *Apert syndrome*: autosomal dominant. Premature closure of coronal sutures, syndactyly, and fusion of fingers and toes. Face deformity similar to Crouzon disease but less severe. May have cerebral malformations and intellectual disability.
- *Carpenter syndrome*: autosomal recessive. Resembles Apert, with additional polydactyly and hypogonadism. May have cerebral malformations and intellectual disability.

Syndromes with recognizable abnormal head shape
- Pear-or light bulb-shaped head: Zellweger syndrome.
- Narrow bifrontal diameter: sulphite oxidase deficiency, molybdenum cofactor deficiency.
- Brachycephaly: Down syndrome.

Large fontanelle
Closure of the anterior fontanelle is complete by 24 months in 96% babies.

Commoner causes of large fontanelle/delayed closure
- Intrauterine growth retardation.
- Prematurity.
- Hydrocephalus.
- Achondroplasia.
- Down syndrome.

Rarer causes
- Hypothyroidism.
- Rickets.
- Osteogenesis imperfecta.
- Congenital rubella.
- Apert syndrome.
- Cleidocranial dysostosis.
- Ring chromosome 20 syndrome.
- Zellweger syndrome.

Head size abnormalities

A common clinical scenario. Consider the child's birth, past medical and family history as well as development, and assess any features of regression. First and foremost measure both parents' heads if possible. Plot current and previous measurements on an appropriate chart (correct for age and sex). Many 'macrocephalic' and 'microcephalic' children are simply (familial) outliers of the normal population.

Large head: >2 standard deviations SDs above mean for age

A large head will be due to either a large brain, a large volume of CSF, or (very rarely) abnormally thick skull vault. Consider whether signs of ↑ ICP present:

- History of headaches or irritability, particularly a steadily worsening picture over weeks.
- Sunset eye sign.
- Full fontanelle, separation of the cranial sutures.
- Presence of venous pulsation on fundoscopy (see Fig. 1.4 in Chapter 1 ➋ p. 18) implies normal ICP; however it is absent in 10% of the normal population!
- Papilloedema is a late and variable feature of ↑ ICP.
- Prominent scalp veins.

If no signs of raised intracranial pressure

- *Familial*: very common. Measure both parents' occipitofrontal circumference (OFC). Note that the OFC of children with familial macrocephaly can rise across centiles during the early months of life. Often associated with benign enlargement of subarachnoid space (see Fig. 3.3 in this chapter ➋ p. 163).
- *Neurocutaneous disorders*: neurofibromatosis type 1, tuberous sclerosis, incontinentia pigmenti.
- *Chromosomal*: fragile X syndrome.
- Cerebral gigantism (Sotos syndrome).
- Achondroplasia.
- Metabolic disorders (the large head is usually *acquired*):
  - mucopolysaccharidoses;
  - glutaric aciduria type 1. Characteristic symmetrical fronto-temporal atrophy with enlarged subarachnoid spaces that may radiologically give appearances confused with non-accidental injury;
  - galactosaemia;
  - leukodystrophies: metachromatic, Canavan or Alexander disease;
  - maple syrup urine disease;
  - storage disorders, especially GM2 gangliosidoses (Tay–Sachs, Sandhoff).
- Undiagnosed neurological disorder: a large head in a child with developmental impairment ± seizures. This is a common clinical scenario although newer genetic techniques are increasing diagnostic yield.
- Due to thickened skull: thalassaemia, osteopetrosis, side-effect of some ASMs.

Benign enlargement of the subarachnoid space
See Figure 3.3.
- Common and often familial.
- Large subarachnoid spaces—especially frontal spaces—normalize by school age although macrocephaly persists.
- Mainstay of management is reassurance and non-intervention.
- In extreme cases there may be a danger of subdural haemorrhage from minor trauma due to 'instability' of the brain in the skull vault.

Chronic subdural effusion
Subdural haemorrhage *due to birth trauma* invariably resolves by 4 weeks. Subdural haemorrhage detected at a later age raises the possibility of inflicted injury or CNS infection.
  If raised intracranial pressure present, consider hydrocephalus due to:
- Post-intraventricular haemorrhage.
- Posterior fossa tumour.
- Aqueduct stenosis (may be X-linked).
- Post-CNS infection.
- Dandy–Walker malformation.
- Klippel–Feil syndrome (dysmorphic with low hairline, short neck, limitation of neck movement).
- Vein of Galen malformation.
- Walker–Warburg syndrome (cerebro-ocular dysplasia).
- Chiari malformation (may be associated with spina bifida).

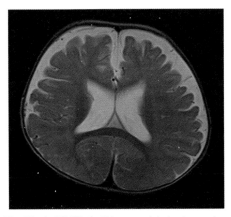

Fig. 3.3 T2 weighted axial MRI in familial macrocephaly showing prominent external subarachnoid spaces particularly in fronto-temporal regions. Note that this can be erroneously reported as 'frontal atrophy' but OFC is large not small; or as 'showing benign external hydrocephalus' but there is no raised pressure! The bridging veins clearly visible in the CSF spaces on this T2 image confirm that it is the subarachnoid space that is enlarged, and permits distinction from enlarged subdural spaces (see below).

Small head <2 SD below mean for age

Indicates a small brain. Development is usually impaired.

Radiologically normal-but-small brain on MRI

Primary microcephaly

If the head has *always been small* (i.e. OFC small at birth) consider:

- Primary genetic microcephalies (autosomal recessive or dominant).
- Chromosomal disorders: aneuploidy of any chromosome, Miller–Dieker syndrome, ring chromosome 20.
- Systemic disease: chronic renal or cardiac disease, malnutrition.
- Undiagnosed neurological disorder: a small head in a child with developmental impairment ± seizures. Investigations are normal. This is a common clinical scenario.

Secondary microcephaly

If microcephaly is of postnatal origin (i.e. birth OFC was normal) consider in addition to the above list:

- Any postnatally acquired cerebral insult (usually clear from history).
- Rett syndrome (girls) and Rett 'mimics' (e.g. *CDKL5*, *FOXG1*, *MEF2C*).
- Angelman syndrome.
- PEHO syndrome.
- GLUT1 deficiency syndrome.
- Sulphite oxidase deficiency; molybdenum cofactor deficiency.

Radiologically abnormal brain

- Anencephaly, encephalocoele, agenesis of corpus callosum, holoprosencephaly, defective cellular migration: lissencephaly, agyria, pachygyria, heterotopia.
- Intrauterine infection: toxoplasmosis, rubella, cytomegalovirus, herpes simplex (TORCH), HIV.
- Perinatal brain injury: HIE, intracranial haemorrhage, CNS infection.
- Toxins: foetal alcohol syndrome, maternal drug ingestion, maternal IDDM, maternal PKU.
- Metabolic disorders: infantile and late infantile neuronal ceroid lipofuscinosis (NCL), Smith–Lemli–Opitz syndrome, tetrahydrobiopterin deficiencies, congenital disorders of glycosylation.

Headache

Headache is common in children and occurs at least annually in approximately 40% of children by 7 yrs of age and 50% of children by 15 yrs.

▶ Most parents who seek help for a child with headache are looking for reassurance that the headache is not due to a serious cause.

The brain itself, most of the meninges, and the skull are not pain sensitive. Pain from supratentorial structures is referred to the front of the head. Pain from posterior fossa structures is referred to the back of head and neck in addition to the forehead. The glossopharyngeal and vagal nerves innervate part of the posterior fossa and pain is referred to the ear and throat. Pain referred to the head can arise from:

- Intracranial or extracranial arteries, large intracranial veins, or venous sinuses.
- Cranial or spinal nerves.
- Basal meninges.
- Cranial and cervical muscles.
- Nasal cavity, sinuses, teeth, mucous membranes, skin, and subcutaneous tissues.

Clinical evaluation

Attempt to characterize the headaches as one of:

- Isolated acute.
- Recurrent acute.
- Chronic non-progressive.
- Chronic progressive.

First (isolated) acute headache

Although a first acute headache may be the initial presentation of a primary headache such as migraine, it is important to consider other possible causes.

- Spontaneous subarachnoid or intracerebral haemorrhage and acute onset hydrocephalus are rare but require immediate management.
- Cranial trauma, meningitis, sinusitis, and dental abscess also require specific treatment but are usually accompanied by other clinical pointers.
- Headache may occasionally be the initial manifestation of hypertension and *blood pressure must be measured*.
- In adolescents, a history of headache related to athletic or other exertion is common and usually benign.
- The most common causes of first isolated headache in routine practice are viral illness, sinusitis, and the primary headaches (see Headache disorders in Chapter 4 ➷ p. 340) of which migraine and tension-type headache are by far the commonest.

Recurrent or chronic headaches

History
- More than one kind of headache? A mixed picture may imply mixed aetiology.
- Describe a typical episode:
  - Any warning?
  - Where does it hurt?
  - What is pain like? (Children, like adults, will find it very hard to describe subtleties of pain type: you may have to ask leading questions: 'is it thumping/crushing/squeezing?')
  - Associated symptoms?
  - Duration?
  - Frequency?
  - Relieving or exacerbating factors?
  - Severity? Prevents activity? Causing school absenteeism?

Refer to Figure 3.4:
  In the context of headache, time-course A might suggest an acute brain pathology such as subarachnoid haemorrhage; B (inexorable progression) would raise important concerns about possible ↑ intracranial pressure; C, with clear symptom-free periods is typical of migraine and other primary headaches; and D, with no symptom-free intervals is typical of chronic daily headache ± analgesia overuse.
- Establishing which of the patterns you are seeing is usually fairly straightforward, particularly over time.
- Distinguishing B and D can be harder when the history is short but in B the key is a chronic progressive picture worsening over days to weeks.

The diagnosis of headache aetiology is *clinical*. The indications for investigation follow from a clinical assessment of the diagnosis.

Pointers to raised intracranial pressure headache
Establishing whether this is a concerning presentation or not is the priority: for you and, of course, the family.

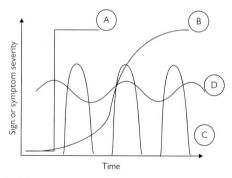

Fig. 3.4 Headache symptom time-courses.

- Aggravation by manoeuvres that raise intracranial pressure.
  - Lying flat, bending, coughing, sneezing, straining at stool.
- Woken from sleep by headache?
  - Physiologic ↑ in intracranial pressure in sleep may result in a child being woken from sleep with a headache, a worrying symptom.
  - It is important to distinguish between those that wake the child out of sleep from those that are noticed after the child has woken normally.
- Recent deterioration in behaviour or school performance.
- See also Primary Headaches/Clinical approach in Chapter 4 ➲ p. 340.

Pointers to a primary headache (migraine, tension-type headache, or mixed)
- Episodicity with clear symptom-free periods.
- Aggravated by bright light or noise?
- Helped by sleep? Resting in dark/quiet?
- Family history of migraine?
  - This may need a little probing: parents may attribute their headaches to other causes such as 'sinusitis'.
  - Additionally their tendency to recurrent headache may have settled with time: did they have headaches when they were younger?

Migraine episodes characteristically show:
- Pain usually asymmetrical, but in younger children can be bilateral.
- Throbbing or pulsatile character.
- Associated autonomic features:
  - abdominal pain, nausea, or vomiting;
  - vasomotor changes: facial pallor and/or 'dark rings under the eyes'? 'Can you tell your child has a headache just by the way they look?'
- Personal or family history of motion sickness.
- Photophobia and/or phonophobia (rarely, osmophobia).
- Association with lack of sleep, menstrual cycle, exertion, school pressure?
  - The importance of dietary triggers is over-emphasized in children. Academic stress is a more important factor than particular foods. Do not condemn children to chocolate or cheese-free lives! Headache susceptibility alters with time (so a trigger may not be a trigger for ever).
- Visual features are characteristic of *migraine with aura* although this is a small minority (perhaps 10%) of all migraine presentations.
  - Visual symptoms are usually +ve, with *added* shimmering, sparkling, and/or coloured distortions.
- Other focal neurological signs and symptoms (e.g. paraesthesia, weakness) can rarely occur before, during, or after the headache phase. Such features tend to be recurrent and stereotyped: it is easier to be relaxed about them after the second or third presentation. At first presentation they are a diagnosis of exclusion and unless there is a very strong family history, e.g. of hemiplegic migraine, MRI will be required.

Tension-type headache is characteristically:
- Diffuse, symmetrical.
- 'Band like' distribution around the head.
- Present most of the time, but there may be symptom-free periods.
- A constant ache, though there may be a partially throbbing character.

Distinction between muscular contraction headache, and migraine without aura is often difficult and it is important to recognize that a mixed migraine/tension headache is very common. The process is often further complicated and perpetuated by analgesia overuse.

Pointers to analgesia overuse headache
Family 'clock-watching', anxious to give the next dose as soon as they can. Can occur with any analgesic including paracetamol and NSAIDs. It is a particular problem with compound analgesics combining paracetamol and codeine which in some countries are available over the counter.

Examination
Neurological examination can be confined to movement patterns and cranial nerves if there are no sensory symptoms.
- Growth parameters, head circumference, and blood pressure.
- Sinuses and teeth.
- Fundoscopy and retinal venous pulsation (see Venous pulsation in Chapter 1 ⤳ p. 18).
  - Confirmation of venous pulsation can be extremely helpful as at unambiguously confirms normal intracranial pressure: however it is absent in 10% normal population.
  - Absence of papilloedema does not exclude ↑ intracranial pressure!
- Visual fields (craniopharyngioma).
- Cranial bruits. Asymmetric 'machinery' bruit may indicate arteriovenous malformation:
  - Innocent cranial bruits are heard in approximately 50% of 5-yr-old and 10% of 10-yr-old normal children.
  - Asymmetry or elimination by compression of the ipsilateral carotid artery is significant.
- Cognitive and emotional status, particularly attitude of child (and family) toward the symptoms, and interaction between family members.

Investigations
- If the history is typical for a 1° headache (migraine, tension-type, or mixed–which is common), and the neurological examination is normal, no imaging is required.
- Occasional families cannot 'move on' without demonstration of a normal MRI but more commonly investigation may undermine the reassurance you are trying to convey.
- If the differential diagnosis includes ↑ intracranial pressure headache, an urgent CT scan will demonstrate nearly all structural causes of headache. MRI may occasionally be necessary for the diagnosis of subtle vascular abnormalities or hypothalamo-pituitary lesions.
- Check blood pressure. A headache due to ↑ intracranial pressure headache may be the only symptom of systemic hypertension.

Hearing loss

- *Conductive*: middle ear. Very common. Typically a high frequency loss selectively affecting discrimination of consonants and intelligibility of speech.
- *Sensorineural*: cochlea, nerve, or brain (incidence approximately 1/1000). Cochlear hearing loss pattern characterized by *recruitment*: a rapid ↑ in sensation of loudness once the hearing threshold is passed.
- Hearing loss in the better ear:
  - <20 dB: normal;
  - 20–40 dB: mild;
  - 40–70 dB: moderate;
  - 70–95 dB: severe;
  - >95 dB: profound.

Causes

See Table 3.9.

Consequences

- *Unilateral hearing loss*. Poor sound localization, difficulties in noisy environments.
- *Bilateral hearing loss*:
  - up to 50 dB: delayed language development;
  - >70 dB: no spontaneous language development;
  - delays in reading and writing skills;
  - delayed psychosocial development;
  - otherwise normal cognition.

History

- Pregnancy, delivery (illnesses, infections).
- Neonatal intensive care: infections, antibiotics (gentamicin), significant jaundice.
- Family history: congenital deafness, consanguinity.
- Development. Important early language/communication milestones:
  - *before 2 months*: startle to sudden loud noise; interest in prolonged noises;
  - *2–6 months*: listen and turn to voice; interest in noises (radio, food being prepared, parent entering room);

Table 3.9 Causes of hearing loss

Congenital	Genetic hearing loss (syndromic or isolated)
	Sporadic
	Malformations of the inner or middle ear
	Intrauterine infections (CMV, Rubella)
Acquired	Prematurity, HIE, BIND (kernicterus)
	Meningitis
	Ototoxic drugs (gentamicin)
	Middle ear disease
	Trauma (especially fracture involving petrous temporal bone)

- *7–12 months*: look toward quiet sounds; talk/babble to parent; say 'ma', 'ba', 'da'; start to understand own name, 'no', 'bye';
- *Second year*: understand simple words and instructions without accompanying gestures; start to use some words.
- Past history of meningitis, head injury.
- Epilepsy:
  - Children with Landau–Kleffner syndrome (see Landau–Kleffner syndrome in Chapter 4 ➲ p. 287) present with a receptive auditory agnosia: they can no longer 'make sense' of sounds, particularly speech. Although not truly hearing impaired, they are often described as behaving 'as if deaf'.
  - By definition, Landau–Kleffner syndrome includes concurrent seizures, although these can lag the onset of the auditory agnosia by a few weeks.

Examination
- Dysmorphism.
- Ear abnormalities (Treacher–Collins, Goldenhaar syndrome).
- Eye disease (Usher, Alstrom, Refsum, Cockayne syndrome).
- Skeletal abnormality (Klippel–Feil, Crouzon, DIDMOAD syndromes).
- Skin nail or hair disorder (Waardenburg syndrome).
- Development and neurology.
- Full ear, nose, and throat examination.

Primary investigations
- Audiogram.
- Audiogram of first-degree relatives.
- ECG (long QTc interval in Jervel–Lange–Nielsen).
- Ophthalmology:
  - for the presence of other diagnostic clues such as retinal pigmentation;
  - for correction of refractive errors to prevent double sensory impairment.
- Urine (microscopic haematuria in Alport syndrome).
- Connexin 26 mutation (common cause of recessive, non-syndromic deafness).
- MRI: visualization of cochlea and internal auditory meati.

Further investigations as indicated
- TORCH screen (CMV, rubella).
- FBC.
- U&E.
- TFT (hypothyroidism in Pendred syndrome).
- Immunology.
- Metabolic: especially mitochondrial and peroxisomal disease.
- Renal USS.
- Chromosomes/array CGH.
- Genetics referral.
- Vestibular investigations/ERG (Usher syndrome).

Refer for assessment if:
- Failed hearing screen.
- Parental worry about hearing.
- Note the child looking for visual clues.

Incontinence

History

- Onset and progression.
- Bladder: retention, frequency, hesitancy, urgency, straining, urge incontinence, pain on urination, abdominal discomfort.
- Bowel: constipation, stool incontinence, abdominal discomfort.
- Sexual: erectile function.

Examination

- Lower limbs: gait, deformities (talipes).
- Perineum: sensation particularly in S2–4 dermatomes (see Fig. 1.7 in Chapter 1 ➔ p. 28), anal tone, anocutaneous reflex, cremasteric reflex. S2–4 function (perianal sensation, anocutaneous reflex) will be absent in conus lesions.
- Spine: tuft of hair, subcutaneous lipoma, dermal sinus, scoliosis.
- Abdomen: palpable bladder, constipation, other abdominal masses (e.g. very rare anterior neural tube defects).
- Micturition: good stream? Leakage when crying? Can 'stop-start' at will?

Investigations

- X-ray spine: spinal deformity (dysraphism, scoliosis).
- MRI spine (dysraphism, low-lying conus medullaris in tethered cord, cord compression, transverse myelitis).
- Urinary tract USS (dilated ureters and pelvic system).
- DMSA (renal cortical scintigraphy; scarring).
- Renal function.
- Video-urodynamic study (pressure/volume study of bladder).
- Cystourethrogram (shape, size, and capacity of bladder, residual urine volume, vesico-ureteric reflux).
- See Table 3.10 for urinary signs and symptoms.

Table 3.10 Urinary signs and symptoms in specific conditions

Neuropathic bladder	Constant severe daytime wetting, constipation, lower limb neurological signs
	Spinal dysraphism (spina bifida, tethered cord)
	Cord compression (discitis, spinal osteomyelitis, trauma, tumour, bleed, etc.)
	Transverse myelitis
Urinary tract infection	Secondary onset wetting, systemic features
Constipation	Secondary urinary problems
Detrusor instability	Daytime urinary frequency, urgency, and urge incontinence
Ectopic ureter	Constant dribble of urine between voidings
Posterior urethral valves	Poor urinary stream, daytime wetting, palpable bladder

(Continued)

Table 3.10 (*Contd.*)

Diabetes mellitus	Weight loss, polyuria, thirst, and polydipsia
Diabetes insipidus	Polyuria, polydipsia, thirst
Emotional and behavioural problems	Secondary onset wetting

For management of continence problems (see Continence in Chapter 4 p. 263).

Movement abnormalities

Motor disorders are central nervous system disorders characterized by abnormalities of posture, movement, tone, and/or power. Within these, the *movement disorders* are disorders in which there is either an *excess of involuntary movement*, or a *paucity* of either voluntary or automatic movement.

Terminology:
- *Hyperkinesia:* excessive involuntary movements,
- *Dyskinesia:* abnormal involuntary movements,
- *Hypokinesia:* poverty and ↓ amplitude of movement,
- *Bradykinesia:* slowness of movements,
- *Akinesia:* loss of movement.

Key features of movement disorders:
- Generally *disappear with sleep* and do not affect consciousness directly (c.f. seizures).
- Traditionally considered *disorders of the basal ganglia* although the involvement of a more distributed motor network is increasingly recognized.
- May arise because of primary (genetic) disorders of neurotransmission or other aspects of motor network function; or as secondary consequences of acquired damage to the motor network.
- By definition movements due to epileptic discharges are excluded, but there can be considerable overlap between epilepsy and movement disorders.

Abnormalities of the *quality* of voluntary movement are usually considered distinct from movement disorders:
- *Apraxia:* inability to perform certain purposive actions.
- *Loss of selectivity* of motor control: inability to isolate and fractionate specific movements.

History
- Family history (consanguinity, dominant conditions).
- Neonatal encephalopathy and neonatal jaundice.
- Age of onset and initial symptoms, temporal course.
- Precipitating and aggravating factors.
- Diurnal fluctuation?
- Association with fasting?

Examination
- Photographs and family video can be very helpful.
- Observation of abnormal movements with limbs in different positions.
- Fine motor skill assessment tasks:
  - drawing and writing in older children;
  - pegboards and threading beads in younger children.
- Allowing the child to rest their hands lightly on the examiner's hands while distracted may be helpful in detecting subtle tremor, myoclonus, or chorea.

- Gait assessment including stressed gait (toe/heel walking), walking backwards, and tandem gait is essential, and may bring out or abolish dystonia.
- The 'striatal toe' or pseudo-Babinski sign may be present in some children falsely localizing the lesion to the pyramidal tract.

Defining the phenotype

The first step in forming a differential diagnosis, planning investigations and management is to define the *phenotype*: what type(s) of abnormal movement is/are present?

- Each body region in turn should be examined for hypo- or hyperkinesia.
- When *hyperkinesia* is present, the type of abnormal movement(s) should be characterized.
- The movement disorder subsequently defined should be considered in the context of other motor abnormalities (e.g. tone, power etc).
- Video recordings are invaluable to this process (allowing off-line rewatching and discussion), and families should be encouraged to document abnormal movements in advance of the first clinic consultation if possible.

Hyperkinesias

A collective term for the common excessive involuntary movements seen in childhood including tics, stereotypies, tremor, myoclonus, chorea, ballismus, athetosis, and dystonia.

Tics

The most common movement disorder in childhood.

- *Stereotyped, involuntary, and irresistible, purposeless* repetitive movements of skeletal, or oropharyngeal muscles causing 'absurd' motor or phonic phenomena.
- Can be suppressed voluntarily to some extent, but often with a rising sense of compulsion and anxiety that is relieved only by 'release' of the tic.
- Exacerbated by anxiety.
- Vary in complexity and range from simple motor tics (e.g. eye closure, shoulder shrugs) through complex tics (such as scratching) to very elaborate or sustained movements.
- *Phonic* tics can also be simple (sniffs) through complex (partial words, animal sounds) to elaborate verbal outbursts (echolalia, palilalia, coprolalia).
- *Sensory* tics are a rare form of tic in which the child suffers episodes of inappropriate sensation (heat, pressure) only relieved by movement of the affected body part. Much more commonly tics are associated with a 'premonitory urge', as if there is an itch they need to scratch, although it can be difficult to separate a pure sensory phenomenon from compulsion in these situations.
- Tics can be difficult to differentiate from other movements, but are typified by the child being able to reproduce them, voluntarily having partial control over them, and their not interfering with voluntary activity.
- Unlike most other forms of movement disorder they *can occur* in sleep.

Stereotypies
- Complex motor tics may be confused with stereotypies—repetitive, rhythmic, and purposeless movements, which may be bizarre, but are characterized by their *absolute voluntary nature*.
- Typical stereotypies include head rolling, arm waving, and head banging.
- Frequent in children with pervasive developmental disorders.

Tremor
Rhythmic oscillation of a body part (usually a limb) resulting from synchronous contraction of reciprocally innervated muscles (i.e. agonist and antagonist pairs that would normally exhibit *reciprocal inhibition*).
- Commonly seen in children with dystonia:
- *Postural tremor*: precipitated by maintenance of the body part position against gravity.
- *Action/intention tremor*: precipitated by voluntary movement and worsens as the limb approaches its target. Usually a result of cerebellar dysfunction.
- *Rest tremor*: occurs when the muscle is at rest, without any active voluntary contraction.

Myoclonus
Brief shock-like jerk due to activation or relaxation of one or more muscle groups:
- *Positive myoclonus*: muscle activation.
- *Negative myoclonus*: muscle relaxation.
- Common feature of many forms of epilepsy–*cortical myoclonus*—with an ictal correlate to the abnormal movement.

Non-epileptic forms can be categorized on the basis of presumed anatomical origin into *subcortical*, *brainstem*, *propriospinal*, or *spinal* myoclonus.

Chorea
Continuing random-appearing sequence of one or more discrete involuntary movements or movement fragments (*chorea* Greek for 'dance').
- Usually affects proximal limbs, trunk, and facial muscles.
- Movements have distinct start and end point, and watched over time, repetition of particular movement fragments can be seen.
- Purposeless. Exacerbated by action or mental concentration.
- May be difficult to differentiate from motor tics and myoclonus.
- The 'milkmaid phenomenon' can be elicited by asking the child to grasp the examiner's fingers who can then feel the 'milking' movements of subtle chorea.

Ballismus is a particularly severe form of chorea characterized by violent, high amplitude involuntary movements of proximal limbs.

Athetosis
Slow, continuous, involuntary writhing movement that prevents maintenance of a stable posture:
- Movements lack a distinct start and end point, and are not composed of recognizable fragments.
- Commonly co-occurs with dystonia and/or chorea.
- Typically involves distal extremities.
- In contrast to dystonia, lacks *sustained* postures.

Dystonia

Characterized by sustained or intermittent muscle contractions causing abnormal, often repetitive, movements, postures, or both:
- Movements typically patterned and twisting, and often tremulous.
- Co-contraction of agonist and antagonist muscle pairs often gives rise to dystonia.
- May also comprise overflow contraction, where muscle contractions spread to muscles not normally involved in the maintenance of a given posture.

Current classification is along two axes: *(i)* clinical features and *(ii)* aetiology.
- On anatomical distribution:
  - *focal* dystonia: involving a single muscle group (blepharospasm, orofacial dystonia, writer's cramp, torticollis);
  - *segmental* dystonia: involvement of two or more adjacent body regions;
  - *hemi-dystonia*: involvement of one-half of the body;
  - *multifocal dystonia*: two or more non-contiguous body segments involved;
  - *generalized* dystonia.

Important mimics of dystonia in childhood include:
- Tonic seizures.
- Sandifer syndrome.
- Hyperekplexia.
- Myotonia.
- Extensor postures due to ↑ intracranial pressure or posterior fossa tumours/masses.

Non-hyperkinetic abnormal involuntary movements

Akathisia

A tic-like dyskinesia, characterized by constant restlessness and changes in posture associated with anxiety:
- Like tics, may be under semi-voluntary control.
- Differs from hyperkinesia, which is characterized by overall ↑ activity, rather than frequent changes in posture.

Mirror movements

Involuntary movements of one side of the body that mirror intentional movements on the other side of the body.
- Normal in infants. Disappear by 8 yrs as the corpus callosum becomes fully myelinated.
- *Obligatory* mirror movements are always abnormal at any age and suggest cervico-medullary junction pathology. Consider Klippel–Feil and Kallmann syndromes, also seen in some children with hemiplegia due to persistence of ipsilateral corticospinal tract projections.

Hypokinetic-rigid syndrome ('Parkinsonism')

Disorders characterized by an overall *paucity and slowness* of movement. Rare in childhood compared with adults. Often associated with dystonia. A combination of:

- *Rigidity*: abnormal tone with ↑ resistance to passive movement that is constant *regardless of the direction or velocity of movement* (so called 'lead pipe' rigidity). This distinguishes it from spasticity: *velocity dependent* ↑ tone.
- *Rest tremor:* 4–5 Hz tremor that occurs in the absence of voluntary movement and is diminished by intentional movement. Superimposed on rigidity, it causes the 'cog-wheeling' phenomenon.

Numbness, pain, tingling, and sensory disturbance

Very rare in child neurology as an isolated phenomenon.

Specific scenarios

- *Unilateral hemi-syndrome*: consider migraine or epilepsy (the duration of disturbed sensation will help differentiate). Dysaesthesia is contralateral to the dysfunctional hemisphere.
- *Distal legs or proximal arms*
  - Extremely distressing paraesthesiae or allodynia (pain brought on by light touch) are often seen with the parainfective neuropathies such as Guillain–Barré syndrome. Distal leg symptoms may *precede weakness*.
  - Paraesthesiae can be an early feature of subacute combined degeneration of the cord due to nitrous oxide abuse (see Nitrous oxide exposure in Chapter 4 ➜ p. 526).
  - Proximal arm/shoulder pain or dysaesthesia often precedes the weakness of *neuralgic amyotrophy* (brachial neuritis), a rare dominantly inherited condition associated with *SEPT9* mutations: pain and motor weakness respond to prompt steroid treatment.
  - *Hereditary neuropathy with liability to pressure palsies* (HNPP) causing pressure related median, or ulnar nerve symptoms. Presentation in childhood very rare (see Hereditary neuropathy with liability to pressure palsies in Chapter 4 ➜ p. 433).
- Concern may be expressed about *apparent insensitivity to pain*. True anaesthesia raises possibility of HSAN conditions such as Riley–Day syndrome (see Hereditary sensory and autonomic neuropathies in Chapter 4 ➜ p. 435). True anaesthesia will lead to injuries and tissue destruction. Much more commonly a child with developmental disability will show *indifference* to pain: he feels (and withdraws automatically from) painful stimuli but shows little emotional distress (i.e. doesn't cry). The histamine flare testing can be useful in ambiguous cases (see Histamine in Chapter 7 ➜ p. 676).
- Patchy sensory loss may accompany demyelinating conditions (e.g. multiple sclerosis) but rarely as an isolated feature.
- Hemidysaesthesia may precede a TIA.
- Dissociated sensory loss (loss of pain sensation but preservation of light touch ± dysaesthesia) particularly in the arms is very suggestive of a syrinx or other central cavity in the cervical cord.
- Acroparaesthesiae in a boy due to Fabry disease (X-linked; very rare).
- Severe abdominal pain with prominent autonomic features (tachycardia, diarrhoea) ± neuropathic pain in limbs occurs in acute porphyrias (see Acute porphyrias in Chapter 4 ➜ p. 487). Essentially only a post-pubertal disease.
- Isolated numbness, tingling, or other sensory disturbance is a relatively common functional complaint (see Functional neurological symptoms in Chapter 4 ➜ p. 335). Such disturbances will typically be reported in patchy distributions that do not correspond to anatomical segmental or

peripheral nerve territory distributions (e.g. in a circumferential 'sleeve' distribution, with normal sensation more proximally and distally).

Reflex sympathetic dystrophy

Also known as causalgia, and complex regional pain syndrome (CRPS). Precise mechanism is unknown although presumed to involve disturbance of the sympathetic nervous system in the affected region. There may also be changes in central representations of sensory input from limbs.

- More commonly presents in girls in adolescence or later.
- Typically involves the distal limb following minor trauma (e.g. ankle sprain).
- Over days to weeks after injury the affected area (usually the distal limb) becomes subjectively severely painful.
- Objective changes suggestive of sympathetic disturbance may occur, e.g. the affected area is flushed and warm, and shows ↑ sweating.
- Management is symptomatic.
  - Gabapentin or pregabalin by mouth may be help neuropathic pain (amitriptyline as second line alternatives).
  - Physiotherapy to maintain the range of movement and prevent secondary deformity.
  - In rare cases consider (in conjunction with specialist pain teams) regional anaesthesia, e.g. nerve blocks.

Secondary emotional morbidity is common and often a significant issue in its own right. Early referral to CAMHS should be considered and may help with FND elements of the presentation.

- Desensitizing such as 'brushing' have become increasingly adopted.
- Other suggested therapies with some biological plausibility include 'mirror box' treatment (positioning the affected limb behind a mirror in such a way that it coincides in visual and proprioceptive space with the reflection of the unaffected limb in front of the mirror, and then brushing the normal limb so that the brain has the visual experience of 'seeing' the affected limb touched without experiencing pain).

Paroxysmal extreme pain disorder

The preferred name for what was previously known as familial rectal pain syndrome.

- Extremely rare.
- Autosomal dominant condition due to mutations in a voltage-gated sodium channel gene *SCN9A* resulting in inability to inactivate after nociceptive stimulus.
- Results in overwhelming severe burning pain typically beginning in eye or jaw or, characteristically, rectum, usually triggered by normally trivial stimuli such as eating, defecation, wiping perineum.
- Pain can become more generalized and has been described by adult women as much more severe than labour pains.
- There may be flushing skin changes in affected region.
- Episodes typically last seconds to a few minutes.
- Presents in infants with paroxysmal flushing and severe inconsolable distress. EEG is normal apart from tachycardia on ECG trace.
- Variable benefit from carbamazepine, gabapentin, topiramate. No benefit from opiates.

Peripheral weakness

Identify the pattern of weakness

Cranial involvement?
- *Facial weakness*: facioscapulohumeral (FSH) dystrophy, myasthenia, myotonic dystrophy, congenital myopathy, congenital MD.
- *Bulbar weakness*: Fazio–Londe (aka Brown–Vialetto–Van Laere syndrome).
- *Ptosis*: myasthenia, myotonic dystrophy, myotubular myopathy.
- *Ophthalmoplegia*: myasthenia, myotubular myopathy, merosin-deficient congenital muscular dystrophy, mitochondrial.
- *Tongue fasciculation*: spinal muscular atrophy, motor neuron disease.
- *Palatal weakness*: (resulting in a nasal voice) myotonic dystrophy.

Proximal?
Difficulties raising head from pillow, combing hair, brushing teeth, shaving, raising arms above head, getting up from chair, climbing stairs (has to use banister), running, hopping, jumping.

Proximal weakness is usually due to muscle disease (Duchenne, Becker, limb girdle, and congenital dystrophies, congenital myopathies) although there are exceptions including spinal muscular atrophies and some neuropathies (CIDP, and neuropathy due to porphyria).

Distal?
Difficulties opening screw cap or doorknob, turning key, buttoning clothes, writing, and in heel walking. There is toe-walking with foot drop and frequent falls and tripping on uneven surfaces.

Distal weakness is usually due to neuropathy (any) but is also a feature of some muscle diseases (Emery–Dreifuss, myotonic dystrophy, dysferlinopathy, Miyoshi myopathy).

Axial?
Difficulties bending forward, lifting head off the bed, respiratory involvement, nocturnal hypoventilation, and diaphragmatic weakness: seen in congenital myopathies and glycogen storage disorders.

Neck extensor weakness ('head drop') is a feature of myasthenia gravis, some inflammatory myopathies (particularly polymyositis, dermatomyositis, inclusion body myositis), chronic inflammatory demyelinating polyneuropathy, facioscapulohumeral dystrophy, myotonic dystrophy, and congenital myopathies.

Identify the symptom time course

Neonatal presentation?
Antenatal onset is suggested by polyhydramnios, reduced foetal movements, contractures (including arthrogryposis and foot deformity), congenital dysplasia of the hip, and unusual 'lies' of the foetus.

Variability?
Diurnal variability (weakness progressively worsening through the day: e.g. evolving ptosis) strongly suggests a *myasthenia*.

Acute onset?
Consider GBS, transverse myelitis, toxic, porphyria, critical illness polyneuropathy.

Episodic or fluctuating? Progressive?
See Fig. 3.5 ➲ p. 181.

Associated features/systems enquiry

- *Toe-walking*: Duchenne, Becker, Emery–Dreifuss, Charcot–Marie Tooth.
- *Falls*: unsteadiness in sensory neuropathy.
- *Myoglobinuria*: dystrophies, metabolic myopathies.
- *Numbness, tingling, pins and needles, burning, pain, 'walking on cotton wool'*: sensory neuropathies.
- Foot deformities (see Foot deformities in this chapter ➲ p. 147).
- *Respiratory involvement* (nocturnal hypoventilation, ineffective cough, diaphragmatic breathing pattern, recurrent infections) important in all neuromuscular disorders.
- *Cardiac involvement*: Emery–Dreifuss, myotonic dystrophy, muscular dystrophies.
- Feeding difficulties.
- Contractures (see Examination).
- Vision (muscle-eye-brain disease).
- Hearing.
- Learning difficulties (some dystrophies).
- Medication and possible toxin exposure.
- Developmental impairment especially delayed walking.
- Family history:
  - Consanguinity, neonatal deaths, still births.

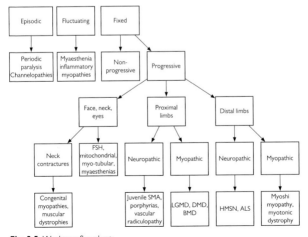

Fig. 3.5 Weakness flowchart.

Examination

Also examine parents and siblings: especially when considering neuropathies, myotonic dystrophy.

- Differentiate between a lesion of the brain, brainstem, cord, root, nerve, neuromuscular junction, muscle (see Table 1.6 in Chapter 1 ➲ p. 40).
- Syndromic features.
- Muscle bulk.
- Atrophy, e.g. of peroneal and intrinsic hand muscles in HMSN.
- (Pseudo-) hypertrophy, e.g. of calves in Duchenne.
- Effects of percussion, grip, and exercise:
  - Myotonia: delayed muscle relaxation after sustained contraction; improvement with repeated contractions (warm-up).
  - Percussion myotonia: prolonged contraction after tapping with a tendon hammer (thenar eminence, forearm, tongue).
  - Paramyotonia: paradoxical myotonia worsening with repeated contractions.
- Reflexes absent in neuropathy, generally present in muscle disorders.
- Fasciculations.
  - *Can be normal!* (Caffeine consumption, fatigue).
  - SMA.
  - Neuropathies.
- Tremor, pseudoathetosis in sensory neuropathies (loss of proprioception).
- Poly-mini-myoclonus in SMA.
- *Contractures/skeletal:*
  - Elbows: Emery–Dreifuss;
  - Achilles tendons: Duchenne, HMSN;
  - Ileotibial band: Duchenne;
  - Knee extension/flexion: sarcoglycanopathies;
  - Fingers, elbows, ankles: Bethlem myopathy;
  - Spine, neck: Ulrich, central core, minicore, lamin A/C (dominant Emery–Dreifuss).
- Foot deformity: neuropathy.
- *Cardiac*
  - Arrhythmias: Emery–Dreifuss, limb girdle muscular dystrophy (LGMD) 1B, myotonic dystrophy.
  - Dilated cardiomyopathy: Duchenne, Becker, LGMD 2 C, D, E, F.
- *Nerve hypertrophy*: hypertrophic HMSN, leprosy, CIDP.
- Functional assessment.
  - Compensatory lordosis;
  - Hyperextension of knees;
  - Consequences of proximal weakness: waddling gait, difficulties with steps, hopping and jumping. Gowers' sign;
  - Timed 10 m (or other convenient standardized distance) walk;
  - Speech;
  - Fine motor function (e.g. pegboard).

Psychomotor regression

Differentiate true regression (unambiguous loss of previously established motor and cognitive abilities) from evolution of signs in a static encephalopathy see also School failure in this chapter ➔ p. 191. There are a number of other conditions that may present with *apparent* regression.

Non-neurodegenerative causes of apparent regression

0–2 yrs
- Infantile spasms.
- Autistic regression.
- Rett syndrome.
- Evolution of signs in a static encephalopathy.

2–5 yrs
- Lennox–Gastaut.
- ↑ intracranial pressure (ICP) (tumour, hydrocephalus).
- Spinal tumour.
- Paraneoplastic.
- Isolated genetic dystonia e.g. DYT-TOR1A, DYT-KMT2B.

School age
- Pseudo-regression due to widening gap between child and peers over time as demands of schooling grow (see also School failure in this chapter ➔ p. 191).
- Landau–Kleffner and DEE-SWAS (see Landau–Kleffner syndrome in Chapter 4 ➔ p. 287).
- Autoimmune, e.g. demyelinating disease.

Adolescents
- Autoimmune.
- Psychiatric disorders.
- Chronic fatigue syndrome.
- Substance abuse.
- Thyroid disorder including Hashimoto encephalopathy.
- Vasculitis, e.g. SLE.

At any age consider
- Epileptic regression (see below).
- Psychosocial deprivation or abuse.
- Factitious or induced illness (see Factitious or Induced Illness in Chapter 4 ➔ p. 332).
- Cerebrovascular events.
- ↑ ICP (space-occupying lesion, hydrocephalus, etc.).
- Toxic (lead, methotrexate, substance abuse, radiotherapy).
- Endocrine (hypothyroidism, Hashimoto encephalopathy).

Psychomotor regression and epilepsy

Regression is often a feature of severe epilepsies ('epileptic encephalopathy') (see Box 4.5 in Chapter 4 ➔ p. 280). This can be a relatively fixed element of a severe 1° seizure disorder (e.g. infantile epileptic spasms and Lennox–Gastaut syndromes); a potentially more reversible seizure disorder (e.g. Landau–Kleffner); or the seizures can be a symptom of a progressive underlying neurological disease. This latter is particularly a consideration in the presence of myoclonic seizures (see The progressive myoclonus epilepsies in Chapter 4 ➲ p. 302).

Approach to diagnosis of neurodegenerative conditions

There is no such thing as a 'general neurometabolic screen': narrow the differential diagnosis, and then focus investigations appropriately. Some of the conditions discussed below are orders of magnitude commoner than others. It is important to have this perspective, but equally to be aware of local ethnicity considerations affecting local 'gene pools' which can create local clusters of particular rare conditions.

A long-running UK surveillance programme for progressive intellectual and neurological decline in children identified a total of 220 diagnoses in 89% of reported cases. The commonest causes differed by age at regression and ethnicity. The majority of cases (81%) developed symptoms before 5 years of age (Table 3.11).

Clues from age at presentation

Ages at presentation is a very useful 'handle' on diagnosis: for common neurodegenerative conditions organized by age at presentation see Tables 3.12–3.16.

Clues from the history:

- *Myoclonus*: gangliosidoses; NCL; Gaucher type 3; Leigh; SSPE; Lafora; vCJD; Unverricht–Lundborg.
- *Early visual impairment*: infantile or juvenile NCL; adrenoleukodystrophy (X-ALD); GM2 gangliosidosis.
- *Behavioural disturbance*: X-ALD; Sanfilippo; Wilson; juvenile Huntington; juvenile NCL.
- *Stroke-like episodes or episodic encephalopathy*: mitochondrial; Leigh; homocystinuria.
- *Gastrointestinal symptoms* (failure to thrive, vomiting, diarrhoea): abetalipoproteinaemia; Leigh; Gaucher type 2; Sanfilippo.

Table 3.11 Ranked order of commonest causes of neurological regression by age in UK PIND study (Dev Med Child Neurol 2021;63(3):287–94). Abbreviations: mito: mitochondrial cytopathies (various); MLD: metachromatic leukodystrophy; NCL: neuronal ceroid lipofuscinoses (various); MPS: mucopolysaccharidosis (type III); NPC: Niemann–Pick type C; X-ALD: x-linked adrenoleukodystrophy

Age at presentation			
<1 yrs	1–4 yrs	5–9 yrs	10–15 yrs
Mito (33%)	NCL (26%)	NCL (31%)	Mito (16.0%)
Krabbe (11%)	MPS Type III (16%)	X-ALD (18%)	X-ALD (11%)
Tay–Sachs (10%)	Mito (12.7%)	Mito (9%)	Lafora body disease (11%)
Zellweger (6%)	MLD (12%)	MLD (9%)	NPC (8%)
Aicardi–Goutieres syndrome (6%)	Rett (9%)	NPC (7.4%)	CJD (8%)

- *Rapidity of regression*: gangliosidoses, neurodegeneration with brain iron accumulation (NBIA), Krabbe, X-ALD, Alpers; Leigh.
- *Family history*: recessive inheritance or X-linked (Pelizaeus–Merzbacher, X-ALD, Hunter).

Ask about history of sudden infant death, unexplained illness, or neurological presentations in family members. Establish ethnicity and ask about consanguinity.

Clues from physical examination
(see also Table 1.1 in Chapter 1 ➲ p. 10).
- *Dysmorphism:* coarse facies of MPS (mild in Sanfilippo), GM1 gangliosidosis, mucolipidoses.
- *Macrocephaly:* Canavan/Alexander, Krabbe, metachromatic leukodystrophy (MLD).
- *Microcephaly:* Rett, infantile NCL.
- *Skeletal abnormality:* MPS, GM1 gangliosidosis, Gaucher.
- *Hepatosplenomegaly:* Gaucher, Niemann–Pick, MPS, gangliosidosis, Wilson.
- *Peripheral nerve involvement:* (absent tendon jerks, abnormal EMG/NCV): MLD, multiple sulphatase deficiency, Krabbe, Refsum, X-ALD, Fabry, Leigh, Friedreich ataxia, infantile neuroaxonal dystrophy (INAD).
- *Pyramidal signs:* leukoencephalopathies, e.g. MLD, Krabbe, X-ALD.
- *Extrapyramidal signs:* Leigh, juvenile Huntington, NBIA/PKAN, Wilson, vCJD.
- *Ataxia:* ataxia telangiectasia, Friedreich ataxia, Leigh, Niemann–Pick, cerebrotendinous xanthomatosis, mitochondrial, MLD, vCJD, Refsum.

Grey or white matter disorder?
See Table 3.12 ➲ p. 185.

Table 3.12 Causes of grey and white matter disease

Grey matter disorders	White matter disorders
Alpers (PNDC)	Krabbe
Gangliosidosis GM1, GM2	Metachromatic leukodystrophy
Mucolipidoses	Adrenoleukodystrophy
Fucosidosis	Pelizaeus–Merzbacher disease
Wilson	Canavan
Lafora body disease	Alexander
Niemann–Pick A, C	Aicardi–Goutières
Gaucher	Sialidosis
Farber	Cockayne
Leigh	Vanishing white matter disease
Menkes	Megalencephalic leukoencephalopathy, subcortical cysts
Huntington	Cerebrotendinous xanthomatosis
Mitochondrial	Mitochondrial
	Multiple sulphatase deficiency
	Sulphatide activator deficiency
	Cobalamin/folate metabolism disorders

- *Grey matter disorders*: suggested by prominent seizures, personality change, and dementia ± movement disorder. Motor features are late.
- *White matter disorders*: suggested by prominent spasticity, ataxia, hearing, and visual impairment. Seizures and dementia are late features.

Clues from imaging, electrophysiology, and ophthalmology examination
For approach to white matter abnormalities (see White matter abnormalities on MRI in Chapter 2 ⊃ p. 77). MRI can support diagnosis of the following conditions:

- Late infantile NCL: cerebellar atrophy with periventricular white matter signal abnormality.
- MLD: symmetrical demyelination with rostro-caudal progression.
- X-ALD: signal abnormality in white matter posteriorly with anterior progression.
- Pelizaeus–Merzbacher disease: signal abnormality in white matter on T2-weighted images, normal on T1.
- Leigh: symmetrical hypointense areas on T1-weighted image, hyperintense on T2, involving basal ganglia (mainly putamen) and brainstem with sparing of the mamillary body.
- Vanishing white matter disease: the signal in the periventricular white matter is similar to CSF; subcortical white matter appears streaky.
- Multifocal leukoencephalopathy with subcortical cysts: diffuse cerebral oedema with cystic changes especially in the parietal and temporal regions.
- NBIA/PKAN: 'eye of the tiger' appearance with signal abnormality in the basal ganglia due to iron deposition.
- vCJD: bilateral pulvinar high signal.

Age at onset: less than 2 yrs
See Table 3.13.

Table 3.13 Neurodegenerative disorders presenting at **less than 2 yrs** of age: suggestive features, diagnostic clues, and investigations

Condition	Clues to diagnosis	Test
PMD	Boys, early eye movement abnormality, hypotonia, head bobbing, dystonia then spastic paraparesis slow cognitive decline	MRI, electrophysiology, DNA testing (some cases)
MLD	Polyradiculopathy (delayed NCV, limb pains) with upper motor signs too, usually present as gait abnormality, high CSF protein	Lysosomal enzyme screen ('white cell enzymes'), MRI
Krabbe	Irritability, myoclonus, hypertonia, opisthotonos, hyperpyrexia, ↑ CSF protein, peripheral neuropathy	Lysosomal enzyme screen

Table 3.13 (Contd.)

Condition	Clues to diagnosis	Test
Gangliosidoses	GM1: dysmorphic, skeletal abnormality, cherry red spot (50%), hepatosplenomegaly. GM2: early visual impairment, cherry red spot (100%), stimulus-sensitive myoclonus, hepatosplenomegaly	Lysosomal enzyme screen
Infantile NCL	Irritable infants with visual loss (early optic atrophy), chorea/dystonia, stimulus-induced myoclonus, microcephaly, EEG: flattened with loss of sleep spindles	Lysosomal enzyme screen, skin electron microscopy: neuronal granular inclusions
INAD	Presentation like MLD (though neuropathy may precede cerebral features) but normal CSF protein, anterior horn cell type denervation on EMG, normal NCV. MRI shows cerebellar atrophy (sometimes with high T2 in cerebellar cortex) ± iron deposition in pallidus	*PLAG26* mutations; Skin biopsy: spheroids in nerve axons
Rett	Acquired microcephaly, loss of speech, and purposeful hand movements, seizures, bruxism in a girl	*MECP2* mutation
Gaucher type 2	Failure to thrive, hepatosplenomegaly, hypertonia with neck extension, stridor, seizures, bone marrow suppression, strabismus, cherry red spot	Lysosomal enzyme screen, Gaucher cells in bone marrow, cytogenetics
Niemann–Pick A	Organomegaly, feeding problems, seizures, cherry red spot	Lysosomal enzyme screen, 'sea blue' histiocytes on bone marrow

Age at onset: 2–5 yrs

See Table 3.14.

Table 3.14 Neurodegenerative disorders presenting at **2–5 yrs** of age: suggestive features, diagnostic clues, and investigations

Condition	Clues to diagnosis	Test
X-ALD	Behavioural/cognitive decline with early visual loss, then motor disorder	VLCFA
NCL—late infantile	Stimulus-induced myoclonus and other seizures, extrapyramidal motor disorder, visual loss later. VEP: giant responses initially. ERG absent later EEG: high amplitude slow, occipital spikes to slow (1 Hz) photic stimulation (=VEP) Electron microscopy of skin: curvilinear inclusions in neurons	Tripeptidyl peptidase (TPP) assay
Mitochondrial	Varied presentations, eye movement abnormality, myopathy, seizures, strokes	Muscle biopsy, respiratory chain enzymes
Sanfilippo	Developmental delay then behavioural disturbance ++, then seizures and motor regression, hip dysplasia, diarrhoea	Urine GAG (heparin sulphate), lysosomal enzyme screen
Alpers	Intractable seizures (myoclonic, akinetic, generalized), liver function abnormality	Mitochondrial respiratory chain activity assay and polymerase gamma mutations
Leigh	Poor suck/swallow, vomiting, irritability, seizures, rapid regression, abnormal eye movements, and early optic atrophy	MRI, mitochondrial studies (skin/muscle), PDH studies
Gaucher type 3	Oculomotor apraxia (failure of upward gaze), supranuclear palsy, myoclonus, ataxia, skeletal abnormality, hepatosplenomegaly, lung involvement	Lysosomal enzyme screen, Gaucher cells on bone marrow biopsy, cytogenetics

Age at onset: 5–12 yrs

See Table 3.15.

Table 3.15 Neurodegenerative disorders presenting at **5–12 yrs** of age: suggestive features, diagnostic clues, and investigations

Condition	Clues to diagnosis	Test
NCL—juvenile	Visual loss (early optic atrophy) behavioural problems, dementia. Later in teens compulsive speech, seizures, motor disorder, ERG: attenuated early in the condition, vacuolated lymphocytes	Lysosomal enzyme screen Electron microscopy of skin: fingerprint inclusions in neurons
NBIA	Extrapyramidal signs (lower then upper limbs), dystonic spasms, retinitis pigmentosa, rapid progression	MRI: Characteristic findings depending upon gene involved (e.g. eye of tiger in PKAN)Genetic testing
Refsum	Ataxia, hepatomegaly, ichthyosis, retinitis pigmentosa, deafness, ↑ CSF protein	Phytanic acid
Niemann–Pick C	Vertical gaze palsy, seizures, ataxia, dystonia, hepatosplenomegaly, cherry red spot	'Sea blue' histiocytes on bone marrow, cholesterol transport/storage in cultured fibroblasts
Unverricht–Lundborg disease	Generalized seizures then stimulus-sensitive myoclonus, ataxia/extrapyramidal signs, cognitive decline is slow, EEG: photosensitivity	*CSTB* mutation
Friedreich ataxia	Ataxia, pyramidal signs with peripheral neuropathy (loss of reflexes, vibration, and proprioception)	Frataxin mutation
HIV dementia	Vertical transmission, immunodeficiency	CD4 counts, viral titres

Age at onset: Adolescence

See Table 3.16.

Table 3.16 Neurodegenerative disorders presenting **in adolescence**: suggestive features, diagnostic clues, and investigations

Condition	Clues to diagnosis	Test
Wilson	Behaviour, psychiatric, and extrapyramidal movement disorders, hepatic involvement	KF rings, penicillamine challenge
SSPE	Behaviour/cognitive decline, optic atrophy, extrapyramidal signs, myoclonus. EEG: synchronous periodic high voltage sharp/slow-wave complexes. History of measles <4 yrs. High CSF protein with OGB	Paired CSF and serum measles IgM; CSF measles PCR
vCJD	Psychiatric, sensory phenomena, then extrapyramidal and cerebellar signs and myoclonus	MRI, post-mortem
Lafora body disease	Rapid dementia, stimulus-sensitive, and resting myoclonus, visual seizures	Axillary skin biopsy with sweat glands (Lafora bodies)
SCA 7	Ataxia, dysarthria, dysphagia, progressive central visual loss	Gene panel
Cerebrotendinous xanthomatosis	Myoclonus, cataracts, xanthelasma, ataxia, slow progression	Cholestanol levels
Juvenile Huntington	Rigidity, seizures, dementia, family history (often paternal)	Genetics after careful counselling

School failure

True, new-onset neurological regression in older children or adolescents is rare. More commonly the problem is in fact longstanding but has come to light due to a sudden ↑ in academic expectations (e.g. a move to a new school). Parental observations should be supplemented by reports from schoolteachers and/or educational psychologists.

Causes
- Non-neurological.
  - previously unidentified learning difficulties, ADHD, autistic spectrum, or pervasive developmental disorders, dyslexia;
  - bullying, stress;
  - chronic non-neurological illness (e.g. renal failure, diabetes) aggravating school absence, emotional issues.
- Drug side effects.
  - prescribed (e.g. ASMs).
  - recreational drugs and alcohol abuse.
- Sensory impairment.
  - evolving hearing or visual impairment.
- Psychiatric.
  - depression, schizophrenia.
- Epilepsy (subtle, unrecognized seizures).
  - absence epilepsy;
  - non-convulsive status;
  - Landau–Kleffner and DEE-SWAS (see Landau–Kleffner syndrome in Chapter 4 ➔ p. 287).

True neurodegenerative disorders presenting in later childhood will eventually manifest neurological signs *as well as* cognitive deterioration.

Conditions in which cognitive failure can be prominent initially include neuropsychiatric SLE, juvenile-onset NCL, Wilson, juvenile Huntington, X-linked adrenoleukodystrophy, SSPE and vCJD (see Table 3.16 in this chapter ➔ p. 190).

History
- Medication and drugs/alcohol?
- Mental state and mood?
- Seizures?
- Exposure to wild measles, tick bites?

Examination
The child will be older and a formal (adult style) neurological examination with assessment of higher mental function should be performed.
- Look at affect, mood, signs of distractibility, and slowness of cognitive processing.
- Cerebellar involvement?
- Pyramidal signs?
- Extrapyramidal signs—involuntary movements, abnormal posturing.
- Handwriting—micrographia (Wilson).
- Eyes: Kaiser–Fleischer rings, pigmentary retinopathy.

- Neuropsychological assessment can be very useful in defining the 'phenotype'.

Assessment and investigation
Depending on impression.

Specific learning difficulty
- Relatively isolated weakness in one domain.
- Further investigation is not indicated: institute appropriate educational assessment and provision.

Mild global learning difficulties
- If clearly longstanding and non-progressive, further investigation is not indicated: institute appropriate educational assessment and provision.

Moderate/severe learning difficulties
- As for global developmental impairment (see Developmental impairment in this chapter **⊃** p. 120).

Psychiatric
- Consider a neuropsychiatric review if a behavioural disturbance or mental illness prominent.

Neurological disease
If there is concern of dementia, test more formally:
- Frontal lobe function: expressive dysphasia, primitive reflexes (palmar-mental, grasp, snout, glabellar), response-suppression (go versus no-go tasks).
- Temporal lobe function: long-term memory recall, receptive dysphasia (three-step command).
- Parietal lobe function: dressing apraxia, constructional apraxia, astereognosis, graphaesthesia, sensory inattention, dyscalculia (serial 7s, etc.).
- Unambiguous findings on formal neurological examination should lead to further investigation guided by imaging (see 'Psychomotor Regression' section).
- Consider EEG (including deep sleep) if LKS or DEE-SWAS is suspected.

Sleep disturbance

There are two physiologically distinct sleep states: rapid eye movement (REM) sleep and non-REM sleep. The latter is further divided into four stages based on EEG/EOG/EMG features. (see Fig. 3.6 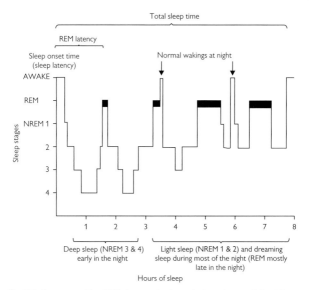 p. 193).

Non-REM sleep

Stage 1 (5–10% of sleep)
- Occurs at sleep onset or following arousal from another stage of sleep.
- Mixed EEG frequencies: reduced α activity, vertex sharp waves.
- Slow rolling eye movements.

Stage 2 (55–60% of sleep)
- Slow EEG activity: sleep spindles and 'K' complexes.

Stages 3 and 4 (25% of sleep)
- Also known as slow-wave sleep: predominantly slow activity on EEG.

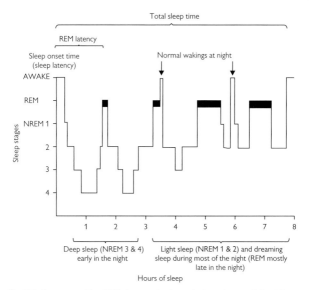

Fig. 3.6 Sleep stages. Non-REM sleep predominates in the early part of the night, with REM sleep predominant in the later part of the night and particularly just before waking.

REM sleep
- Physiologically very different.
- Brain metabolism is high.
- Low voltage, non-alpha EEG.
- Spontaneous rapid eye movements.
- Skeletal muscle almost completely paralysed (EMG activity absent).

The sleep cycle
Non-REM and REM sleep alternate cyclically throughout the night starting with non-REM for 80 min followed by REM for 10 min. The whole cycle repeats itself about 5–6 times. Each REM typically ends with a brief arousal or transition into light non-REM (Fig. 3.6).

History
- Is this a problem of getting to sleep, staying asleep, or both?
- Is this a problem of being too sleepy during the day?
- Is this a problem of disturbed episodes at night?

Specific features in history
- 24 h sleep–wake schedule.
- Sleep log/diary.
- Systems review.
- Caffeine intake.
- Psychiatric/psychological/learning difficulties.
- Snoring or noisy breathing in sleep.

In relation to parasomnias
- Timing:
  - Night terrors tend to occur at a fairly regular time.
  - Events occurring in the early part of the night are probably non-REM-sleep-related (night terrors, confusional arousal, sleep walking).
  - Events occurring later in the night are more probably REM-sleep-related (nightmares, REM sleep behaviour disorder).
  - See Sleep disorders in Chapter 4 ➲ p. 493.
  - *Multiple events per night* are very suggestive of frontal lobe epilepsy (see Box 4.9 in Chapter 4 ➲ p. 495).

> ❗ Serious consideration should be given to the possibility that events occurring more than once per night, and/or clustering with several per night for a few nights at a time are nocturnal frontal lobe seizures.

Examination
Pay particular attention to physical factors that may disturb sleep (e.g. upper airway obstruction).

Video
Video recording of arousals can be very useful; however, 'half-hearted' attempts where parents only start filming once woken will miss the most informative first part of the arousal. Continuous filming throughout the night is ideal (preferably at home as this is more likely to capture representative

sleep behaviour). Many more sophisticated home baby monitors offer video recording.

Assessment

Difficulty getting to sleep or staying asleep

Consider developmental issues (see Development and sleep disorders in Chapter 4 ➲ p. 493) and the effect of primary neurodevelopmental disorders on sleep.

Excessive daytime sleepiness

Likely to be due to poor nocturnal sleep hygiene but consider obstructive sleep apnoea, narcolepsy (under-recognized) (see Narcolepsy in Chapter 4 ➲ p. 497) and adolescent delayed sleep syndrome (see Adolescence in Chapter 4 ➲ p. 493).

Disturbed episodes related to sleep (parasomnias)

These are recurrent episodes of behaviour, experiences, or physiological changes that occur exclusively or predominantly during sleep. Decide whether these are primary, or secondary to neurodevelopmental or neuropsychiatric issues (see Parasomnias in Chapter 4 ➲ p. 493).

If a primary parasomnia, the differential depends on whether it is occurring at sleep onset, out of non-REM sleep (i.e. particularly in the early hours of the night), or in REM sleep (later in the night). (Compare Fig. 3.6.)

Investigation

Formal investigation of sleep is resource intensive. Consider for investigation of excessive daytime sleepiness, difficult parasomnias, and objective checks on diagnosis and treatment. Options include: *actigraphy* (use of a wristwatch-like motion detector that logs periods of movement and stillness—i.e. sleep—over several days) providing an extremely helpful, low-cost initial evaluation in establishing sleep patterns; and *polysomnography*. The latter collates multi-channel information on the physiological changes of sleep including EEG, EMG, and EOG. This allows the stages of sleep to be categorized into a formal hypnogram. Analysis of the results is complex. Some of the possible parameters are:

- Sleep continuity.
- Total time in bed.
- Time to go to sleep (sleep latency).
- Number of brief and longer awakenings.
- Time fully awake.
- Total time asleep and awake and sleep efficiency (total time in asleep/ total time in bed × 100).
- Non-REM measures:
  - actual and percentage times in stages 1–4;
  - total slow-wave sleep.
- REM measures:
  - time between first falling asleep and start of first REM period (REM latency);
  - actual and percentage time in REM;
  - total REM.

- The *Multiple Sleep Latency Test* (MSLT) quantifies daytime sleepiness, particularly in the context of suspected narcolepsy. Using conventional EEG, the time taken to reach REM sleep is noted during five opportunities at least 2 h apart during the day. Practicability in younger children (<8 yrs), and paediatric normative data, are limited.
- Where access to MSLT is limited or it is difficult to perform (e.g. in younger children) *CSF hypocretin* may be used. Levels are very low in narcolepsy and are not affected by use of stimulant medication, so symptomatic treatment can be initiated pending diagnostic confirmation. Hypocretin measurement is not necessary when MSLT is diagnostic.

Speech difficulties

Neurological disorders that affect speech commonly also affect swallowing (see Swallowing and feeding problems in this chapter ➜ p. 201) and vice versa, although they may occur in isolation and as such are discussed separately.

Conceptual framework

Speech and language disorder
- Secondary to cognitive disability, hearing impairment, or environmental adversity.
- For primary developmental language disorders (see Specific language impairment in this chapter ➜ p. 123).

Sound and speech production disorders (dysphonia)
- *Abnormal voice quality*: due to allergies, vocal abuse, chronic reflux, hypothyroidism, papilloma viruses (HPVs 6 and 11), trauma, recurrent laryngeal nerve palsy, Chiari malformation (recurrent laryngeal nerve palsy reported), psychological disorders.
- *Orofacial structural abnormalities*: nostril patency, enlarged adenoids, dental malocclusion, cleft lip/palate, macroglossia, significant tongue-tie.
- Neuromotor disorders.

Neuromotor speech disorders

Apraxia
Abnormal planning, sequencing, and coordination of articulation not due to muscle weakness.

Dysarthria
Weakness/paralysis of the musculature of speech (larynx, lips, tongue, palate, and jaw). Breathing and feeding/swallowing may also be affected. There are several different types of dysarthria:

Spastic dysarthria
- Due to hemispheric disease (a cerebral palsy e.g. Worster–Drought syndrome; acquired brain injury including stroke, tumour, neurosurgery; cytotoxic and other drugs, e.g. metoclopramide) or bilateral pontine injury ('pseudobulbar palsy').
- Characterized by slow slurred speech, drooling, reduced movement of muscles of lips and tongue, exaggerated jaw jerk, and gag.

Ataxic dysarthria
- Due to cerebellar lesions.
- A characteristic presentation of Friedreich ataxia (see Friedreich ataxia in Chapter 4 ➜ p. 425).
- Characterized by slow articulation, soft monotonous voice. May be preceded by cerebellar mutism (see Cerebellar mutism ('posterior fossa syndrome' in Chapter 4 ➜ p. 520) at the time of the acquired insult.

Dyskinetic
- Due to basal ganglia lesions.
- Characterized by slow laboured speech ± stuttering, extraneous tongue movements evident, grimacing.

Lower motor neuron
- Flaccid bulbar palsy due to lower motor neuron injury to cranial nerves V, VII, IX, and X or their nuclei.
- Moebius syndrome, spinal muscular atrophy variants, bilateral VII palsy, brainstem pathology, Arnold–Chiari malformation.
- Voice is of low volume and monotonous.

Mixed upper and lower motor neuron lesion patterns
- Neuromuscular junction, e.g. myasthenia gravis.
- Primary myopathic (uncommon, e.g. FSH dystrophy).

Secondary dysarthria
Children with SeLECTS (see Childhood onset epilepsy syndromes in Chapter 4 ➔ p. 282) may present with episodes of transient dysarthria. Dysarthria may also be the presentation of metabolic (e.g. Wilson disease) or neurodegenerative disorders (e.g. Huntington disease and Friedreich ataxia).

The stiff infant

Stiffness (better described as hypertonia) is a common, relatively non-specific feature of the cerebral palsies (see Management of hypertonia and contractures in Chapter 4 ➔ p. 243) and some movement disorders (see Disorders associated with hypokinetic-rigid syndrome in Chapter 4 ➔ p. 415). Here we concentrate on the assessment of the unexpectedly stiff neonate or young infant.

As ever, the 'where'—the site(s) of the pathology—comes from clinical examination. In this context, imaging may also provide valuable additional localizing information. Important clues to the 'what'—the nature of the problem— will come from the history.

Examination

The key aims of the examination are to delineate:

- Is this a central or a peripheral problem (i.e. a reflection of CNS or peripheral neuromuscular disease respectively)? As with the *floppy* infant, an important clue is any presence of associated encephalopathy.
- The anatomical extent of the involvement in patterns of abnormal tone (Upper and lower limbs? Symmetrical?)
- The nature of the tone abnormality, specifically distinguishing *spasticity* (indicative of corticospinal tract involvement) from *dystonia* and/or *rigidity* (indicating involvement of the extrapyramidal system and basal ganglia). This often not easy in practice!
  - Remember that the hallmark of spasticity is *velocity-dependent* variability in tone: limbs feel tighter if you attempt to move joints more rapidly and may demonstrate the characteristic *catch* if moved fast enough.
  - Established spasticity is unusual in infancy: corticospinal pathology often presents initially with hypotonia with the spasticity evolving over time.
  - Resistance to movement with dystonia is variable, depending particularly upon level of arousal. In contrast to rigidity, limbs affected by dystonia will return to an involuntary posture when manipulation ends.
  - In contrast, the resistance to movement felt in rigidity is constant, throughout the range of movement of a joint and irrespective of speed of passive movement.
  - In practice, dystonia, rigidity, and spasticity are often all present in a mixed presentation.

If rigidity is a feature also look for evidence of *hypokinesia*—reduced levels of spontaneous movement—particularly evident on the face. The combination of hypokinesia and rigidity implies a *neonatal Parkinsonism* phenotype. Other relevant points:

- Dysmorphism?
- Contractures? (Implies antenatal onset).
- Jaw rigidity? (Suggesting tetanus).
- OFC and fontanelle (↑ intracranial pressure?).
- Excessive startle to noise or tactile stimulus, particularly tapping the nose (a feature of hyperekplexia).
- Examine both child and mother for myotonia and myokymia (channelopathies).

- Eye movement abnormalities? (Examine by doll's eye manoeuvre)—suggesting e.g. hydrocephalus. Aicardi–Goutières syndrome, or sepiapterin reductase deficiency.
- Reflexes.

History

Note the timing of rigidity onset. If stiffness presents within 24 h of delivery consider hypoxic–ischaemic encephalopathy (HIE); however, this attribution must be evidenced and warranted (see Box 4.2 in Chapter 4 ➲ p. 230 for robust criteria). If evidence for HIE is equivocal, *or stiffness persists more than first 24–48 h*, think carefully about alternatives as the early stiffness of HIE is usually transient.

Conversely, however, MRI evidence of mild/moderate acute HIE can be subtle and occasionally a child will be worked up for an alternative cause of early hypertonia only for a retrospective attribution to HIE to be made based on subtle thalamic changes on MRI evident at 2 or 3 yrs of age.

- Pointers to *antenatal onset* include presence of contractures/arthrogryposis.
- Obviously a full obstetric, family, and pregnancy history is also important.

Investigations

Early (first 24 h) and/or acute presentations
- MRI.
- EEG (? tonic seizures).
- Ca^{2+}, $Mg2+$.
- Biotinidase.
- Amino acids.
- CSF neurotransmitters, amino acids.
- TORCH screen if imaging and/or history suggestive.
- Consider therapeutic trial of benzodiazepines if hyperekplexia suspected.

If no diagnosis made, proceed to further investigations:
- Paired blood and CSF lactate, amino acids, glucose (and neurotransmitters if not already done).
- aCGH and genetics review. Consider WGS/WES.
- Consider muscle and skin biopsies for mitochondrial studies.

Suspected peripheral cause
- EMG/NCS.
- K^+, Ca^{2+}, Mg^{2+}.
- Skeletal survey for skeletal dysplasias.

Treatment

In all unexplained hypertonia, a trial of L-DOPA (see Levodopa in Chapter 7 ➲ p. 682) should be considered although CSF neurotransmitter sampling should ideally be performed first. In suspected *peripheral*-origin rigidity consider trials of carbamazepine or phenytoin (ion-channel dysfunction).

Further reading: See Hart *et al*, *Dev. Med. Child Neurol.* 2015;57: 600–610 for a review of the approach to the hypertonic neonate.

Swallowing and feeding problems

Mechanism of normal swallowing

- *First stage*: oral (voluntary). Tongue pushed against the palate, forcing food into the pharynx. Problems with this stage are usually due to impaired control of the tongue during swallowing causing difficulty keeping liquid in the mouth, difficulty chewing food, pocketing of food in the vestibule of the mouth, or aspiration of food during inhalation.
- *Second stage*: pharyngeal (involuntary). Receptors with afferents in V and IX trigger efferent signals via V, IX, X, and XII to elevate the soft palate, seal the nasopharynx and close the glottis, and move the larynx under the base of tongue. Food is passed into the oesophagus. Problems with this phase may lead to retention of food in the pharynx and aspiration.
- *Third stage*: oesophageal (involuntary). Liquids usually fall by gravity; peristaltic waves push solids along (innervated by X). Problems with this phase can occur when there are motility disorders, mechanical obstruction, or impaired opening of the lower oesophageal sphincter.

Causes of swallowing disorders in children

Neurological disorders that affect swallowing commonly also affect speech (see Speech difficulties in this chapter ➜ p. 197) and vice versa, although they may occur in isolation and as such are discussed separately.

- *Structural abnormality*: oesophagitis, gastro-oesophageal reflux, oesophageal strictures (e.g. secondary to ingested caustic material), tracheo-oesophageal fistula, impaction of a foreign body, cleft palate, or velopharyngeal insufficiency (e.g. 22q11 deletion syndrome).
- *Neurological disorders*: (see Speech difficulties in this chapter ➜ p. 197).
- Motility disorders.
- Connective tissue diseases, e.g. dermatomyositis.
- Functional.
- *Iatrogenic*: large unpalatable tablets (calcium and iron supplements in particular); anticholinergic agents, calcium channel blockers and drugs that ↑ fatigue or oral secretions.

Assessment of disordered swallowing

A multidisciplinary team approach is beneficial in the assessment and management of children with swallowing problems: speech pathologist, dietician, occupational therapist, physiotherapist, psychologist, ENT specialist, neurologist, gastroenterologist, and dentist.

History

- Feeding history: onset of problem (acute or chronic), severity (drooling, choking, coughing with feeds), voice change, nasal regurgitation, retention of food in the mouth, symptoms of gastro-oesophageal reflux.
- Problems with certain textures and consistencies (typically worst with thin liquid, e.g. water).
- Weight, nutritional status, caloric intake, centiles.
- History of medical comorbidities, e.g. recurrent pneumonia, stridor.

Examination
- Physical examination: respiratory and neurological systems (including jaw jerk and gag reflex), ENT (macroglossia, tonsillar hypertrophy, para- or retro-pharyngeal masses, head and neck masses, e.g. goitre), nasal patency (e.g. choanal atresia), cardiovascular system (atrial hypertrophy).
- A water swallow test may be used to check for abnormal drooling or coughing.
- Observe feeding: posture, self-feeding ability, pace of feeding, ability to handle oral secretions, tongue and jaw movements, coughing, the number of swallows required to clear a bolus of food, and noisy airway during swallowing.

Investigation
(See Investigations for aspiration in Chapter 4 ⬆ p. 254).
- Videofluorographic swallowing study.
- Cervical auscultation.
- Functional endoscopic evaluation of swallowing.
- Other tests may be indicated, e.g. oesophagogastroduodenoscopy (OGD), pH study, barium swallow, oesophageal motility studies.

Toe-walking

Toe-walking may be associated with developmental impairment of multiple aetiologies. The usual presentation, however, is of isolated toe-walking in a child with normal development.

Causes

- Primary Idiopathic/Habitual.
- Manifestation of cerebral palsy.
- Transient dystonia of infancy.
- Early DMD or other neuromuscular disease (NB a normal CK only excludes dystrophies, not other non-dystrophic myopathies).
- HMSN.
- Hereditary spastic paraplegia.
- Spinal pathology—tethered cord, occult spinal dysraphism.
- Early leukodystrophy (X-ALD, MLD).

History

- As for 'foot deformities', (see Foot deformities in this chapter **⊃** p. 147).
- Diurnal variation?
- Autistic behaviours, sensory processing disorders.
- Family history.

Examination

- Spine.
- Is it correctible? (Voluntarily, or passively correctible only?)
- Is there Achilles shortening?
- Intrinsic foot deformities?
- Range of movement of joints including upper limbs.
- Long tract signs?
- Diminished reflexes?
- Weakness and/or atrophy? (Proximal—hip extension and abduction; distal—ankle dorsiflexion and eversion).
- Ligamentous laxity—often associated with toe-walking.
- The most sensitive discriminator of idiopathic from secondary forms of toe-walking is the dynamic gait posture (e.g. on Fog testing; see Fog's test in Chapter 1 **⊃** p. 47) which may indicate corticospinal or extrapyramidal dysfunction.

Investigation

- Imaging of brain ± cord if long tract signs are present.
- **❶** Check CK in boys particularly if they are late walking.
- DNA tests for HMSN1 if the child and parent are areflexic. Nerve conduction studies if DNA screen –ve and then proceed to genetic panels of neuropathies.

Empiric treatment (independent of cause)
- Conservative, e.g. accommodative footwear, stretches.
- Casting.
- Botulinum toxin injection to calves (not for lower motor neurone/neuromuscular disorders).
- Surgery, e.g. gastrocnemius recession, tendon lengthening/transfers, osteotomies.

Unsteadiness and falls

▶ Do not make the mistake of assuming a complaint of *unsteadiness* neces-sarily implies or equates to *ataxia*!
   Other causes include:
- Weakness: myopathic (generally proximal) or neuropathic (peripheral).
- Clumsiness (dyspraxia).
- Limb *pain* (particularly exercise-related cramps and discomfort).
- Visual impairment.
- Syncope and other 'funny turns' (see Table 3.5 p. 151) causing altered awareness.
- True vertigo (vestibular or labyrinthine disease).
- Labyrinthitis is occasionally misdiagnosed as ataxia. Labyrinth or vestibular disease will not be associated with past pointing.
- Non-neurological causes.
- Musculo-skeletal factors including leg-length and alignment problems.

History

Time course of symptoms
- Fixed or episodic?
- Duration of episodes?
- Progressive?

Precise nature of symptoms experienced
Complaints of 'dizziness' must be unpacked carefully. True vertigo is much more rare than pre-syncopal 'light-headed' feelings.
- *Pre-syncope*: older children and parents will be familiar with the light-headed sensation associated with suddenly standing up (e.g. after a hot bath).
- *True vertigo*: much rarer. Explicit sensation of motion (usually as if the world is spinning).
- Very rarely 'ship's deck' ataxia (as if the world is 'rolling' side to side), associated with cerebellopontine angle disease.

Associated features?
- Fine motor skills (dressing, ball catching, writing).
- Worse in dark? (implies disordered proprioception).
- Speech (cerebellar dysarthria?).
- Headaches, travel sickness, family history of migraine? (May suggest susceptibility to migrainous processes though such findings are common and may be misleading!)
- Position-dependence (made worse by turning over in bed? Symptoms improved or worsened if head elevated on pillows etc.?)
- Epilepsy?
- Several seizure types can result in fall (see Table 3.7 p. 155).
- Failure to attain motor and speech developmental milestones.

Examination

- Skin (telangiectasia).
- Eye movements (disordered smooth pursuit is a sensitive indicator of cerebellar disease).
- Speech articulation.
- Cerebellar function.
  - Assess truncal coordination (heel–toe-walking) reflecting midline cerebellar (vermis) function and peripheral coordination (finger–nose) that reflects cerebellar hemisphere function (if asymmetrical implies ipsilateral disease).
- Pyramidal tract signs.
  - Subtle pyramidal tract signs can result in falls if the child is catching the tip of their shoe on uneven ground. Examine shoes for evidence of scuffing and wear at the toe.
  - Observe for pronator drift (see Power in Chapter 1 ◆ p. 25).
  - Perform Fog's test (see Real world examination of a grossly normal older child in Chapter 1 ◆ p. 47).
- Joint position sense (proprioception).
  - Romberg sign (↑ body sway in standing when eyes closed).
  - Difficulty touching own nose with finger with eyes closed.
- Fine motor coordination.
  - Finger–thumb movement sequences;
  - Throw ball and clap hands before catching;
  - Handwriting (observe pencil grip).
- Examine for motion-sensitivity by rotating child slowly in chair, shaking head from side to side slowly while looking ahead.

Falls and unsteadiness due to phenomena other than ataxia

Dyspraxia

- Also known as *developmental coordination disorder*.
- Refers to the very common picture of relatively isolated fine motor sequencing problems resulting in clumsiness.
- Affects dressing (shoelaces), writing, and drawing, and (typically) hand–eye coordination tasks such as ball catching.
- ❶ Formal cerebellar signs (e.g. past pointing, or disordered pursuit eye movements) are *incompatible* with a diagnosis of dyspraxia.
- A period of observation may be necessary to distinguish a progressive ataxic disorder from 'mere' dyspraxia—be particularly suspicious if the child is female (male:female ratio in dyspraxia = 4:1).

Vestibular disease

- Associated with true vertigo ± nystagmus.
- Seek ENT opinion.
- Consider opsoclonus–myoclonus syndrome in toddler/pre-school age group (rare: see Opsoclonus–myoclonus ('dancing eyes and dancing feet') syndrome in Chapter 4 ◆ p. 395).

Channelopathies and metabolic myopathies

Consider particularly in the case of exercise-related unsteadiness:
- Periodic paralyses.
- Congenital myotonia.

- GLUT1 deficiency.
- Other metabolic myopathies.

Ataxia

- Cerebellar.
- Sensory.
  - Due to large fibre neuropathy or dorsal column disease;
  - Impaired joint position sense and vibration sense;
  - Worse in the dark due to loss of compensatory visual information on body position. Romberg test will be +ve.
- *Mixed* ataxias (with both cerebellar *and* sensory ataxia) occur in Friedreich ataxia (a spino- and cerebellar degeneration), and in children who have received vincristine for posterior fossa tumours (the posterior fossa surgery causing the cerebellar ataxia and the vincristine the sensory ataxia).

Consider whether ataxia is acute or chronic, progressive, or non-progressive, or episodic.

Acute ataxia

- *Onset over hours*: consider intoxication as very probable.
- *Onset over hours to days*: consider parainfective processes including acute disseminated encephalomyelitis.
- *Onset over days to weeks*: consider expanding posterior fossa space-occupying lesion.

Causes of acute, subacute, and acute recurrent ataxia

- Post-infectious cerebellitis.
  - A parainfective subacute onset ataxia is particularly characteristic 7–14 days post-varicella. Conservative treatment only is required (see Acute post-infectious cerebellitis in Chapter 4 ⟳ p. 370).
- Miller–Fisher syndrome (see Miller–Fisher syndrome in Chapter 4 ⟳ p. 436).
- Episodic ataxias type 1 and 2 (see Episodic ataxias in Chapter 4 ⟳ p. 326).

Recurrent ataxias

Good spells and bad spells, lasting days or weeks. Consider:

- Paraneoplastic: particularly opsoclonus–myoclonus (see Opsoclonus–myoclonus ('dancing eyes and dancing feet') syndrome in Chapter 4 ⟳ p. 395) typically with nystagmus and involvement of the arms and hands ± upper trunk.
- NARP (neuropathy ataxia and retinitis pigmentosa with the 8993 mtDNA mutation). Recurrent ataxia without nystagmus. Retinal findings can be subtle.

Slowly progressive ataxias (over months to years) with initial symptom-free period

- Nearly all genetically determined progressive ataxias of older childhood are both (i) extremely rare and (ii) dominantly inherited with high penetrance so that a family history will be informative (see Spinocerebellar ataxias in Chapter 4 ⟳ p. 426).

- Friedreich ataxia (FA, see Friedreich ataxia in Chapter 4 🔂 p. 425) is the most important *recessively* inherited progressive ataxia (i.e. where family history is –ve).
- In toddlers consider ataxia telangiectasia (AT; see Ataxia telangectasia in Chapter 4 🔂 p. 468).

Congenital, non-, or slowly progressive ataxias with no initial symptom-free period

- If imaging suggests unilateral or very asymmetric cerebellar involvement, the cause is probably acquired (e.g. vascular) insult.
- Identification of the anatomical pattern of cerebellar involvement (e.g. distinguishing a pan-cerebellar process from one primarily affecting the vermis and midline) can help narrow the differential (see Congenital, non-progressive ataxias with no initial symptom-free period in Chapter 4 🔂 p. 423).

Suggested approach to initial investigation of chronic non-progressive or slowly progressive cerebellar disorders

See also Congenital, non-progressive ataxias with no initial symptom-free period in Chapter 4 🔂 p. 423.

- MRI.
- Fasting cholesterol/triglycerides and lipoprotein profile.
- Blood film (acanthocytes, vacuolated lymphocytes).
- LFT and CK.
- Transferrin isoforms.
- Amino and organic acids.
- Capillary pH, plasma lactate, mitochondrial DNA deletions.
- α-fetoprotein.
- Vitamin E.
- Consider EMG/NCV for evidence of peripheral neuropathy.
- Consider increasingly available 'ataxia gene panels' or equivalents.
- See also 🔗 www.ataxia.org.uk for current guidance in a fast-moving field.

Visual disturbance

Visual impairment (VI) may be:
- Congenital or acquired.
- Of sudden or progressive onset.
- Isolated, with a purely ocular basis, or associated with neurological or other systemic disease in a setting of multiple impairments.

VI profoundly impacts a child's development, social, education, and employment opportunities. In low income countries, around 50% of children die within a few years of the onset of blindness. Even in high income countries, 10% of children die within 1 year of diagnosis of severe VI.

Visual acuity

- Conventional 'Snellen' acuities such as 6/60 imply 'patient can only see at 6 metres distance letters that general population can read at 60 metres'. Normal vision is thus '6/6' (or in North America '20/20 (yards)').
- More commonly nowadays expressed as 'logarithm of the Minimum Angle of Resolution (logMAR)'.
  - logMAR acuity charts address several technical limitations of traditional Snellen charts.
- logMAR effectively a measure of *visual loss*:
  - Normal vision is 0 logMAR (Snellen 6/6 =1; $\log_{10}1=0$).
  - A value <0 implies better than normal vision.
  - A value >0 implies reduced acuity: 6/60 = 1 logMAR ($\log_{10}(60/6) = 1$).
  - Counting fingers corresponds to ~2 logMAR and perceiving light to ~3 logMAR.
- WHO definition of blindness: best-corrected acuity >1.3 logMAR.

Normal visual development milestones

See Table 3.17.

Table 3.17 Normal visual development milestones

Reliably present from 31 weeks gestation	Pupillary light reflex, blink response and dazzle response (eyelid remains closed in presence bright light) NB these reflexes only depend on brainstem structures: they do not indicate cortical vision
By 6 weeks post-term	Fixing and following (human face at 30 cm is best target)
From 3 months post-term	Visually directed grasping (needs concurrent motor development)
By 5 months post-term	Blink in response to threat

VEP: see response from 30 weeks gestational age, mature flash/pattern response by 3–4 months post-term; response to orientation reversal later.

Age of child and mode of presentation

See Table 3.18.

Table 3.18 Age of child and presentations of visual disease

Infant	**Take parental concerns seriously**
	***Persistent* squint is abnormal at any age** (see Eye movement abnormalities in this chapter ➐ p. 130)
	Not fixing and following, poor eye contact
	Epiphora, photophobia (will be less apparent if born in winter)
Pre-school	Fails to imitate others. Delayed development, distractible, immature
	Sits too close to TV; prefers toys with sounds.
	New squint, scared in dim light, photophobia.
	Clumsy, falling, 'ataxic', acute refusal to walk
School age	Gradual onset visual impairment may present as school failure
	Specific complaints of blurred or weak vision
	In acute onset 'grey-black curtain descending' or fogging

Key points on history taking
- First episode or recurrent?
- Unilateral or bilateral?
- Painless loss of vision in one eye like a 'wall developing' after trauma? (Retinal detachment).
- Photophobia?
- Headache, nausea (symptoms of ↑ intracranial pressure)?
- Tearing, painful eye, nausea, and vomiting (symptoms of ↑ intraocular pressure (IOP)/glaucoma)?
- Medical history: hypertension?
- Drugs: vigabatrin (field defects), phenytoin (blurred vision in toxicity), chemotherapy?
- Abnormal colour vision (optic neuritis)?

Careful history and stepwise examination of the visual pathway from anterior to posterior will suggest specific ophthalmological, electro-diagnostic, laboratory, and radiological investigations.

Localizing value of visual field defects
See Figure 3.7.

Children may report a visual symptom 'in one eye' but mean 'to one side of my visual world'.

❶ A visual field deficit (or indeed any visual sign or symptom) that is truly confined to one eye (i.e. it disappears when that eye is closed) is due to pathology anterior to the optic chiasm (A).

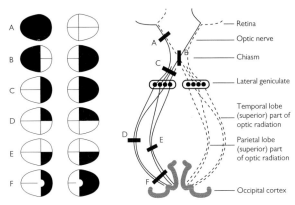

Fig. 3.7 Localization of visual field defects.

- Chiasmatic lesions (B) typically give bi-temporal hemianopia.
- A homonymous hemianopia (C) arises from a lesion in the contralateral optic tract.
- Temporo-parietal lobe lesions result in partial deficits, rarely precisely quadrantanopic (D, E).
- A branch of the middle cerebral artery supplying the area of occipital cortex relating to the macula allows posterior cerebral artery lesions affecting the occipital cortex to result in 'macular sparing' (F).

Key points on examination from anterior to posterior
- External inspection: microphthalmia, dysmorphism, coloboma?
- Visual acuity: light and movement perception, fixing and following?
- Visual fields?
- Eye movements: dysconjugate gaze, nystagmus, cranial nerve palsies, squint? (See Cranial nerves III, IV, and VI in Chapter 1 ⤵ p. 17).
- Pupils: retinal (red) reflex; light and accommodation reflex; relative afferent pupillary defect (RAPD); leukocoria; fixed mid-position pupil in ↑ IOP?
- Roving eye movements? (Strong indicator of pathology anterior to chiasm).
- A *red and painful eye* needs dilated slit lamp examination with fluorescein by an ophthalmologist to exclude keratopathy, ulcer, infection, ↑ IOP, or an intraocular foreign body.
- Cornea and lens: cloudy cornea, cataract.
- Fundoscopy: swollen optic nerve disc (papillitis)? Central retinal artery occlusion (causing sudden painless and unilateral blindness)?

❶ Optic neuritis (papillitis) and papilloedema have very similar fundoscopic appearances but distinguishing them should not be difficult.
• *Visual loss is prominent in papillitis* and is the usual presenting complaint (only in the mildest cases is it confined to loss of colour vision).
• Visual impairment in papilloedema occurs as a result of chronic optic nerve ischaemia and as such usually only occurs in very longstanding situations (e.g. mis-managed idiopathic intracranial hypertension, see Idiopathic intracranial hypertension in Chapter 4 ➸ p. 347) or fulminant situations with severe elevation of ICP (where prompt intervention may save vision).

Visual impairment from birth

All babies with apparent visual impairment (VI) should be seen by an ophthalmologist.

Clues from history
• High-risk baby? Prematurity, family history of squint, amblyopia, or VI; perinatal infection; maternal medications.
• Development? VI interferes with all areas of development (social and fine motor more than language or gross motor). Forty per cent of children with VI have learning difficulties and/or CP.
• Behaviour? Blind babies may eye-poke; VI babies may wave their hands in front of a light source.

Clues from examination
• *External*. Microphthalmia, aniridia, albinism, buphthalmos, dysmorphism, colobomata.
• *Cornea*. Clouding seen in mucopolysaccharidoses and Fabry disease; less commonly in GM1 gangliosidosis, Pelizaeus–Merzbacher, Zellweger, and foetal alcohol syndrome.
• *Lens*. High myopia, cataract, dislocation (Ehlers–Danlos, Marfan, homocystinuria).
• *Fundoscopy*:
  • Abnormal vitreous: haemorrhage, retinoblastoma, persistent primary hyperplastic vitreous, retinopathy of prematurity;
  • Abnormal disc: optic nerve hypoplasia, optic atrophy;
  • Abnormal retina: normal ERG (toxoplasmosis); abnormal ERG (Leber congenital amaurosis, retinal dystrophy).

If all examination findings are normal, consider:
• Cortical blindness. Occipital lobe injury: abnormalities on MRI.
• Delayed visual maturation. Visually unresponsive in early months of life then develop normal vision; other developmental domains may be affected.
• Congenital idiopathic.

Leber congenital amaurosis
- Most common inherited cause of congenital VI, usually autosomal recessive.
- Rod-cone dystrophy and retinal degeneration.
- Presents at birth or in the first months of life with roving eyes or upbeat nystagmus, photophobia, day-blindness, and eye-poking.
- Sluggish pupillary light responses.
- The retina in infancy may appear normal; pigmentary retinopathy and disc pallor develop with age.
- ERG and VEP are usually undetectable from the outset.
- Associated features include cerebellar atrophy and learning difficulties.

Cataracts in childhood
Less than half are idiopathic; all warrant a vigorous search for aetiology.
- Congenital infections (rubella).
- Inborn errors of metabolism (galactosaemia, Morquio).
- Chromosomal abnormalities (trisomies 13, 18, 21, Turner syndrome).
- Maternal drugs and exposure (corticosteroids, chlorpromazine, radiation, malnutrition, diabetes).
- Biochemical derangement (hypocalcaemia, pseudohypoparathyroidism).
- Inherited conditions (hereditary spherocytosis, neurofibromatosis type 2, myotonic dystrophy).

Cerebral visual impairment
VI due to visual pathway or occipital cortical injury or dysfunction is a common feature of both developmental and postnatally acquired brain injury (see Vision in Chapter 4 ➲ p. 258).

Acquired visual impairment
For sudden onset monocular visual loss (see Sudden onset visual loss in Chapter 6 ➲ p. 634).

Acquired VI in childhood is likely to have a primary ocular cause, in contrast to adults, in whom occipital cortical ischaemia and emboli are common.

Differentiating acute from progressive onset may not be straightforward. Slowly progressive loss may be perceived as of abrupt onset (e.g. progressive visual field restriction is usually only reported once it involves the macula at which point a 'sudden deterioration' is reported). Progressive visual loss is usually noticed by a teacher or parent rather than by the child. It is therefore best to consider both acute and progressive causes in every child (Tables 3.19 and 3.20). In addition, the causes of progressive loss overlap with the causes of congenital blindness.

Anterior visual pathway (pre-chiasmatic and chiasmatic)

Posterior visual pathway (post-chiasmatic)

Progressive visual impairment
Leber hereditary optic neuropathy (LHON)
See Leber hereditary optic neuropathy in Chapter 4 ➲ p. 409.

Table 3.19 Causes of visual loss: **pre-chiasmatic** sites and mode of presentation

Site	Acute		Progressive	
	Pathology	Condition	Pathology	Condition
Cornea	Scarring	Vitamin A deficiency; harmful traditional medicines		Keratoconus (trisomy 21)
Lens				Cataract, dislocation
Macula		Photic damage		Dystrophy
Retina	Trauma	Non-accidental injury (NAI), detached retina	Intraocular tumour	
	Vascular	Migraine, central retinal artery occlusion	Tapeto-retinal degeneration	Metabolic disease, NCLs, Laurence–Moon–Biedl, Refsum, Usher, Cockayne
Optic nerve	Inflammation	Optic neuritis, papillitis	Optic atrophy	LHON, other neuropathies
	Compression	↑ ICP, ↑ IOP, trauma, orbital, and extraocular tumour, bone disease (osteopetrosis), infection (abscess, sinusitis)	Ischaemia	Idiopathic intracranial hypertension, ↑ ICP, ↑ IOP, tumour aneurysm, arteriovenous malformation
	Trauma			
	Tumour			Optic glioma
	Ischaemia	Hypotension, systemic vascular disease		
Chiasm	Tumour	Craniopharyngioma, pituitary, hypothalamic tumour		

Table 3.20 Causes of visual loss: **post-chiasmatic** sites and mode of presentation

Site	Acute		Progressive	
	Pathology	Condition	Pathology	Condition
Optic radiation	Inflammation, trauma, tumour, radiation		Tumour	
Visual cortex	Inflammation	Acute disseminated encephalomyelitis	Inflammation	Rasmussen syndrome
	Compression	Trauma, tumour, hydrocephalus	Compression	Tumour, hydrocephalus
	Infection	Abscess, meningitis, cerebral malaria		
	Vascular	Migraine, cluster headaches, haemorrhage, infarct, anoxia		
	Epilepsy	Childhood onset visual epilepsy		
	Post-traumatic transient cerebral blindness			
Systemic	Hypoglycaemia	Glycogen storage disease, insulin therapy		
	Hypo-/ hypertension			
	Toxicity/ nutritional	Anti-TB drugs, sulphonamides, chloramphenicol, desferrioxamine, penicillamine, vincristine and BCNU, ciclosporin, heavy metals, and solvents		
Other	Functional			Stimulus deprivation amblyopia
				Chronic progressive external ophthalmoplegia (mitochondrial)

Compressive optic neuropathies
Refer to Table 3.21.

Table 3.21 Causes of compressive optic neuropathies

Region	Clinical features
Intraocular tumours	Always diminish visual acuity
	New squint: impaired acuity (sighted eye fixes, blind eye deviates)
	Leukocoria: ('white pupil'—absence of normal red ocular light reflex) should prompt immediate referral for potentially life-saving recognition of retinoblastoma
Retro-orbital tumours	Strabismus and proptosis
	Visual field defects occur late
Tumours around the chiasm	Craniopharyngioma: associated growth failure and endocrinopathies
	Bi-temporal hemianopia in 50%
	I, III, or VI nerve involvement if anterior extension
	Pituitary adenomas: only 1–2% of childhood intracranial tumours, 1/3 secrete ACTH, 1/3 secrete prolactin, 1/3 are silent

Stimulus deprivation amblyopia
- Reduced visual acuity in one eye.
- Adverse consequence of untreated cataract, squint, or refractive error.
- Age-dependent: highest risk up to 3 yrs, little risk after 6 yrs.

Toxic, nutritional
- Usually present with ↓ acuity and colour vision, especially if there are central scotomata.
- Usually dose related (see Table 3.20 ➲ p. 215). Reduce the dose or withdraw the causative drug. Consider B12/folate therapy.

Idiopathic intracranial hypertension
See Idiopathic intracranial hypertension in Chapter 4 ➲ p. 347.

Inborn errors of metabolism
Juvenile NCL is an important cause of progressive visual loss in primary school age children (see School age (5–12 years) in Chapter 4 ➲ p. 478). Most other metabolic disorders do not usually *present* with visual disturbance, although eye features are common (see Table 1.2 Chapter 1 ➲ p. 20).

Specific conditions

Acquired brain injury

The term 'acquired' brain injury (ABI) comprises a very heterogeneous group of conditions (stroke, hypoxic–ischaemic injury, inflammation, trauma etc.) with very different acute management approaches. The value of the ABI concept, as with 'cerebral palsy', is primarily operational. These children share:

- The consequences of injury after a period of normal development that will *interact with ongoing development* in complex ways.
- Patterns of injury that are often *focal or multifocal* leading to idiosyncratic and unusual combinations of impairments.
- Having to address needs *acquired 'overnight'* in a system (particularly within education) built to support children with slowly evolving, developmentally related needs.
- The 'bereavement' of *losing the 'child that was'* (both family and child remember that things used not to be this way).
- A sudden need to learn how to navigate *'The System'*.
- In some cases (particularly traumatic injury acquired through 'misadventure'), additional challenges created by pre-existing behavioural traits and family/social factors.

Recognition of 'low-level' states

Consciousness can simplistically be envisaged as having two components:
- *Arousal* (i.e. eyes open, not asleep): largely a function of *brainstem* structures (particularly the pontine reticular activating system).
- *Awareness*: evidence of sensory and cognitive processes reflecting function of the cerebral *cortex*.

These can be dissociated: arousal without any awareness occurs in unresponsive wakefulness syndrome (UWS: a less pejorative synonym for vegetative state).
- Arousal can be readily assessed: the eye-opening scale of the Glasgow Coma Scale (GCS) is essentially a measure of arousal (pontine integrity).
- Awareness can only be established by the observation of *behaviours that occur consistently in response to external events* (with eye movement and speech considered as specialized forms of behaviour).
- If a child has very limited reliable voluntary control of movement, he/she may not be able to demonstrate their awareness. This can occur in so-called 'locked-in' syndrome although some preservation of eye movement is usual.
- Pure locked-in syndrome is extremely rare. MRI findings (pontine lesions with sparing of cortex) and/or preservation of relatively normal EEG rhythms may alert the team to the possibility.
- Much more commonly a child's voluntary movements are present but are very delayed or inconsistent.
  - The term minimally conscious state (MCS) refers to the spectrum of very severe impairment but with some limited demonstrable awareness. Identifying low levels of awareness requires careful and skilled multidisciplinary assessment to identify movements (typically blinks, eye movements, vocalizations, or limb movements) that are

under some voluntary control, although responses may be delayed by many seconds, and inconsistent.
- Suitable 'control' requests are important to avoid false +ve situations (e.g. to avoid the danger of issuing a command — 'squeeze my hand'—repeatedly until the action occurs by chance).
- Use of a mirror to allow a child to see his or her own face is the most potent stimulus for visual fixation.

Acute medical management of ABI

- Early fluid management.
  - May have been fluid-restricted on PICU;
  - Insensible losses may be high if agitated and/or pyrexial;
  - Hyponatraemia can be iatrogenic (hypotonic fluids), or due to SIADH or cerebral salt wasting: see Hyponatraemia in a neuro-intensive care setting in Chapter 5 ➲ p. 581.
- Management of early agitation: see Acute behavioural disturbance in Chapter 6 ➲ p. 610.
  - Common after severe injury.
  - Environmental interventions are the primary approach: nurse in a well-lit, quiet setting (preferably cubicle). Consider nursing on a floor mattress if at risk of coming out of bed (although also need to consider lifting and handling issues for nurses).
  - Paradoxically, stimulant therapy (e.g. methylphenidate) can be effective.
  - Avoid benzodiazepines (chlorpromazine acceptable if no alternative).
  - In the context of traumatic injury, extracranial fractures may occasionally be missed during the PICU phase. Evaluate carefully for bony injury if there is unexplained distress on movement.
  - Monitor skin integrity carefully: a degree of muscle wasting, and weight loss can be seen post-PICU, and agitation can result in friction abrasions: consider pressure-relieving mattress.
- Aggressive prevention of contractures (splinting, botulinum toxin).
  - High-dose enteral baclofen may be required but watch for unwanted sedative effects complicating assessment of awareness.
- Heterotopic/ectopic calcification in muscle bellies: calcification of micro-haemorrhages and tears resulting from severe spasticity and/or physiotherapy stretches.
  - Consider if passive stretching becomes painful after a period.
  - Ossification identified on plain X-ray or muscle ultrasound.
  - Treat with NSAIDs: stretching and maintenance of range of movement (ROM) is likely to still be a priority.
- Involvement of appropriate colleagues in assessment of bulbar function; early mobilization; and evaluation of hearing and vision as a prelude to the re-establishment of communication.
- Nutrition and appropriate feeding strategies.
  - Constipation is very common and can be distressing.
  - Gastro-oesophageal reflux disease (GORD).
  - Hyperalimentation has been shown to improve neurological outcome.

- Consider evaluation of pituitary function particularly in context of fractures of the skull base (due to risk of trauma to pituitary stalk). Routine screening is not justified.
- Treatment of seizures.
  - *Prophylactic* ASM therapy is unwarranted.
  - Exclude hyponatraemia.
- Treat respiratory disease (e.g. aspiration due to impaired bulbar function).
  - Liaise over closure of tracheostomy if performed during the PICU phase.

Central dysautonomia syndrome
- Also known as hypothalamic-midbrain dysregulation, paroxysmal sympathetic hyperactivity, or central hyperpyrexia.
- Characterized by tachycardia, marked hyperpyrexia (often >40°C), severe muscle stiffness and hyper CK-aemia, profuse agitation, sweating, and hyperventilation.
  - Associated with severe (particularly brainstem) injury and poor outcome;
  - Requires HDU care;
  - Maintain hydration status and monitor fluid balance (high insensible fluid losses; risk of renal impairment from high plasma CK levels);
  - Treat with opiates; clonidine and propranolol also useful.

Age at injury and time since injury

Manifestations of ABI result from a complex interaction between age at injury, time since injury, and the domain of outcome under consideration. While a static concept of 'complete recovery' of a previously fully established function after injury is meaningful in an adult (see Fig. 4.1, left), it is ambiguous in the context of a young child in whom the function was not fully established at the time of injury. Returning to pre-injury levels of function (point A) is not 'full recovery': reaching point B as an adult is. It is

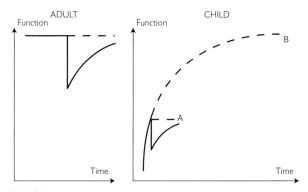

Fig. 4.1 Age at injury.

generally easier to regain previously established function than to establish *de novo* function after injury. It follows that late outcome is generally better for functions that were fully or nearly fully established at the time of injury. In crude terms, motor development completes before language development, which in turn completes before cognitive development: hence the particular concern about late cognitive outcomes in children injured at a young age.

Interdisciplinary working and goal setting

The distinguishing feature of rehabilitation is a process of working together. Multidisciplinary working can become problem based, and focused on impairments, with each professional seeing one part of the picture (dysphasia, contractures, seizures) and addressing it in isolation. In contrast, rehabilitation is characterized by a cross-disciplinary, forward-looking setting of specific, relevant, and measurable goals, ideally involving child and family. This can result in interdisciplinary cooperation.

Typical goals might include:
• Prevent physical deformity.
• Achieve safe, effective means of nutrition.
• Establish a means of communication.
• Get to cousin's wedding next month.
• Identify suitable educational provision.

Medium and long-term medical management

In practice cognitive/behavioural issues and educational liaison/advocacy roles often predominate.
• Fatigue and timing of return to school.
  • arrange graded return to school.
• Behavioural change due to:
  • disordered sleep.
  • post-traumatic stress disorder (PTSD)-like processes.
  • disrupted parenting responses.
  • impulsiveness.
  • inability to perceive sarcasm, teasing, or irony in others' speech, leading to literal ('concrete') interpretation of others' remarks.
  • resulting social isolation.
• Specific cognitive deficits.
  • attentional difficulties.
  • executive (self-organization) difficulties.
  • struggling at times of transition (e.g. to secondary schooling) with sudden jumps in expectations of self-direction and management.
  • arrange for formal neuropsychological assessment: see Neuropsychological testing in Chapter 2 p. 109.

Other issues include:
• Epilepsy.
  • May not manifest until as late as a decade post-injury.
  • Do not assume a causal relationship: check that the EEG is consistent with focal onset at sites of known radiological change and not an entirely unrelated idiopathic generalized epilepsy!
  • Usually fairly-readily controlled with reasonable remission rates.

- Headaches.
  - post-traumatic migraine.
  - post-whiplash.
- Dysgeusia (food tastes 'metallic') usually due to anosmia because of fracture of the cribriform plate. Improves with time.
- Late neuro-endocrine complications of acquired brain injury.
  - Consider testing anterior and posterior pituitary function if suggestive symptomatology, particularly if history of fracture to skull base.
  - Precocious puberty a non-specific late complication of brain injury (particularly hypoxic) in early childhood: may require referral to endocrinology for management.

Psychiatric/emotional issues

A major problem for both child and the rest of the family.
- Siblings often 'side-lined' in family's concern for injured child and can experience feelings of isolation.
- In cases of severe injury, family have a daily reminder of the child they lost and need support to grieve.
- Normal parenting 'boundaries' (i.e. normal disciplining of unacceptable behaviour) are often understandably relaxed in the aftermath of the injury and can be difficult to re-establish.
- Child may experience PTSD symptoms (intrusive flashbacks, etc.) particularly if recall of the event is preserved.
- Secondary behavioural morbidity may occur due to new experiences of educational failure and social isolation if not adequately addressed.

Prognosis

Outcome relates to both *mechanism* and *severity* of the insult.
- Outcome from traumatic brain injury (TBI) is generally considerably better than for anoxic injury, and recovery can continue to be seen for months after injury with rehabilitation.
- In general, younger children make better *motor* outcomes than adults do. This tends to lead a misplaced optimism that 'plasticity' allows the young brain-injured child greater scope for recovery in general. TBI tends to result in predominantly cognitive patterns of morbidity with relatively little residual motor disability (children who 'walk and talk and look reasonably OK'). The cognitive effects of injury (which are ultimately major determinants of functioning in adulthood) tend to compound over the remaining period of development, and deficits tend to become more apparent with time. Typical areas of difficulty include *new learning* (what the child knew at the time of injury is retained but learning efficiency for new material is reduced requiring more repetition: a struggle to 'make a year's progress every year') and *frontal lobe functions* including attention, impulse control, and executive skills: see Executive Functions in Chapter 2 ➋ p. 110.
- Outcome after TBI is notoriously variable and cognitive/behavioural outcome especially late after injury is affected by many injury-independent variables.

- If a child has moved school in the interim the fact of a past TBI may not have been communicated (because the child was thought to have 'recovered') resulting in misattribution of the late difficulties being seen.
- Crude estimates of injury severity can be made using the GCS motor score (see Table 6.1 in Chapter 6 ⊃ p. 613) and particularly duration of post-traumatic amnesia (PTA). This is defined as the period that ends with the restoration of orientation (awareness of time, place, and person) and the ability to form and correctly recall new memories ('Who came to visit you this morning? Who won the football match on Saturday?'). Formal instruments for the assessment of PTA in children exist although they are time-consuming.
- Hypoxic–ischaemic injury has a worse prognosis than traumatic injury of similar apparent initial severity (see Table 4.1).

Table 4.1 Outcome in children still in unresponsive wakefulness (i.e. vegetative state) 30 days after insult (from Heindl. Neuropediatrics. 1996; **27**: 94)

		3 months	6 months	12 months	18 months
Traumatic	Recovered at least low-level consciousness	40%	65%	80%	84%
	Vegetative	60%	35%	20%	15%
	Dead	0%	0%	0%	1%
Hypoxic	Recovered at least low-level consciousness	20%	25%	50%	55%
	Vegetative	76%	70%	40%	27%
	Dead	4%	5%	10%	18%

Acquired spinal cord injury

For emergency management of paraparesis, see The child who suddenly stops walking in Chapter 6 ➲ p. 636.

Causes

Trauma
- Falls and road-traffic accidents with no, or poorly adjusted, seat belts (particularly cervical trauma in young children).
- A flexion-extension injury that doesn't disrupt vertebral alignment can be remarkably inapparent radiologically, an entity described as SCIWORA (spinal cord injury without radiological abnormalities).

Inflammatory
- Post-infectious processes (transverse myelitis, acute disseminated encephalomyelitis: see Demyelinating syndromes in this chapter ➲ p. 265).
- Abscess, tuberculoma.

Infarction
- The anterior spinal artery supplies the ventral two-thirds of the cord. It originates from branches of the vertebral arteries and descends the anterior aspect of the cord, fed variably by branches from segmental arteries at various levels including the artery of Adamkiewicz at around T10. Acute anterior spinal artery infarction can occur spontaneously, reflecting this variable and somewhat insecure blood supply. Onset is typically over several minutes. Sparing of the dorsal parts of the spinal cord (different blood supply) leads to classic picture of paralysis, with *loss of spinothalamic but preservation of dorsal column sensation* (vibration, joint position) (see Fig. 2.11b in Chapter 2 ➲ p. 70).
- Axial spinal imaging may show 'owl's eye' sign: symmetric circular areas of high T2 signal in the metabolically active ventral horns of the grey matter with a corresponding 'pencil-like' linear high T2 signal over several segments in sagittal imaging. (Recall that neuroradiological convention, with dorsal columns at the bottom, is the inverse of images in neuroanatomical textbooks).
- Infarction may be caused by fat embolism following trauma or bone marrow infarction in the context of sickle cell disease.

Compression
- Tumours and other space-occupying lesions: may be *intrinsic* (arising from cord substance) or more commonly extrinsic. Compression due to expansion of a paraspinal neuroblastoma through a vertebral foramen is an important cause.
- Extra-axial haematomas from inflicted injury or rupture of spinal AVM.
- Vertebral disc disease.
- Syringomyelia: expansion of the central canal causing a slowly evolving deficit. May arise as a secondary complication of other spinal diseases.

Acute management
For emergency management, see Spinal cord compression in Chapter 6 ➲ p. 643 and Box 4.1.

Box 4.1 Autonomic dysreflexia

- This is an important problem characteristic of complete lesions above T6.
- Noxious stimuli *below* the level (as trivial as a full bladder or constipation, of which the child has no subjective awareness) lead to ↑reflex sympathetic activity in the disconnected lower cord, vasoconstriction, and sometimes dangerously severe hypertension.
- This is sensed by the CNS *above* the lesion, resulting in ↑vagal tone and (sometimes severe) bradycardia. Above the lesion, vasodilatation results in pounding headache, sweating, and red blotches on the skin.
- Emergency treatment involves the relief of the cause (e.g. catheter blockage) and sitting upright. Extreme care must be taken in administering enemas and other potentially noxious stimuli below the level of the lesion. Glyceryl trinitrate may help relieve the excess vasoconstriction seen in acute attacks.

- Emergency neurosurgical evaluation to consider surgical decompression of cord and/or spinal stabilization by external fixation following traumatic cord injury.
- High-dose steroid therapy to minimize aggravation of cord compression by oedema; typically for 72 h.
- Ventilatory support for high lesions.
- Urinary catheterization and management of constipation.

Prognosis

Depends on aetiology.
- Recovery from extrinsic compression is typically good, but dependent on prompt recognition and decompression.
- Inflammatory injury: 1/3 excellent recovery, 1/3 incomplete, 1/3 poor.
- Vascular injuries (particularly anterior spinal artery syndrome) and severe trauma have the worst prognoses.

Long-term management

Many long-term management issues are shared with children with spina bifida, and these clinics (if available) may be best suited to meet the needs of a child with an acquired paraplegia.

Motor
- Intrathecal baclofen therapy (see Intrathecal baclofen in this chapter ➲ p. 249) may be particularly useful for severe lower-limb spasticity.
- Aggressive contracture prevention.
- Monitor spinal deformity and respiratory disease.
- Correct postural abnormalities.
- Treat and prevent pathological fractures.

Sensory
- Careful skin care: absence of nociception risks skin breakdown with pressure (not being turned), friction (ill-fitting shoes etc.), scalds, cold weather.

Sphincters
- Aggressive management of constipation/faecal incontinence.
- Ensure complete bladder dysfunction: risk of renal failure if 'unsafe' bladder is not managed: see Continence in this chapter ➲ p. 263.

Emotional
- Address lack of independence, depression in teenagers and adults.
- Sexual dysfunction is an important issue after puberty.

Syringomyelia

- Important, potentially reversible cause of spinal cord injury.
- Can arise secondary to craniocervical junction pathology (e.g. Chiari malformation).
- Expansion of central cavity of the cord due to abnormal CSF flow and pressure (symptoms can sometimes be precipitated by a cough, sneeze, or other Valsalva manoeuvre).
- Early signs can be subtle: initially presents with loss of *pain* (pinprick, temperature) but preserved *sensation to light touch*, and normal motor function.
  - Because the fibres of the *spinothalamic tracts* that cross just anterior to the central canal cavity (see Fig. 2.11b in Chapter 2 ➲ p. 70) are the most vulnerable to an expanding central cavity.
- Early syringomyelia is only going to be detected if pain sensation is specifically examined!

Cerebral palsies

Definition

A group of disorders of the development of control of movement and posture attributed to non-progressive events that occurred in the foetal or infant brain. Although the cause is non-progressive, the pattern and severity of the movement disorder may evolve during childhood mimicking a progressive neurological disorder—investigate further if in doubt (see below). Prevalence relates strongly to gestational age and socioeconomic factors and varies internationally: average rate (across all gestations) is approximately 1.5 per 1000 live births but rises markedly to >60 per 1000 live births in children <1500 g birthweight. Many research teams have confirmed a *slowly declining* incidence in CP of pre- and perinatal origin in high income countries over the last decade.

- The plural term 'cerebral palsies' highlights heterogeneity in aetiology, severity of motor impairment, comorbidities, functional ability, and prognosis.

▶ The value of the concept and term 'cerebral palsy' is regularly questioned as an ever-increasing number of primary neurogenetic, neurodevelopmental, and neurometabolic causes are identified. The main justification for its retention is a pragmatic one relating to planning and provision of services: these children tend to have similar clinical courses and needs whatever the cause.

Classic descriptions of the cerebral palsies

Classic categories are based on the predominant movement disorder (spasticity, athetosis, etc.) and the pattern of limb involvement. This is a useful framework for epidemiological studies, but inadequate for clinical management of the individual child.

- Unilateral (upper limb involvement usually > lower limb): 33–38%.
- Bilateral (usually lower-limb predominant): 35–43%.
- Total-body involvement: 6%.
- Dyskinetic, dystonic and athetoid: 7–15%.
- Ataxic: 6%.
- Monoplegia: lower-limb spasticity typical, often presenting late. Poorly represented in epidemiological studies.
- Worster–Drought phenotype:
  - prominent orobuccopharyngeal palsy with marked feeding, speech, and cognitive problems and epilepsy, often due to bilateral perisylvian pathology;
  - under-represented in epidemiological studies.

Classifications for clinical care

A *multiaxial* description of a child with a cerebral palsy is important to facilitate inter-professional communication and therapies, guide investigations, and formulate a prognosis.

The following scheme is suggested for routine clinical care, e.g. to complement the problem list in clinic letters. Evaluate and record the findings along each of the following axes.

Types of movement disorder
- Presence not only of spasticity but often under-recognized concurrent dystonia, dyskinesia/athetosis/hyperkinesia, ataxia, hypotonia.
- Re-evaluate classification at regular intervals, e.g. at annual review.
  - Classifying children below 2–3 yrs age may be inaccurate.
  - Axial and limb hypotonia may evolve to dystonia, dyskinesia, and/or ataxia.
  - Limb spasticity is more difficult to assess than early limb preference.

Pattern of anatomical involvement
- Body parts involved, degree of symmetry.

Severity of motor impairment
- Distinguish and individually quantify spasticity, strength, presence of fixed contractures, and coordination.
- The Gross Motor Function Classification System (GMFCS, ➔ see Gross motor function scales, in this chapter p. 245) provides a widely used and understood functional severity scale.
- The Manual Ability Classification Scale (MACS) describing manual function (➔ see Manual Ability Classification System in this chapter p. 247) is a five-point ordinal scale comparable to the GMFCS.
- The combination of MACS and GMFCS scores usefully describes functional impact of motor impairment.
- Motor impairment scales are less reliable in infants.

Comorbidities
- Create a neurological and systemic problem list, e.g. learning disability, epilepsy, visual impairment, chest infections.
- Cognitive development is difficult to ascertain in young infants.

Functional abilities of daily living
- Transfers; self-cares, etc. Standard measurement tools are available.

Known aetiologies and risk factors
- Nature and timing: prenatal, perinatal, or postnatal/neonatal.

Known neuroimaging findings
- Periventricular leukomalacia, cerebral malformations, hypoxic–ischaemic encephalopathy at term, etc.

Aetiology and risk factors for a cerebral palsy

Multiple risk factors and aetiologies often interact hence it may be more appropriate to talk in terms of a 'causal pathway'. Ascertain risk factors from history, examination, and investigations, particularly MRI.
- 50–60% children with cerebral palsy are born at term: they tend to be more severely impaired than children born pre-term.
- 20% children with cerebral palsy born at <32 weeks.
- Conversely, 14% of survivors of <32 week delivery develop a motor disorder (9% at 31–32 weeks; 32% at 26–26 weeks).
- Risks higher in ♂'s and in lower socioeconomic status families.

Risk factors relevant to >60% of term-born children and >15% of pre-term.

Risk factors at all gestational ages
- Twin pregnancy and twin–twin transfusion.
- Small-for-gestational age.
- Placental dysfunction or abnormalities including placenta praevia.
- Maternal infection or pyrexia.
- Intrauterine infections, e.g. TORCH, HIV.
- Major and minor birth defects including genetic disorders of neuronal proliferation, migration, and organization.
- Kernicterus (rare at term in high income countries; consider in pre-term born infants who develop dyskinetic cerebral palsy).

Risk factors for term infants
Prenatal risk factors
- Maternal disease in pregnancy: hypertension, perinatal infection (especially chorioamnionitis), pre-eclampsia.
- Maternal epilepsy (consider teratogenic risks), intellectual disability, thyroid disease.
- Second or third trimester haemorrhage.

Intrapartum risk factors
- Second stage of labour >1 h duration.
- Induction of labour.
- Meconium-stained liquor, meconium aspiration.
- Delivery method: caesarean section, vacuum extraction, forceps delivery, breech.
- Birth asphyxia.
  - Cooling significantly reduces mortality and major neurodevelopmental disability: see Therapeutic cooling for neonatal encephalopathy in Chapter 5 p. 560.
- Sentinel events:
  - cord prolapse.
  - placental abruption.
  - haemorrhage/shock.

Neonatal risk factors
- Neonatal seizures.
- Hypoglycaemia.
- Infections including meningitis and sepsis.
- Respiratory distress syndrome.
- Hyperbilirubinaemia.
- Perinatal thrombophilia leading to intracranial arterial or venous stroke (consider in hemiplegic cerebral palsy, especially if porencephaly is found on MRI).
- Perinatal cerebral haemorrhage (consider *COL4A1* mutations if there is a family history).

Neonatal encephalopathy
- 24% of term-born children with cerebral palsy had neonatal encephalopathy.
- Development of a cerebral palsy is dependent on the severity of encephalopathy (see Box 5.3 ➲ p. 561):
  - ~25% of those with Sarnat grade II.
  - ~75% fo those with Sarnat grade III.
- Ascribing a cerebral palsy to 'perinatal asphyxia' or 'hypoxic–ischaemic encephalopathy' has medico-legal implications: see Box 4.2.

Box 4.2 Identifying intrapartum hypoxic aetiology

To provide strong evidence that the cerebral palsy is due to an intrapartum hypoxic event in the term infant, look for a history of moderate or severe neonatal encephalopathy (Sarnat grade II or III: see Box 5.3 ➲ p. 561) *in association with:*
- Near-term (>34 weeks) delivery.
- Cerebral palsy with corticospinal involvement or dyskinetic type in keeping with MRI findings.
  - After acute and profound hypoxia-ischaemia: early signal change in deep grey matter and basal ganglia bilaterally; progressing to involvement of pre- and post-central gyri, followed by more widespread hemisphere injury progressing to encephalomalacia in late imaging.
  - After chronic partial injury hypoxia-ischaemia: signal change in parasagittal subcortical white matter ('watershed' regions), again progressing to encephalomalacia.
- Umbilical arterial acidosis (pH <7.0 and base deficit >12 mM) or foetal scalp pH of a similar degree.
- Any combination of the following indicators of an intrapartum event:
  - abnormal foetal heart rate on tocograph;
  - difficult delivery or other history suggestive of a hypoxic event around the time of labour;
  - low Apgar scores (<7 at 5 min);
  - need for resuscitative measures at delivery;
  - early multiorgan dysfunction;
  - early imaging suggestive of acute cerebral injury, e.g. cerebral oedema on cranial ultrasound and ↓resistance index in cerebral Doppler studies.

Evidence *against* intrapartum hypoxia as the main cause
- History of only mild neonatal encephalopathy (Sarnat grade I).
- Family history of cerebral palsy (particularly a sibling).
- Predominantly ataxic movement disorder.
- Congenital microcephaly or other major anomalies.
- Intrauterine growth retardation.
- Presence of significant prenatal risk factors e.g. amnionitis, major abruption.

(Continued)

Box 4.2 *(Contd.)*

- CNS or systemic infection.
- Significant postnatal risk factors, e.g. prolonged hypoxia and hypotension.
- Inherited coagulopathy.
- Early imaging findings suggestive of long-standing injury, e.g. ventriculomegaly, cystic encephalomalacia.
- Neuroimaging findings atypical for injury at term: schizencephaly or other malformations of cortical development; periventricular leukomalacia (see MRI and brain development in Chapter 2 ➋ p. 71).
- Progression of motor signs (note however that ataxia and dyskinesia *are* often preceded by a period of hypotonia in infancy).
- Normal MRI brain: consider trial of L-DOPA to identify DOPA-responsive dystonia.

Pre-term aetiological risk factors
Neonatal risk factors
- Chorioamnionitis (the most important).
- Gestational age.
- Respiratory distress syndrome.
- Hypocarbia.
- Pneumothorax.
- Intraventricular haemorrhage.
- Hypoglycaemia.
- Hyperbilirubinaemia.

Post-neonatal-onset cerebral palsies
By convention children sustaining insults in the first 24 months of life are regarded as having a cerebral palsy, rather than an acquired brain injury, although this is obviously an arbitrary threshold.
Causes include:
- Meningoencephalitis.
- Traumatic head injury (especially inflicted brain injury).
- Hypoxic–ischaemic events, e.g. near-drowning, prolonged hypotension.
- Arterial ischaemic/haemorrhagic stroke.

The prevalence of post-neonatal-onset cerebral palsy (acquired between 28 days and 2 yrs) in developed countries is ~1 per 10,000 live births, accounting for only 5% of cerebral palsy. It is more prevalent in developing countries.

Investigations and differential diagnosis
Cerebral palsy is a clinical diagnosis. In a child with a consistent clinical picture, and an explanatory history, investigations may not be necessary. It is usually possible to make a 'positive' diagnosis of cerebral palsy: it is not normally a diagnosis of exclusion unless no known risk factor can be identified. There may be a role for investigations in understanding 'why' cerebral palsy has happened. Investigations may also have a role in identifying specific comorbidities.

When to consider an alternative diagnosis than cerebral palsy
- Absence of known risk factors in history.
- Family history of progressive neurological disorders.
- Any loss of previously attained ability (i.e. regression).
- Development of unexpected focal neurological signs.
- MRI findings not in keeping with a clinical diagnosis of cerebral palsy including those of progressive neurological disorders.

Conditions that can mimic a cerebral palsy

Any pattern
- Intracranial space-occupying lesion.
- DOPA-responsive dystonias.
- Mitochondrial disorders (very slow progression possible).
- Metabolic leukodystrophies.
- Urea cycle disorders—mild OCT deficiency (particularly in ♀s), argininosuccinic aciduria.

Predominantly lower-limb spastic weakness (diplegia)
- Spinal cord lesion (ask about continence, check sensation).
- Hereditary spastic paraplegias: see Hereditary spastic paraparesis in this chapter ➔ p. 481.
- Cerebral folate deficiency, arginase deficiency, biotinidase deficiency, Sjögren–Larsson, HIV.

Ataxia

▶ Treat all diagnoses of 'ataxic cerebral palsy' with suspicion!

- Genetic disorders.
- Biotinidase deficiency, infantile neuroaxonal dystrophy, Pelizaeus–Merzbacher, ataxia telangiectasia (tend to be progressive).
- Other non-progressive genetic ataxias (see Congenital, non-progressive ataxias with no initial symptom-free period in this chapter ➔ p. 423).
- Cerebellar mass lesions.

Dyskinesia/dystonia
- DOPA-responsive dystonia.
- GLUT1 deficiency syndrome.
- Glutaric aciduria type 1.
- *GNAO1* related encephalopathy.
- *ADCY5* mutations.
- Lesch–Nyhan.
- Mitochondrial disorders.
  - PDH deficiency.
- NBIA/PKAN.
- In older children consider:
  - Wilson disease (treatable);
  - Isolated genetic dystonia (e.g. DYT-TOR1A, DYT-KMT2B);
  - Juvenile Huntington and Parkinsonism.

Hypotonia
- May precede ataxic and dyskinetic cerebral palsy, but also neuromuscular disorders.
- Common feature in global developmental impairment.

Specific diagnostic investigations for mimics of Cerebral Palsy

When a clinical diagnosis of cerebral palsy is insecure (e.g. lack of clear risk factors; incompatible findings on clinical examination) MRI is the single most useful investigation and will focus subsequent investigations. In addition:
- CT brain may be occasionally useful as focal or diffuse calcifications can be missed on MRI (neurophakomatoses, TORCH, pseudo-TORCH, Aicardi–Goutières).
- MRI spine (in all cases of diplegia where MRI brain is normal).
- Consider MR spectroscopy in mitochondrial disorders, creatine deficiency disorders.
- EEG where epilepsy is suspected clinically (characteristic findings in Rett syndrome, infantile neuroaxonal dystrophy).
- aCGH.
- WES/WGS should particularly be considered in children with 'idiopathic' dyskinetic cerebral palsy as a number of monogenic causes of CP (e.g. *TUBA1A*, *CTNNB1*, *FBXO3*, *RHOB*) have been identified, some of which are amenable to symptomatic treatment.

Where appropriate (e.g. if above investigations have been either suggestive or non-informative) *consider*:
- TORCH—CMV, Toxoplasma, HIV. Guthrie card blood spot PCR test.
- Blood acylcarnitines.
- Ammonia: ↑in urea cycle disorders (can be intermittent in arginase deficiency although arginine always ↑).
- Lactate.
- Urine organic acids, amino acids, muco/oligopolysaccharides, sulphite.
- Plasma aminoacids and total homocysteine.
- Plasma uric acid.
- Lysosomal enzymes.
- VLCFA (adrenoleukodystrophy, or other peroxisomal disorders).
- Biotinidase (see Biotinidase deficiency in this chapter ➋ p. 525).
- Coagulopathy screen can be considered in hemiplegia associated with unilateral MRI lesion although yield in the commonest scenario of straightforward large-vessel middle cerebral artery territory ischaemic stroke will be very low (this typically due to embolism from placental clot via right-to-left foetal circulation connection).
- Transferrin isoelectric focusing: congenital disorders of glycosylation (CDGs), particularly CDG1a (phosphomannomutase 2 Deficiency) can present with hypotonia and ataxia.
  - Note that transferrin isoforms can give a false –ve, i.e. be misleadingly normal, in the first 3–4 weeks of life.
- Serum copper and caeruloplasmin (low in Menkes, Wilson); urine copper ↑in Wilson.
- CSF studies:

- • ↓CSF: blood glucose in GLUT1 deficiency syndrome;
  - • CSF lactate for mitochondrial disorders;
  - • CSF neurotransmitter studies, including CSF folate, for DOPA-responsive dystonias, cerebral folate deficiency;
  - • CSF glycine and serine if neonatal seizures and progressive microcephaly (non-ketotic hyperglycinaemia (high levels) and 3-phophoglycerate dehydrogenase deficiency (low levels)).
- • Nerve conduction studies (hereditary neuropathy can present with toe-walking and tight Achilles tendons).
- • Investigations for causes of developmental impairment as indicated: see Developmental Impairment in Chapter 3 ➔ p. 120.
- • Ophthalmological, auditory, and speech and language evaluation.

MRI brain findings: diagnostic and prognostic implications

(See also MRI and brain development in Chapter 2 ➔ p. 71).

No brain lesions

Approximately 10% of children in historical cohorts have no brain lesions; well-described in ataxia and dyskinesia-predominant cerebral palsy.

Consider:

- • Progressive or genetic disorders.
- • Performing MRI spine if spasticity present.
- • Repeating MRI brain if first MRI was done before 2–3 yrs of age or if a higher magnet-strength scanner is now available.
- • CT brain for calcification if SWI sequences were not performed (or repeat MRI with SWI).
- • Trial of L-DOPA: see L-DOPA in Chapter 7 ➔ p. 682.

Periventricular leukomalacia (PVL)

See Figure 4.2.

This clinical-radiological picture is typically associated with pre-term delivery although occasionally reported after ischaemic injury at term and is associated with predominantly lower-limb spasticity. There is predominant dystonia in some pre-term infants. Can be asymmetrical. Epilepsy is less common than in cortical lesions. Assess for visual impairment and specific learning deficits.

Several risk factors for PVL have been identified although precise mechanism is not established.

- • Results from injury to oligodendroglia between 26- and 34-weeks' gestation.
- • Radiological evidence of gliosis implies injury occurred after the establishment of a foetal glial cell population, i.e. from beginning of third trimester onward.
- • Cerebral Blood Flow (CBF) instability appears important (pre-term infants have very poor CBF autoregulation). Risk factors include:
  - • mechanical ventilation;
  - • hypotension;
  - • hypoxaemia;
  - • acidosis;
  - • hypocarbia;

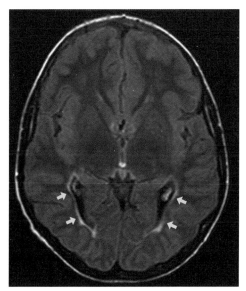

Fig. 4.2 Typical FLAIR appearances of PVL: irregular lateral ventricle enlargement and reduced white matter thickness are seen particularly posteriorly (arrows): deep sulci nearly reach the ventricle; increased T2 signal in white matter reflecting gliosis. The latter typically implies third trimester injury. Fewer features are seen in mild PVL.

- patent ductus arteriosus;
- predictive indices based on exposure to risk factors have been developed.
- Cytokine release due to chorioamnionitis or maternal infection is probably also important.
- Other risk factors include: placental vascular anastomoses, twin pregnancy, antepartum haemorrhage, maternal cocaine abuse.
- Many infants have no identifiable risk factors.

Consider:
- Leukodystrophies if there is an atypical distribution of white matter changes; or if marked cerebral or cerebellar atrophy/hypoplasia are present.

Delayed myelination, hypomyelination
Appearances can range from local peri-trigonal changes to widespread changes. Associated with delayed developmental milestones, hypotonia, and ataxia. May also result from a perinatal ischaemic event. A thin

juxta-ventricular rim of normal myelination should be visible posteriorly—if not, suggests a leukodystrophy: see White matter abnormalities on MR imaging in Chapter 2 ⊃ p. 77.

- *Consider*: biotinidase deficiency and cerebral folate transport defects (both rare but importantly, treatable), 3-phosphoglycerate dehydrogenase deficiency, Pelizaeus–Merzbacher, congenital disorders of glycosylation, Menkes, Sjögren–Larsson, other metabolic leukodystrophies. Repeat the MRI scan at 2–3 yrs of age.

Basal ganglia and thalamic lesions

Bilateral infarctions in the putamen (posterior) and thalamus (ventrolateral nuclei) can result from perinatal acute, severe hypoxic–ischaemic injury at term. The typical association is with dystonia and dyskinesia. Spasticity and total-body involvement is present if the internal capsule and cortex are affected. Kernicterus is now more common in pre-term infants—look for globus pallidus lesions. A unilateral lesion suggests thrombo-embolic stroke.

▶ Term HIE characteristically causes an early high T2 signal and later atrophy in the putamen and thalamus. Involvement of the *globus pallidus* or *caudate* is suspicious for metabolic disease (especially mitochondrial disease and organic acidurias).

- *Consider*: mitochondrial disorders (Leigh syndrome), biotinidase deficiency, other rarer metabolic disorders, post-encephalitis, or toxins if there were no prenatal risk factors or late presentation.

Porencephaly

This is a focal peri-ventricular cyst or irregular lateral ventricle enlargement, often a remnant of foetal/neonatal periventricular haemorrhagic venous infarction. There is typically no gliosis as the insult is usually in the second trimester (the gliotic response is only present from beginning of third trimester) but extensive unilateral lesions are possible after arterial ischaemic or haemorrhagic stroke at term. Results in upper limb-predominant hemiplegia.

- *Consider*: coagulopathy screen; *COL4A1* gene mutation in familial cases.

Cortical infarctions

- Symmetrical parasagittal and parieto-occipital/fronto-parietal watershed lesions can result in spastic quadriparesis and suggest hypoperfusion typically due to hypotension, at term.
- Focal symmetrical infarctions in perisylvian areas can lead to the Worster–Drought phenotype.
- Unilateral lesions suggest a thrombo-embolic cause; they result in spastic hemiplegia (usually upper limb-predominant).
- If infarcts do not respect vascular boundaries (see Fig. 2.8 in Chapter 2 ⊃ p. 65), consider mitochondrial disorders, e.g. MELAS (deletions and point mutation test available).

Cystic encephalomalacia

Multiple subcortical cysts and gliosis (↑T2 signal in remaining white matter) with septation in the cysts. This suggests perinatal injury near term, or early postnatal injury.

- If diffuse, consider neonatal/infantile meningitis;
- If there are watershed areas, consider severe perinatal ischaemic injury;
- If focal and predominantly cortical, suggests thrombo-embolic stroke.

Schizencephaly

This is a neuronal migration disorder: specific genes are implicated. It is an *early gestation insult*—distinguish from porencephaly. Type I (closed lip) and type II (open lip, often associated with polymicrogyria). Type II is more commonly associated with early unilateral or severe bilateral involvement and ↑risk of learning disability and epilepsy (see also MRI and brain development in Chapter 2 ⟐ p. 71). *Check for septo-optic dysplasia.*

Other malformations of cortical development

- Disorders of neuronal proliferation, migration, and organization including heterotopias, lissencephalies, and hemimegalencephaly.
- ↑risk of epilepsy, and learning disability if extensive.
- Bilateral perisylvian polymicrogyria may result in Worster–Drought phenotype.
- Many specific genetic causes but can also be caused by early to mid-gestational teratogens, e.g. CMV: See also MRI and brain development in Chapter 2 ⟐ p. 71.

Box 4.3 Radiological signs of malformations of cortical development (see also MRI and brain development in Chapter 2 ⟐ p. 71)

In simple terms, brain development occurs in three phases:
- Massive neuronal proliferation from progenitor cells in the periventricular ependymal layer.
- Successive waves of migration of neurons from this central periventricular zone out to the cortex (counter-intuitively, the latter waves migrate further, passing the earlier waves to reach the surface in an 'inside out' manner).
- Consolidation and organization of intracortical neuron-to-neuron connections.

Corresponding radiological indicators include:
- Ectopic grey matter: subcortical 'islands' of grey matter that never made it all the way to the cortex.
- Band heterotopias: bands of grey matter representing arrested migration of a neuronal 'wave' (can result in 'double cortex' appearances with a layer of white matter sandwiched between two grey matter layers).
- Abnormally thick cortex due to failure of organization and 'pruning' (pachygyria).
- Abnormally simple cortex without sulcation (lissencephaly).

Hypoplasia and agenesis of the corpus callosum

A thin/hypoplastic corpus callosum may be secondary to PVL and extensive cortical lesions.

- Agenesis of corpus callosum suggests an early gestation insult, typically genetic malformations of cortical development.
  - Consider Aicardi syndrome in ♀s: see Epilepsies with imaging abnormalities in this chapter ⊃ p. 294.
- *If septum pellucidum is absent, consider* septo-optic dysplasia (check pituitary MRI scans, endocrine and visual function). Consider pyruvate dehydrogenase deficiency (skin fibroblasts for enzyme studies) and amino acid synthesis defects.
- Any myelination disorder may be associated with callosal hypoplasia.

Cerebellar hypoplasia and atrophy

A non-progressive lesion (hypoplasia) may be indistinguishable from a progressive lesion (atrophy)—check antenatal ultrasound for clues. Hypotonia may precede ataxia. Inferior cerebellar hemisphere atrophy in extreme pre-term survivors is associated with ↑disability. Vermis atrophy may follow severe perinatal ischaemic injury—associated cortical, basal ganglia, and brainstem lesions should be visible. *Consider* genetic and metabolic disorders, e.g. mitochondrial disorders, congenital disorders of glycosylation, pontocerebellar hypoplasia type I, Joubert, infantile neuroaxonal dystrophy, Menkes.

Diffuse cortical atrophy

A thin cortex/subcortex results in ventriculomegaly. It is the result of a severe neonatal encephalopathy due to an intrapartum hypoxic event. It is associated with spastic total-body involvement cerebral palsy and cognitive disability. It may also result from post-neonatal hypoxic events. If there is no clear history of risk factors, consider a progressive disorder.

Brainstem atrophy

This is associated with severe, acute perinatal/postnatal ischaemic injury in term-born children. Corticospinal/bulbar injury leads to spastic total-body involvement. It has a poor prognosis if there is bulbar weakness or a tendency to aspiration pneumonia.

Consider Pontocerebellar hypoplasia type 1 (PCH1) and CDG1a if there are no historical risk factors.

Prognosis in the cerebral palsies

See Table 4.2.

Estimating prognosis (e.g. life expectancy, ambulation) in the individual child is an inexact art. Recent studies have utilized severity grading such as the GMFCS, rather than mere patterns of limb involvement and movement disorder (such as spastic unilateral, dystonic cerebral palsy) to stratify cohorts. Multiaxial classification (e.g. including neuroimaging findings in stratification of cohorts) should improve accuracy in the future.

Table 4.2 Typical profile of impairments and activity limitation across cerebral palsy motor subtypes

	Unilateral Cerebral Palsy	Bilateral Cerebral Palsy	Bilateral Cerebral Palsy
Typical GMFCS levels (see Fig. 4.4)	I or II	III	IV or V
Epilepsy	~30% (50% after perinatal stroke). Focal. Epilepsy surgery consideration. Often late onset. Associated with lower IQ	~30%	90%; less frequent in dyskinetic. GTCs. Early onset
Other medical issues (age-dependent)	Minimal	Drooling, GORD, incontinence, enuresis	Hydrocephalus (15%), dysphagia, caries, chest infections, GORD, constipation, incontinence, malnutrition, drooling, osteopaenia, precocious puberty with delayed completion
Upper limb	Wrist flexion and pronator contractures; thumb adductor spasticity; fall-related fractures	Fine motor functions affected (handwriting, cutlery); proximal weakness may limit self-propelled wheelchair use	Shoulder, elbow flexion contractures; wrist flexion/extension contracture; thumb-in-palm and intrinsic hand muscle deformity; poor hand use
Lower-limb orthopaedic of functional consequence	Calf/ankle contracture; leg length discrepancy; flexion at the knee	Foot deformity; hip and knee fixed flexion; hip subluxation; patella alta; torsional lower limb; spondylolysis	Scoliosis, pelvic obliquity, hip dislocation, long bone pathological fracture
Vision	Visual acuity usually normal; visual field/lateralized attention deficit	Strabismus, hypermetropia, astigmatism. Higher visual deficits.	Visual impairment and blindness frequent (ocular and cerebral causes)
Hearing	Normal range	No severe hearing loss	5% have severe hearing loss (higher after kernicterus)

(Continued)

Table 4.2 (Contd.)

	Unilateral Cerebral Palsy	Bilateral Cerebral Palsy	Bilateral Cerebral Palsy
Neuropsychology	Low normal range (20% have IQ<70); performance IQ most affected; worse with epilepsy. Focal deficits	50% have IQ <70; usually pre-term. Visual-perceptual deficits.	80% have IQ <70
Speech and language	Delayed speech; overall in line with IQ	Mild dysarthria	Majority non-verbal; severe dysarthria in dyskinetic
Behaviour and psychological	ADHD-like (20%), anxiety (25%), peer problems, autistic spectrum (3–15%)	↑emotional and peer problems.	Sleep disturbance; generalized pain/agitation
Academic/ education	Mainstream school often without support. Dyslexia, dyspraxia, dysgraphia-like problems may become evident in later years	Mainstream school with support. Specific learning problems may become evident.	Special school typical

Life expectancy
- Most children with a cerebral palsy (80–90% overall) survive into adulthood, including those with severe disability (60–70%): paediatricians need to anticipate transfer to adult services (see Transition to adult services in Chapter 5 ⊘ p. 606).
- Current survival data by definition reflect medical care of 20–30 years ago. There has been clear evidence of improved survival in previous decades although whether this can be sustained remains to be seen.
- Cognitive and visual impairment are independent predictors of mortality.
  - IQ <20 (50% survival to adulthood) vs. IQ >85 (>95% survival to adulthood).
- Causes of death: respiratory infections, aspiration, status epilepticus, other infections.
- For reviews see ⊘ http://www.lifeexpectancy.com.

Walking and mobility
Predictors include the pattern of limb involvement and movement disorders.
- Spastic unilateral CP: majority walk before 2 yrs.
- Spastic bilateral CP: majority unlikely to walk.
- Other predictors for ability to walk by the age of 6 include development achieved at age 3 yrs.
  - If unable to roll, only a minute percentage will walk with assistance.
  - If able to roll, but not sit (GMFCS level IV) then ~25% will walk with assistance.
  - If able to roll and sit, ~50% will walk, most with assistance.
  - If able to roll, sit, pull to stand (GMFCS level II), ~70% will walk, many unassisted.

- As a simple rule of thumb, children with CP who will be 'community walkers' (i.e. will walk outdoors and not just in therapy sessions or around the house) are sitting well by age 2. A child not sitting by 4 will not walk.
- The ability to do standing transfers is a pre-requisite for independent living as an adult.
- These predictions assume normal vision.

See Figure 4.3.

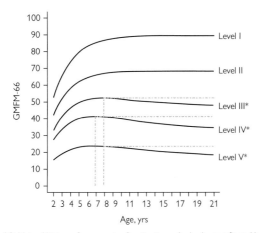

Fig. 4.3 Natural history of gross motor function in cerebral palsy as reflected by Gross Motor Function Measure (GMFM-66). Note that in more severely impaired children (GMFCS levels III to V) it is normal for function to peak late in the first decade and then show a modest decline.

Reproduced from Hanna SE, Rosenbaum PL, Bartlett DJ, Palisano RJ, Walter SD, Avery L, et al. Stability and decline in gross motor function among children and youth with cerebral palsy aged 2 to 21 years. *Developmental Medicine and Child Neurology*, Volume 51, Issue 4, p295–302, Copyright © 2009 Mac Keith Press.

▶ Be aware of the phenomenon of 'going-off feet' in adolescence. Increases in limb length and body and limb weight have adverse biomechanical effects on children with precarious mobility. Gross motor skills are often best late in the first decade (see Fig. 4.3) and a child who was just walking may cease to: recognizing this prevents unwarranted hunts for neurodegenerative disease.

Prediction by aetiology

The cause of a cerebral palsy is a significant predictor of outcome. Neonatal encephalopathy as a cause of a cerebral palsy tends to result in a higher incidence of:

- Severe motor disability (47% vs. 25% for all other causes).
- Epilepsy (53% vs. 29%).
- Cognitive impairment (75% vs. 43%).
- Being non-verbal (47% vs. 22%).
- Early mortality (death by 6 yrs 19% vs. 5%).

Cerebral palsy due to grey matter pathology (developmental malformation or damage) is associated with a higher incidence of epilepsy than that associated with periventricular leukomalacia.

Prediction by mode of presentation

Children presenting early in infancy, e.g. from follow-up in a high-risk neonate clinic, tend to have a more severe cerebral palsy, e.g. bilateral spastic CP.

Children presenting in late infancy/early childhood, e.g. from health visitor concerns, have a milder cerebral palsy. Children may already be walking, e.g. toe-walking in unilateral spastic CP. Mild cognitive impairment is more likely.

Care of the disabled child

Models of disability

The current WHO model of disability (the International Classification of Functioning, ICF) envisages multilevel effects:

- *Impairment* refers to effects at the level of the *structure and function* of a body organ such as weakness in a limb or poor vision in an eye.
- *Activities* are description of functioning at the level of the person in a standardized or idealized environment (e.g. in a physio gym with a smooth floor).
- *Participation* is involvement in 'real-life' situations, including the performance of social roles. It is seen as 'what matters' about disability.

Key to the ICF model is the realization that while participation is affected by impairment, it is also determined by impairment-independent *contextual* factors. Change the child's environment (address discriminatory attitudes or legislation, or the lack of adapted facilities or appropriate services) and a child's participation could dramatically improve without any change in impairment. The ICF is a qualitative synthesis of two different concepts of disability. Extremes of the medical and social models of disability exaggerate respectively the importance of intrinsic impairment and environmental context on the disadvantage experienced by disabled people.

- The extreme medical model sees disability as arising from the biological nature of a disease and emphasizes diagnosis: disability is something you 'have'.
- The extreme social model sees 'the process of disablement' as arising from discriminatory attitudes and policies within society: disability is something 'done to you'. It regards medical diagnosis as largely irrelevant.
- This also drives a usage debate, with arguments that both 'disabled person' and 'person with disability' reflect enlightened attitudes.

The basic ICF conceptual framework is a useful guide to practice. Clinicians tend to focus on and treat impairments. Demonstrating an improved range of movement at a joint after botulinum toxin (i.e. reduced impairment) is not enough: has this improved participation?

In situations where we can do little to reduce impairment, devoting energy to improving the environment in which the impaired child lives may have much greater effects on participation.

Management of hypertonia and contractures

▶ Hypertonia—an increased resistance to passive movement.

This may be due to:

- Changes in the viscoelastic properties of muscle and soft tissue.
- Involuntary and inappropriate muscle contraction.

Involuntary muscle contraction can be characterized as:

- *Spasticity*: A velocity-dependent increase in tone (i.e. resistance to stretch depends on how quickly you attempt to move the body part) due to dis-inhibition of the spinal reflex arc. Spasticity is often associated with exaggerated tendon reflexes and clonus.

- *Dystonia*: Intermittent or sustained muscle contractions causing abnormal, often repetitive, movements and postures. Tone as examined is variable, and body parts affected with be observed to move into abnormal postures.
- *Rigidity*: 'lead-pipe' tone (i.e. does not vary by speed or direction of stretch), often associated with Parkinson Disease. Does not cause abnormal postures.

In practice, hypertonia is almost always due to a combination of these elements, which may be difficult to distinguish clinically.

Hypertonia can complicate cerebral palsy, acquired brain injury, and neuromuscular disorders. Consequences include:
- Pain and discomfort.
- Difficulty with care, e.g. washing in the groin area because of hip adduction.
- Loss of function, e.g. mobility.
- Contractures.

Hypertonia is treated *to ameliorate one or more of these consequences*, not as an end in itself. Realistic treatment goals should be agreed prior to treatment and these goals are the criteria against which treatment success is assessed.

Assessment
History
Pain, discomfort, and ease of care, and the impact of these on the life of child and family.

Examination
- Tone (attempting to discriminate between elements of soft tissue change and involuntary muscle contraction), power, and deep tendon reflexes.
- Opportunities for examination under anaesthesia are invaluable for identifying static elements (e.g. fixed contracture).
- Reasonably objective rating scales (see below) can be used to monitor change over time.

Clinical measures of motor impairment and function
Assessment of motor impairment and function should be interdisciplinary, involving physiotherapists, occupational therapists, and orthopaedic surgeons. Structured analysis of videotaped movements may aid decision making.

Identify and measure, if possible:
- Different components of hypertonia.
- *Fixed* tendon, bone, and joint problems, e.g. Achilles contractures, scoliosis.
- Muscle weakness.
- Gross motor function (do this at the very least).
- Coordination and selective motor control (fine motor).
- Perceptual and cognitive problems, e.g. visual impairment.
- Abilities and disabilities in daily living, e.g. self-care.

Numerous structured observational scales and questionnaires exist for measuring motor impairments and functions of daily living. The focus here is on cheap, rapid, and/or well-validated measures.

Spasticity scales
Modified Ashworth Scale
A six-point ordinal scale. Simple and widely used but not very reliable as the speed of movement at which to evaluate resistance to stretch is not specified.
- 0 = no increase in muscle tone.
- 1 = slight increase in tone, with catch and release, or minimal resistance at end of range.
- 2 = minimal resistance through range following catch, but body part is easily moved.
- 3 = more marked increased tone throughout range.
- 4 = considerable increase in tone, passive movement difficult.
- 5 = affected part is rigid in flexion/extension.

Reprinted from *Physical Therapy*. Bohannon Rand Smith M, In-terrater reliability of a modified Ashworth scale of muscle spasticity, 1987, Volume 67, Issue 2, p. 206–7, of the American Physical Therapy Association. © 1987 American Physical Therapy Association.

Dystonia scales
Measurement scales for dystonia are not as well established as for spasticity. The Barry–Albright dystonia scale was developed for children with severe generalized dystonia. Five-point ordinal scale, scored for the eyes, mouth, neck, trunk, and each limb separately.
- 0 = normal.
- 1 = slight, body part affected less than 10% of the time.
- 2 = mild, body part affected less than 50% of the time; not interfering with function.
- 3 = moderate, body part affected more than 50% of the time and/or interferes with function.
- 4 = severe, body part affected more than 50% of the time; prevents or severely limits function.

Reproduced with permission from Barry MJ, Van Swearingen JM, and Albright AL. Reliability and responsiveness of the Barry–Albright Dystonia Scale. Developmental Medicine and Child Neurology, Volume 21, Issue 6 pp 401–11.

Other scales include the Burke-Fahn Marsden Dystonia Rating Scale (BFMDRS) for isolated dystonia, and the more recently developed Dyskinesia Impairment Scale (DIS) for children with CP.

Gross motor function scales
Gross Motor Function Classification System (GMFCS)
- A very simple and well-recognized classification of mobility in cerebral palsy.
- Five-point ordinal scale describing levels I mild to V severe (see Fig. 4.4).
- Routine use in clinics is feasible.
- More reliable in children over 2 yrs old.

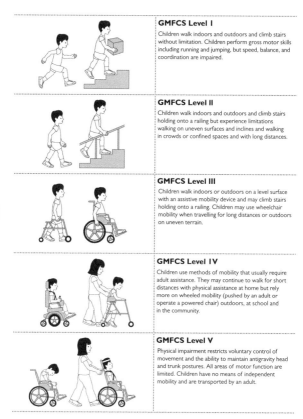

GMFCS Level I

Children walk indoors and outdoors and climb stairs without limitation. Children perform gross motor skills including running and jumping, but speed, balance, and coordination are impaired.

GMFCS Level II

Children walk indoors and outdoors and climb stairs holding onto a railing but experience limitations walking on uneven surfaces and inclines and walking in crowds or confined spaces and with long distances.

GMFCS Level III

Children walk indoors or outdoors on a level surface with an assistive mobility device and may climb stairs holding onto a railing. Children may use wheelchair mobility when travelling for long distances or outdoors on uneven terrain.

GMFCS Level IV

Children use methods of mobility that usually require adult assistance. They may continue to walk for short distances with physical assistance at home but rely more on wheeled mobility (pushed by an adult or operate a powered chair) outdoors, at school and in the community.

GMFCS Level V

Physical impairment restricts voluntary control of movement and the ability to maintain antigravity head and trunk postures. All areas of motor function are limited. Children have no means of independent mobility and are transported by an adult.

Fig. 4.4 Descriptors and illustrations of GMFCS levels at age 6–12. Similar illustrations of function at other ages available at same resource.

Descriptors reproduced from Palisano R, Rosenbaum P, Walter S, Russell D, Wood E, and Galuppi B. Development and reliability of a system to classify gross motor function in children with cerebral palsy. *Developmental Medicine and Child Neurology*, Volume 39, Issue 4, p. 214, Copyright © John Wiley and Sons.

Illustrations reproduced from Kerr Graham, Bill Reid, and Adrienne Harvey, The Royal Children's Hospital, Melbourne, Copyright © 2016 Kerr Graham, Bill Reid, and Adrienne Harvey.

- Ignores *quality* of performance, and upper limb function.
- Part of its value is that the longitudinal 'trajectory' of children in each band has been defined: if you know a child's current GMFCS level, you can predict with some confidence levels of future function expected of young people in that level.

Manual Ability Classification System (MACS)
Developed to compliment the GMFCS, this is a 5-level ordinal scale describing the manual ability of a child. It is also easily applied in clinic, and more reliable over 2 years of age:
- Level I: Objects are handled easily and successfully.
- Level II: Handles most objects, but with some reduced quality and/or speed.
- Level III: Handles objects with difficulty—the child will need help to prepare and/or modify activities.
- Level IV: Handles a limited selection of easily managed objects and always requires some help from others.
- Level V: The child is not able to handle objects or to complete even simple actions with their hands.

Reproduced from Eliasson, A., et al (2006). The Manual Ability Classification System (MACS) for children with cerebral palsy: Scale development and evidence of validity and reliability. *Developmental Medicine and Child Neurology*, 48(7), 549–54.

Gross Motor Function Measure (GMFM)
This is sometimes confused with the GMFCS. It is a somewhat time-consuming assessment consisting of up to 80 standardized motor tasks assessing lying and rolling; sitting; standing; walking, running, and jumping tasks. The GMFM-66 version gives a 'Gross Motor Ability Estimate': a single number on a continuous 0–100 scale that can detect change over time, used for detecting response to therapy.

Other measures
A wide variety of specialist scales exist to assess specific constructs. Their use is generally restricted to research or formal evaluation exercises as they are time-consuming (typically 20–30 min). Examples include:
- Fine motor coordination, e.g. Movement Assessment Battery for Children (Movement ABC), Gross Motor Performance Measure (GMPM), Quality of Upper Extremity Skills Test (QUEST).
- Visual perception and motor coordination, e.g. Developmental Test of Visual–Motor Integration.

Limitations in daily living are not just due to motor impairments. Disability measures integrate the effects of comorbidities (e.g. scoliosis), cognitive deficits, perceptual deficits (e.g. visual impairment), and behavioural disorders. Examples include the Pediatric Evaluation of Disability Inventory (PEDI) and WeeFIM (paediatric Functional Independence Measure).

Physical management
Problems to be addressed encompass weakness, fatigue, and abnormal tone, abnormal posturing, reduced movement control, and muscle contractures. The aims of physiotherapy are to retain and improve function, and to preserve muscle length.

- *Muscle strengthening exercises* are controversial. They could potentially worsen spasticity although others emphasize the importance of maintaining muscle strength. Recent studies suggest training antagonists of shortened muscles may improve function.
- *Muscle stretching exercises* comprise slow manual stretching aimed at preventing shortening of the muscle and stiffness of the joint. Fast stretching may damage the muscle. Animal data suggest that several hours of stretch per day are probably necessary which is only feasible with splints.

Positioning
Frequent repositioning can prevent contractures. If this is not possible, prolonged periods of immobility should be in an optimal position (maintained by sleep systems, seating, and standing frames). Weight bearing enhances bone density and promotes joint remodelling in weight-bearing joints. This can help to prevent dislocation of the hips.

Splints
Night splints provide prolonged stretching to prevent contractures. Day splints may prevent contractures but are also intended to improve function by joint stabilization and support. Static splints limit the joint range of movement. Dynamic splints limit the joint range of movement in one plane only (e.g. an ankle foot orthosis preventing in- and eversion, while allowing plantar and dorsiflexion).

Serial casting
Casting has a similar effect to splinting but ensures compliance. Serial casting can help lengthen muscles, sometimes in combination with botulinum toxin injections; however, the duration of wearing a cast should be limited to prevent muscle atrophy during immobilization. During serial casting, 2–4 casts are applied in succession for 4–5 days each. The foot is positioned just past the point of resistance to passive movement, and the angle of correction is increased with every cast.

Medical management of spasticity and dystonia
Pharmacological interventions may potentially reduce involuntary muscle contraction but will have no impact on soft tissue properties. Baclofen and diazepam are the most used oral medications for spasticity, with baclofen and trihexyphenidyl most commonly used for dystonia. The use of oral medications to treat hypertonia is often limited by unwanted effects. Common side effects include impaired alertness, attention, and, importantly, oromotor function. When used intrathecally, much higher CSF levels of baclofen can be achieved without systemic side effects (see Surgical management of spasticity and dystonia in this chapter ❷ p. 249).

Botulinum toxin
Derived from *Clostridium botulinum*. The toxin weakens the muscle by inhibiting the release of acetylcholine at the neuromuscular junction. The effect reverses slowly over weeks to months, probably through sprouting of new nerve terminals. There are several subtypes, of which botulinum toxin A is mostly used. This is commercially available in two forms: Botox® (Allergan) and Dysport® (Ipsen).

❶ It is vital to be aware that the dosage units of the various commercial products are *not equivalent* and care must be taken to specify the brand intended when specifying doses (see Botulinum toxin A in Chapter 7 ➋ p. 656).

- Botulinum toxin can reduce dynamic contraction, and regular injections may delay formation of fixed contractures and the need for surgery.
- It has little role in management of established contractures.
- It may be used for both spasticity and dystonia.
- The effect of the toxin starts around 12–72 h after injection and lasts between 3 and 6 months.
- Injections typically must be repeated every 6–12 months to maintain the effect.

Common sites of injection are calf muscles, hamstrings, and hip adductors. The injection site can be identified by vision and palpation, although ultrasound guidance is often very helpful. Injection can be given after application of topical local anaesthetic cream, with oral sedation in younger children or nitrous oxide inhalation. In some children, and for injection of ileopsoas, general anaesthesia may be needed.

It is paramount that splints and physiotherapy are in place at the time of injections.

Adverse effects
- Local pain at the injection site.
- Falls due to imbalance and fatigue.
- Loss of function if muscles have been weakened too much (e.g. ability to weight-bear for transfers, or walk).
- Incontinence especially after hip adductor injections.
- Swallowing problems and bulbar dysfunction have been reported after cervical injections for torticollis.

The effect of the toxin, however, is temporary and all these problems resolve over time.

Surgical management of spasticity and dystonia

Intrathecal baclofen
Baclofen acts on the GABA-B receptors in the spinal cord but crosses the blood–brain barrier very poorly.
- with intrathecal administration, higher CSF concentrations are possible without systemic effects: effective intrathecal doses are of the order of a few hundred micrograms per 24 h, c.f. typical enteral doses of tens of milligrams per day.
- intrathecal baclofen can be extremely effective in combatting severe total-body spasticity and/or dystonia in children in GMFCS IV or V, improving seating and general care.
- its role in more able children (GMFCS I–III) is less clear: reduction of lower-limb hypertonicity may paradoxically worsen ambulation by reducing weight-bearing strength.

A battery-operated, programmable, subcutaneous, and fully enclosed pump (usually placed on the anterior abdominal wall) is connected to a tunnelled subcutaneous catheter delivering baclofen directly into the intra-thecal space. The infusion rate is *very slow* (typically less than a mL *per day*) and consequently issues of dead-space and priming become very important. The pump is refilled every few months percutaneously and its rate and other parameters can be set using a remote-control wireless programmer.

Assessment for pump implantation, and the management of implanted pumps, should only be performed in specialist centres.

- A 25–50 microgms test dose may be given to assess sensitivity of muscle tone to baclofen although this step may be omitted if there is a clear history of responsiveness to oral baclofen.
- Maximal effect is seen ~4 h after injection with reversal by ~8 h. CSF pressure is measured. Pressures >20 mmHg are a relative contraindication to an intrathecal catheter because of the risk of a CSF leak.
- Subsequently a pump can be implanted, and the dose titrated.

Complications
- Infection, CSF leak, wound breakdown.

Effects of baclofen withdrawal
- Interruption of intrathecal baclofen delivery in chronically treated children can cause withdrawal symptoms with itching, extreme spasticity, fever, hallucinations, psychosis, and seizures.
- In severe cases rhabdomyolysis and dehydration can lead to renal and/or multiorgan failure.
- Cases of suspected acute baclofen withdrawal should be managed aggressively with high-dose enteral baclofen and enteral and/or parenteral benzodiazepines (if necessary with ventilator support) until intrathecal delivery can be re-established.
- Monitor treatment adequacy by CK levels.

❶It is vital that families and professionals are aware of the potentially life-threatening dangers of acute total baclofen withdrawal due to pump or (much more commonly) catheter failure and the need to seek experi-enced emergency medical advice in the event of apparent loss of effect.

Adverse effects of overdose
- Mild overdose can cause hypotonia, listlessness, trouble concentrating, and urinary retention and/or constipation, readily reversed by reducing the dose.
- Severe overdose can cause hypotonia, respiratory depression, and coma necessitating intensive care.
- Loss of trunk tone may accelerate progression of scoliosis if seating inadequate.

Outcome
Reduction of hypertonicity, with prevention of contractures and delay of surgery. There may be improved function.

Selective dorsal rhizotomy

Selected dorsal rootlets are transected, diminishing sensory input and feedback to anterior horn cells, and reducing spasticity. This procedure cannot reduce dystonia. The procedure is performed in only a few centres and is usually restricted to potential walkers aged 3–10 with severe spastic diplegia with no associated ataxia, dystonia, or athetosis; nor severe established contractures. Side effects may include paraesthesia and bladder problems.

Deep-brain stimulation (DBS)

Fine electrodes are stereotactically inserted into the deep nuclei of the brain (most commonly the *globus pallidus interna*) and connected to a subcutaneous neurostimulator placed in the abdomen or chest delivering a continuous electrical stimulus. DBS can improve dystonia and chorea but will have no impact on spasticity. Significant spasticity is typically a contraindication to DBS.

- DBS can dramatically reduce dystonia due to some genetic causes (e.g. DYT-TOR1A, DYT-KMT2B, *GNAO1* related encephalopathy), but more modest changes in dystonia are seen in acquired brain injury (including cerebral palsy).
- Expert multidisciplinary assessment is required to identify suitable patients, with careful consideration of goals for the intervention.
- Risks:
  - <1% chance of significant intracranial event during surgery.
  - ~5% risk seizure at the time of surgery.
  - ~10% chance of implant infection requiring removal of the device in most cases.
- Adverse effects of stimulation include unwanted activation of the corticospinal tract or optic tracts, and typically resolve with device reprogramming, or following discontinuation of stimulation.

Orthopaedic surgery

Orthopaedic soft tissues and bony surgery will be needed to address fixed deformities. Aims must be clearly defined and weighed against anaesthetic risk. Timing is of importance, and problems often recur after surgery if performed too early in life. Post-operative management with intensive physiotherapy and splinting is paramount.

Surgery for gait abnormalities

- Past approaches of sequences of single operations (so-called 'birthday syndrome': another year, another operation) have given way to single-stage multilevel surgery.
- Several deformities are corrected in one session, which might include any of: psoas, Achilles tendon, or hamstring lengthening, hip adductor release, rectus femoris transfer, or subtalar arthrodesis.
- Planning of these operations is complex and gait analysis can be helpful.
- Botulinum toxin injections can help predict the results of an operation.
- In general, it is preferred to postpone the surgery until at least 8 yrs of age, as prior to this the risk of recurrence of deformities is high. Vigorous conservative treatment is thus essential to maintain a child until surgery is appropriate.

Surgery to correct hip deformity/dislocation
- Problems with the hips can cause difficulty with seating, hygiene, and/ or pain.
- It is important to have a surveillance system in place with regular reviews and 6–12 monthly X-rays to monitor for hip (sub-) luxation.
- Once the femoral head is 50% uncovered, hip dislocation is inevitable.
- When 25–40% uncovered, adductor and psoas release may prevent luxation. Adductor release may also be needed to ease hygiene.
- Once the femur head is more than 40% uncovered this often has to be combined with bony procedures (e.g. femoral osteotomy).
- When the hip is dislocated, more elaborate surgery may be needed (e.g. hip replacement, acetabular reconstruction, femoral head resection, hip arthrodesis).

Surgery for upper limbs
Interventions for the upper extremity are limited, although there is a rising interest in this. As improvement in muscle control is usually not achievable, the aim of surgery is to obtain functional positions of joints. Release of a pronator contracture, or tendon transfers can have a functional benefit in selected cases. Some families will opt for surgery to improve appearance.

Scoliosis surgery
Scoliosis, like hip problems, can interfere with seating. It also greatly adds to the risk of respiratory complications (see Respiratory disease in neurodisability in this chapter ➲ p. 260). Management of scoliosis can include spinal bracing and supportive seating. In general, the scoliosis will progress slowly despite these measures, and spinal fusion may still be needed.

Feeding

Most experience has been gained in children with cerebral palsy, however children with other neuromuscular conditions experience similar problems. Problems of feeding tend to be in the following areas:
- Time. Feeds can be extremely time-consuming, taking several hours.
- Poor intake. Consequently, caloric intake may be poor, resulting in poor growth, nutritional status, and general health.

▶ A report that 'he'd eat all the time if I let him' may not reflect excessive appetite and intake, but rather a permanently hungry child with slow feeding and inadequate intake!

- Vomiting and gastro-oesophageal reflux. This can again lead to poor intake but can also cause discomfort.
- Aspiration. Problems with swallowing related to bulbar or pseudobulbar involvement can occur both during swallowing, and after vomiting or reflux.

Assessment

Nutrition

Dietetic input is required to assess adequacy of intake both of calories and other nutrients. Weight and height (absolute, centile, or Z-scores), upper arm length, lower leg length, and skinfold thickness have been used to monitor progress, although there are few population standards for children with cerebral palsy. There is an ↑risk of low bone mineral density: dietary intake of calcium and vitamin D must be carefully evaluated, and supplementation may be necessary. General health, in particular the frequency of chest infections and admissions, is another important guide.

Aspiration

An experienced speech and language therapist (SALT) can often assess whether aspiration is occurring. Assessment includes history and a test feed. Apart from chewing, bolus formation, and swallowing, attention is also paid to aversive responses and persisting primitive reflexes, e.g. rooting and tongue thrust. Coughing during feeds is a strong indicator of aspiration. Usually, thin liquids cause greater problems than thickened fluids or puréed solids. Further supportive evidence can come from various techniques (see Investigations for aspiration in this chapter ⊃ p. 254) although correlation between them is poor.

Reflux

A history of recurrent vomiting or positing, especially if there is haematemesis, is very suggestive of GORD. Regular spasms and arching after feeds suggests Sandifer syndrome (see Gastro-oesophageal reflux in this chapter ⊃ p. 546). Reflux is also an important cause of pain and distress, with secondary aggravation of spasticity or dystonia. Investigations include barium meal, endoscopy, and pH probe. Sometimes a treatment trial is warranted.

Investigations for aspiration

Videofluoroscopy

Provides ciné-radiographic record of the preparatory oral and pharyngeal phases as well as the involuntary oesophageal phase of a swallow. Barium-containing contrast agent is mixed with food: the ability to compare different food consistencies and seating positions is useful; however, the technique involves a high radiation exposure.

Specific attention is paid to movement of the tongue and palate, bolus formation, nasal regurgitation, swallow, failure to clear from valeculae, laryngeal penetration, and frank aspiration (passage of feed in the trachea beyond the larynx).

Salivogram

Normal saline with radioactive technetium is inserted in the mouth of the supine child, after having been fasted. Scintigraphic evidence of radioactivity in the lungs after a few hours indicates aspiration.

Milk scan

The child is given their usual milk or other drink, mixed with technetium, after fasting. Again, radioactivity in the lungs indicates aspiration.

Cervical auscultation

Listening to airway sounds by auscultating neck with stethoscope. Simple and non-invasive and can readily be repeated but requires experienced assessor.

Fiberoptic endoscopic evaluation of swallowing (FEES)

Real-time observation of the pharynx by endoscope passed through a (locally anaesthetized) nostril. Allows observation over a prolonged period of the handling of secretions, but does require child's cooperation so not always feasible.

Management

Treatment of swallowing problems

- Maintain adequate nutrition, may require NGT or PEG.
- Modify diet (textures, thickening liquids, etc.) to optimize swallow.
  - Aspiration is often worst with thin liquid (water, juice).
- Protect the airway: balance the convenience of oral feeding versus the potential risks for aspiration, consider changes in posture/position (e.g. seating provision for feeding).
- Treat underlying or associated conditions that may affect swallow, e.g. gastro-oesophageal reflux.
- Ongoing monitoring of the child's respiratory status is essential.

An upright, well-supported posture is paramount during feeding, and an occupational therapist may help with this. The SALT can advise on optimal food textures and help with desensitization of overactive mouth reflexes. A dietician can advise on supplementary feeds.

If oral intake is deemed dangerous, or inadequate, enteral feeding will be necessary via an NGT or gastrostomy. Long-term feeding via an NGT can be acceptable, especially with less irritant modern silk tubes; however, they can be uncomfortable, and cause ↑salivation, bronchial hypersecretion, retching, heaving, and erosion of the nasal septum, as well as being cosmetically unacceptable. Parents' perceptions can vary considerably and should be taken into account.

The decision to insert a gastrostomy should always be interdisciplinary and include parents. Although safer than many surgical procedures, insertion of a PEG is not risk-free, especially in malnourished children with multiple disabilities. A period of NGT feeding is often initiated to improve nutrition and health before the procedure. There are benefits to physical health and quality of life. The gastrostomy 'takes the stress out of feeding', and drug administration becomes easier. Oral intake can continue for pleasure, but there is no pressure to get calories in.

Reflux

With an upright posture, gravity will help prevent reflux. Medical treatment includes reduction of acid production (ranitidine, omeprazole), prokinetics (domperidone, erythromycin), and thickening agents (Gaviscon, carobel). If gastrostomy is contemplated, and reflux is severe, the procedure can be combined with (laparoscopic) fundoplication.

Drooling

Children with quadriplegic cerebral palsy tend to drool. This is mainly due to poor bulbar function and is aggravated by problems with head control, lip closure, tongue control, dental malocclusion, chewing, sucking, swallowing, intraoral sensitivity, and dysarthria. Reducing secretions by means of hyoscine patches or glycopyrrolate (see Glycopyrronium in Chapter 7 ➋ p. 673) often helps this. Other options include a palatal plate, botulinum toxin injections into the parotid glands, and surgical transplantation of salivary ducts posteriorly.

Tube feeding

Percutaneous endoscopic gastrostomy (PEG)

An endoscope is passed into the stomach. The stomach and abdominal walls are perforated, and a gastrostomy tube passed through the resulting hole, from inside out. After about 6–12 months, the tube is replaced with a skin-flush button device. Benefits include ↑weight, improved growth and skinfold thickness, less time spent feeding, improved health (reduced admissions for chest infections), and improvement in quality of life, improvement in social functioning, mental health, energy, vitality, and general health perception.

Children being assessed for a PEG are at high risk of significant GORD, which will typically remain largely unaddressed if not actually worsened by a move from nasogastric to PEG feeding (which merely removes the tube descending through the cardia). An important part of assessment for PEG insertion is therefore whether it should be combined with a surgical anti-reflux procedure (typically fundoplication).

Complications
- Risk of anaesthesia.
- Laceration of the oesophagus.
- Pneumoperitoneum.
- Peritonitis.

- Colonic perforation.
- Local site infection.
- Vomiting, worsened GORD.
- Aspiration, pneumonia.
- Stoma leakage.
- Skin erosion, granulations.
- Tube blockage, tube migration.

Jejunal feeding
- Nasojejunal feeding can be a useful short-term feeding solution in situations of gastric dysmotility and GORD as feed is delivered distal to the pylorus.
- *Percutaneous endoscopic gastro-jejunostomy (PEGJ)* involves the endoscopic 'threading' of a feeding tube into the jejunum through the pylorus via a PEG: separate lumens allow delivery into jejunum or stomach (typically medications into the stomach, and feed to the jejunum).
- *Percutaneous endoscopic jejunostomy* (PEJ) may be offered as a longer-term solution in situations of extremely challenging gastric dysmotility.
- Specialist individualized pharmacy advice should be sought on jejunal delivery of a child's medication.
  - For many drugs there is little information on effects on bioavailability of the changed route of delivery.
  - Jejunal feeding is typically continuous: some medications (e.g. phenytoin) are conventionally given 'on an empty stomach'.
  - Some drugs are known to require exposure to acidic pH.
  - Tube blockage by thick 'syrups', sediment from ground tablets, and granules can be troublesome. Blockages should be dissolved with liquid preparations (water, cola, proprietary enzyme-containing products) and not cleared mechanically with guidewires because of the risk of perforation.
  - The tip of a jejunal tube can silently 'flip' and double-back through the pylorus into the stomach rendering the child once again vulnerable to reflux: tube tip position should be checked (by confirming *alkaline* pH on aspirate) before use.

Late gastrointestinal problems in children with cerebral palsy.

The GI tract has a complex, largely parasympathetic, intrinsic nervous system under CNS control, and neurogenic gut dysmotility is an important consequence of neurodisability that is aggravated by medication (particularly use of anticholinergics for dystonia). In severely impaired (GMFCS V) children there is often a progressive element with gut dysmotility, ileus and secondary gut-driven dystonia developing in the second decade (see 'GI Dystonia' in Chapter 5 p. 547 and 'Late Intestinal Failure in Severe Neurodisability' in Chapter 5 p. 547).

Communication

Requires the understanding of received communication, and the ability to conceive and convey a reply.

Receptive communication (understanding) therefore requires adequate hearing (for verbal communication) or vision (for gestural or symbolic communication) and the cognitive ability to interpret this information.

Expressive communication ultimately requires the ability to perform at least some movements voluntarily, with reasonable consistency. Speech production is, of course, a particularly versatile form of complex movement, but in situations where speech is not possible, other voluntary movements can be recruited for purposes of communication.

- Children with neurological impairments may find hand and limb gestures easier to perform than speech production: hence the existence of gesture-based communication systems such as Makaton.
- Specialist communication systems exist, e.g. picture-exchange communication system (PECS) for children with autistic spectrum disorders.
- For the non-verbal child cognitively capable of more complex forms of expressive communication, the key is to provide *access* (through appropriate sound-, gesture- or eye movement-controlled *switches*) to an *assistive (or augmentative) communication (AAC)* device.
- Benefiting from a sophisticated AAC system requires significant cognitive abilities (to form messages for communication and to learn the operation of the device); however, the greater danger is in underestimating a child's ability to use such devices.

▶ Dystonic cerebral palsy and acquired dystonias are important causes of severe motor impairment with relatively preserved cognition, i.e. children who may particularly benefit from specialist AAC assessment.

Special senses

Hearing

Traditional assessments (e.g. distraction testing at 10 months and/or audiometry sweep test at school entry) unreliable and increasingly replaced by universal newborn screening for severe hearing impairment (i.e. no longer restricted to selected high-risk groups).
- Oto-acoustic emissions (a sound stimulus produces an acoustic emission from the cochlea) confirm cochlear function but will miss auditory nerve dysfunction proximal to the cochlea.
- Consider brainstem auditory evoked potentials if clinical concerns raised.

Investigation aims to:
- Identify associated conditions.
- Aid genetic counselling.
- Support habilitation.
  - Speech and language therapy; peripatetic specialist teacher of the deaf, partially hearing unit in mainstream schooling or specialist school.

Two distinct communication strategies are available, with the widespread use of cochlear implants in severe hearing impairment increasing the importance of the first:

Oral–aural strategy
- Based on spoken language.
- Hearing aids including consideration of a cochlear implant (after bacterial meningitis, progressive otosclerosis may occur within months: urgent assessment for a cochlear implant is required).
- Early amplification and auditory training may improve the outcome in language speech and development.

Manual–visual strategy
- Training in sign language, lip-reading, reading facial expression, and social situation cues.

Vision

Some processes that cause general neurological disease will also cause primary ocular (particularly retinal) disease and/or refractive errors. More commonly, however, CNS damage affects vision via disruption of visual pathways or damage of cortical areas involved in visual processing perception. The term *cerebral* (or *cortical*) *visual impairment* (CVI) describes this common, under-recognized, and underestimated problem.
    Typical CVI behaviours include:
- Light gazing.
- Apparent eccentric gaze (i.e. looking to one side of the person speaking).
- Striking day-to-day variation in apparent visual abilities.

Visuoperceptual problems

As well as conventional visual field defects and visual inattention problems, other more or less discrete visuoperceptual disorders may occur in focal brain injury.

- Visual post-processing beyond the primary visual cortex takes place in two streams.
  - The dorsal stream (in occipital and parietal lobes) performs analysis of position and the visuomotor planning of reaching ('where and how').
  - The ventral stream (occipital and temporal lobes) performs orientation and recognition ('what').
- These streams may be differentially affected and result in a variety of relatively discrete visual-perceptual problems such as with figure–ground discrimination (the recognition of an object against a complex background), perception of motion, size, etc.

Appropriate multidisciplinary assessment of these issues is likely to include specialist paediatric ophthalmology and neuropsychology or occupational therapy input.

Respiratory disease in neurodisability

There are many reasons why a child with severe neurodisability is at risk of respiratory complications. Consideration of which may be at work in an individual child is important in identifying potential interventions, realistic assessments of long-term respiratory prognosis and in informing always-difficult decisions about appropriateness of intensive care.

Disturbed control of respiratory rate/rhythm

Central hypoventilation

Signs may be minimal when awake. Associated conditions:
- *Chiari malformation*: central, obstructive, or mixed sleep apnoea.
- *Prader-Willi syndrome*. Obstructive and central sleep apnoea.
- *Congenital central hypoventilation syndrome*: hypoventilation mainly in sleep. Developmental impairment and seizures common. Other clues: absence of tears, Hirschprung disease. 90% have de novo *PHOX2B* mutation.
- *Brainstem damage* (ADEM, syringobulbia, traumatic, tumour).
- *Leigh syndrome*: hypoventilation ± apnoea both awake and asleep.
- *Hypothalamic damage* e.g. post-encephalitis.
  - Other indicators may include temperature instability, or disturbance of the hypothalamopituitary axis.
- *Epileptic seizures:* temporal lobe focal seizures, epilepsy of infancy with migrating focal seizures (see Epilepsy of infancy with migrating focal seizures in this chapter ➲ p. 278).
- *Prolonged expiratory apnoea*: poorly understood but probably an extreme form of toddler cyanotic breath-holding (see Blue (cyanotic) breath-holding attacks in this chapter ➲ p. 330). Appears more common in children with profound neurological disability.
- Secondary to *cardiac* problems e.g. arrhythmias.
- *Medication* side effects e.g. benzodiazepines, chloral, phenobarbital, morphine.

Hyperventilation

May be interspersed with apnoeas.
- *Joubert*: hyperventilation alternating with apnoea typically more severe when awake.
- *Rett*: periodic breathing interspersed with profound hyperventilation and Valsalva. Associated with collapses. Respiration in sleep may be normal.
- Children with tumours in the floor of the third ventricle have been described presenting with a respiratory pattern similar to Rett.
- *Pitt-Hopkins*: hyperventilation and apnoea: see Rett syndrome, Rett-like syndromes, and *MECP2*-associated phenotypes in this chapter ➲ p. 297.

Disturbed anatomy and control of upper airways

- Anatomical malformations (congenital or acquired).
- Neuromuscular control of the airway (both awake and during REM sleep, i.e. obstructive sleep apnoea).

Classic indicators
- Snoring, stridor/stertor, apnoeas, open mouth breathing, drooling, feeding difficulties, recurrent chest infections, nocturnal arousals, recurrent otitis media.
- Poor sleep efficiency may worsen comorbid epilepsy.

Associated conditions:
- Down syndrome.
- Mucopolysaccharidoses.
- Mid-face hypoplasia (e.g. Russell–Silver, Treacher Collins).
- Syndromic craniosynostosis (e.g. Apert, Pfeiffer, Crouzon).
- Choanal atresia (CHARGE).
- Laryngomalacia in generalized hypotonic disorders, cerebral palsy, congenital myasthenic syndrome.
- Laryngospasm (acute, intermittent) due to GORD/aspiration-induced reflex.
- Velopharyngeal insufficiency, e.g. Worster–Drought, brainstem lesions.
- Oromotor dyskinesia.
- Vocal cord paralysis e.g. dystonias, neuromuscular disorders (*DOK7*, *CMT2C*).
- Obesity-related syndrome.
- Medication side effects e.g. baclofen, benzodiazepines, chloral hydrate.

Lung and lower airways problems
- Turbulent airflow through partially obstructed oro- and nasopharynx 'dislodges' bacteria which are carried to the lungs.
- Immobility can cause orthostatic pneumonia.
- Reduced FVC.
  - Reduced ability to generate inspiratory and expiratory pressure reduces cough flow velocity. This can increase tendency to infection through ineffective clearance of secretions and atelectasis.
- Aspiration due to oromotor dysfunction or severe GORD/oesophageal motility:
  - poor clearance of secretions may be exacerbated by seizures and medications;
  - may be clinically 'silent' until presentation with chronic lung disease;
  - classic indicators: recurrent infections, wheeze, productive cough, oxygen requirement.

Associated conditions:
- Tracheobronchomalacia e.g. in ex-premature infant, Hunter, Crouzon.
- Tracheoesophageal fistula, particularly H-type.
- Kyphoscoliosis leads to a restrictive lung defect.
- High spinal cord injury.
- Chronic lung disease of prematurity.
- Early diaphragm involvement in *SMARD1*, CMT variants, adult-variant Pompe. Reduced FVC lying compared to sitting. Reduced sniff nasal pressure. May occur in walking patients.
- Remember a child with neurodisability may also have asthma, cystic fibrosis, etc. like any other child!
- Medication side effects: glycopyrrolate (thickened secretions), morphine (cough suppressant).

Syndrome specific considerations

- *Ataxia telangiectasia*: interstitial lung disease, bronchiectasis.
- *Cockayne* syndrome: chest infections.
- *MECP2 duplication*: recurrent severe chest infections.
- *Benign hereditary chorea* (*TTF1* mutation): respiratory distress syndrome in neonatal period, chronic interstitial disease, respiratory infections.
- *Hereditary haemorrhagic telangiectasia*:
  - pulmonary AVMs, lung haemorrhage, right-to-left shunting, dyspnoea.
- *Tuberous sclerosis*: lymphangioleiomyomatosis (diffuse, small, thin-walled cysts) in young ♀ adults, progressive dyspnoea.

Chronic nocturnal and diurnal hypoventilation

Usually late complication of neuromuscular disease, e.g. Duchenne, Ullrich congenital muscular dystrophy, congenital myaesthenias (e.g. slow channel syndrome).

Classic symptoms and signs
- Morning headache.
- Non-refreshing sleep.
- Difficulty rousing (e.g. after elective GA).
- Excessive daytime sleepiness.
- Nocturnal sweating.
- Recurrent chest infections.

Severe nocturnal hypoventilation can cause overnight atelectasis and secondary infection. Daytime hypoventilation may follow due to ↓response to chronic hypercapnia. May result in ↑intracranial pressure (ICP) and cor pulmonale if left untreated.

Interventions
- Medication review, e.g. glycopyrrolate; prophylactic antibiotics; anti-reflux; reduce sedatives.
- Preventative immunizations against e.g. influenza, COVID-19.
- Chest physiotherapy.
- Oxygen.
- Suction.
- Cough assist machine.
- Upper airways surgery, e.g. adenotonsillectomy.
- Non-invasive ventilation: see Long-term ventilation in Chapter 5 p. 600.
- Tracheostomy and invasive ventilation.
- Anti-reflux surgical procedures.
- Feeding strategies (occult aspiration).

Continence

A neuropathic bladder can be contractile or acontractile, and *safe* or *unsafe*. The latter refers to the extent that the kidneys are subject to obstruction with back pressure and/or infection through vesico-ureteric reflux and thus whether the **child is at risk of chronic renal failure**.
- Contractile, reflex bladders are *usually unsafe*.
- Acontractile bladders are *sometimes* safe.

General principles:
- Avoid constipation.
- Prevent UTI (prophylactic antibiotics in reflux or recurrent infections).
- Only treat *symptomatic* UTIs (no treatment for asymptomatic bacteriuria).

Contractile, reflex type bladder
- An 'upper motor neuron' picture in the bladder. S2–4 are intact but descending inhibitory pathways lost due to brain or spine damage.
- Detrusor sphincter dyssynergia: bladder and sphincter contraction occur simultaneously, preventing normal voiding and transmitting back pressure to the kidneys.
- Small volume, hyperreflexic bladder.
- Intermittent reflex emptying—usually incomplete bladder voiding.
- Brisk anal reflex.

Management
- Anticholinergics (oxybutynin) and catheterization.
- In severe cases: sphincterotomy, pudendal neurectomy, or urinary diversion to reduce outflow obstruction, cystoplasty to augment bladder capacity.

Acontractile bladder
- A 'lower motor neuron' picture due to involvement of S2–4.
- Large weak bladder: does not contract.
- Weak sphincter, leakage with cough, cry.
- Patulous anus.

Management
- Bladder expression, intermittent catheterization, continence with an artificial urinary sphincter.

Safe bladder
- <20 mL residue after voiding (assessed by post-micturition bladder ultrasound), normal upper tract, normal renal function, no pressure transmission.

Management
- Toilet training, suprapubic pressure.

Unsafe bladder
- Large bladder residue after voiding, outlet obstruction, high back pressure to kidneys, hydronephrosis.

- Clean intermittent catheterization has revolutionized management of unsafe neuropathic bladders. It can be performed by carers or taught to older children (developmental age >6 yrs). Technique is not *aseptic*, just *clean*. Complications: infection, trauma.
- Continuous (indwelling) catheterization may be considered in situations of severe upper renal tract dilatation or in severely disabled children but has much higher rates of infection.

Bowels

The same spinal pathologies that cause bladder problems can cause bowel problems and will need a similar approach. Usually the bladder problems are more pronounced and bowel habits can often still be trained.

- High spinal lesion: intact reflex, absent sensation (continence can be gained):
  - stimulation with bisacodyl, finger, microenema.
- Low lesion: absent reflex, sensation present (incontinence more likely).
  - abdominal pressure, straining, manual evacuation, bulking agents.
- Other:
  - high fibre diet, stool softeners, and bowel stimulants for hard stools.

Demyelinating syndromes

Acquired demyelinating syndromes (ADS) are acute neurological illnesses characterized by clinical deficits persisting for at least 24 hours, involving the optic nerve, brain, or spinal cord, and associated with areas of ↑T2 signal on MRI.
- Affect 1–2/100 000 paediatric patients per year.
- Clinical manifestations include: monofocal optic neuritis (ON) or transverse myelitis (TM); or multifocal involvement either *with* (acute disseminated encephalomyelitis, ADEM) or *without* encephalopathy.
- May occur as a monophasic illness or as a chronic disease such as multiple sclerosis (MS), Aquaporin-4 antibody (AQP4-Ab) neuromyelitis optica spectrum disorder (NMOSD) or relapsing myelin oligodendrocyte glycoprotein antibody (MOG-Ab) associated disease (MOGAD).

▶▶Relapsing demyelination does not necessarily imply one of these diagnoses: children with recurrent demyelination who do not meet criteria for MS, NMOSD or MOGAD should be investigated for both inflammatory and non-inflammatory mimics (such as genetic autoinflammatory syndromes).

- Persistently undiagnosed patients should be managed empirically for neuroinflammation depending on risk of relapse and disease progression.
- Around 20% of individuals with an ADS will go on to have further episodes. The risk of relapse is related to the specific clinical syndrome.
- Patients presenting with a first ADS should be investigated with MRI brain and spine with contrast, oligoclonal bands, and serum MOG and AQP4 antibodies.

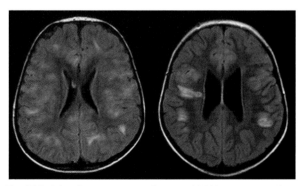

Fig. 4.5 Radiological appearances in two three-year old children presenting with first episode of ADEM. 'Typical' appearances on left. Child on right shows 'atypical' radiological features (well defined, periventricular, perpendicular to corpus callosum); had family history of MS and went on to develop relapsing-remitting MS.

Acute disseminated Encephalomyelitis (ADEM)

- Typically, a disease of young children with a peak incidence around ~ 5y. Slightly more common in ♂'s.
- Frequently a clear history of viral illness (or less frequently, immunization) in the preceding 2 weeks.
- MRI shows either single or multiple areas of 'fluffy' demyelinated plaques (high T2 signal): these can be anywhere in the hemispheres (neocortex, white matter and/or deep grey matter), brainstem, and/or cerebellum. Lesions are often asymmetrical. Some lesions may demonstrate contrast enhancement and/or restricted diffusion (see Fig 4.5).
- Optic nerve and spinal cord involvement can be seen and may be asymptomatic.
- Radiological appearances lag clinical course in about 30% of patients: rarely patients have normal MRI at presentation with changes developing over few days (and persisting after clinical recovery).
- MOG-Ab are detected in about 50% of children with ADEM.
- CSF lymphocytosis may be seen and does not preclude the diagnosis.
- Oligoclonal bands are frequently –ve (in about 90%): if +ve they typically show a Type 3 pattern (see Table 2.4 in Chapter 2 ➜ p. 99).

Treatment of ADEM

- Pulsed intravenous methylprednisolone (typically 30 mg/kg maximum 1 g daily for 3–5 days) followed by 4–6 weeks weaning course of oral prednisolone.
- If no/minimal response, consider escalation to plasma exchange and/ or IVIG.
- Even if MOG-Ab +ve, maintenance immunosuppression is not recommended following a first attack.

Outcome of ADEM

- Typically, complete recovery from initial episode, particularly when treated acutely. A small proportion of patients have residual cognitive and behaviour problems.
- Risk of relapse is ~10–30%.
- Relapse can occur decades later.

▶▶Relapses are predominantly seen in MOG-Ab +ve patients.

- Relapse can be resemble the initial presentation or involve new sites. Radiological evidence of new lesions or evidence of new optic neuritis is required to diagnose relapse.
- Treatment decisions are influenced by (i) timing of relapse (ii) recovery from attack (iii) response to treatment (iv) antibody positivity (see Paediatric MOGAD in this chapter ➜ p. 270).

Optic neuritis (ON)

- Visual loss usually occurs over hours to days, typically reaching a nadir within days.
- Pain with eye movement is reported in 33–77% of paediatric cases.

- Decreased visual acuity (VA), abnormal colour vision, particularly red colour desaturation, and visual field deficits.
- Unilateral presentation at onset may be followed rapidly by bilateral involvement. Three patterns are distinguished:
  - *Bilateral simultaneous* ON: involvement of second side within 2 weeks.
  - *Bilateral sequential* ON: involvement of second side 2–12 weeks after first.
  - *Bilateral recurrent* ON: involvement of second side >12 weeks later.
- Children <10 years of age more likely to present with bilateral ON, whereas children ≥10 years present more frequently unilaterally.
- Some children may complain of headaches and other symptoms of ↑intracranial pressure.
- VA at onset: 20% better than 20/40; 20% between 20/50–20/190; 60% worse than 20/200.
- While ON may be clinically limited to one eye, neurophysiological studies often identify bilateral involvement.
- When ON is the first presentation of relapsing-remitting multiple sclerosis (RRMS), MRI brain usually already demonstrate lesions typical of RRMS. Children presenting with optic neuritis and normal brain MRI are unlikely to be subsequently diagnosed with MS.
- ON due to MOGAD very rarely involves the chiasm, unlike ON due to AQP4.

Treatment
- No clinical trials have been performed for paediatric ON.
- In adults, recovery after IV steroid administration was more rapid than with placebo or oral steroid if given within 15 days of onset. Little difference between groups at 7 weeks.
- Treatment does not reduce risk of relapse in MS.
- If AQP-Ab are +ve more aggressive ongoing immunosuppression is required.
- Typical regime 30 mg/kg per day IVMP, maximum 1 g daily, for 3–5 days. Followed by weaning course of oral prednisolone.
- If presenting visual loss is very severe rapid escalation to plasma exchange is recommended.

Outcome
- Vision returns to almost normal high contrast visual acuity in the majority of children (particularly in MOGAD and RRMS); however, children often report subjective residual visual abnormalities.
- Poor recovery more commonly seen in children presenting with AQP4-Ab NMOSD.
- May be left with clinical optic atrophy (despite normal acuity).
- Time to treatment influences final visual outcome in antibody-mediated demyelination.

Acute transverse myelitis

- Demyelination of one or more segments of the spinal cord resulting in acute or subacute onset symptoms and signs of severe spinal cord dysfunction with motor, sensory, and sphincter disturbance.

- 'Transverse' refers to the presence of a sensory level.
- All children will require urgent MRI to exclude surgically remediable causes of cord compression.
- Lesion distribution varies:
  - *Longitudinally extensive transverse myelitis* (LETM), defined as involvement of ≥3 contiguous levels, more commonly seen in MOG-Ab and AQP4-Ab disease.
  - *MOG-Ab lesions* are more likely to be central with 'H-shaped' involvement on axial imaging (H-sign) and may involve conus.
  - *AQP4-Ab lesions* typically extend to the dorsal brainstem (area postrema).
  - *MS lesions* are typically short and peripheral.
- When transverse myelitis is the first presentation of RRMS, MRI brain will typically have lesions typical of RRMS.
- Most children with isolated LETM (no brain lesions) are antibody -ve but antibody testing is recommended in all patients.

Treatment
- Treatment is typically with high-dose IV methylprednisolone followed by a weaning course of oral prednisolone.
- Plasma exchange and/or IVIG needs to be considered if response to steroids is poor.
- If AQP4-Ab are +ve long-term immunosuppression is recommended at first presentation.
- Rehabilitative spinal care is crucial (see Acquired spinal cord injury in this chapter ➲ p. 224).

Outcome
- Approximately 1/3 make a full recovery, 1/3 partial recovery (often residual urinary dysfunction) and 1/3 left with significant or severe impairment.
- Time to treatment and early escalation influence final outcome.
- Most cases of transverse myelitis are monophasic outside context of RRMS.

Paediatric multiple sclerosis (MS)

▶▶Paediatric multiple sclerosis (MS) is associated with higher relapse rates, more rapid MRI lesion accrual and worse cognitive outcome and physical disability in the long term compared to adult-onset disease.

- Predominantly a disease of adolescence but has been reported in children as young as 2 years. Presentation in the pre-pubertal age group is rare with many previously reported cases now known to be relapsing MOGAD and not relapsing-remitting (RR) MS.
- Aetiology is a complex interplay between environment, genetics, and infection. Vitamin D levels and EBV infection appear to be important.
- Signs are often relatively focal: e.g. unilateral optic neuritis; weakness and spasticity; or sensory symptoms (paraesthesia and abnormal vibration testing).
- Encephalopathy is *absent* (c.f. present by definition in ADEM).

- The diagnosis of MS in children, as in adults, requires evidence of CNS inflammatory activity in more than one CNS location (i.e. *dissemination in space*, DIS) and recurrence over time (i.e. *dissemination in time*, DIT).
  - The term Clinically Isolated Syndrome (CIS) is used for a first episode of demyelination unless and until DIS and DIT occur.
  - The 2017 McDonald diagnostic criteria permit the diagnosis of MS at first presentation in a child (i.e. accept radiological evidence of DIS *and DIT*, the latter implied by lesions of different ages) provided that the MRI features demonstrate lesions in areas typical for MS (periventricular white matter, juxtacortical, brainstem, and spinal cord) and there are ≥2 clinically silent lesions, ≥1 of which enhances with gadolinium.
  - Oligoclonal bands positivity if present is also evidence of DIT.
- MS in children is usually RRMS although primary progressive has been reported.

▶▶As in adults, consideration and exclusion of differential diagnoses is fundamental to the diagnosis of MS in children. This includes exclusion of antibody-mediated disease (MOG and AQP4) and consideration of monogenic disorders with relapsing-remitting clinical course, such as Haemophagocytic Lymphohistiocytosis (HLH, see Haemophagocytic lymphohistiocytosis (HLH) in this chapter ➋ p. 402), leukodystrophies, and mitochondrial disease.

Treatment in MS
- As with other ADS, steroids are typically used in the acute phase and appear to shorten relapse duration but with no evidence of an effect on longer-term course.
- Early initiation of disease modifying therapy has been shown to improve long-term outcome.
- The more aggressive course of paediatric-onset MS justifies early use of the more effective treatments typically used for 'highly active' disease in adults, e.g. anti-CD20 therapies rather than interferons.
- 6 monthly brain MRI monitoring is recommended with treatment escalation if radiological disease activity is noted.
  - 'No evidence of disease activity' (NEDA), i.e. the absence of both radiological and clinical signs of relapse is used as the primary endpoint for evaluation of treatment efficacy.
  - Monitoring brain volume is also important in paediatric MS.

Paediatric neuromyelitis optica spectrum disorder (NMOSD)
- An antibody-mediated demyelinating disease.
- Relapsing disease in the majority.
- Distinct clinical and radiological phenotype from MS.
- In contrast to MS, accumulating disability is thought to result from the attacks themselves with little inter-relapse neurodegeneration.

- Antibodies against the astrocyte water channel protein, aquaporin-4 (AQP4) are disease specific and can be measured in serum using cell-based assay.
  - AQP4-Ab seropositivity otherwise rare in children presenting with a first ADS episode (0.7–4.5%).
- Clinical and MRI features of NMOSD in children resemble adults'.
- NMOSD diagnostic criteria depend on AQP4 antibody status:
  - If AQP4-Ab +ve only one core clinical feature is required to make the diagnosis, from: optic neuritis; acute myelitis; area postrema syndrome; acute brainstem syndrome; acute diencephalic clinical syndrome (including narcolepsy) together with NMOSD-typical diencephalic MRI lesions; or any symptomatic cerebral syndrome with NMOSD-typical brain lesions.
  - If AQP4-Ab –ve (or unknown) at least two core clinical features are required alongside supportive MRI findings.

Supportive MRI findings
- *Features supportive of acute ON:*
  - brain normal or only non-specific white matter lesions;
  - optic nerve T2-hyperintense or T1 GAD enhancing lesion extending >50% optic nerve length or involving chiasm.
- *Features supportive of acute myelitis:*
  - associated lesion extending over ≥ 3 contiguous segments (i.e. LETM);
  - or ≥ 3 contiguous segments of focal cord atrophy in patients with prior history of acute myelitis.
- *Features supportive of area postrema syndrome (APS):*
  - dorsal medulla/area postrema MRI lesion.
- *Features supportive of acute brainstem syndrome:*
  - peri-ependymal brainstem lesions.

Treatment
- Acute episodes treated aggressively with IV methylprednisolone and prolonged oral steroid weaning course over six weeks.
- Low threshold for adding PLEX ± subsequent IVIG.
- Treatment with anti-CD20 treatment (e.g. rituximab) recommended following the first clinical attack.
- Several conventional MS therapies such as interferon β are associated with disease *worsening* in NMOSD.

Paediatric MOGAD
- MOGAD is a specific entity distinct from both MS and AQP4-Ab NMOSD.
- MOG-Ab seropositivity is common in children: present in >30% children with first ADS episode and >50% of those presenting with ADEM.
- Two-thirds of children will have a monophasic disease: full recovery is commoner in young children.
- Age-dependent phenotypes:
  - ADEM more frequently seen in younger children (under 10).

- Optic neuritis or NMOSD (without brain involvement) in older children.
- MOGAD can also cause an encephalitic illness resembling 'viral meningitis' with prominent seizures (see Anti-MOG antibody encephalitis in this chapter **⊃** p. 394); and also fulminant intracerebral hypertension.
- About 10% of children with MOG-Ab appear to have a more aggressive disease course, refractory to most treatments:
  - typically young, with a Multiphasic Disseminated Encephalomyelitis (MDEM) phenotype;
  - accumulate disabilities, cognitive decline, cerebellar features, visual problems, and seizures;
  - MRI may demonstrate a leukodystrophy-like phenotype.
- Antibodies typically measured in *serum*: utility of measuring CSF antibodies being evaluated.
- When antibodies are measured using fixed-cell assays, at least one supportive clinical or MRI feature is required to make the diagnosis:
  - *Optic neuritis supportive features*: bilateral simultaneous involvement; longitudinal optic nerve involvement (>50% length); optic sheath enhancement; papillitis of optic disc.
  - *Myelitis supportive features*: LETM; central cord lesion or H-sign; conus lesion.
  - *Features supporting brain, brainstem, or cerebral syndrome*: multiple ill-defined T2 hyperintense lesions in supratentorial and often infratentorial white matter; deep grey matter involvement; pons, middle cerebellar peduncle, or medulla involvement; cortical lesion with or without lesional and overlying meningeal enhancement.

Acute treatment

- Typically, intravenous methylprednisolone (IVMP) for 3–5 days. Steroids thought to be very useful in reduction of inflammation, sealing of the blood–brain barrier and overall reduction of antibody production.
- Many patients with MOGAD are extremely steroid responsive and may achieve complete and dramatic symptom remissions following a short course of IV steroids. Consider steroid tapering with oral prednisolone for a maximum of 3 months.
- Where improvement with IVMP is not seen, or in severe attacks (complete visual loss, paralysis, severe encephalopathy requiring ICU admission), escalate treatment with plasma exchange (PLEX) and/or intravenous immunoglobulins (IVIG, total of 2 g/kg over 2 or 5 days).
  - PLEX with five exchanges on successive days is the best way of reducing antibody levels if urgently required, but not all centres will have the facilities.
  - IVIG should be given *after* PLEX as otherwise PLEX will remove it!

Maintenance treatment

- Possible benefits of maintenance therapy need to be weighed against the risks of long-term immunosuppression.
- Current guidance does *not* recommend maintenance therapy after a first episode of demyelination even if MOG-Ab +ve (assuming they do not fulfil criteria for MS and are AQP4-Ab –ve).

- Where needed maintenance with MMF, azathioprine, rituximab, or IVIG may be considered.
  - MMF and azathioprine have delayed onsets of action and the first few months should be covered with steroids.
- If relapse or progression occurs e.g. on MMF or azathioprine, escalate to rituximab and/or monthly IVIG (some reports of life-threatening relapses on rituximab in contrast to AQP4-Ab NMOSD).
- Decisions to discontinue maintenance therapy need to consider severity of previous attacks and residual disability; challenges of evaluating treatment benefits vs regression to the mean; and side effect and risks of ongoing medication.
- In contrast to AQP4-Ab NMOSD, in which withdrawing maintenance treatment is risky, the relapses in MOG-Ab associated disease are milder and some patients and clinician will consider stopping treatment after 2 yrs' stability.

Outcome
- Most paediatric patients make a good recovery with an Expanded Disability Status Score (EDSS) <2 at 2 years.
- It is estimated that about 40% of adults and 30% of children with MOGAD present with a second clinical attack within five years.
- Approximately 60% of adult patients develop permanent neurological deficits, including motor and visual symptoms.
- About 50% of children with relapsing MOGAD and brain involvement develop cognitive problems.

Prediction of disability based on characteristics of the first attack remains unsatisfactory: antibody titres, even when measured longitudinally, do not correlate with disability outcomes. Similarly, baseline MRI parameters are not predictive of risk of relapse or disability.

Epilepsy

Remember the essential steps:
- Is it epilepsy? See Funny turns: likely epilepsy? in Chapter 3 ➲ p. 153.
- What seizure type(s) are present?
- Do I understand the cause of the epilepsy?
- Do the features constitute an epilepsy syndrome?

Thinking about causes

As in many areas of paediatric neurology, approaches to thinking about causes of epilepsy have been frequently revised in recent years in attempts to reflect rapidly advancing knowledge in epilepsy genetics while at the same time remaining of pragmatic clinical value. The current classification of epilepsies published by the International League Against Epilepsy (ILAE) (2017) divides aetiologies under the following headings:
- Genetic.
- Structural.
- Metabolic.
- Immune.
- Infectious.
- Unknown.

A child's epilepsy may fit two or more headings. For example, there may be a *structural* pathology such as a cortical dysplasia of known *genetic* origin (such as a *DCX* mutation); or a *metabolic* mechanism such as GLUT1 deficiency syndrome or non-ketotic hyperglycinaemia with an identified *genetic* basis.

Genetic

This heading includes both known monogenic epilepsies (such as those due to *SCN1A* mutations); but also the epilepsies where there is strong empiric evidence of a genetic origin (e.g. through studies of familial aggregation) even if the precise mechanisms of that genetic basis have not yet been identified. This includes the large, important group of *Idiopathic Generalized Epilepsies* (IGEs) accounting for perhaps a third of all cases of epilepsy: see Idiopathic generalized epilepsy syndromes in this chapter ➲ p. 288.

Conversely note that *genetic* need not imply *inherited*: many children with epilepsy due to tuberous sclerosis will have *de novo* mutations.

Structural

Epilepsies with radiologically evident structural abnormalities that can reasonably be assumed to be causative. While these abnormalities may be acquired (e.g. stroke), as stressed above these abnormalities may themselves be of genetic origin. See also MRI and brain development in Chapter 2 ➲ p. 71.

Metabolic

Including a number of individually rare vitamin-responsive conditions. Note that by convention seizures associated with an acute, temporary biochemical disturbance (e.g. hypoglycaemia, hyponatraemia, uraemia) would not normally be regarded as 'an epilepsy'. The term '[recurrent] acute symptomatic seizures' is available for this situation.

Immune
Including epilepsies due to autoimmune encephalitides: see Autoimmune encephalopathy in this chapter ⮞ p. 391.

Infectious
Probably the commonest aetiology of epilepsy globally.

Deprecated terms
Various terms in previous approaches to classification of epilepsy causation are now deprecated: however as they may still be met in clinic letters it is useful to understand the ideas that they were trying—imperfectly—to convey:

- 'Symptomatic' was used to convey situations of readily identifiable aetiology (often, in practice, the presence of radiological abnormalities). Such children would now typically be regarded as having *structural* or *structural-genetic* epilepsy.
- 'Cryptogenic' (meaning 'hidden cause') and its successor 'presumed symptomatic' represented the children for whom the aetiology of their epilepsy was unknown. This group is, of course, steadily shrinking with time although an 'unknown' category remains in the current ILAE scheme.
- 'Idiopathic' is particularly confusing term: in epilepsy it is being used in the etymologically correct sense of the cause being within the person (idios: Greek for 'personal' or 'private'; pathos: 'disease'), rather than the 'can't find a cause' (i.e. 'unknown') meaning in some other areas of medicine: it is *not* the 'dustbin category'! It is the positive recognition of one of a number of specific epilepsy pictures where the cause is believed to be polygenic and further investigation and imaging is generally not required. The term is currently reserved for idiopathic generalized epilepsies (IGEs) which are a subcategory of genetic generalized epilepsies (GGEs) and includes four specific epilepsy syndromes: childhood absence epilepsy; juvenile absence epilepsy; juvenile myoclonic epilepsy and generalized tonic–clonic seizures alone.

Epilepsy syndromes

The idea and identification of epilepsy *syndromes* (Greek *syn* meaning 'together' and *dromos*, 'running') has been a fruitful concept in progressing epileptology, but it is important to appreciate that the approach has limitations.

- Epilepsy syndromes were initially defined entirely *phenotypically* based on observable features, such as age at onset, seizure type(s), EEG features, natural history, family history, neurodevelopmental outcome, response to drugs, and so on.
- In recent years, the genetic basis of an ever-increasing proportion of epilepsies has been identified and it is clear that genotype–phenotype relationships can be complex: one gene can cause multiple syndromes and one syndrome can have multiple genetic causes.
- Syndromic approaches to epilepsy diagnosis have proven pragmatic value: knowing what epilepsy syndrome one is dealing with can guide decisions relating to the need for investigation, ASM selection, and aspects of counselling. Whether genotypic perspectives will ultimately

prove more useful in clinical practice remains to be seen but for the time being phenotypic perspectives are probably still predominant.

- Some epilepsy syndromes are very characteristic and specific; in others a degree of variability is recognized and boundaries are less well defined. Deciding on a syndromic diagnosis can take time: with the passing of a few months, increased clarity in the history, and where appropriate repeat EEGs, the definition of the syndrome becomes possible in most cases.

▶ It is important to appreciate that some of the syndromes are very much commoner than others. Some (e.g. particularly SeLECTS and the idiopathic generalized epilepsies) will be seen regularly even in general paediatrics: others are rare even in specialist paediatric neurology practice.

- The notion of 'epilepsy epochs', considering the age at which a child's epilepsy begins, is a useful one. Different age-groups are associated with particular epilepsy syndromes. For example, neonatal-onset epilepsies are often (though not always) severe and intractable and associated with genetic or structural-genetic aetiologies; in contrast, in epilepsies of adolescent onset the idiopathic generalized epilepsies predominate.

The description of epileptic syndromes here follows the 2017 International League Against Epilepsy (ILAE) classification and the 2022 ILAE Task Force on Nosology and Definitions paper.

Neonatal and infant-onset epilepsy syndromes

Many neonatal seizures reflect serious pathologies such as stroke or infection (see Neonatal seizures in Chapter 5 ⟳ p. 551). In cases where no obvious cause is immediately identifiable, consider:

Self-limited epilepsy syndromes
Self-limited (familial) neonatal epilepsy (SeLNE)

- Previously known as benign familial neonatal seizures.
- Brief clonic seizures in the head, face, and limbs that may progress to sequential features. Associated with autonomic features in ~1/3 of cases. May alternate sides within or between episodes. The infant is normal between seizures.
- Clusters of seizures may occur over hours or days.
- Resolve spontaneously by 6 months of age, the majority by 6 weeks.
- Development is normal.
- Around a third of patients have seizures later in life.
- Sporadic cases have a *de novo* pathogenic variant while an autosomal dominant inheritance is found in familial cases.
    - Family is often surprisingly relaxed about their seizing infant as grandmother has reassured mother it also happened to her!
- *KCNQ2* in ~80% of cases. Other genes: *KCNQ3, SCN2A*.
- Typically respond well to carbamazepine.
- Need to exclude other causes.

Self-limited familial neonatal-infantile epilepsy (SeLFNIE)
- Onset within first two years (mean: 11 weeks).
- ♂=♂.
- Semiology similar to SeLNE.
- Focal clonic or focal clonic seizures, with head and eye deviation, with apnoeic spells and staring. Seizure may last up to 4 min and may occur in clusters.
- Seizures typically readily controlled with ASM. Normal development.
- Remit by 12–24 m of age, with no reappearance later in life.
- Autosomal dominant inheritance or de novo pathogenic variants (in nonfamilial cases) usually in *SCN2A* gene.

Self-limited (familial) infantile epilepsy (SeLIE)
- Relatively common. Previously known as benign familial infantile seizures.
- Onset 3–20 months (peak: 6 months).
- Brief focal seizures with behavioural arrest, impaired awareness, cyanosis, automatisms, head/eye version, and clonic movements.
- May change sides between seizures and evolve to bilateral tonic–clonic seizure.
- Seizures can be frequent and difficult to control at onset, but usually resolve with a year of onset.
- A minority develop epilepsy in later life.
- Genetic aetiology is found in 80%, usually *PRRT2*; more rarely on *SCN8A*, *SCN2A*. Familial cases: autosomal dominant inheritance.

Generalized epilepsy with febrile seizures plus (GEFS+) spectrum
GEFS+ is an entity that sits awkwardly within the syndromic approach in that the hallmark is a family history rather than characteristic clinical features. There is a pedigree consistent with autosomal dominant inheritance with high penetrance (60% or more) and a strong flavour of seizures being fever-associated; however the actual seizure types can vary within pedigrees. GEFS+ is more a diagnosis for a family rather than for an individual!
- Individuals in the pedigree may have Dravet syndrome, myoclonic-atonic seizures, IGE, focal epilepsies, febrile seizures plus (FS+), or classic febrile seizures. FS+ is the most common phenotype.
- Generalized or focal afebrile seizures present at different ages and are responsive to ASM (not all need medication). Usually remit by puberty.
- Due to *SCN1A* mutations in many pedigrees.
  - As such related to Dravet syndrome (see Dravet syndrome in this chapter ➔ p. 278) although typically much less severe.
- Other genes identified: *SCN2A, SCN1B, STX1B*, and GABA receptor subunit genes.

Myoclonic epilepsy in infancy (MEI)
- Rare, accounting for only 1% of genetic generalized epilepsies.
- Onset 4 months to 3 yrs (peak: 16–18 m). ♂: ♀= 2:1.
- Myoclonic seizures affecting trunk and upper limbs (e.g. brief nodding movements of the head) but only rarely the lower limbs, sometimes occurring in brief clusters of a few at a time, which can lead to falls.

- No drop attacks.
- Children are otherwise normal.
- May be confused with infantile spasms until EEG available.
- Interictal EEG usually normal. Myoclonic jerks are associated with spike–wave or polyspike–wave discharges at frequencies >3 Hz.
- ASM can be stopped in most children (those with photosensitivity may be more difficult to control).
- Usually remit 6 months to 5 years after onset. Later epilepsy risk is ~10%.
- No causal genes as yet identified.

Developmental and epileptic encephalopathies (DEEs)
Early infantile developmental and epileptic encephalopathy (EIDEE)
Previously known as Early Infantile (Ohtahara) and Early Myoclonic Epileptic Encephalopathies but combined into a single entity in the latest ILAE framework.

- Characterized by epilepsy onset before 3 months (adjusted for prematurity), abnormalities on EEG and on neurological examination from the moment the seizures begin, and evolution to moderate to severe developmental delay.
- Seizures are typically drug resistant and can be tonic, myoclonic, epileptic spasms or sequential seizures, and occur independent of the sleep cycle (except for the epileptic spasms that are often on awakening) .
- Tonic seizures are common and usually asymmetric in the neonatal period. Typically sustained longer than an infantile spasm and occur in clusters.
- Focal or multifocal myoclonus is frequent, can be erratic (asynchronous, asymmetric, and random) or massive and bilateral. When present consider metabolic etiologies such as non-ketotic hyperglycinaemia or (importantly) pyridoxine-dependent epilepsy.
- Neuroimaging, metabolic, and genetic investigations identify the aetiology in about 80% of cases.
- May be associated with severe structural abnormalities, some of which may be amenable to resective surgery.
- In those with normal imaging, a rapidly increasing number of single-gene causes of EIDEE are now recognized including *KCNQ2*, *SCN2A*, *SCN8A*, *STXBP1*, *CDKL5*, *KCNT1*, and *UBA5*. This is a group for whom investigation through early onset epilepsy gene panels can be particularly useful: see Role of genetic investigation in this chapter p. 294.
- Metabolic investigations required especially when neuroimaging is normal or suggests a particular metabolic disorder.
- EEG may show a suppression-burst pattern, multifocal spikes/spike waves/sharp waves with or without slowing, discontinuity, and/or diffuse slowing. Ictal EEG depends on seizure type.
- Poor prognosis for development and ↑mortality. Often later evolution into infantile spasms or Lennox–Gastaut syndrome (LGS) (see Box 4.4).
- Resistant to ASM treatment unless a structural abnormality can be resected, or a specific metabolic therapy instituted.

> **Box 4.4 Epilepsy syndromes, development, and aetiology**
>
> It is important to remember that epilepsy syndromes are often defined *phenotypically*, and can have multiple causes. Confusion can arise from textbook statements that, for example, 'West syndrome is a cause of Lennox–Gastaut syndrome'.
>
> It is useful to recognize that there are a limited number of ways the brain can manifest dysfunction from an underlying pathology, and that this repertoire is age-dependent (e.g. constrained by myelination status). In the same way that absence seizures are only a feature of epilepsies in a particular age band, epileptic spasms are to an extent 'what seizures look like' in a 6–12 month old. The manifestations of any given primary pathology may change with age and development. For example, a child with severe birth asphyxia can sequentially move through several phenotypically described syndromes with time, e.g. from EIDEE to West and then to Lennox–Gastaut syndrome over time, *all as manifestations of the same primary pathology.*

Epilepsy of infancy with migrating focal seizures (EIMFS)
- Rapidly evolving epilepsy comprising very frequent (at least hourly) focal motor clonic or tonic seizures of multifocal origin (i.e. no single focus) usually starting in first 6 months of life.
- Although EEG may be initially normal it develops characteristic features:
  - *interictally*, multifocal spikes;
  - *ictally*, independent, uni-hemispheric foci that move ('migrate') between hemispheres *during a seizure*, correlating with a clinical shift of focus.
- Associated with extreme drug resistance, very poor neurodevelopmental outcome, and reduced life expectancy.
- Genetically heterogeneous; 50% with de novo abnormalities in *KCNT1* potassium channel gene; other genes associated: *SCN1A*, *SCN2A*, *SLC12A5*, *BRAT1*, and *TBC1D24*.

Dravet syndrome
- Relatively common and increasingly recognized: probably 1–3% of all epilepsies beginning before 1yr of life.
- The label Severe Myoclonic Epilepsy of Infancy (SMEI) has previously been regarded as synonymous with Dravet however a picture similar in all respects save for the absence of myoclonic seizures can arise from the same mutations, so the term Dravet syndrome may be preferable.
- Presents typically between 3 and 12 months with recurrent episodes of *febrile status epilepticus* (often focal/lateralized).
  - Many of the children previously regarded as having had pertussis vaccine-related encephalopathy are now recognized to have Dravet syndrome: the apparent relationship with vaccination reflected susceptibility to seizures with pyrexia.

- Consider in any infant who has been admitted more than once to PICU in febrile status.
- Prior development is normal.
- Multiple seizure types develop in second year of life with prominent myoclonus emerging at >18 months of age.
- Heat (febrile illness or even a hot bath) characteristically remains a precipitant of seizures.
- Family history of epilepsy and/or febrile seizures in 30–50% (consider GEFS+, see Generalized epilepsy with febrile seizures plus (GEFS+) spectrum this chapter ➋ p. 276).
- Interictal EEG shows generalized, focal, and multifocal abnormalities and may show photosensitivity.
- Up to 85% of cases are associated with *SCN1A* sodium channel mutations.
  - Other identified causative genes in some *SCN1A* –ve cases include *GABRG2*, *GABRG1*, *STXBP1*, and *SCN1B*.
  - Genotype–phenotype relationships are complex.
- Valproate remains first-line treatment of choice despite concerns about valproate use (see Contraception and reproductive health in this chapter ➋ p. 320); together with a benzodiazepine (usually clobazam) plus stiripentol and/or topiramate.
  - Carbamazepine, lamotrigine, oxcarbazepine, and phenytoin typically *worsen* seizures.
  - Some children respond well to ketogenic diet: see Ketogenic diet in this chapter ➋ p. 315.
  - Consider cannabidiol, fenfluramine.
- Loss of neurodevelopmental progress typically begins from 12 to 60 months after onset of seizures, with consequent moderate to severe intellectual disability.
  - It is unclear whether early recognition and prompt aggressive ASM therapy improve the long-term developmental outcome.
- There can be a slight delay in walking (mean: 16–18 months). A gait instability evolving to crouch gait typically occurs around puberty.
- ↑risk of SUDEP: see Death in epilepsy in this chapter ➋ p. 322.

Infantile epileptic spasms syndrome (IESS)

IESS includes West syndrome, which strictly refers to the combination of (i) epileptic spasms, (ii) hypsarrhythmia on EEG, and (iii) developmental stagnation or regression (see Box 4.5); but also infants who don't fulfil all these criteria.

- A very characteristic, recognizable clinical-EEG picture.
- Peak onset between 6 and 12 months but can occur at any time in first two years of life.
- If onset <3 months, consider other epileptic encephalopathies.
- Tonic spasms—sudden jerks with posture 'held' for a second or so occurring in clusters or runs especially on waking.
  - A history of several weeks, or even months, of subtler seizures prior to presentation is common, so recognition and treatment is often delayed.

- Child typically *cries* at end of run of spasms, sometimes leading to mistaken diagnoses of 'infantile colic'.
- Spasms may be either predominantly flexor, extensor, or mixed.
  - Focal brain pathology may cause *asymmetrical* spasms.
- Typically associated with a degree of *encephalopathy* (see Box 4.5): often loss of visual attentiveness and smile. The child may be irritable and is distressed by the spasms.
- Note that hypsarrhythmia (see Fig. 2.21 Hypsarrhythmia in Chapter 2 ➋ p. 89) develops over time and is not necessary for the diagnosis of infantile spasms.
  - Strictly, 'West Syndrome' refers to the combination of the spasm-type seizures, the encephalopathy (regression), *and* hypsarrhythmia on EEG.
- The most common *ictal* EEG pattern is a broad slow-wave followed by voltage suppression in association with the spasm (a so-called electrodecremental response: see Fig. 2.21 Hypsarrhythmia in Chapter 2 ➋ p. 89).
- Prognosis for seizure remission and neurodevelopment is strongly determined by the underlying aetiology: see Infantile epileptic spasms syndrome in this chapter ➋ p. 279.
- Neuroimaging abnormalities are found in ~50% and a genetic aetiology is found in up to 40% of the cases (Trisomy 21, *de novo* pathogenic variants in *ARX*, *CDKL5*, *STXBP1*, *IQSEC2*, *TSC1*, *TSC2*, and other genes).

Treatment
One of the few areas in paediatric neurology where practice can be informed by Level 1 RCT evidence!

Box 4.5 Developmental and epileptic encephalopathy

The term 'epileptic encephalopathy' relates to situations where epileptiform activity *additionally* contributes to neurologic dysfunction (e.g. reduced awareness or cognitive deficits) alongside the underlying aetiology.

Seizures - - - → Cognitive effects

Primary pathology

The implication is that such dysfunction might be at least partially reversible with ASM therapy although this is often difficult in practice. This concept is particularly applied to EIDEE (see Early infantile developmental and epileptic encephalopathy in this chapter ➋ p. 277), West, Lennox–Gastaut, and Landau–Kleffner syndromes, as well as to non-convulsive status epilepticus.

Epileptic encephalopathy is a feature in ~40% children with epilepsy first presenting at between 1 month and 3 yrs of age.

- Traditional options have included steroids in the form of high-dose oral corticosteroids, ACTH or tetracosactide (a synthetic ACTH analogue); and/or vigabatrin.
- Data from the International Collaborative Infantile Spasms Study (ICISS) indicated higher spasm-cessation rates with steroids *and* vigabatrin (72%) than hormonal therapy alone (57%); however, there was no difference in developmental or epilepsy outcomes between the groups at 18 months. This study confirmed the importance of timely diagnosis.
- Vigabatrin monotherapy remains first-line treatment in spasms due to tuberous sclerosis.
- There is significant morbidity associated with both treatments.
  - *Steroids*: hypertension, diabetes, immunosuppression (rarely, overwhelming sepsis), sometimes severe irritability. Monitor BP and urine for glycosuria weekly while on treatment.
  - *Vigabatrin*: irreversible visual field deficits associated with prolonged use (see Vigabatrin in Chapter 7 **⮞** p. 707). Aim to wean and replace vigabatrin over several months. (In some contexts, e.g. a child with known prior severe disability and cortical visual impairment in whom vigabatrin has proven very effective, this risk may be less pertinent and in informed agreement with family a decision to continue the treatment may be appropriate.)
  - A therapeutic trial of pyridoxine should be considered where no aetiology is evident.

Aetiology-specific syndromes

This is a new and rapidly growing group of neonatal and infantile-onset epilepsies, mostly associated with Development and Epileptic Encephalopathy (DEE). The ILAE emphasizes pictures with a distinct phenotype, associated with specific anomalies on EEG, neuroimaging findings, or genetic tests.

KCNQ2-DEE

- Seizure onset in the first days of life.
- Tonic seizures with autonomic features resemble SeLNE but are more frequent and associated with abnormalities on neurological exam and EEG (~60% with burst-suppression pattern).
- Although some achieve seizure control with sodium channel blockers (carbamazepine, phenytoin) there is no impact on the moderate to severe developmental delay.
- There is a severe loss of K^+ channel function caused by *de novo* missense variants in *KCNQ2* gene.

PD-DEE and P5PD-DEE

- Pyridoxine-dependent and pyridoxamine 5'-phosphate oxidase deficiency developmental and epileptic encephalopathies (PD-DEE and P5PD-DEE, respectively) are rare epilepsies due to metabolic defects within the lysine degradation pathway. See Vitamin B6 in this chapter **⮞** p. 524.

CDKL5-DEE
- X-linked disorder, ♀:♂ = 4:1 with ♂ more severely affected.
- Seizures start <3 months of life (median of 6 weeks).
- Tonic seizures and clusters of epileptic spasms alongside other seizure types.
- Hypotonia and cortical visual impairment, evolving to severe intellectual disability and other comorbidities such as movement disorders.
- Refractory epilepsy.

PCDH19 clustering epilepsy
- X-linked. Almost all ♀: rare mosaic ♂s described.
- Epilepsy starts <1 yr (mean 10 months).
- Clusters of focal seizures (sometimes prolonged) with fever sensitivity.
- Initially refractory seizures but improve in adolescence and ~¼ become seizure-free.
- Intellectual disability, autism, and psychiatric symptoms in adulthood.

Gelastic seizures with hypothalamic hamartoma
- Epilepsy onset in infancy or early childhood.
- *Gelastic* seizures: short episodes of odd, emotionless, and inappropriate laughter with retained awareness.
- Some also have *dacrystic* seizures (crying, sobbing, or grimacing).
- Multiple seizures per day, resistant to ASM.
- Hypothalamic hamartoma on MRI.
- Early surgical resection is important for seizure control and to prevent neurocognitive deterioration however morbidity related to damage of the chiasm (visual field defects, diabetes insipidus) is an important risk: refer to highly specialized centres.
- 5% associated with Pallister Hall syndrome (*GLI3* mutation).

Others
See also:
- Glucose transporter 1 deficiency syndrome (see Glucose transporter-1 deficiency syndrome (GLUT1-DS) in this chapter ⊃ p. 301).
- Sturge–Weber syndrome (see Sturge–Weber syndrome in this chapter ⊃ p. 467).

Childhood-onset epilepsy syndromes
Self-limited focal epilepsies of childhood

Self-limited epilepsy with centrotemporal spikes (SeLECTS)
(Previously known as Rolandic epilepsy or benign epilepsy with centrotemporal spikes).

▶ The most common focal onset epilepsy in childhood, yet often under-recognized. The value of making the diagnosis is that it allows you to convey a good prognosis from the outset.

- More common in ♂s.
- Onset between the ages of ~ 4–10 yrs.

- Key to recognition is that it is a *focal to tonic–clonic bilateral seizure with a perioral onset*. Seizure onset is from sleep up to 80% of the time (so initial perioral features may not be experienced or witnessed) and these features will only be elicited by direct questioning.
- The clues to a focal, perioral onset will be reflected either in the aura (the very earliest features of the seizure, although as seizures often arise from sleep this may not be available), or in *temporary post-ictal signs or symptoms*.
  - Typical features include unilateral numbness or paraesthesia of the tongue, lips, gums, or cheek; guttural sounds or speech arrest, hypersalivation, poor swallowing, or drooling post-ictally; involuntary movements or tonic contractions of the tongue or jaw; or clonus affecting one side of the face. It may evolve to a tonic–clonic seizure of the ipsilateral upper limb, followed by a hemiclonic or even a bilateral tonic–clonic seizure.
- The characteristic EEG finding is diphasic sharp-waves in the central-midtemporal area that have an orientation tangential to the cortex with a frontal +ve dipole. These are often activated by drowsiness or sleep, though might appear only unilaterally in any given EEG recording.

▶ Incidental centrotemporal spikes in people who have never had seizures are well recognized (e.g. in first-degree relatives of children with SeLECTS). Thus the presence of spikes is sensitive, but *not specific*, for a diagnosis of SeLECTS, and can only *support* a diagnosis of SeLECTS in the context of an appropriate history.
▶ If history, developmental, and/or EEG features are not entirely typical then consider MRI imaging to exclude a lesional epilepsy.

- Treatment is required only if seizures are frequent or long.
- Typically respond well to lamotrigine, levetiracetam, carbamazepine, oxcarbazepine or zonisamide (in more severe forms with DEE-SWAS/EE-SWAS carbamazepine may cause atonic and myoclonic seizures).
- 90% achieve remission around puberty.
- May be associated with language impairment, memory dysfunction, and auditory processing difficulties.
- A small proportion of cases have very frequent epileptiform discharges in sleep, sometimes approaching (D)EE-SWAS (see (Developmental) epileptic encephalopathy with spike-and-wave activation in sleep in this chapter ➲ p. 286); which should prompt an evaluation of language and cognitive impairments. Some authorities regard these children as being on a spectrum between straightforward SeLECTS and Landau–Kleffner syndrome: see DEE or epileptic encephalopathies with onset in childhood in this chapter ➲ p. 287.

Self-limited epilepsy with autonomic features (SeLEAS)
- Formerly known as Panayiotopoulos syndrome.
- Presentation 3–5 yrs (75% cases), but may range from 1 to 14 yrs.
- Seizures typically occur with sleep onset.

- Lateral gaze deviation and vomiting or other autonomic features, often with impaired consciousness. These can be very prolonged (tens of minutes) and it is common for children to be admitted (even to PICU) and treated for suspected encephalitis.
- Most become seizure-free before 10 yrs of age, and ¼ only ever have a single seizure.
- As with SeLECTS, there is commonly a family history of seizures and interictal EEG abnormalities in first-degree relatives.
- EEG shows focal or multifocal occipital epileptiform abnormalities suppressed by eye opening and activated by sleep.
- MRI should be performed if there is persistent focal slowing on the EEG, an atypical presentation, or frequent seizures.

Childhood occipital visual epilepsy (COVE)
- Formerly known as Gastaut syndrome.
- Onset 7–9 yrs (range: 1–19 yrs).
- Brief diurnal visual symptoms (typically, multicoloured circles) and retained consciousness, with a diffuse post-ictal headache, nausea, and vomiting.
- Additional versive seizures (turning to the seizure onset hemisphere), sensory abnormalities, dysphasia, automatisms, hemiclonic, or focal to bilateral tonic–clonic seizure.
- Has a slightly poorer prognosis for seizure cessation than SeLEAS. There is some phenotypic overlap with both migraine with aura and migraine with brainstem aura.
- MRI should be done to exclude a focal lesion.
- Good response to ASM used for focal seizures, such as levetiracetam, oxcarbazepine, or carbamazepine.

Photosensitive occipital lobe epilepsy (POLE)
Rare syndrome, with onset between 4 and 17 yrs; most cases ♀.
- Family history of epilepsy in 1/3.
- Brief focal sensory visual seizures, associated with head deviation, triggered by photic stimuli (flickering lights, or video game).
- Headache and vomiting during the seizure can cause confusion with migraine with aura.
- Rarely, seizures occur during sleep without photic stimulation.
- May evolve to impaired awareness or to bilateral tonic–clonic seizure.
- EEG with occipital abnormalities facilitated by eye closure and intermittent photic stimulation. MRI is normal.
- Good response to ASM.

Genetic Generalized epilepsy syndromes of childhood
Epilepsy with eyelid myoclonia (EEM)
- Previously known as Jeavons syndrome.
- Onset between 2 and 14 yrs : peak onset at 6–8 yrs.
- Commoner in ♀.
- Brief seizures (3–6 s duration) either spontaneously or precipitated by eye closure in light (but not in darkness).
- Upward gaze deviation and head retropulsion.
- Eyelids make repetitive myoclonic or fluttering movements.

- Most patients have infrequent generalized tonic–clonic seizures.
- EEG shows brief, generalized 3 Hz spike–waves and photosensitivity.
- There is usually a family history of epilepsy.
- Is often resistant to ASM and a life-long condition.

Epilepsy with myoclonic absence
- Very rare. Onset between 2 and 13 yrs; most cases ♂.
- Half of cases have normal development at onset.
- Seizures typically comprise an abrupt onset of absences with severe, bilateral, and synchronous rhythmic myoclonic jerks of upper limbs. Tends to involve the mouth and chin rather than the eyes or eyelids. Seizures typically last less than 1 min.
- Frequent prolonged generalized tonic–clonic seizures, pure absence seizures, and atonic seizures occur in one-third of cases, typically where the myoclonic absences persist.
- Family history of epilepsy in 25%. Appears to be polygenic involving the same genetic variants as IGEs.
- Some children with GLUT1DS (see Glucose transporter-1 deficiency syndrome in this chapter ⊇ p. 301) can present with this picture: because of the potential of the ketogenic diet in this situation, have a low threshold for GLUT1DS testing.
- With the exception of GLUT1DS children on the ketogenic diet, prognosis for development and seizure control is generally poor.
  - Typically treated with combined, high-dose sodium valproate (see Contraception and reproductive health in this chapter ⊇ p. 320) and ethosuximide.
  - Steroids may be helpful.

Childhood absence epilepsy (CAE)
- See Idiopathic generalized epilepsy in this chapter ⊇ p. 288.

Epileptic encephalopathies with onset in childhood
Epilepsy with myoclonic-atonic seizures (EMAtS)
- Previously known as Doose syndrome.
- A rare syndrome slightly more common in ♂s. Family history in one-third of cases.
- Onset at 2–6 yrs, with frequent drop attacks. These can be due to the hallmark myoclonic-atonic seizures ('jerk and immediately drop'), and/or pure atonic seizures.
- Myoclonus sometimes involves ocular or oral muscles. One-third develop non-convulsive status epilepticus, characterized by frequent facial twitching, drooling, and impaired consciousness; and ~2/3 develop GTC seizures at some stage. Tonic seizures can occur later.
- Initially seizures are drug resistant, and a stagnation or regression in development is seen during this phase.
- EEG may be normal in the early stages, later developing biparietal slowing, generalized slow spike-and-wave discharges, and irregular spike–wave discharges accompanying the myoclonic-atonic attacks.
- Treatments options include levetiracetam, valproate (see Contraception and reproductive health in this chapter ⊇ p. 320), clobazam, ethosuximide, topiramate, and zonisamide.

- Prognosis is variable: 2/3 achieve remission within a few years, with EEG and cognition improvement.
- A polygenic inheritance occurs in the majority, but pathogenic single gene variants are found in some children.
- GLUT1DS is responsible for 5% EMAtS cases and must be excluded (see Glucose transporter-1 deficiency syndrome in this chapter ➔ p. 301).
- Some authorities question the distinction between EMAtS and LGS (see Lennox–Gastaut syndrome in this chapter ➔ p. 286). The 'splitters' emphasize the family history and sometimes better prognosis of EMAtS (also reflected in a trend to better preservation of background rhythms on EEG than LGS).

Lennox–Gastaut syndrome (LGS)

Severe DEE usually presenting between 3–5 yrs. Multiple aetiologies, including structural and genetic causes. Cause remains unknown in up to 1/3 cases.

Characterized by:

- Multiple refractory seizures with hallmark *tonic* seizures, more prevalent in sleep; also atonic, atypical absence, myoclonic, focal impaired awareness, and GTC seizures, non-convulsive status epilepticus, and epileptic spasms.
  - more severe tonic seizures may have a vibratory component.
  - If myoclonic seizures are prominent consider EMAtS: see Epilepsy with myoclonic-atonic seizures in this chapter ➔ p. 285).
- Abnormal EEG with widespread slow (2–2.5 Hz) spike-and-wave discharges interictally on EEG: commonly frontally dominant. Other background slowing is common. The most characteristic pattern in sleep is paroxysmal fast discharges with a frequency of 10–12 Hz.
- Intellectual and behavioural impairment.
- Can be difficult to confirm in the early stages of the disease, before clinical and EEG findings have fully evolved.
- Can also evolve from earlier epileptic syndromes (see Box 4.4).
- Initial treatment typically is with sodium valproate (see Contraception and reproductive health in this chapter ➔ p. 320), though lamotrigine, clobazam, and topiramate can also be effective. Other treatments include cannabidiol, ketogenic diet, and vagus nerve stimulation.
- The prognosis for cognitive development, behaviour, and seizure control is generally poor.
- Seizures and epileptic encephalopathy tend to worsen in drowsiness and sleep: excessively sedating ASM regimes may paradoxically worsen seizure control.

(Developmental) epileptic encephalopathy with spike-and-wave activation in sleep ((D)EE-SWAS)

New terms for the picture previously known synonymously as either electrographic status epilepticus in sleep (ESES) or continuous spike–wave in sleep (CSWS).

- EE-SWAS refers to the triad of continuous or near-continuous spike–wave EEG activity during sleep, with seizures and developmental

regression. DEE-SWAS refers to the same picture in patients with previous neurodevelopmental disorder.
- Associated with regression of memory and cognitive skills with hyperactivity.
  - Epileptic activity disrupts the normal memory consolidation functions of deep sleep (see Box 4.5).
- SeLECTS, SeLEAS (see Self-limited focal epilepsies of childhood in this chapter ➲ p. 282), and structural focal epilepsies may evolve to EE-SWAS.
- The most common initial event is a focal to bilateral tonic–clonic seizure in sleep, but focal motor seizures, with or without impaired awareness also occur, in some cases resembling SeLECTS.
- As EE-SWAS develops, it is common to see atypical absences, focal motor seizures with –ve myoclonus, and atonic episodes.
- MRI is recommended to exclude structural lesions.
- Treatment is often difficult and a variety of ASMs are often tried. Sodium valproate (see Contraception and reproductive health in this chapter ➲ p. 320) may be helpful for overt clinical seizures.
  - Other options include clobazam, ethosuximide, levetiracetam, zonisamide, lacosamide.
  - Corticosteroids: high-dose prednisolone (e.g. 2 mg/kg/day) for several weeks before tapering. If there has been a response, prolonged steroid treatment can be achieved with minimized toxicity using a 4 mg/kg once weekly regime.
  - Carbamazepine may exacerbate the condition.
- Some children may be suitable for ketogenic diet or surgical intervention, but results are variable.
- Intellectual and behavioural improvement typically accompanies resolution of the SWAS, but many remain with residual impairment.
- Mutations in *GRIN2A* have been identified in some patients: L-serine may be beneficial.

Landau–Kleffner syndrome
Landau–Kleffner syndrome (LKS) is a subtype of EE-SWAS where regression primarily affects language, and the child behaves 'as if deaf'. There are fluctuating but rapidly progressive problems with comprehension of language: failure to understand everyday noises (so-called auditory agnosia: e.g. failing to recognize the significance of a ringing telephone) and an acquired expressive aphasia. Other cognitive and behavioural problems are common.

Febrile infection-related epilepsy syndrome (FIRES)
- Super-refractory sudden-onset *status epilepticus* that starts after a febrile infection in the previous 2 weeks typically in a school-aged child.
- During the acute phase (1–12 weeks) the child is encephalopathic, with refractory status. Mortality is ~10%.
- In the late phase a variable degree of intellectual and language impairment and motor dysfunction is observed, in addition to drug-resistant multifocal epilepsy.

- Investigation to exclude toxic, infection, metabolic, or autoimmune encephalopathies.
- Cause unknown. Possible genetic predisposition to an anomalous neuroinflammation response.
- Possible therapeutic role for anakinra.

Hemiconvulsion-hemiplegia-epilepsy syndrome (HHE)
- Uncommon consequence of focal motor status in young children (typically <4), usually during a febrile illness.
- Remains hemiplegic (± aphasic if dominant hemisphere involved).
- Acute MRI shows oedema of the affected hemisphere, progressing to late atrophy.
- After an initial period of seizure freedom, a drug-resistant focal epilepsy may develop, and the child should be evaluated for surgical approaches (see Surgical Treatment of epilepsy in this chapter → p. 312).

Idiopathic generalized epilepsy (IGE) syndromes

The most important epilepsies presenting in late childhood or early adolescence (previously known as 'genetic' and 'primary' generalized epilepsies).

Although CAE, JAE, JME, and GTCA phenotypes are delineated, there is considerable overlap, and it is probably better to regard these phenotypes as being points on a continuum.

Childhood absence epilepsy (CAE)
- Brief arrest of speech and activity (typically <5 s). Manual automatisms, subtle peri-oral, or periocular flickering may be seen.
- May occur tens or even hundreds of times per day.
- Events usually reliably precipitated by 1–2 min of well-performed hyperventilation in an untreated child. Routinely tested in EEG but may also be useful diagnostically in the outpatient setting.
- More common in ♀. Onset typically at 4–8 yrs (onset <3 yrs is rare).
- Strong genetic component, with a family history in one-third of cases and a risk of seizures in siblings of around 10%. In around 10% of cases, there will be a history of febrile seizures preceding onset of absences.
- GLUT1DS is found in 10% of children with onset of absence seizures <4 yrs of age (see Glucose transporter-1 deficiency syndrome in this chapter → p. 301).
- GTC seizures do occur, if rarely: families must be forewarned of this.
- EEG shows a 3 Hz generalized spike-and-wave pattern.
- Treatments: ethosuximide (may not prevent GTC seizures), valproate in ♂ (see Contraception and reproductive health in this chapter → p. 320) or lamotrigine. Carbamazepine will usually aggravate and is contraindicated.
- Prognosis for resolution of absences in early adulthood is very good, but GTC seizures may continue, which may be part of the evolution to another IGE syndrome, like JME, JAE, or GTCA.

Juvenile myoclonic epilepsy (JME)

▶A very common and important epilepsy syndrome to recognize!

Onset usually between the ages of 12 and 18 yrs.
- Characterized by a combination of absence, myoclonic, and GTC seizures.
- It is typically the first GTC seizure that prompts medical attention: the absences and myoclonus may have been happening unrecognized for some time although the child will have reputation for clumsiness and accidents first thing in the morning.
- Awareness is retained during the myoclonic jerks: a history of dropping objects while preparing breakfast ('not being a morning person') is common.
- GTC seizures are often preceded by a crescendo of myoclonic jerks: effectively a myoclonic–tonic–clonic seizure. Absence seizures occur in up to one-third.
- Excessive tiredness, sleep deprivation, alcohol, and marijuana are strong triggering factors.
- EEG typically shows polyspike discharges followed by irregular slow waves with a frequency of between 1 and 3 Hz. Absences are associated with polyspike–wave complexes at 4–6 Hz that slow to 3 Hz. These epileptiform discharges are far less regular than those with CAE and JAE.
- First-line treatment with lamotrigine or levetiracetam. Valproate is a second-line option in ♂ (see Contraception and reproductive health in this chapter ⊃ p. 320 in relation to use in ♀).
- Carbamazepine is contraindicated.
- Prognosis for seizure control is generally good, but the consensus is that ASM treatment should be maintained well into adulthood due to very high risk of relapse if treatment is withdrawn.

Juvenile absence epilepsy (JAE)
Essentially 'JME without the myoclonic jerks'.
- Peak age of onset is 12 yrs, typically near or soon after puberty.
- In contrast to CAE, there are typically only a few episodes per day, and consciousness seems to be less impaired even though the electrographic seizures tend to be longer.
- Around 90% will develop generalized tonic–clonic seizures. Some patients may have myoclonus during an absence seizure (more subtle than those in JME, though there is some clinical overlap between these syndromes).
- EEG shows a 3 Hz generalized spike-and-wave pattern often induced by hyperventilation, but photosensitivity is unusual.
- Most respond to ASM, though long-term seizure cessation is less likely than with CAE.
- Ethosuximide is not recommended because of the high prevalence of GTC seizures.

Absence status epilepticus
- Commonest form of non-convulsive status.
- Rarely seen before 10 yrs of age but occurs in up to 20% of JAE.
- ASM drug treatment changes are the commonest precipitating factor:
  - introduction of tiagabine and levetiracetam in particular;
  - over-rapid withdrawal of ASM medication.
- Associated impairment of consciousness variable.

- Presents as slow cognition, poor memory, confusion, inappropriate behaviour, experiencing strange sensations and feelings.
- May be associated with minor motor disturbances:
  - clonic jerks of eyelids or mouth;
  - atonic head or trunk drops;
  - lip-smacking, swallowing, fumbling, or other automatisms;
  - autonomic features: pallor, pupil dilatation.
- Characteristic EEG: generalized discharges 1–4 Hz.
- In most cases oral or parenteral benzodiazepines will be effective.
  - buccal midazolam;
  - oral clonazepam especially if myoclonic jerks present;
  - IV lorazepam or midazolam infusion with continuous EEG monitoring.
- Recent reports suggest oral ketamine to be useful.

Epilepsy with generalized tonic–clonic seizures alone (GTCA)
- 'JME without the absences *or* the jerks'.
- Again, very much part of the IGE spectrum with JME and JAE.
- Age at presentation, EEG features, ASM selection, vulnerability to lifestyle-related seizure triggers (alcohol, fatigue, sleep deprivation), need for treatment into adulthood all as for JME.

Epilepsy syndromes with onset at variable age

Sleep-related hypermotor (hyperkinetic) epilepsy (SHE)
- A rare syndrome, commoner in ♂. Onset usually during adolescence though very variable.
- Formerly named nocturnal frontal lobe epilepsy, but now appreciated that extra-frontal foci are common; and about a third of patients report at least some seizures while awake!
- Brief motor seizures with abrupt onset and offset, preserved awareness if awake, and clustering in sleep.
- Parents report tonic/dystonic posturing or a hyperkinetic pattern with pedalling, pelvic thrusting, beating, or rocking movements.
- Prognosis depends on the aetiology, which can be genetic (*de novo* or familial), genetic-structural, or acquired. Structural causes can be drug resistant, but patients with focal cortical dysplasia are good candidates for surgery.

Familial mesial temporal lobe epilepsy (FMTLE)
- Common focal epilepsy with onset usually in adolescence or adulthood (range 3 to ~60 yrs). More frequent in ♀.
- Presentation is typically after the first focal to bilateral tonic–clonic seizure. A history of other phenomena (not typically recognized as seizures by the family) should be sought. These can include déjà vu, other 'dream-like' states, sensations of fear, visual or auditory illusions, or autonomic symptoms.
  - a family history of similar symptoms in relatives is a major clue.
- EEG is normal in ~60%. MRI is usually normal, but some show hippocampus atrophy or sclerosis (associated with treatment resistance).
- Most patients have infrequent seizures and respond well to ASMs. Few require epilepsy surgery.

Familial focal epilepsy with variable foci (FFEVF)

- Rare syndrome that usually starts in adolescence, but ranging from 1 month to ~50 yrs.
- Autosomal dominance inheritance with incomplete penetrance. Location of foci and severity varies within pedigrees.
- MRI typically unremarkable but can show focal cortical dysplasia.
- Up to a third can be drug resistant: refer early to epilepsy surgery centres.
- Pathogenic gene variants in *DEPDC5*, *NPRL2*, and *NPRL3* have been reported. These are all part of the *GATOR1* complex involved in regulation of mTOR and cell division providing a unifying mechanism between these epilepsies, focal cortical dysplasias, and tuberous sclerosis.

Epilepsy with auditory features (EAF)

- Previously known as autosomal dominant partial epilepsy with auditory features and autosomal dominant lateral temporal lobe epilepsy.
- Onset usually in adolescence or adulthood, $♀ = ♂$.
- Focal aware seizures with auditory symptoms and/or receptive aphasia; comprising buzzing, murmuring, or ringing, or distortions in auditory perception. Reflex seizures precipitated by a sound may also occur.
- MRI required to exclude structural causes.
- Prognosis very variable.
- Mostly are *de novo* but there are familial cases with autosomal inheritance and incomplete penetrance.

Mesial temporal lobe epilepsy with hippocampal sclerosis (MTLE-HS)

- One of the most common focal epilepsies in adults. Onset usually in adolescence or early adulthood.
- Hippocampal sclerosis on MRI: hippocampal atrophy on T1-weight images ± gliosis on T2 and FLAIR.
- Mostly an acquired aetiology. There is a history of an initial insult (usually a prolonged febrile seizure, <4 yrs of age) followed by a latent period, after which a refractory epilepsy develops.
- Focal awareness seizures are described as viscerosensory (often epigastric sensation): fear, *dèjá vu*, and dream-like states. Some evolve to behavioural arrest, oral and ipsilateral automatisms, and impaired consciousness, with prolonged post-ictal confusion.
- Deficits in verbal or visual memory occur when the MTLE-HS affects the dominant or nondominant temporal lobes, respectively.
- Resistant to ASMs. Epilepsy surgery in selected cases can lead to full remission of seizures.

Rasmussen syndrome (RS)

- A rare disease with unknown but presumed inflammatory aetiology usually starting before 10y (see Rasmussen encephalitis in this chapter ➜ p. 400).

- Initially subtle focal motor seizures increasing in frequency and severity and often evolving to *epilepsia partialis continua* (EPC).
- EEG shows hemispheric slowing with epileptiform abnormalities.
- Hemispheric atrophy develops over time accompanying a contralateral hemiparesis and cognitive impairment.
- Highly resistant to ASMs. Hemispherectomy or hemispheric disconnection surgery usually required to control seizures (see Surgical Treatment of epilepsy in this chapter → p. 312).

Progressive myoclonus epilepsies (PME)
See The progressive myoclonus epilepsies in this chapter → p. 302).

Investigating epilepsy

Epilepsy as a symptom

To assess a child's epilepsy fully, correct assessments must be made at least four levels.

- *Disease*: am I sure this is epilepsy and not either a disease causing recurrent acute symptomatic seizures, or events that are not seizures at all? See Funny turns: episodic events (paroxysmal episodes) in Chapter 3 ⊋ p. 148.
- *Seizure types:* what seizure type(s) am I seeing? Some seizure types increase the likelihood that there is an underlying cause for the epilepsy (e.g. myoclonic seizures in the appropriate clinical context).
- *Epilepsy syndrome* See Epilepsy syndromes in this chapter ⊋ p. 274.
- *Aetiology*: structural, genetic, infectious, metabolic, immune, or unknown.

▶ If a child's epilepsy treatment is proving ineffective, review at each of these four levels: am I sure it is epilepsy? Have I misinterpreted seizure descriptions and selected the wrong drug? Have I missed a (possibly progressive) underlying cause?

- Epilepsy comorbidities should also be considered at each step— associated problems with cognition, behaviour and mood, and their resultant effects on life and schooling: see Epilepsy and daily life in this chapter ⊋ p. 317.

Role of EEG

EEG is overused at the level of disease (i.e. asking 'Is this epilepsy or not?' where its predictive value is poor) and underused as a means of defining epilepsy syndrome and aetiology. Many epilepsy syndromes have, by definition, characteristic EEG features. A small number of primary causes of symptomatic epilepsy (e.g. infantile neuronal ceroid lipofuscinosis, SSPE) have EEG hallmarks. Other EEG findings are less specific.

Role of imaging

Indications for imaging cause much confusion amongst novice epileptologists. The key to understanding the need for imaging is to make a syndromic diagnosis.

▶ Imaging is *not* normally required if a diagnosis of an idiopathic generalized epilepsy (IGE) (including Childhood Absence Epilepsy), or Self-limited Epilepsy with Centrotemporal Spikes (SeLECTS) is supported by clear clinical and EEG features and a good response to appropriate ASMs.

In most other situations there is likely to be a role for imaging. Other than in an emergency where CT imaging may be more practicable, MRI is the preferred imaging modality. Typical indications include:

- New-onset focal epilepsy in a previously developmentally normal child, to rule out acquired lesions (e.g. infarction, neoplasia, inflammation).

- A history implying a possible remote symptomatic cause for the epilepsy (e.g. previous asphyxia, meningitis).
- Children (typically pre-school age) with aggressive epilepsy with multiple seizure types (e.g. LGS)—although the diagnostic yield is relatively low where there is no significant past medical history.
- Any new-onset seizure disorder in the neonatal period or infancy.
- Loss of previously established seizure control or change in seizure pattern.
- Any focal neurological signs on examination.
- Current NICE guidelines recommend imaging within 6 weeks of first presentation of a seizure disorder.
- 3T (Tesla) MRI preferred where available.

Role of genetic investigation

- Investigation for genetic causes has been revolutionized by epilepsy gene panels and other newer techniques (see Molecular genetics in Chapter 2 ❯ p. 81).
- Particularly in severe epilepsies beginning in the first year of life with unremarkable imaging, early molecular genetic analysis is increasing demonstrating its value as the most cost- and time-effective route to an aetiological understanding of a child's epilepsy. Although this does not as yet always lead to more effective treatment, some monogenic epilepsies have specific therapeutic approaches that improve seizure control: e.g. carbamazepine or phenytoin for KCNQ2-DEE, and ketogenic diet for GLUT1DS.
- Some children have a *structural-genetic* epilepsy with imaging demonstrating distinctive structural features that strongly suggest candidate genes (see Fig. 2.14 Radiological appearances of developmental brain abnormalities in Chapter 2 ❯ p. 73).

Epilepsies with imaging abnormalities

Congenital brain malformations
Seizures often present in first month of life.
- Malformations of cortical development (common):
  - focal cortical dysplasia, schizencephaly, hemimegalencephaly, lissencephaly, polymicrogyria;
  - some of these malformations can be a part of a complex syndromic disorder, e.g. Miller–Dieker, linear sebaceous naevus syndrome;
  - some radiological phenotypes now recognized to be due to defined single-gene mutations: see Recognizable genetic brain malformation syndromes in Chapter 2 ❯ p. 72;
  - genetic counselling is advised.
- Aicardi syndrome:
  - relatively common (1–4% of infantile spasm series);
  - affects ♀s only (isolated case reports in XXY ♂s; presumed lethal in XY ♂ fetuses);
  - sporadic; no familial cases reported;
  - characteristic MRI features include agenesis of corpus callosum (with an elevated third ventricle), areas of dysplastic cortex, periventricular heterotopic grey matter, choroid plexus cysts, and vermian agenesis;

- characteristic chorioretinal 'punched out' lesions ('lacunae') on fundoscopy ± colobomata;
- May also see vertebral abnormalities and microphthalmia.

CNS features of neurocutaneous disorders
- Tuberous sclerosis, neurofibromatosis, Sturge–Weber, etc.

Acquired lesions
Tumours
- Dysembryoplastic neuroepithelial tumour (DNET).

Vascular malformations
- Cavernous angioma.
- Acquired ischaemic lesions, e.g. porencephalic cyst.

Inflammation
Seizures can occur as feature of autoimmune and autoinflammatory diseases of the CNS and MRI evidence of inflammation is often an important clue.
- Acute disseminated encephalomyelitis: see Acute disseminated encephalomyelitis in this chapter ➔ p. 266.
- Autoimmune encephalitides: see Autoimmune encephalopathy in this chapter ➔ p. 391.
- Rasmussen encephalitis: see Rasmussen encephalitis in this chapter ➔ p. 400.

Metabolic disease
- It is important to recognize that some inborn errors of metabolism also give rise to anatomical/structural features on MRI. For example, agenesis of the corpus callosum can be seen in non-ketotic hyperglycinaemia) thus demonstration of structural brain abnormalities does not obviate the need for metabolic investigation.

Epilepsies with findings on genetic testing
Chromosomal abnormalities
Clues to a chromosomal disorder associated with epilepsy may include dysmorphic appearances and learning difficulties. aCGH has largely replaced conventional karyotyping even in first-line genetic testing and beyond the classical syndromes resulting from large-scale deletions and rearrangements an increasing number of distinctive microdeletion syndromes are recognized: consultation with clinical geneticists is advised.

Wolf–Hirschhorn syndrome
- Deletion of 4p.
- 'Greek helmet' facial appearance, cleft palate, cerebral abnormalities, developmental impairment, and seizures.

Miller–Dieker syndrome
- Submicroscopic distal deletion of 17p13.3 involves the *LIS1* gene.
- Facial features, seizures/infantile spasms, visceral abnormalities, and type 1 lissencephaly: see Recognizable genetic brain malformation syndromes in Chapter 2 ➔ p. 72.

Ring chromosome 20
Cytogenetic abnormalities resulting in ring-form chromosomes can cause epilepsy.
- Severe epilepsy, learning, and behaviour problems (often bordering on the psychotic) without obvious dysmorphism.
- Cytogenetic abnormality can be *mosaic* so the laboratory should be asked to examine a large number of mitotic figures (typically 50; some sources suggest 200).

Single-gene disorders and epilepsy gene panels
Seizures are a feature of several single-gene disorders associated with other features including developmental impairment and additional neurological signs (e.g. tuberous sclerosis, NF1, Fragile X). Generally, these disorders will be diagnosed because of their other (including neuroradiological) features.

Single-gene disorders showing conventional Mendelian inheritance are responsible for only 1% epilepsies without other clinical features; however, they often present in infancy and early onset epilepsy gene panels/WES/WGS are becoming increasingly useful in the evaluation of children with early onset epilepsy.
- It is increasingly clear that a given phenotype (epilepsy syndrome) can have multiple causes (the number of genes associated with developmental and epileptic encephalopathies is now over 100!)
- Perhaps more interestingly some genes are capable of a range of presentations, suggesting much yet to understand about the factors that determine this (e.g. *SCN1A* mutations can cause EIDEE, epilepsy of infancy with migrating focal seizures, West, Dravet, *and* GEFS+ syndromes!)

Current gene panels can screen up to 600 relevant genes at a single sitting. Recent epidemiological studies suggest 25% children with seizure onset before 3 years will have a monogenic cause.

Angelman syndrome
- In contrast to the traditional Mendelian model, it is now realized that genes may be labelled by methylation (known as *imprinting*) that distinguishes maternally and paternally derived copies.
- Arises from lack of maternally derived chromosome 15q11-13:
  - 70% have deletion; 2–3% are due to paternal uni-parental disomy; imprinting centre mutations within 15q11-13 in 3% and mutation of the maternally derived *UBE3A* gene in 11%.
- The classic phenotype is of seizures, happy facial expression, and developmental impairment.
- In 10% of cases with typical clinical features, there is no identified genetic cause.
- For ♀s with an Angelman phenotype but apparently –ve genetic studies, consider *MECP2* analysis.
- See also Pitt-Hopkins syndrome below.
- Investigations: 15q11-13 methylation studies, *UBE3A* sequencing. If uninformative proceed to multigene panel (with *MECP2*, *TCF4*) and consider WES, WGS, and mitochondrial DNA studies.

Rett syndrome, Rett-like syndromes, and MECP2-associated phenotypes
Epilepsy is a common later feature of typical Rett syndrome (see Rett syndrome in this chapter ➽ p. 297) however an increasing range of *MECP2*-associated phenotypes is now recognized. Consequently, *MECP2* is commonly included in early epilepsy gene panels.

- *MECP2 point mutations* are increasingly recognized in ♂'s, typically giving rise to a severe neonatal-onset epileptic encephalopathy with severe hypotonia, abnormal movements, and breathing patterns. They should be sought in ♂'s with neonatal epileptic encephalopathy, severe hypotonia, or in families with a pedigree consistent with X-linked learning disability.
- *MECP2 duplications* are causative in a few percent each of severe developmental impairment in ♂'s and X-linked severe developmental impairment.
  - Note that *duplications* have to be specifically sought and are missed by standard sequencing techniques used to identify mutations *including next-generation sequencing techniques* (see Molecular genetics in Chapter 2 ➽ p. 81).
- Some additional genes cause Rett-like pictures and should be considered particularly in ♀s where Rett syndrome was considered and excluded:
  - *CDKL5* should be considered in ♀s with a Rett-like picture in whom aggressive early onset (<6 months) seizures are prominent.
  - In 'congenital Rett' pictures with no clear early 'normal' phase consider *FOXG1*.
- Pitt-Hopkins syndrome (due to 18q deletions or microdeletions involving the *TCF4* gene) causes a picture with some Rett- and Angelman-like features (severe learning disability, Rett-like hyperventilation, Angelman-like distinctive wide-mouthed facies); however, seizures are not usually prominent.

Fragile X
- Common: ~1:4000 ♂'s and 1:8000 ♀s.
- Distinctive features become progressively apparent over time (characteristic tall, narrow face with large ears and prominent jaw), hyperextensible fingers, macroorchidism (in ♂'s) after puberty.
- Consider in SeLECTS-like epilepsy presentations in a child with learning difficulties.
- Note that the genetic basis (triplet repeat expansion in *FMR1* gene) will not be identified on WES/WGS panels.

Am I missing an underlying cause?

Neonatal seizures

See also Neonatal seizures in Chapter 5 ➲ p. 551.

The epilepsy syndrome approach has limited application in neonatal seizures.

Common causes

- Hypoglycaemia, hypomagnesaemia.
- Hypoxic–ischaemic encephalopathy.
- Infection.
- Structural.
- Note that structural brain abnormalities are seen in some metabolic disorders, e.g. non-ketotic hyperglycinaemia (NKH) and peroxisomal disorders, so further evaluation and investigation may still be necessary.
- Maternal drug withdrawal.
- Metabolic.
- Genetic.

If the initial evaluation has not identified a cause, consider a large number of—individually rare but collectively important—neurometabolic and neurogenetic conditions; see Neonatal seizures in Chapter 5 ➲ p. 551 and Neonatal and infant-onset epilepsy syndromes in this chapter ➲ p. 275 for further details: this is an important indication for an appropriate urgent gene panel (see Single gene disorders and Epilepsy Gene Panels in this chapter ➲ p. 296).

Infants

Infantile epileptic spasms syndrome (IESS)

IESS sits rather awkwardly in the ILAE classification: it is a syndrome with many causes. Since both optimal treatment and prognosis are strongly influenced by aetiology, there is a case for seeing this as a heterogeneous group of conditions sharing a non-specific phenotype constrained by development (see Box 4.4). A cause will be identified in approximately 80% of the broad phenotype (i.e. epileptic spasms associated with either typical or atypical ('modified') hypsarrhythmia). Typical causes include:

- Perinatal asphyxia and HIE.
- Cerebrovascular events.
- Congenital brain malformations: tuberous sclerosis and Aicardi syndrome.
- Malformations of cortical development (lissencephaly, schizencephaly, polymicrogyria, megalencephaly, grey matter heterotopia, and focal cortical dysplasias: see Recognizable genetic brain malformation syndromes in Chapter 2 ➲ p. 72).
- Pre-, peri-, or postnatal infection, particularly herpes encephalitis.
- Metabolic disorders.
- Degenerative disorders including PEHO: see Rare causes of severe epilepsy and severe developmental impairment in this chapter ➲ p. 300.

The UK Infantile Spasms (UKISS) study identified aetiology in 61%: HIE in 10%, chromosomal abnormalities, brain malformations, and stroke in 8%

each, tuberous sclerosis in 7%, periventricular leukomalacia or haemorrhage 5%. Monogenic causes are being increasingly recognized as predisposing to IESS, including *SCN1A*, *CDLK5*, *ARX*, *PAFAH1B1/LIS1*, *DCX*, *TUBA1A*, *STXBP1*, *KCNQ2*, *SPTAN*, and *GRIN2A*, among many others.

It follows that the most useful investigations are MRI, careful neurocutaneous and neuro-ophthalmological examination, and targeted metabolic investigations, with early epilepsy gene panel/WES/WGS testing for those in whom first-line investigation is uninformative. Specific considerations include:

- Pyridoxine- and P5P-dependent DEE (see Vitamin B6 in this chapter ➜ p. 524). These usually present with seizures in the neonatal period but can occasionally present as *de novo* infantile spasms.
- PKU.
- The phenotypic spectrum of glucose transporter deficiency (see Glucose transporter-1 deficiency syndrome (GLUT1DS) in this chapter ➜ p. 301) is now recognized as being broader than initially described and this diagnosis should be considered in any child with onset of seizures before the first birthday.
- Maple-syrup urine disease.
- Biotinidase deficiency.
- Menkes disease (consider in a ♂ with occipital changes on DWI).
- Hyperammonaemia.
- Non-ketotic hyperglycinaemia (NKH).
- Leigh disease.
- Krabbe disease.
- *MECP2* deletions/duplications are commoner than point mutations as a cause of epileptic encephalopathies in ♂s: remember deletions/duplications are *missed* by many next-generation sequencing methods.
- *ARX* gene mutations in ♂s and *CDKL5* gene mutations in ♀: included in most gene panels.

Metabolic and neurodegenerative disorders associated with epilepsy in infants and children

🚹 Seizures accompany a vast number of neurodegenerative and neurometabolic diseases. There are, however, relatively few conditions in which seizures are likely to be the sole presenting sign, long pre-dating other features.

- The important *neonatal-* and *infant-*onset examples are NKH, sulphite oxidase/molybdenum cofactor deficiency, Menkes disease (♂ in status with high lactate and occipital changes on DWI in first few months' life), pyridoxine- and P5P-dependent DEE, and biotinidase deficiency.
- In *older* children, important considerations are Alpers disease/PNDC, late infantile NCL, GLUT1DS, and the progressive myoclonic epilepsies.

Conditions in which other features are more dominant than, or present before, seizure disorder

- Glutaric aciduria type 1 (now detected by newborn screening).
  - Typically presents between 6 and 18 months with an acute encephalopathy and seizures precipitated by mild intercurrent illness.

- Late-onset urea cycle disorders.
  - Predominantly present with recurrent encephalopathy associated with hyperammonaemia. Possible family history of unexplained death in ♂ siblings.
- Multiple carboxylase deficiency.
  - Classically has dermatological features as well as seizures, although these can be subtle: rash and alopecia appearing around 3 months of age.
- Neurotransmitter metabolism defects: see Neurotransmitter disorders in this chapter ➲ p. 488.
- Mitochondrial disorders: see Mitochondrial disease in this chapter ➲ p. 404.
- Lysosomal disorders including neuronal ceroid lipofuscinoses: see Late infantile neuronal ceroid lipofuscinosis in this chapter ➲ p. 476.

Rare causes of severe epilepsy and severe developmental impairment
- 3-Phosphoglycerate dehydrogenase deficiency:
  - Microcephaly, severely impaired development. Intractable epilepsy and severely abnormal EEG. MRI: reduction in white matter.
- Creatine deficiency disorders (CDD):
  - *Treatable* inborn errors of creatine metabolism or transport: guanidinoacetate methyltransferase (GAMT), arginine-glycine amidinotransferase (AGAT), and creatine transporter (CRTR) deficiencies.
  - Developmental impairment (notably speech and language) and intellectual disability are common to all.
  - Intractable epilepsy, behaviour disorder, and extrapyramidal symptoms are seen in GAMT and CRTR.
  - Initial clue may be a *low* plasma creatinine, (which would not normally regarded as abnormal!); however, this is a non-specific finding common in small infants with reduced muscle mass. Note that in CRTR plasma creatinine is normal or *high*.
  - An absent creatine peak on brain MRS is the radiological hallmark of CDD.
  - Before the genetic result is known, CDDs can be distinguished by urine guanidinoacetate levels, and urine creatine:creatinine ratios.
  - GAMT and AGAT are autosomal recessive. CRTR is X-linked recessive with ♀s at most mildly affected.
  - Improve with creatine administration (poor response in CRTR).
- PEHO (progressive encephalopathy, peripheral oedema, hypsarrhythmia, and optic atrophy):
  - Sometimes now referred to as Neurodegeneration and Spasticity with or without Cerebellar Atrophy or Cortical Visual Impairment (NESCAV).
  - Severe neurodevelopmental disorder caused by mutations in *ZNHIT3* with other genes (*CCDC88A, KIF1A, GNAO1*) recently implicated in PEHO and PEHO-like pictures.
  - MRI shows atrophy of the temporal lobes and folial atrophy of the cerebellum.

Glucose transporter-1 deficiency syndrome (GLUT1DS)

- A disorder of brain energy metabolism caused by impaired GLUT1-mediated glucose transport into the brain with several recognized phenotypes:

Classical early onset (80%)

- Neonatal period *may be normal.*
- Seizures are the main presentation, usually associated with fasting: semiology can include cyanotic attacks.
- Mean age at seizure onset 26 weeks with 80% of all first seizures in first 6 months.
- Paroxysmal eye-head gaze saccades (sometimes mistaken for opsoclonus-myoclonus) are the most frequent symptom in infants after seizures.
- Global developmental impairment, especially affecting speech.
- OFC decelerates after 3 months, in ~50% of infants.
- Complex movement disorder including ataxia, dystonia, and pyramidal tract signs.

Classical late-onset (18%)

- Seizure onset 2–10 yrs (seen in 40%):
  - A phenotype resembling epilepsy with myoclonic absences (see Epilepsy with myoclonic absence in this chapter ➲ p. 285) is particularly characteristic.
- Movement disorder in 10%.
- CSF:plasma glucose not as low as early onset.
- All have learning difficulties (mild in 70%).
- Microcephaly in 29%.

Rarer presentations

- Mental retardation and movement disorder but no epilepsy; mild intellectual disability in 50%.
- Familial or sporadic paroxysmal, exercise-induced movement disorder, with or without seizures.
- Also minimal symptom pictures (adult clumsy on prolonged fasting).

Biochemistry

- Fasting CSF:plasma glucose ratio ≤50% (with 4 to 6h of fast).
- CSF glucose ≤2.2 mM.
- Decreased or normal CSF lactate (a low CSF glucose with high lactate has been reported in biotinidase deficiency: pyruvate carboxylase is a biotin-dependent enzyme).

Neurophysiology

- EEG may show ictal focal slowing or discharges, 2.5–4 Hz spike and wave, aggravated by fasting, and improved by food intake.

Genetics

- Autosomal dominant heterozygote mutations in *SLC2A1* gene encoding GLUT1 seen in ~90%.
- Usually sporadic although familial transmission is reported.

Treatment
Ketogenic diet, from infancy to at least adolescence.
- Seizures are controlled at lower blood levels of β–hydroxybutyrate than needed to nourish the brain.
- Avoid inhibitors of GLUT1 function (phenobarbitone, valproate, diazepam, general anaesthesia, chloral hydrate, methylxanthines, caffeine, green tea, ethanol).

Neurodegenerative conditions that may present with epilepsy in older children
- SSPE: see Slow-viral and prion infections in this chapter ⮕ p. 375.
- HIV: see HIV and HIV-associated progressive encephalopathy in this chapter ⮕ p. 367.
- Alpers/PNDC: see Alpers-Huttenlocher syndrome (PNDC) in this chapter ⮕ p. 409.
- Niemann–Pick type C (see Niemann–Pick type C in this chapter ⮕ p. 479).
- Huntington disease: see Juvenile Huntington disease in this chapter ⮕ p. 480.

The progressive myoclonus epilepsies
Of all indicators that an epilepsy may be symptomatic of a progressive underlying neurological disease, the presence of *myoclonic seizures* is perhaps the most sensitive—although it is *very non-specific*.

> ❗ Although myoclonic seizures may indicate a progressive underlying cause, most children experiencing myoclonic seizures—even as part of severe epilepsies—will have a syndrome such as Dravet or Lennox–Gastaut rather than a metabolic underlying primary cause.

Progressive myoclonus epilepsies (PMEs) are characterized by the triad of multiple seizure types (including myoclonic seizures), abnormal neurological signs (typically with ataxia and dementia) and *progressive deterioration* (although the latter may be slow). See Figure 4.9.

PMEs presenting in infancy
- Early infantile NCL: see Early infantile neuronal ceroid lipofuscinosis in this chapter ⮕ p. 474.
- Tay–Sachs: see Tay–Sachs disease in this chapter ⮕ p. 474.
- Sandhoff: see Table 4.20.
- Tetrahydrobiopterin deficiencies: see Tetrahydrobiopterin synthesis defects in this chapter ⮕ p. 474.
- Alpers disease: see Alpers-Huttenlocher syndrome (PNDC) in this chapter ⮕ p. 409.
- Acid ceramidase deficiency due to *ASAH* mutations is a cause of PME associated with spinal muscle atrophy.

PMEs presenting in early childhood
- Juvenile myoclonic form of Huntington disease: see Juvenile Huntington disease in this chapter ⮕ p. 480:
  - onset >3 yrs: regression with cerebellar signs, rigidity, and dystonic posturing; eventually seizures;

- dominant transmission always from the *father* (although the father may be undiagnosed at the time of the child's presentation).
- Late infantile NCL: see Late infantile neuronal ceroid lipofuscinosis in this chapter ⊃ p. 476.

PMEs presenting in childhood and adolescence
- Juvenile NCL: see Juvenile NCL in this chapter ⊃ p. 478.
- Juvenile Gaucher (see Juvenile Gaucher type 3 (neuronopathic) in this chapter ⊃ p. 477):
  - hepatosplenomegaly precedes neurological deterioration and myoclonic epilepsy;
  - lymphocytes: low levels of glucocerebrosidase.
- Sialidosis (see Table 4.20).
- Galactosialidosis (see Table 4.20).
- Lafora body disease: see Lafora disease in this chapter ⊃ p. 481.
- Myoclonus epilepsy with ragged-red fibres: see Myoclonic epilepsy with ragged-red fibres (MERRF) in this chapter ⊃ p. 410.
- Unverricht–Lundborg disease: see Unverricht–Lundborg disease in this chapter ⊃ p. 479.
- Dentato-rubral-pallido-luysian atrophy (DRPLA; very rare). Dominantly inherited—mimics Huntington Disease.
- Action myoclonus renal failure syndrome (AMRF), *PRICKLE-1* related progressive myoclonus epilepsy with ataxia—both exceptionally rare.

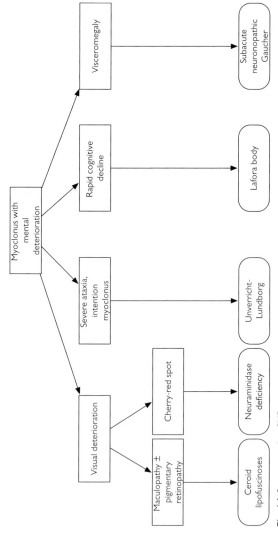

Fig. 4.6 Basic approach to PMEs.

Treatment of epilepsy

Principles of therapy with antiseizure medications (ASMs)

Decide whether or not treatment is appropriate or necessary.

- Generally considered after two or more seizures; however, the epilepsy syndrome (see Epilepsy syndromes in this chapter ➋ p. 274) should be considered. Treatment may be unnecessary in self-limiting conditions such as SeLECTS and SeLEAS.
- Although animal models of epilepsy have demonstrated the phenomenon of *kindling* (a 'vicious circle' cycle of seizure-related neuroplasticity changes particularly in the hippocampus making further seizures more likely) there is no evidence in clinical practice that delaying treatment affects prognosis.
- The choice of ASM must be tailored to the child's age, gender, comorbidities, co-medication, and child and carer choice, based on the risk–benefit ratio.
- Identification of seizure type and/or epilepsy syndrome is invaluable in choosing the most suitable ASM.
- Aim for seizure control without unacceptable unwanted effects.
  - Err on the side of living with seizures rather than unwanted 24/7 drug effects that may be far more deleterious developmentally.
  - Monotherapy should be used if possible.
  - Start low and go slow.
  - In general, combination therapy should only be used if monotherapy is ineffective since combinations tend to be associated with more unwanted effects.
- If the first ASM is unsuccessful, the second ASM should be started and built up to a therapeutic dose before the first ASM is slowly withdrawn.
- Consider ASM withdrawal after 2 seizure-free years but again consider the epilepsy syndrome (e.g. would not normally consider discontinuation in JME; would be cautious in epilepsy of known structural cause), and child and family psychosocial factors.
- ASM withdrawal must take place gradually (see specific drug entries in Chapter 7). Withdraw one ASM at a time.
- Avoid 'brand switching' between manufacturers where possible to minimize variation in bioavailability: particularly for phenytoin, phenobarbital, and carbamazepine.

The antiseizure medications

- As prescriber you must be aware of the current licenced indications for ASMs in children. A significant proportion of ASM prescription in children with severe epilepsy remains 'off-licence': families must be made aware of this.
- In the UK, there is guidance on drug choice, based on seizure type(s) and epilepsy syndrome, from the National Institute for Health and Clinical Excellence (NICE) (Tables 4.3, 4.4).

Table 4.3 Medication choice by seizure type

Seizure type	Monotherapy	Add-on Treatment	Second-line Add-on	Drugs to be avoided (may worsen seizures)
Generalized tonic–clonic	Lamotrigine Levetiracetam	Clobazam Lamotrigine Levetiracetam Perampanel Valproate† Topiramate	Bivaracetam Lacosamide Phenobarbital Primidone Zonisamide	Carbamazepine Gabapentin Lamotrigine* Oxcarbazepine Phenytoin Pregabalin Tiagabine Vigabatrin
Focal	Lamotrigine Levetiracetam Carbamazepine[2] Oxcarbazepine[2] Zonisamide[2] Lacosamide[3]	Carbamazepine Lacosamide Lamotrigine Levetiracetam Oxcarbazepine Topiramate Zonisamide	Brivaracetam Cenobamate Eslicarbazepine Perampanel Pregabaline Valproate† Phenobarbital# Phenytoin # Tiagabine # Vigabatrin #	

Seizure type	Monotherapy	Add-on Treatment	Second-line Add-on	Drugs to be avoided (may worsen seizures)
Absence	Ethosuximide	Valproate[12] Lamotrigine[3] Levetiracetam[3]		Carbamazepine Gabapentin Oxcarbazepine Phenobarbital Phenytoin Pregabalin Tiagabine Vigabatrin
Absence with other seizure types	Lamotrigine[2] Levetiracetam[2]	Lamotrigine Levetiracetam Valproate[12]	Ethosuximide	Carbamazepine Gabapentin Oxcarbazepine Phenobarbital Phenytoin Pregabalin Tiagabine Vigabatrin

(Continued)

Table 4.3 (Contd.)

Seizure type	Monotherapy	Add-on Treatment	Second-line Add-on	Drugs to be avoided (may worsen seizures)
Myoclonic	Levetiracetam	Levetiracetam Valproate†	Brivaracetam Clobazam Clonazepam Lamotrigine* Phenobarbital Piracetam Topiramate Zonisamide	Carbamazepine Gabapentin Oxcarbazepine Phenytoin Pregabalin Tiagabine Vigabatrin
Tonic or atonic‡	Lamotrigine	Lamotrigine Clobazam Rufinamide Topiramate Valproate†	Ketogenic Diet Felbamate	Carbamazepine Oxcarbazepine Gabapentin Pregabalin Tiagabine Vigabatrin

† UK MHRA guidance updated in 2023 imposes major restrictions on the use of valproate (see Contraception and reproductive health in this chapter ⟳ p. 320). In most situations lamotrigine or levetiracetam can be considered as alternatives.

* May worsen myoclonic seizures

‡ Second-line monotherapy; § Third-line monotherapy; # Third-line add-on therapy

Table 4.4 Medication choice by epilepsy syndrome

Epilepsy syndrome	First-line treatment	Second-line treatment	Third-line treatment	Further options	Drugs to be avoided (may worsen seizures)
Idiopathic Generalized Epilepsy	Lamotrigine Levetiracetam	Lamotrigine Levetiracetam Valproate‡	Perampanel Topiramate		
Dravet Syndrome‡	Valproate‡ Valproate‡ with Stiripentol and clobazam	Cannabidiol& with clobazam		Ketogenic diet Levetiracetam Topiramate Potassium bromide	
Lennox–Gastaut syndrome‡	Valproate‡	Lamotrigine	Cannabidiol& and clobazam Clobazam Rufinamide Topiramate	Ketogenic Diet Felbamate¶	Carbamazepine Gabapentin Lacosamide Lamotrigine Oxcarbazepine Phenobarbital Pregabalin Tiagabine Vigabatrin
Infantile spasms syndrome‡	High-dose oral prednisolone and Vigabatrin◇	Ketogenic Diet Levetiracetam Nitrazepam			

(Continued)

Table 4.4 (Contd.)

Epilepsy syndrome	First-line treatment	Second-line treatment	Third-line treatment	Further options	Drugs to be avoided (may worsen seizures)
Self-limited epilepsy with centrotemporal spikes	Lamotrigine Levetiracetam	Valproate Topiramate	Sulthiame		Carbamazepine Oxcarbazepine Lamotrigine
Epilepsy with Myoclonic- Atonic seizures‡ (Doose syndrome)	Levetiracetam	Valpro ate† Ketogenic Diet	Clobazam Ethosuximide Topiramate Zonisamide		Carbamazepine Gabapentin Oxcarbazepine Phenytoin Pregabalin Vigabatrin

† UK MHRA guidance (2023) imposes major restrictions on the use of valproate (see Contraception and reproductive health in this chapter ⟳ p. 320). In most situations lamotrigine or levetiracetam can be considered as alternatives although valproate remains a first-line choice in Dravet, and probably in Lennox–Gastaut.

‡ Should be assessed by neurologist with expertise in epilepsy

◇ Start with vigabatrin alone in tuberous sclerosis or in children at high risk of steroid-related side effects.

˙ May worsen myoclonic seizures

¶ Not licenced in the UK, but available by importation

ª In children over 2 years

For further Guidance see: NICE guideline NG217: Epilepsy in adults and children, young people and adults (April 2022); www.nice.nhs.uk

Adapted from National Institute for Health and Care Excellence. Clinical guideline [NG217]: Epilepsies in children, young people and adults: diagnosis and adults, https://www.nice. org.uk/guidance/ng217, accessed 11 Feb. 2023, Copyright © NICE 2022.

Very general rule of thumb for first-line ASM
- Generalized epilepsies and syndromes: levetiracetam or lamotrigine.

▶ Due to the increased risk of birth defects and neurodevelopmental disorders in children born to ♀ who take valproate during pregnancy, NICE guidelines (2022) contraindicate valproate in ♀ over 10 years old (see Contraception and reproductive health in this chapter ➋ p. 320). For this reason lamotrigine and levetiracetam are now the first-line ASM choices in most situations.

- Focal seizures with or without generalization: lamotrigine or levetiracetam should be considered as first-line monotherapy.
- Infantile spasms: high-dose oral prednisolone with vigabatrin.

Role of ASM blood level measurement

The main problem with blood monitoring is slavish adherence to quoted laboratory 'therapeutic ranges'. Drug monitoring gets you 'downstream' of pharmaco*kinetic* sources of variation in therapeutic response (those factors that affect the drug concentration at the receptor for a given administered dose such as absorption and metabolism) but not pharmaco*dynamic* sources of variability (differences in the effects of a given drug concentration at the receptor: largely genetically determined). A population therapeutic or 'target' range is only useful for drugs where pharmacokinetic variability outweighs pharmacodynamic: the only drugs for which this is true are phenytoin, and, to a lesser extent, phenobarbital. For other drugs quoted 'therapeutic ranges' are population-derived statistical averages of little relevance to the individual child: some children's seizures will be well-controlled at lower levels and other children may tolerate and require higher levels for complete seizure control.

Relative indications
- Detection of non-adherence (trough levels should be taken).
- When toxicity is suspected (level should be taken at around time of the maximum symptomatology).
- Adjustment of phenytoin and phenobarbital doses: see Phenytoin in Chapter 7 ➋ p. 691.
- Management of pharmacokinetic interactions.
- Specific clinical conditions (pregnancy, organ failure).

Role of routine monitoring of haematological and biochemical parameters

Although some sources recommend regular monitoring of full blood counts, liver function, and other parameters, there is no evidence for this practice. Parents should be advised of possible effects of drugs (e.g. valproate-related thrombocytopaenia) and monitoring should be targeted to children with suggestive presentations.

▶ Correct attribution of cause and effect is a major challenge in the management of refractory epilepsy. Good and bad periods come and go without apparent reason: sometimes spontaneously without changes in medication, but more problematically sometimes when a change *has* recently been made.

Bear in mind the phenomenon of *regression to the mean*: there will be an average severity and frequency around which fluctuation occurs over time. Since treatment and management changes are generally made when things are worse than average, many such changes will be followed by improvement even if there is no truly causal relationship with the symptoms. It is worth reminding families that chance might be at play and that attribution of effects should not be automatically assumed.

Complaints such as poor concentration might be due to undertreatment (incomplete seizure control), overtreatment (drug toxicity), or completely unrelated to treatment (due to the primary cause of the epilepsy), or any combination of these factors! In such situations it is all too easy to seek and find apparent patterns and 'reasons' for changes in a child's situation, only for families to become exasperated when a pattern they thought they had found ceases to hold.

The only practical solution to these dilemmas is to change one thing at a time; to make changes infrequently (resist the temptation to fiddle—a particular danger during hospital admissions); and assess the effects of a change over a period of weeks (to allow random fluctuations in the condition to manifest themselves).

Surgical treatment of epilepsy

Epilepsy surgery referral is currently indicated in drug-resistant epilepsies (more than 20% of patients continue to have seizures after two tolerated and appropriately selected ASMs), in patients with intolerable side effects from ASMs and, in seizures where a structural lesion is detected and ASM resistance is likely.

- *Curative* surgery removes or disconnects the brain parenchyma that is considered to be the source of seizures (the epileptogenic zone), and as a result can *sometimes* eliminate seizures.
- *Palliative* surgery aims to reduce the frequency and intensity of seizures with no expectation of 'cure'.

Selection of surgical candidates

It is well recognized that children have been coming to surgery too late, delaying potentially curative treatment and exposing children to prolonged periods of unsatisfactory seizure control and exposure to unwanted effects of ASMs, typically at a critical period in terms of neurodevelopment.

The ideal candidate for resective surgery is a child with:

- A focal (preferably unifocal) epilepsy.
- A radiologically evident abnormality at the identified epileptogenic zone (desirable but not essential).
- No evidence that seizures are also originating from other foci (although under some circumstances a very dominant seizure focus might be removed in the knowledge that other foci remain).
- Where the predicted morbidity of resection is minimal, or at least acceptable.

Referral should be early particularly for hemimegalencephaly and Sturge–Weber syndrome where the prospects of medical control are known to be poor and the neuro-developmental impact of continuing seizure activity is undesirable.

Common indications for epilepsy surgery
- Focal cortical dysplasias (FCD).
- Focal epilepsy associated with structural causes such as perinatal stroke or cavernomas.
- Diffuse unilateral hemispheric syndromes (Sturge–Weber, Rasmussen, hemimegalencephaly).
- Glioneural tumours.
- Mesial temporal lobe epilepsy with hippocampal sclerosis (MTLE-HS).
- If a child is not suitable for resective surgery, palliative procedures may still be considered.

Contraindications to resective surgery
- Generalized genetic epilepsies.
- Neurodegenerative or progressive systemic diseases.
- Location of the epileptogenic zone (EZ) in an eloquent area of the brain (e.g. language or dominant hemisphere motor cortex).
- Psychiatric morbidity (may compromise post-surgical outcome).

Workup
There must be an acceptable risk–benefit ratio for the proposed surgery and anatomical and electroclinical location of the EZ must be concordant. The pre-surgical workup should be carried out in the specialized centre where the surgery will be performed.
- Non-invasive EZ-locating investigations include, as appropriate:
  - clinical semiology.
  - video-surface EEG.
  - MRI.
  - fMRI.
  - PET (especially in 'MRI-negative' cases).
  - SPECT.
  - Neuropsychological and psychiatric evaluation.
- When non-invasive approaches fail to localize the EZ, invasive investigations can be performed:
  - Subdural electrodes: a grid or strip of electrodes placed on the brain surface at craniotomy.
  - Stereo-EEG: placement of fine intracerebral electrodes deep in the suspected EZ under with light sedation.

Likely effects of resection (e.g. of eloquent cortex) should also be carefully evaluated. fMRI can be used to assess if the remaining lobe can sustain memory and language function in older children.

Curative surgical techniques
- Surgical resection: tailored cortical resection removes the EZ. Examples include temporal lobectomy (cortico-amygdalo-hippocampectomy or selective amygdalo-hippocampectomy).

- Disconnection: tailored disconnection isolates the EZ without removing it. Examples include:
  - hemispherotomy (e.g. for Rasmussen, hemimegalencephaly, Sturge–Weber): disconnects the pathological cerebral hemisphere by division of the corpus callosum and peduncles.
  - Stereo-EEG-guided radiofrequency thermocoagulation (good results on MTLE-HS, FCD, hypothalamic hamartomas).
  - MRI-guided laser-induced interstitial thermal ablation (less invasive and an alternative in small EZ).

Palliative surgery
- Callosotomy (for atonic seizures; divides the corpus callosum, preventing the spread of seizures).
- Neurostimulation: vagus nerve stimulation (VNS), deep-brain stimulation (DBS) and responsive neurostimulation (RNS).
  - Of these only VNS is in widespread used currently.
  - Important to establish a child is not a candidate for resective surgery before implanting VNS: potential for seizure freedom is greater with resection and VNS complicates subsequent specialist neuroimaging.

Vagus nerve stimulation

The VNS is an implantable pulse generator placed subcutaneously beneath the left clavicle and a lead wire that is connected to the left vagus nerve (mainly afferent fibres therefore fewer cardiac or gastrointestinal effects). Mechanism of action is unclear, but modulates activity of the limbic system, locus coeruleus, thalamus, and cortex.
- Output current, frequency, pulse duration, and duty cycle can be adjusted.
- Programmed with pre-defined stimulation sequences. Can also be activated acutely by swiping a magnet over the device. Recent models have a sensing component and respond automatically to ictal tachycardia detection.
- Indicated as adjunctive therapy for children with refractory focal and generalized epilepsies and who are not candidates for surgery.

Efficacy
- 25–50% of children experience a 25–50% reduction of seizure frequency (parents should be counselled that prospect of total seizure freedom is less than with ketogenic diet).
- Decreases SUDEP risk, and improves quality of life (alertness, general behaviour).
- The rate of response improves over time.

Adverse effects of implantation
- Vocal cord paralysis.
- Facial nerve palsy.
- Hemidiaphragm paralysis.
- Infection.
- Hyperaesthesia.

Adverse effects of stimulation

Dose-dependent and usually decrease or disappear with readjustments in the VNS parameters.
- Hoarseness.
- Cervical paraesthesia.
- Dyspnoea (caution when used in patient with obstructive sleep apnoea).
- Cough.
- Throat pain.
- Dyspepsia.
- Dysphagia (turning off or adjust the parameters during mealtime may help).

Ketogenic diet treatment (KD)

The mode of action is unclear: ketones are thought to cause neuronal inhibition indirectly but there are probably multiple mechanisms. A trained dietician must create an individualized dietary plan. The child's weight, growth, pubertal status, and mobility must be taken into account. Diets are described in terms of the ratio of fat calories to carbohydrate and protein calories:
- The classic diet is based on high proportions of saturated dairy fat. A child will typically be on a 3 or 4:1 ratio.
- The MCT diet uses medium chain triglyceride oil (highly ketogenic) that allows inclusion of more carbohydrates and proteins and is thus slightly less restrictive.
- Modified Atkins Diet and Low Glycaemic Index Treatment are less restrictive and may be recommended for adolescents, due to better adherence.

There is no evidence of difference in efficacy between classic and MCT diet in older children. In children <2 years of age the classic diet appears superior.

Clinical efficacy
- RCTs confirms efficacy.
- Very variable but significant *complete seizure-freedom* rate that are higher than for vagus nerve stimulation.

Candidate selection
- Treatment of choice in children with GLUT 1 deficiency syndrome and pyruvate dehydrogenase deficiency.
- Particularly useful in the management of Dravet syndrome, EMAtS, TSC, FIRES, EIDEE, and super-refractory status epilepticus.
- Should be considered in a child who has failed two ASMs.
- Contraindicated in pyruvate carboxylase, fatty acid oxidation disorders, and porphyria. **Check acylcarnitines before institution.**

Problems
- Time-consuming.
- Requires motivation of staff, family, and child.
- Requires expert staff and education of family.

- Socially restrictive in terms of permitted foods.
- May require hospital admission to enable establishment.
- Requires regular blood and urine tests to ensure safety and efficacy.

Adverse effects
- Hypoglycaemia especially at onset.
- Dehydration.
- Nausea and vomiting.
- Metabolic acidosis especially with intercurrent infection and some ASMs such as topiramate, zonisamide, and acetazolamide.
- Kidney stones—again, more likely with topiramate.
- Constipation with the classical and diarrhoea with the MCT diets.
- Poor growth and weight gain.
- Lethargy and fatigue.
- ↑blood fat levels.
- Vitamin, calcium, trace element, and carnitine deficiencies; thus need regular monitoring and supplements.

Epilepsy and daily life

For some children the psychosocial consequences of epilepsy can be more debilitating than the seizure disorder itself. Such difficulties may affect mental health and themselves further exacerbate seizure control.

Epilepsy is an individual condition, so informed choices about activities need to be made on a personal basis depending on the type and frequency of seizures as well as the level of control with medication. The aim should be to maximize participation in all age-appropriate aspects of life while taking a realistic approach to risk management: err on the side of inclusion.

Mental health affects quality of life for young people with epilepsy more than seizure frequency.

Schooling

Most children with epilepsy will attend mainstream school; however, there is evidence for underachievement.

- Poor progress is associated with early age at onset and long seizure history particularly if seizure control is poor.
- Intractable seizures are often associated with disorders of cognitive function, memory, or attention. Neuropsychometry is recommended to define educational strengths and weaknesses and aid tailoring of educational support.
- Dominant hemisphere disturbances are likely to affect language-related skills.
- Other mechanisms of adverse impact on schooling include:
  - absence from school;
  - low self-esteem;
  - drug toxicity;
  - anxiety due to poor adjustment and stressors at home;
  - nocturnal seizures and poor sleep;
  - brief undetected epileptic discharges;
  - DEE-SWAS disrupting memory consolidation.

It is important that pupils with epilepsy participate fully in school life and achieve their full potential.

- The provisions of the Disability Discrimination Act in the UK and equivalent legislation elsewhere cover children with epilepsy. Effective communication between the teacher, parents, doctor, and child are important. School staff may need training, often from an epilepsy specialist nurse.
- For children with no additional physical or learning difficulties or medical problems, the aim must be to enable full participation in school life with provisions made for their safety. For some other children, epilepsy is part of a wider spectrum of problems needing appropriate provision either in mainstream schooling with support or in a specialist educational setting.

Education of school personnel involves
- Basic knowledge of epilepsy.
- Awareness of medical management including regular ASMs.

- First aid management including administration of rescue medication and when to call an ambulance.
- Special considerations including swimming (see In and around water in this chapter p. 319) and photosensitivity (see Photosensitivity in this chapter p. 319).
- Awareness of potential for bullying and low self-esteem.
- Awareness of issues surrounding epilepsy, learning, and behaviour.

Emotional adjustment

Adjusting to a diagnosis of epilepsy involves living with unpredictability. Some families must also cope with additional 'hidden' deficits such as language and memory problems or learning disability.

- The unpredictability of seizures erodes self-esteem and confidence. Families may prefer to live with a predictable pattern of seizures (e.g. occurring reliably first thing on waking while child is still at home) than risk ASM manipulations in an attempt to improve control.
- Ill-informed and prejudicial attitudes may be experienced.
- Unwanted effects of medication, e.g. weight gain or facial hair may be very detrimental to self-esteem.
- Highs and lows of successive treatment failures may be particularly hard to cope with, especially failure of epilepsy surgery.
- Rates of anxiety, depression, agoraphobia, and suicide are ↑in children with epilepsy.

Responses

- Establish good communication between health, education, and the family.
- Consider a family-held child health care record.
- Education about epilepsy for teachers, school peers, family, and child.
- Encourage self-esteem.
- Avoid unnecessary restrictions.
- Minimize time off school for clinic appointments.
- Minimize disruptive responses to seizures (e.g. the school calling an ambulance following a seizure a child has recovered from, not realizing this will mean a several hour wait in the Emergency Department).
- Ensure full education:
  - Encourage tertiary education.
  - Provide informed career advice: some careers (e.g. uniformed services) are unavailable or only available on restricted basis to people who have, or *who have ever had*, active epilepsy. Refer to national policies on these issues to avoid young people experiencing refusal.
- Sensitive monitoring:
  - detect difficulties early;
  - detailed neuropsychological assessment.
- Avoid seizure triggers:
  - Photic stimuli (flickering light sources, see below).
  - Fatigue, late nights, excessive alcohol, and recreational drug use are recognized triggers particularly in JME and other idiopathic generalized epilepsy syndromes.

In and around water

- A child with poorly controlled seizures should be accompanied at all times in and around water. This includes bathing as well as water sports.
  - Showering is a strongly recommended alternative to bathing that will allow privacy.
- For a child with well-controlled seizures, it is good practice for a designated person (with knowledge of how to manage a seizure and capable of effecting a rescue) to be in the vicinity when child is swimming.
  - If no qualified life-saver is present, then the child should not be allowed to swim any deeper than the supervisor's shoulder height.
  - A 'buddy' system where all children swim with a partner makes the child less conspicuous.
- Although UK recreational underwater ('scuba') diving precautions are guidelines and do not have regulatory force they are likely to be applied by diving schools. They are currently very restrictive and require an individual to have been seizure-free off medication for 5 yrs.

Cycling

A child with poorly controlled seizures should cycle away from traffic under supervision. As for any cyclist, a helmet should be worn!

Photosensitivity

Misinformation frequently leads to unwarranted restriction of IT lessons and other computer-based activity.

- Photosensitivity is uncommon, affecting 5% of young people with epilepsy, of whom about 40% only ever have photic-induced seizures.
- Identified by the advent of a triggered seizure or on photic stimulation during a standard EEG.
- Sources include natural (e.g. sunlight on water, travelling past sunlit trees), and artificial (e.g. strobe) sources of flickering light.
- Typical provoking flicker rates are 10–50 Hz.
  - Old cathode ray tube (CRT) TVs (the ones with a prominent 'bulge' on the back) are in this range and did pose a potential trigger source but are largely obsolete. Nearly all computer monitors—even the CRT type—have much higher, safe, refresh rates.
  - All flat screen displays are flicker free: there is no need to limit access to IT lessons at school.
- Stroboscopic lights in nightclubs etc may be an issue.
- Some seizures occurring during computer games may result from repetitive/geometric patterns in the image, or excitement, arousal, or fatigue rather than display flicker.
- Nearly all patients with clinical pattern sensitivity show photo-paroxysmal responses on testing.
- Aim to reduce the intensity of the flickering light source relative to other steady illumination. Watch CRT type TV in a well-lit room: consider putting a small lamp on top of the set to 'dilute' the flickering light source, avoid getting too close to the screen: use the remote control.

Alcohol

- Excessive alcohol can cause seizures particularly in juvenile myoclonic and other idiopathic generalized syndromes.
- The frequency of seizures is ↑in the 'hangover' period.
- However, abstinence not required!

Driving

- Current UK legislation requires 12 months' seizure freedom (with ongoing ASM treatment if necessary) or 3 yrs' demonstration of a seizure disorder's restriction to sleep, before an ordinary driving licence can be given.
  - It is 'recommended' (but not mandatory) that individuals refrain from driving for 6 months after any substantial change to medication (including ASM withdrawal).
- Occurrence of a seizure resets the clock and driving must be suspended until event free for a further 12 months.
- Some specialist vocational driving licences (bus, coach, heavy goods vehicle) require the driver to have been event free and off medication for 10 yrs.
- Legislation applies to any cause of paroxysmal event that incapacitates (e.g. recurrent syncope) not just epilepsy.
- Similar legislation applies in other countries.

Contraception and reproductive health

Epilepsy treatment and contraception

- Adolescence is an important time to review the implications of ASM for a ♀'s daily life. Advice on contraception should ideally be given before a young woman becomes sexually active.
- Enzyme-inducing ASMs —carbamazepine, eslicarbazepine, oxcarbazepine, topiramate (>200 mg/day), phenytoin, phenobarbital, rufinamide, perampanel — enhance the clearance and reduce the effectiveness of hormonal contraception by any route: oral, transdermal, or vaginal.
- When it's not possible to change to a non-enzyme-inducing ASM, young ♀ should receive counselling about possible risks:
- Medroxyprogesterone acetate depot injection, levonorgestrel-releasing intrauterine devices (IUD) and copper-IUD may be suitable alternative options.
- Non-enzyme-inducing ASMs do not influence hormonal contraceptive metabolism so there's no risk of OCP failure.
- Combined OCPs increase the clearance of lamotrigine, which may worsen seizure frequency (monitoring of lamotrigine plasma levels may be useful) and dosage increases may be advisable.
  - Progestogen-only OCP may be a better option.

Use of sodium valproate

- There are number of implications for reproductive health of valproate use by young women of reproductive age:

- Polycystic ovarian syndrome and menstrual irregularity appear to be a risk with valproate use; however, the mechanism involves weight gain and most young women will insist on discontinuing valproate anyhow if significant weight gain is occurring.
- The risk of birth defects and n eurodevelopmental disorders in children born to ♀ who take valproate during pregnancy are now well established.

▶ UK Medicines and Healthcare Products Regulatory Agency (MHRA) advice (2023) states that:

- Valproate must not be started in new patients (male or female) younger than 55 years, unless two specialists independently consider and document that there is no other effective or tolerated treatment, or there are compelling reasons that the reproductive risks do not apply
- At their next annual specialist review, women of childbearing potential and girls should be reviewed using a revised valproate Risk Acknowledgement Form, which will include the need for a second specialist signature if the patient is to continue with valproate and subsequent annual reviews with one specialist unless the patient's situation changes

▶This guidance adds to previous MHRA (2021) and Commission on Human Medicines (CHM 2022) recommendations that valproate should only be prescribed in ♀ <10 years and when treatment is expected to be short-term. Valproate should not be prescribed to ♀ >10 years of age unless other treatments are ineffective or not tolerated.
▶Valproate use is also associated with (reversible) reduced fertility in ♂'s.
▶ If valproate is strictly necessary, a Pregnancy Prevention Programme should be implemented in line with BPNA and RCPCH joint guidance (2019).

ASMs in pregnancy
- There is evidence of ↑risk of adverse outcomes in children exposed to carbamazepine, phenytoin, phenobarbital, and high-dose topiramate *in utero*.
- The latest MHRA report (2021) reinforced that lamotrigine and levetiracetam are safer in pregnancy than other ASMs (no increase in rates of foetal growth restriction, pre-term birth, or congenital malformations; nor of adverse neurodevelopmental outcome), which makes them first-choice treatment options in many epileptic syndromes in young women.

Individualized advice
The appropriate course of action for a young woman with epilepsy wishing to conceive depends on individual consideration of:
- Risks of discontinuing, reducing, or changing ASM considering epilepsy syndrome.

- Risk to fetus of maternal seizures (especially convulsive status epilepticus).
- Options for mitigating risks of foetal exposure to ASMs:
  - Prefer lamotrigine or levetiracetam.
  - Choose monotherapy and the lowest dose, whenever possible.
  - Monitor ASMs levels, especially lamotrigine.
  - Periconceptual high-dose folate use may mitigate risks of neural tube defects.

❶ Optimal management requires prospective planning: above all avoid unplanned pregnancy.

Air travel

All regular and rescue medication is to be carried on the person. A letter to explain to security and customs personnel may be necessary.

Death in epilepsy

Epilepsy-related death in a child may be due to:
- Complication of seizure, e.g. aspiration, suffocation, injury, or drowning.
- Convulsive status epilepticus.
- Related underlying condition, e.g. neurodegenerative disease or cerebral palsy.
- Sudden unexpected death in epilepsy (SUDEP) (see below).

Risk factors for epilepsy-related death:
- Epilepsy with onset in the first 12 months of life.
- Structural epilepsy, e.g. cerebral malformation.
- Severe myoclonic epilepsies of infancy and early childhood.
- Infantile spasms treated with steroids.
- Severe developmental impairment present at the onset of epilepsy.

SUDEP

Defined as a sudden, unexpected, non-traumatic, and non-drowning death in children with epilepsy, with or without evidence for a seizure, excluding documented status epilepticus, in which a post-mortem examination does not reveal a toxicological or anatomical cause for death. Tentative explanations include primary or secondary cardiac arrhythmias and/or a primary respiratory dysfunction.

For bereaved relatives, the shock of SUDEP is often greater because they had not realized this could occur. They may also implicitly believe that the death could have been prevented. When and how to raise these matters with children and their families requires careful clinical judgement: the concern is for the potential −ve effects on active participation in life of ↑anxiety, more restrictive supervision, and possible demands for more aggressive ASM treatment.

It is clear that the very large majority of paediatric epilepsy-related deaths are in children with significant associated neurodisability: in this group there is likely to be greater prior recognition of the presence of a life-limiting situation. The exact rate of SUDEP is still unknown but in children with genetic primary epilepsies with no additional neurological problems is less than 65 per 100 000 patient years (comparable to the rate of sudden death in diabetes).

Increasingly families bring up this subject themselves—sometimes at first consultation. Concise factual data to inform but not frighten families is a constructive approach. If appropriate comparative realistic rates of other causes of death in children (such as asthma) and in the general population may bring things into perspective.

Risk factors for SUDEP
- Young adult ♂.
- Living alone.
- Early age of onset of seizures.
- GTC seizures.
- ↑frequency of seizures.
- Polytherapy and poor adherence to ASM.

Non-epileptic paroxysmal phenomena

As emphasized in Chapter 3 (see Funny turns (paroxysmal episodes) in Chapter 3 ➲ p. 148), paroxysmal episodes in children have a wide differential diagnosis and misdiagnosis is an ever-present risk. Hazards of a false +ve diagnosis of epilepsy include exposure to inappropriate investigations, but more particularly treatment failure. It is important to be familiar with the wide range of non-epileptic processes that can give rise to paroxysmal or episodic signs or symptoms.

> ❶ The most important example of the reverse error (mistaking an epileptic condition for a non-epileptic one) arises in the context of (often nocturnal) frontal lobe seizures being mistaken for night terrors: see Night (or sleep) terrors in this chapter ➲ p. 495.

Episodes without prominent alteration of awareness

The following conditions are arranged in approximate order of age at presentation.

Benign neonatal sleep myoclonus

Typically, a healthy infant presenting at a few weeks of age with quite dramatic myoclonic movements confined entirely to sleep. The jerks which can be quite violent typically occur in flurries and migrate, involving first one limb and then another in clusters of a few per second. The child is not woken or distressed by the episodes and the abnormal movements do not involve the face. They may be precipitated by gently rocking the sleeping infant.

While the diagnosis can usually be made from history, it is important to ensure that ictal EEG is normal. No treatment is required: the phenomenon stops automatically, usually within a few months, and there are no long-term neurodevelopmental implications.

Gastro-oesophageal reflux

Gastro-oesophageal reflux disease (GORD) enters the differential diagnosis of paroxysmal disorders in two ways.
• Occult GORD in an infant is an important cause of apnoea, a phenomenon for which epileptic aetiologies are also sometimes considered.
• In older children, particularly children with significant neurological disability (but not confined to this group), GORD can precipitate episodic dystonic movements resulting in bizarre posturing particularly of the head and neck, a condition sometimes referred to as Sandifer syndrome.

Shuddering (juddering) attacks

This is a common, under-recognized variant of normal infant behaviour. Presenting the child with an interesting or novel object such as a toy (or dinner!) typically precipitates episodes. The child typically holds his or her arms out and shows an involuntary shiver or shudder sometimes involving most of the body.

The condition is entirely benign and requires no intervention.

Hyperekplexia

In its severe form this is a rare differential of neonatal seizures.
- Causes a marked susceptibility to startle:
  - Sudden sounds, and particularly being touched or handled, precipitate episodes of severe total-body stiffening;
- In the severe neonatal forms, these can result in life-threatening apnoea:
  - Well-intentioned attempts to encourage respiration by stimulation make the situation worse!
  - The spells (and apnoea) can be terminated by forcibly flexing the neck: a potentially life-saving manoeuvre family and carers should be taught.
- Tapping the nose is a particularly sensitive stimulant for this phenomenon and is a useful bedside test.
- Event severity tends to lessen with time and so long as hypoxic complications are prevented, prognosis is good.
- Clonazepam (0.01–0.2 mg/kg/day) is first-line treatment.
- Typically due to *GLRA1* mutations or in other genes related to glycinergic neurotransmission system with failure of inhibitory neurotransmission: recessive and dominant variants described.

Paroxysmal tonic upgaze of infancy

- Prolonged episodes (hours at a time) of sustained or intermittent upward tonic gaze deviation, with down-beating nystagmus on down gaze, and compensatory neck flexion.
- Horizontal eye movements are normal and the phenomenon disappears in sleep.
- Onset usually before 10 months of age.
- Episodes may worsen with fatigue or intercurrent illness.
- Diagnosis of exclusion: MRI is required.
- Mutations in *CACNA1A*, and *GRID2* have been identified in some cases. Condition tends to resolve by approximately 3 yrs of age.
- L-DOPA may be effective if indicated.

Benign myoclonus of early infancy

A rare disorder of early infancy with spasms closely resembling infantile epileptic spasms syndrome (IESS). Onset is between 1 and 12 months, and movements settle by the end of the second year. A presumptive diagnosis of IESS is commonly made before it becomes apparent that the EEG is normal between and during the episodes.

Long-term neurological development is normal.

Benign paroxysmal torticollis

- Rare.
- Recurrent episodes of cervical dystonia occur resulting in a head tilt or apparent torticollis.
- Events typically last several hours to a few days in duration.
- Accompanied by marked autonomic features (pallor and vomiting).
- Typically starts in infancy, resolving within the pre-school years, but children often go on to develop hemiplegic migraine in later life.
- There is usually a family history of (hemiplegic) migraine, and many cases are associated with calcium channel mutations (e.g. *CACNA1A*).

Benign paroxysmal vertigo
- Resembles benign paroxysmal torticollis. Children present with sudden-onset signs consistent with vertigo (poor coordination and nystagmus). The picture, however, is dominated by an impression of fear and distress.
- Children are often strikingly pale and may be nauseated and distressed but not encephalopathic.
- It may be a migraine variant (ion channel disorder).
- The condition should not be confused with the similarly named benign paroxysmal *positional* vertigo, a condition of adulthood caused by debris in the utricle of the inner ear.

Self-comforting phenomena (self-gratification, masturbation)
Common in normal toddlers, and in older children with neurological disability.
- Typical setting is highchair or car travel seat with a strap between the legs and a tired or bored child.
- Older children often lie on the floor, prone or supine, with tightly adducted or crossed legs.
- Child will typically extend the legs at the hips and press thighs together.
- May continue for prolonged periods, the child often becoming flushed and quite unresponsive to attempted interruption.
- Typically diminishes when children become ambulant.
- Behaviour is self-limiting and no treatment is required. Parents sometimes require considerable reassurance that such behaviour is commonplace, normal, and simply a source of comfort, not a sign of sexual deviancy.

Tics
Isolated 'fragments' of gestures or movements repeated compulsively, sometimes in conjunction with vocal tics as part of Tourette syndrome: see Tic disorders and Tourette syndrome in this chapter p. 421.
    Older children can by definition at least briefly suppress the desire to tic although they will often report a sense of rising tension, which only resolves by 'releasing' the movements.

Ritualistic movements and behavioural stereotypies
These are relatively common in young children, and older children with neurological disability particularly autistic spectrum disorders.

Hyperventilation and anxiety attacks
The respiratory alkalosis resulting from hyperventilation is a potent cause of sensory phenomena (particularly peri-orally) and tetanic contraction of the muscles of the forearm and hand resulting in carpopedal spasm. Severe hyperventilation can sometimes result in syncopal collapse.

Episodic ataxia type 1
Caused by a potassium channel gene (*KCNA1*) mutation. Onset of paroxysmal attacks is from 5 yrs of age: sudden weakness, unsteady and blurred vision, lasting minutes to hours. The child will eventually develop myokymia. Acetazolamide or carbamazepine may reduce the frequency of episodes.

Episodic ataxia type 2

Onset is in later childhood due to *CACNA1A* mutation. Unsteadiness and ataxia are associated with nausea and vomiting. Attacks become milder and less frequent with age, but cerebellar signs may persist (cerebellar vermis atrophy on imaging); usually acetazolamide responsive.

Paroxysmal dyskinesias

A range of individually rare paroxysmal movement disorders is recognized including paroxysmal dystonias and choreoathetosis. They are generally grouped into paroxysmal kinesiogenic, non-kinesiogenic, and exertional dyskinesias (PKD, PNKD, and PED, respectively; Table 4.5). Episodes of involuntary movement in PKD are triggered by volitional movement (with no such trigger in PNKD). Episodes of dyskinesia in PKD are generally shorter and more responsive to ASM (particularly carbamazepine) compared to PNKD. PKD is often caused by *PRRT2* mutations. Episodes of dyskinesia in PED occur following periods of exercise and are most commonly due to glucose tranporter-1 deficiency syndrome (GLUT1DS). Dyskinesias occurring before meals or after fasting should raise suspicion of GLUT1DS: see Glucose transport-1 deficiency syndrome in this chapter ⬧ p. 301.

Secondary paroxysmal movement disorders

Paroxysmal dyskinesias can arise because of drugs (phenytoin, gabapentin), acquired brain injury (trauma, stroke, infections, perinatal hypoxic–ischaemic injury), metabolic disease (hypoparathyroidism, thyrotoxicosis, maple-syrup urine disease, non-ketotic hyperglycinaemia), and infections (HIV-AIDS, SSPE).

They generally respond to ASMs.

Episodes with altered awareness

Syncopal mechanisms

Involve loss of awareness due to a temporary inadequacy of cerebral blood flow. There is prominent early pallor. As stressed in Chapter 3 (see Funny turns (paroxysmal episodes) in Chapter 3 ⬧ p. 148), 'seizure-like' jerking limb movements and even incontinence of urine can result in the late phases of a syncopal episode, raising the risks of a misdiagnosis of epilepsy. The context in which the episode occurred, and its earliest features are the most telling.

Cardiac disease

The importance of correctly identifying an intermittent cardiac dysrhythmia or structural cardiac disease as the cause of episodic loss of awareness is self-evident. Historic clues will include the relationship to exercise and, as stressed, prominent early pallor.

▶ Any apparent syncope coming on in a lying position must be presumed to be cardiac in origin until proven otherwise.

▶ A history of *exertional* syncope should prompt search for prolonged QT syndromes (see below) but also HOCUM (hypertrophic obstructive cardiomyopathy) particularly if there is a family history (dominantly inherited). Note that ECG is insensitive to the presence of cardiomyopathy and echocardiography is required if this is suspected.

Table 4.5 Paroxysmal dyskinesias: phenotypes and treatment

	Paroxysmal non-kinesiogenic dyskinesia	Paroxysmal kinesiogenic dyskinesia	Paroxysmal exertional dyskinesia	Paroxysmal hypnogenic dyskinesia
Movement	Dystonia or choreoathetosis. May be unable to communicate during episode. Episodic ataxia	Dystonia often with prodromal sensation. May have chorea or ballismus.	Dystonia or chorea	Dystonia, chorea, or ballism
Localization	Face, limbs, either unilateral or bilateral.	Legs, unilateral	Leg, unilateral, or arm if being exercised	Any, generalized, REM sleep
Duration	Minutes–hours	Seconds to <5 min	Minutes	Minutes
Frequency	3/day to 2/yr	100 s/day	2/day to 1/month	5/night to 5/yr
Age at onset	Infancy	Infancy to 30 s	Childhood	Childhood
Inheritance	AD	AD, sporadic	AD, sporadic	Heterogeneous
♂:♀ ratio	2:1	4:1	1:4	Variable
Treatment	Avoid triggers Clonazepam May be refractory	Carbamazepine (sensitive to very low doses) Phenytoin	Avoid triggers Ketogenic diet in GLUT1DS Clonazepam but may be refractory L-DOPA Acetazolamide	Short attacks usually responsive to CBZ, VPA, or LEV. Longer attacks may respond to L-DOPA or acetazolamide

	Paroxysmal non-kinesiogenic dyskinesia	Paroxysmal kinesiogenic dyskinesia	Paroxysmal exertional dyskinesia	Paroxysmal hypnogenic dyskinesia
Precipitants	Fatigue, alcohol, caffeine, stress	Sudden initiation of movement	Prolonged exercise, cold, vibration	REM sleep
Genes	Myofibrillogenesis regulator (MR-1)	PRRT2	SLC2A1	Heterogenous: related to SHE

NaChR: neuronal nicotinic acetylcholine receptor gene; SHE: Sleep-related hypermotor epilepsy

Reflex asystolic syncope

The term reflex asystolic syncope (RAS) has replaced 'reflex anoxic seizure' as it better conveys the fundamental mechanism. The phenomenon has also been referred to as 'pallid syncope' and in the old paediatric literature— extremely confusingly—as a pallid breath-holding spell (a complete mis- nomer for reasons that should be apparent).

In understanding the process, it is helpful to realize that children with RAS grow into adults who faint at the sight of needles and blood. A sudden unexpected shock or pain results in a vagally mediated severe bradycardia or even asystole with consequent hypotension, pallor, and loss of con- sciousness that may then lead to episodes of limb stiffening or clonic jerks. An accurate history identifies the triggers that consistently precede these episodes.

Episodes are self-limiting and generally require no specific treatment. Children should be evaluated by 12-lead ECG to exclude prolonged QT syndrome. Occasionally, severely affected children have come to cardiac pacemaker implantation.

▶ Long QT syndromes are estimated to have a prevalence of around 1 in 2000 live births. Long QT1: associated with exercise, particularly swim- ming, with fairly frequent events but a relatively low risk of sudden death. Long QT2: events occurring in response to emotional stress or auditory stimuli, such as alarm clocks, but also occur at rest. Long QT3: most of events occur at rest and have a higher mortality.

Vaso-vagal syncope

In older children, this is probably the condition most frequently misdiag- nosed as epilepsy. Common triggers include intercurrent illness, hot wea- ther, missed meals, inadequate fluid intake, and prolonged standing. It is typically a disease of adolescents who will be able to report a prodromal awareness of feeling cold, clammy, and unwell. They may be able to report sounds becoming distant or their vision 'greying out'. If the event is not terminated by lying down in the prodromal phase, the child goes on to fall stiffly to the ground or slump and may exhibit brief tonic or clonic move- ments or urinary incontinence. These movements often raise concerns about possible GTC seizures for family and carers witnessing episodes and care is required to obtain a detailed description of events.

Blue (cyanotic) breath-holding attacks

There has in the past been a lot of confusion between this and RAS (see above). They are quite distinct processes. RAS is a primarily cardiac phe- nomenon. Blue breath-holding spells are primarily hypoxic in origin due to disordered respiration. Typically, a toddler who has become angry or frustrated begins to cry and becomes 'stuck' at the end of a period of pro- longed sobs (i.e. the condition is more accurately described as a prolonged end expiratory apnoea). As a result, the child becomes predominantly *blue*, limp, and may briefly lose consciousness; again, this may result in subse- quent jerking limb movements.

Daydreaming

Daydreaming enters the differential of absence seizures as a cause of 'vacant spells'. The history often differentiates the two. Daydreaming typically occurs when bored, tired, or absorbed in watching TV, and is characterized by reports from a parent or teacher of 'having to call his name three times before he responds'. The flavour is very different from an absence or other seizure that actively interrupts and cuts across normal activity.

Non-epileptic attacks

Non-epileptic attack disorder (NEAD) is a common functional neurological symptom and important differential of generalized seizures occurring usually in ♀s. It is common for the onset of NEAD to be quite explosive with repeated urgent requests to see an adolescent previously unknown to the service with a sudden and dramatic onset of many episodes per day. They are typically briefer and less stereotyped than epileptic seizures. Movements may include pelvic thrusting, rolling, reciprocating kicking or flailing movements. None of these occur as part of the repertoire of epileptic seizures. Typically, there is a lack of post-ictal drowsiness or confusion. It is often possible to make a positive diagnosis of NEAD on the basis of a review of video recordings of the episode. Capturing episodes on an EEG/videotelemetry for confirmation is not mandatory. *Pseudosyncope* ('swooning') is a similar condition. See Functional neurological symptoms in this chapter ➜ p. 335.

Narcolepsy and cataplexy

Narcolepsy is an under-recognized cause of excessive daytime sleepiness (see Narcolepsy in this chapter ➜ p. 497). Cataplexy is a sudden loss of muscle tone typically precipitated by laughter or startle that is a common feature of narcolepsy particularly by early adulthood (although there are other causes).

Factitious or induced illness

Factitious or induced illness (FII) refers to the range of ways in which the healthcare system can be manipulated to harm children, with healthcare workers unwitting instruments of the harm. FII is preferable to previous terms including 'Munchausen syndrome by proxy'. There are pointers that are suggestive of an FII situation, but none are intrinsically diagnostic and there is always a differential diagnosis. Clinical features can vary widely, and the conclusion that they are due to FII can only be reached after careful multidisciplinary assessment.

A spectrum of problems exists from fiction (reporting something that is not occurring), through fabrication of documentation and charts, ultimately to direct causation of symptoms or signs in a child.

FII can present to most if not all paediatric subspecialties. Common neurological symptoms include reported seizures, collapse, drowsiness, and developmental impairment.

Verbal fictions are much more common than induced physical signs of illness: this poses particular problems in the context of reported seizures, which by their nature are typically unobserved. Lack of independently observed seizures (e.g. at school), demonstrated non-adherence to drug treatment (e.g. prescription refill records, undetectable blood levels), and repeatedly normal EEGs despite descriptions of aggressive epilepsy may all raise concerns. However, as with non-epileptic attack disorder, FII and genuine epilepsy can co-exist, perhaps in up to 5% of cases.

The long-term effects on children (e.g. as future parents) of distorting understandings of themselves and health and illness (even if the situation is not likely to lead to serious immediate harm such as surgery) are unclear.

Thinking the unthinkable

The possibility of FII has first to be entertained, if only to be discounted. FII often implies a *folie à trois* between child, parent, and misled professional, and it can be uncomfortable to acknowledge that one has been deceived. Any senior professional will, however, acknowledge that it has happened to them. The key is a story that does not hang together: symptoms not congruent with known diseases; symptoms, signs, and investigation results that do not correlate; treatments that do not produce the expected results. Repeated presentations to multiple specialties, the reporting of new symptoms following resolution of the previous ones, and particular reported symptoms (stopping breathing, loss of consciousness, seizures, choking, or collapse) are concerning.

If you have concerns as a trainee under supervision, these must be discussed with the child's named paediatrician at the earliest opportunity.

Initial concerns: questions to ask yourself

- Are there child welfare concerns that might explain discrepancies in the child's symptoms or response to treatment?
- Is it clear that factors other than natural disorders may be operating?
- What are the needs of the child?
- Is the child coming to quantifiable harm?

- Are the parents able to respond appropriately to the child's needs? Is the child being adequately safeguarded from significant harm, and are the parents able to promote the child's health and development?
- Is action required to safeguard and promote the child's welfare?

Source: data from Department for Education and Skills and Her Majesty's Stationery Office. *Working Together to Safeguard Children: A guide to inter-agency working to safeguard and promote the welfare of children*, ℘ https://www.gov.uk/government/publications/working-together-to-safeguard-children--2; ℘ https://assets.publishing.service.gov.uk/government/uploads/system/uploads/attachment_data/file/942454/Working_together_to_safeguard_children_inter_agency_guidance.pdf, accessed 20 Sept 2023, London: HMSO, Copyright © 2018 Crown Copyright.

The 2021 RCPCH Document 'Perplexing Presentations (PP) / Fabricated or Induced Illness in Children RCPCH Guidance' suggests additional 'warning signs':

- In the child:
  - Reported physical, psychological, or behavioural symptoms and signs not observed independently in their reported context.
  - Unusual results of investigations (e.g. biochemical findings, unusual infective organisms).
  - Inexplicably poor response to prescribed treatment.
  - Some characteristics of the child's illness may be physiologically impossible e.g. persistent −ve fluid balance, large blood loss without drop in haemoglobin.
  - Unexplained impairment of child's daily life, including school attendance, aids, social isolation.
- In the parent/carer:
  - Insistence on continued investigations instead of focusing on symptom alleviation when reported symptoms and signs not explained by any known medical condition in the child.
  - Repeated reporting of new symptoms.
  - Repeated presentations including to Emergency Departments.
  - Inappropriately seeking multiple medical opinions.
  - Providing reports by doctors from abroad in conflict with UK medical practice.
  - Child repeatedly not brought to some appointments, often due to cancellations.
  - Not able to accept reassurance or recommended management, and insistence on more, clinically unwarranted, investigations, referrals, continuation of, or new treatments (sometimes based on internet searches).
  - Objection to communication between professionals.
  - Frequent vexatious complaints about professionals.

Source: data from Royal College of Paediatrics and Child Health. Perplexing Presentations (PP): Fabricated or Induced Illness (FII) in children. https://childprotection.rcpch.ac.uk/wp-content/uploads/sites/6/2022/06/FC59055-Perplexing-Presentations-FII-Guidance-updated.pdf. Accessed 2 June. 2023
Copyright © 2021 RCPCH.

Persisting concerns

If concerns cannot be allayed, further assessment is mandatory. Procedures will vary by jurisdiction, and local policies should be followed, but it is clear that adequate assessment must involve other agencies able to evaluate concerns in the context of familiarity with the wider family background.

Specific investigations

Suspected hypoglycaemia

- If hypoglycaemia is suspected or documented, measure true blood glucose (fluoride oxalate) and draw 2 mL of blood (in lithium heparin or serum) for C-peptide and insulin. High insulin with low C-peptide implies administration of exogenous insulin.
- Insulin/C-peptide samples have to be handled urgently: speak to on-call biochemist.
- 'Rebound' hyperglycaemia may occur after hypoglycaemia.

Suspected intoxication

- 'Blind' toxicology screens are unhelpful. The preferred sample (blood, urine) and handling requirements depend on the substance of interest. Discussion with Toxicology colleagues can greatly enhance the utility of testing.
- Collect all urine samples voided within 6 h of any collapse, and any vomitus or other samples available in plain containers. Arrange for their accurate labelling and careful freezing and storage to enable retrospective analysis if concerns regarding a particular intoxicant arise.

Seizures

- Prolactin levels typically rise after significant tonic–clonic seizures but may not, so that the value of normal levels is limited. Sample needs to be collected within 15 min (which severely limits their usefulness) and compared with a control sample taken exactly 24 h later (to allow for the normal circadian rhythm in the levels).
- Repeated prolonged/video EEGs may be required.

Functional neurological symptoms

Children presenting with symptoms or signs that are not of a conventional pathophysiological origin are well recognized in many subspecialties, and paediatric neurology is no exception. Recognition and appropriate management of functional symptoms is a frequently needed skill for the child neurologist. Keep in mind that functional symptoms often co-exist with non-functional neurological disease (e.g. non-epileptic attacks with epilepsy).

Terminology

This is a sensitive and important issue if a successful outcome is to be achieved. It is important to realize that families may be accessing professional or patient support group material on the internet, and they need to understand that although a variety of terms are in widespread use, they are referring to essentially the same phenomenon. Terms in current use include 'conversion disorder', 'psychogenic', 'dissociative', 'medically unexplained symptom'; and in specific relation to seizures, 'non-epileptic attack disorder'.

- Individual perceptions of the acceptability or offensiveness of particular terms will vary.
- In the context of seizures, the terms non-epileptic seizure and non-epileptic attack disorder are in widespread use (though again limited as the emphasis is on what the episodes 'are not' rather than what they are).
- We would argue 'medically unexplained' is unhelpful in engendering lack of confidence in the physician and therapeutic process, and suggesting (incorrectly) that we have no insight as to why these processes occur.
- At least at present Functional Neurological Disorder (FND) appears to be widely accepted by patient and families and we will use this term here.

Successful resolution of FND symptoms involves at least three steps:
- Accurate recognition and diagnosis by the medical team.
- Successful communication of the diagnosis and of the concept of functional symptoms to the family in ways they find acceptable and that keep them 'on board' so that they can access …
- … appropriate therapeutic input including but not necessarily limited to psychological support.

The middle step is often the hardest.

Presentations and diagnosis

▶ Functional symptoms frequently co-exist with non-functional brain disease (e.g. functional seizures in children with epilepsy).

▶ Onset of symptoms can often be linked to an initial non-functional event, (e.g. a severe syncope or migraine) particularly if the index event occurred in an unusual setting or manner or provoked a dramatic response from others.

▶The hallmark of functional symptoms is the *role of attention*: symptoms occur or worsen when they are attended to and ameliorate when they are not being thought about. It is this feature that gives the impression to the untutored eye that symptoms are intentionally and knowingly feigned which is very rarely the case.

Functional symptoms in neurology may include weakness or paralysis, numbness, or pain, disturbed gait or balance, and seizures. Diagnostic pointers to a functional basis include the following:

Paralysis
- Variable loss of function.
- Hoover sign. In situations of asymmetric leg weakness the examiner places his hand under the heel of the more affected foot as the child lies supine and is asked to raise the other, stronger leg off the bed against resistance. Even if the movement is not performed, there is typically an involuntary postural adjustment anticipating supporting the weight of the lifted leg, felt as ↑downward pressure of the held heel into the couch.
- Collapsing weakness, ipsilateral sternocleidomastoid weakness, lack of ipsilateral facial weakness, weakness with normal tone and reflexes.
- Drift without pronation of the weak arm.

Gait and stance
- Variability.
- Dragging an everted or inverted foot.
- Excessively slow movement.
- 'Astasia-abasia' (i.e. inability to stand steadily, violent lurchings to the side but without actual falls).
- Romberg test '+ve' with the child always falling toward examiner irrespective of position.
- Unsteadiness of stance may be no worse with eyes closed compared to eyes open (i.e. not true Romberg).
- Uneconomical gait.
- Walking 'as if on ice'.

Sensory
- 'Sleeve', 'stocking' or whole-limb patterns of sensory loss; hemisensory loss for all modalities to the midline.
- Cylindrical, rather than conical, restriction of peripheral vision (field boundary a fixed distance from, rather than a constant angle to, the visual axis).

Tremor
- *Entrainment.* In situations particularly of asymmetric involuntary movements they lessen when the examiner asks the patient to perform a repeated rhythmic movement (e.g. tapping, finger movement) with the other hand and become at least partially synchronized with the latter.

Tic-like phenomena
Repetitive outbursts of dramatic movement ± vocalizations (often expletives) may superficially resemble Tourette syndrome (see Tic disorders and

Tourette syndrome in this chapter ➲ p. 421) and differentiation may be challenging however:

- Symptom onset in Tourette is usually in pre-adolescent ♂'s whereas functional tics usually present in adolescent ♀s.
- Functional tics are more variable, elaborate, and extended movement sequences c.f. Tourette where there is typically a rather limited repertoire of stereotyped movement 'fragments'.
- Similarly phonic tics in Tourette are more commonly simple sniffs, coughs, or throat-clearing: more complex vocalizations such as swearing (coprolalia) is rare.
- A strong premonitory 'urge' to move that can however be temporarily controlled and suppressed, and comorbidities including obsessive-compulsive traits are more suggestive of Tourette.
- There is a rostrocaudal distribution to Tourette tics: involvement of eyes, face, neck, and shoulders is much commoner than arms, trunk, or legs.
- As with epilepsy and non-epileptic attacks, tics and functional tic-like movements may co-exist.

Seizures

- Contextuality (e.g. happening predominantly at school).
- Precipitated by an immediate stressor.
- Long duration (e.g. >5 min), waxing and waning activity during the event.
- Eloquent, elaborate accounts of subjective features (c.f., trying to articulate the subjective experience of epileptic seizures is typically very difficult).
- Presentation as seizure status, or prolonged limp unresponsiveness.
- Reciprocating movements (including side to side movements of the head and alternating rather than synchronous movements of the limbs).
- Pelvic thrusting.
- Ictal or post-ictal crying.
- Partial responsiveness during events.
- Closed eyes/resistance to eye opening, unexpectedly rapid recovery.

Source data from Reuber M, Mitchell AJ, Howlett SJ, Crimlisk HL, and Grünewald RA. Functional symptoms in neurology: questions and answers. *Journal of Neurology, Neurosurgery and Psychiatry*, Volume 76, p. 307, Copyright © 2005 BMJ Publishing Group Ltd.

Suggested communication approaches

- Emphasize that we see this commonly in paediatric neurology practice ('I've seen this many times') and the outcome is generally excellent.
- Diagnosis of FND is one of *positive recognition, not exclusion.*
  - It's FND *because the symptom/sign is attention-dependent*, not because scans and EEGs have been −ve. The latter rationale only begs the question of whether more tests are needed.
- *Specifically draw attention to the role of attention.* If Hoover's sign is positive for example demonstrate it: these various test manoeuvers are not 'trade secrets'.

- 'Have you noticed — can I show you— how your symptoms aren't so bad when you're not thinking about them and not paying them attention? That's how we're going to get them better'.
- *Don't* predicate the diagnosis of FND on identifying a psychological stressor.
  - Such approaches tend to elicit angry 'she's not stressed!' protests from parents.
  - Latest versions of DSM and ICD no longer require a stressor to be identified for diagnosis.
  - Notions of 'conversion' of anxiety into physical symptoms often make little sense to families.
  - If present, psychological drivers will emerge in subsequent therapeutic work: the presence of clear, accepted stressors tends if anything to be protective (faster resolution).
- 'FND is due to your brain putting an incorrect interpretation on what it's sensing'.
  - Optical illusions provide a useful metaphor of how our brains can be misled: even if we know what we're perceiving is inaccurate the illusion is compelling ('real, but wrong').

Therapeutic principles

- Establishing that symptoms or signs are functional is the beginning, not the end, of the child neurologist's role.
- With experience, recognition that symptoms are functional is often relatively straightforward and can be made with confidence. It is rare for a functional diagnosis to be subsequently revised to a somatic condition.
  - Probably the most problematic areas relate to unwitnessed seizures (video footage or direct observation are extremely helpful), and bizarre postures that may turn out to be dystonia.
  - Pursuit of 'diagnostic certainty' through exhaustive investigation may create further iatrogenic anxiety and delay or even prevent the family's engagement with psychosocial issues.
- Explicitly call out and challenge the feelings of irritation or anger that these children can evoke in all members of the healthcare team as 'time wasters'. Such feelings are rapidly sensed by families and tend to exacerbate and perpetuate symptoms.
- Look forward, not backwards: it is more constructive, and often easier to achieve consensus between child, family, and professionals, if discussion focuses on where one wants to be in x months time rather than how the present situation arose.
- Establish any specific fears the child or family may have as to what the symptoms may represent and explain how these can be discounted.
- Earn acknowledgement by the child and family that you have 'heard' and understand any psychological, emotional, or other current pressures.
- Acknowledge the strong possibility of a non-functional 'kernel' to symptoms (e.g. migraine, syncope) while stressing if appropriate that it is not responsible for the majority of symptoms. In the case of functional seizures, keep open the possibility that a (small) proportion of events may be due to epilepsy.

- Consider the appropriateness of continuing to see them in neurology outpatients.
  - Potential advantages include acknowledgement of the 'legitimacy' of the symptoms, the frequent co-occurrence of non-functional disease (requiring ongoing specific management), and reassurance that the functional diagnosis and possibility of alternatives will be regularly reviewed.
  - In some situations, however, it may be more appropriate to hand over ongoing management to other services.
- Acute presentations promptly and appropriately managed may not require child psychiatry involvement; however, skilled psychology input is invaluable in severe or prolonged cases.
- f possible copy all correspondence to the family to avoid perception (and reality) of agencies 'talking behind the family's back'.
- Be particularly careful to respect confidentiality in discussions with school.
  - Prolonged school absence creates specific considerations. There is a statutory legal requirement in UK for children under 16 yrs to receive schooling and educational agencies may be seeking to apply legal sanctions for truancy.
  - Establish if absence from school is being instituted by family or school.
  - Identify perceived reasons for absence/exclusion from school.
- Perceptions of the illness by other professionals involved with the child need to be addressed e.g. legal, health, and safety concerns of school staff to allow school re-integration; local therapy teams; local child and family mental health team; social services.
- A multidisciplinary physical-psychosocial-schooling rehabilitation approach may be useful for complex situations.
- Provide appropriate information about FND symptoms: pamphlets or websites (e.g. ℘ https://neurosymptoms.org/).

Headache disorders

The International Headache Society (IHS) distinguishes primary from secondary headaches due to a defined disease process. The IHS primary headaches include migraine, tension-type headache (TTH), cluster headache with other trigeminal autonomic cephalalgias, and others. Figures in brackets in this section refer to the International Classification of Headache Disorders (ICHD, currently in its 3rd Edition) .

Mechanisms of pain perception

Although the brain itself is not sensitive to pain, large cerebral vessels, pial vessels, venous sinuses, and the dura mater are all innervated by small diameter myelinated and unmyelinated neurons serving nociception. Nociception is modulated by arousal state, anxiety levels, memory, cognition, local pathology, and genes. This complexity is presumed to underlie the misperception as pain of normal sensory input such as light or sound (allodynia).

Primary headaches

Pathophysiology

- The pathophysiology of primary headache remains poorly understood. Previous vasomotor hypotheses of migraine have been discredited.
  - TTH is characterized by reduced inhibitory activity of brainstem interneurons, presumably reflecting abnormal endogenous pain control mechanisms.
  - The mechanism of cortical spreading depression appears additionally important in migraine resulting in activation of trigeminal neurons leading to sterile neurogenic inflammation and plasma extravasation with mast cell degranulation and platelet aggregation.
  - Despite its name, there is no evidence of a primary role for anxiety or scalp muscle contraction in TTH.
- The headache of migraine depends on activation and sensitization of trigeminal nociceptors innervating large meningeal blood vessels. Sequential activation of second and third order trigeminovascular neurons may then activate different brain stem and forebrain areas producing attendant discomfort or other symptoms. Whether brainstem grey matter structures are generators, sustainers, or merely transmitting disordered neural signal traffic is unclear. Calcitonin Gene Related Peptide (CGRP) has emerged as a key component of this process, with benefit demonstrated in adults of anti-CGRP monoclonal antibodies.
- 50–80% of children with primary headache have an affected parent suggesting important, as yet unidentified, genetic factors (the parent's headache disorder may have remitted so absence of a current headache history may be misleading).
- Single-gene aetiologies have been identified in some rarer migraine subtypes: 50% cases of familial hemiplegic migraine are associated with mutations of *CACNA1A* and 20% with *ATP1A2*. These and other findings suggest channelopathies may compromise neurotransmitter homeostasis causing aura and other neurological manifestations.

- There is evidence for considerable overlap in the pathophysiology of migraine and TTH, concurring with clinical observations that all primary headache types show very similar premonitory symptoms, and that a child's headache can move between migraine and TTH phenotypes (in either direction).
- Although many clinical presentations do not fit tidily into the IHS classification, it remains essential for research into causation and treatment. A pragmatic approach is often required in clinical practice.

Prevalence (% experiencing a 'current headache disorder')
- Any headache 51%.
- Migraine 3% prepubertally (♂ = ♀); post-pubertally 3% ♂, 7% ♀.
- TTH 31%.
- Chronic daily headache 1.2%.

Clinical approach
Screen for 'red-flag' features that require urgent imaging to rule out structural causes of ↑ICP.
- Headache worsened by lying down, bending over, coughing, or straining.
- Visual symptoms on bending over, coughing, straining, etc.
- Persistent, or morning, nausea, or vomiting.
- Symptoms that are progressively worsening over days to weeks with increasingly rare symptom-free intervals.
- Being woken at night by headache (note the difference between this and headache present on or soon after normal waking which is not uncommon in migraine).
- Any change in personality, behaviour, or educational performance.
- Any abnormality on physical examination, to include visual field defect, short stature, cranial bruit, cerebellar signs, or fundoscopic signs of ↑ICP: see Optic nerve (II) fundoscopy in Chapter 1 ⟴ p. 17.

Occipital headache is more commonly secondary in nature, although it can occur in primary headache due to the involvement of the trigeminal nucleus with the dorsal horns of C1 and C2 (remember how long the nucleus is!).

Usually there are no red-flag features, and no physical signs. The episodes have a distinct start and finish and the child is well in between. At this point consider a primary headache syndrome.

Primary headache types
The IHS Classification identifies hundreds of headache types! In practice the common primary headache types are:

Tension-type headache (ICHD 2.1–2.4)
- Episodes lasting minutes to days; the pain typically bilateral and mild/moderate pain without nausea (although photo-/phonophobia may be present).

Migraine without aura (ICHD 1.1)
- Previously known as common migraine.
- Responsible for 80% of migraine.

- Uni- or bilateral, throbbing headache with nausea and/or autonomic features (e.g. pallor). Differentiating between migraine without aura and infrequent episodic TTH may be difficult.

Migraine with aura (ICHD 1.2)
- Previously known as classical migraine.
- Complete absence of signs and symptoms between episodes, and the frequent presence of a prodrome with tiredness, difficulty concentrating, and autonomic features are emphasized.
- The aura lasts 5–20 min before headache onset and can be the sole manifestation of the episode. Aura is usually visual: flashing, sparkling, or shimmering lights; fortification spectra (zigzags); black dots, and/or scotomata (field defects). Rarely there is distortion of size (micropsia/ macropsia).
- Some specific forms of aura are recognized as subtypes.
  - Migraine with brainstem aura (ICHD 1.2.2) (previously known as 'Basilar type' migraine) is characterized by symptoms referable to the posterior circulation: vertigo, ataxia, tinnitus, hyperacusis, and visual disturbance. More common in adolescent or young adult ♀s.
  - Hemiplegic migraines (ICHD 1.2.3) (familial and sporadic) presenting with aura including motor weakness, which generally last <72 hours, often with sensory loss which can be difficult to distinguish from weakness.
  - Retinal migraine (ICHD 1.2.4) presenting with repeated attacks of monocular visual disturbance including scintillations, scotomata or blindness (though monocular visual loss is rare, and other causes should be considered).
- Clinically these episodes resemble transient ischaemic attacks (reversible focal neurological deficits lasting tens of minutes to a few hours). As such, migraine enters into the differential diagnosis of a wide range of episodic neurological symptoms and signs.
  - At first presentation the differential often includes more serious pathologies including stroke (see Stroke in this chapter ➔ p. 500) and causes of confusional states (see Acute behavioural distrubance in Chapter 6 ➔ p. 610).
  - MRI is typically entirely normal although scattered punctate T2 hyperintensities in white matter are described particularly in adults. Prominent *autonomic* signs (nausea, vomiting, sweating, vasomotor changes in skin) are also suggestive.
  - With subsequent presentations it is easier to be confident of the diagnosis. Individuals may establish a particular pattern of complicated migraine with a characteristic neurological deficit that may also be familial, in which case no further investigation of an otherwise typical episode will be required.

Triggers
Migraine episodes may be triggered by a variety of factors including stress, relaxing after stress (e.g. exams), lack of sleep, excitement, and menstruation. Food triggers (chocolate, hot dogs, smoked and spiced meats, Chinese food containing monosodium glutamate, cheese, cola drinks, bananas, yeast and beef extract, wine) are much less common in children than

adults. Remember triggers may not consistently trigger; the child's threshold for attacks will itself show periodicity.

Chronic daily headache

Reported in 0.9% of UK children and up to 4% in some US studies with ♀:♂ ratio of 3:1. Almost 75% had chronic TTH (ICHD 2.3) and nearly 7% had chronic migraine (ICHD 1.3). These families present a diagnostic and management challenge.

- Consider and exclude space-occupying lesions and idiopathic intracranial hypertension:
  - Demonstration of venous pulsation (see Venous pulsation in Chapter 1 ➔ p. 18) is extremely useful in this context.
  - If normal ICP cannot be verified clinically further investigation may be required (imaging ± ICP measurement).
- Refractive errors are an uncommon cause of headaches but visual acuity should be checked. Refraction should be performed if there is a clear history of reading-related headache, relieved by rest.
- More commonly psychological factors (particulary unacknowledged educational support or other mental health needs) are important drivers.
- Migraine prophylaxis (see below) and/or amitriptyline may be a useful adjunct alongside psychological approaches.

Chronic analgesia overuse headache (ICHD 8.2)

Paradoxical aggravation and perpetuation of headache through analgesia overuse *commonly* contributes to chronic daily headache pictures.

- Under-recognized in children.
- Occurs with NSAIDs and paracetamol (i.e. not just opiates).
- Compound analgesics (especially codeine-containing) are particular culprits.
- Suspect in any situation where the family are watching the clock to see 'when he can have another dose'.
- Explain the problem and the need to change the pattern of analgesia —use for severe incapacitating episodes only. Migraine prophylaxis (e.g. topiramate, amitriptyline) and/or clinical psychology may be helpful.

Episodic Disorders that may be associated with migraine (ICHD 1.6)

Recurrent disorders regarded as migrainous in that they commonly precede the establishment of a more conventional migraine picture. Symptom complexes may overlap. The child is well in between episodes.

- *Cyclical vomiting (ICHD 1.6.1.1)*: recurrent stereotyped episodes of vomiting and intense nausea associated with pallor and lethargy.
- *Abdominal migraine (ICHD 1.6.1.2)*: episodic midline abdominal pain of moderate to severe intensity lasting 1–72 h, associated with vaso-motor symptoms, nausea, and vomiting.
- *Benign paroxysmal vertigo of childhood (ICHD 1.6.2)*: brief and sudden episodes of vertigo, difficult for the child to explain, often associated with nystagmus, ataxic gait, and a fearful expression in infants. See Benign paroxysmal vertigo in this chapter ➔ p. 326.
- *Benign paroxysmal torticollis (ICHD 1.6.3)*: see Benign paroxysmal torticollis in this chapter ➔ p. 325.

Cluster headache and other trigeminal autonomic cephalalgias (ICHD 3.1–5)
Uncommon in adolescence and very rare under 10 yrs. Described symptom complexes include cluster headache, chronic paroxysmal hemicranias (CPH) and short-lasting unilateral neuralgiform headache attacks with conjunctival injection and tearing (SUNCT).
  Key features:
- Distressing episodes of severe unilateral pain in orbital, supra-orbital, or temporal location (or any combination of these):
  - SUNCT characterized by stabbing or burning eye pain.
- Different characteristic timings:
  - SUNCT episodes very short and frequent;
  - cluster headache typically lasting up to 3 h or so;
  - paroxysmal hemicrania bouts may occur at the same time daily.
- Associated with ipsilateral autonomic disturbance such as conjunctival injection, lacrimation, nasal congestion, rhinorrhoea, forehead and facial sweating, myosis, ptosis, or eyelid oedema.
- 90% are ♂.
- Verapamil has replaced more traditional approaches to prophylaxis with methysergide or lithium. Short course (1–2 week) corticosteroids may be useful 'bridging' therapy while verapamil is titrated up.
- Acute episodes can be treated with sumatriptan, indomethacin, or by inhalation of high-flow 100% oxygen. Indomethacin is first choice for CPH and regarded by some as a diagnostic test.

Painful cranial neuropathies and other facial pains (ICHD 13)
Recurrent painful ophthalmoplegic neuropathy (IHS 13.9)
- This term preferred to *ophthalmoplegic migraine* although the latter still widely used.
- Repeated episodes of paresis of (in this case) the oculomotor (III) nerve with ipsilateral headache. Headache can precede the ophthalmoplegia by up to 2 weeks.
- Episodes last several days: treatment with oral steroids shortens episode duration and reduces the risk of residual paresis (i.e. incomplete recovery).
- MRI with gadolinium during an attack shows oculomotor nerve oedema and enhancement confirming an inflammatory basis.

Tolosa-Hunt syndrome (IHS 13.7)
- A similar condition of unilateral orbital pain associated with paresis of one or more of cranial nerves III, IV, V (usually Va), VI, VII, or VIII.
- Caused by granulomatous inflammation in the cavernous sinus, superior orbital fissure, or orbit demonstrated by MRI or biopsy.
- Requires exclusion of other causes of painful ophthalmoplegia including tumours, vasculitis, basal meningitis, sarcoid, or diabetes mellitus.
- Pain and paresis resolve with corticosteroids.

Management of primary headaches
Intervention should include:
- A simple explanation of the nature of the primary headache disorders, and reassurance they are not 'damaging' the brain. The more the child and family understand, the less they worry.

- Explanation of the periodicity (good and bad spells).
- Help to identify precipitating and exacerbating factors.
- Ample opportunity for the asking of questions (particularly to elicit anxieties about tumours or other sinister causes). The family's consultation agenda may not match your own.
- Unnecessary investigation may undermine reassurance although occasionally a family may need to see a normal scan result before being able to proceed.
- Discussion of how young people with head pain might behave once fear of underlying disease or illness is abated:
  - encouragement of behaving well rather than behaving ill;
  - help for children to feel in control of their headaches rather *vice versa*.
- Pharmacological intervention.
  - Rescue treatment to lessen the frequency, duration, and intensity of acute symptoms.
  - Consideration of prophylactic treatment (only required in very few).
  - When the subject is raised, discussion of the place of complementary alternative interventions.

General lifestyle advice
- The importance of dietary triggers is generally over-estimated and probably only ever relevant during a bad spell (do not condemn children to lives without chocolate and cheese!)
- Excessive consumption of caffeine (in many colas and tea as well as coffee) can be an issue.
- Good sleep hygiene is helpful. Avoiding long periods of fasting may also help.
- Understand the different roles of prophylactic and acute medication (cf. preventative and rescue inhalers in asthma).
- Sleep (if feasible in the context) will often cure a migraine episode.

▶▶Combined hormonal contraceptives should not be prescribed for ♀s with migraine with aura because of the ↑risk of cerebrovascular events.

Rescue treatment
Limited evidence base: most studies have been under-powered and none address a paediatric population.
- Paracetamol and the NSAIDs are similar in their efficacy (personal choice often reflects personal efficacy). Advise families to take analgesia early in a bout to promote absorption before the onset of significant nausea and gut dysmotility.
- There is no role for codeine, codeine-containing compound analgesics, or opiates.
- Aspirin should not be given to children under 10 yrs of age to avoid the risk of triggering Reye syndrome and hepatic failure.
- Prochlorperazine in combination with caffeine and indomethacin are as efficacious as a triptan.

- For children with a lot of nausea, prochlorperazine is available in tablets absorbed through the buccal mucosa.
- Zolmitriptan is available as a well-tolerated oral preparation.

Prophylactic treatment

Only consider when headaches are becoming intrusive and affecting daily life, e.g. missing significant time from school, sports activities, etc. As a rule of thumb, only consider in situations where children are experiencing headache fortnightly or more frequently.

Again, limited evidence base: some evidence for propranolol, even less for pizotifen and others. Options include propranolol, pizotifen, topiramate, amitriptyline, and flunarizine.

- Propranolol probably first choice so long as no history of bronchospasm or asthma.
- Start with a low dose and build to a target dose over at least 2 or 3 weeks. Maintain until in remission for at least 6 weeks; withdraw over a further 6 weeks.
- Though widely used the overall evidence base for complementary and alternative medicine is poor.
- For ♀s with menstruation-related migraine, frovatriptan or zolmitriptan can be taken on the days migraine is anticipated.
  - Use of an oral contraceptive pill may be warranted.
- Antibodies directed to Calcitonin Gene Related Peptide (anti-CGRP monoclonal antibodies) are of proven efficacy in adults and under investigation in children.

Behavioural and cognitive approaches

Once a more chronic pattern has established, non-pharmacological approaches are more likely to be effective.

- Assessment should be directed towards identifying the predisposing, precipitating, and perpetuating factors operating in the child's home and school environment.
- Unrecognized academic difficulties, difficulties with peers, and home-related stress are the most common causes.
- 'Perfectionist' traits in high-achievers may respond well to cognitive-behavioural approaches.
- Depression may also be a contributing factor to daily headaches in some children and may require appropriate treatment.
- Chronic analgesic overuse may be complicating the picture.

Prognosis

Migraine/tension-type headache may be periodic with bad spells lasting weeks to months separated by good spells lasting months or years. In long-term follow-up of 9000 Swedish school children with migraine:

- One-third had been migraine-free for >1 yr at 6-yr follow-up.
- Two-thirds had been migraine-free for >2 yrs at 16-yr follow-up.
- At 40-yr follow-up, 30% were experiencing at least one migraine a year; half were migraine-free.

Idiopathic intracranial hypertension

Also known as pseudotumour cerebri.

▶ The label 'benign' is misleading and should be outlawed! Idiopathic intracranial hypertension (IIH) is an important, preventable cause of visual loss.

A clinical syndrome of symptoms and signs of ↑ICP in the absence of any space-occupying pathology on imaging. The clinical picture is indistinguishable from ↑ICP due to tumour or hydrocephalus.
- Persisting, worsening headaches worsened by straining, coughing, sleep.
- Persistent vomiting.
- Papilloedema.
- Sixth cranial nerve palsy as a 'false localizing' sign. See Figure 1.6 in Chapter 1 ➋ p. 22.

Diagnosis
- Normal CT sufficient to proceed with LP.
- Subtle MRI findings include prominent sleeves on optic nerve sheaths and 'reverse cupping' of optic nerve heads indenting backs of globes, downward displacement of the pituitary and floor of the third ventricle, and slim lateral ventricles.
- Documented elevation of ICP at lumbar puncture (>30 cm H_2O).
  - Beware of making the diagnosis on ambiguous history and borderline ICP elevation. (Upper limit of normal ICP in children under general anaesthesia probably ~28 cm H_2O; Avery et al. N Engl J Med (2010) 363 (9) p. 891).
- Beware false-+ve elevation of ICP:
  - Struggling/distress during lumbar puncture.
  - Use of inappropriate anaesthetic agents if LP is done under GA: **ensure end-tidal CO_2 is normal** (hypercarbia will elevate ICP).
- Exclusion of venous sinus thrombosis (if history suggestive) may require MRI/MRV (very similar clinical picture but by convention would not be regarded as IIH).

▶ In a largely asymptomatic child referred with isolated 'papilloedema' consider the possibility of pseudo-papilloedema due to optic nerve Drusen (can be distinguished by careful ophthalmological evaluation, OCT, or ultrasound of the optic nerve head).

Associations
Cause uncertain (impaired CSF resorption?). Association with:
- Adolescent and older ♀s.
- Obesity.
- Tetracycline use.
- Steroid use.
- Oral contraception.
- Excessive vitamin A consumption (can be seen after correction of fat malabsorption by supply of pancreatic enzymes in newly diagnosed cystic fibrosis due to sudden reversal of vitamin A malabsorption).

Management

> ❗ The risk of inadequately managed IIH is permanent visual loss due to chronic optic nerve ischaemia. Unfortunately lack of headache or other symptoms cannot be taken as reassurance. Long-term, regular (at least annual) ophthalmological review (particularly of visual fields) is required to detect early signs.

Normal CSF production rates are ~30 mL/h: the volume of CSF removed at a single LP (irrespective of 'closing pressures') will be replaced within a few hours. The symptomatic benefit gained results from the *CSF leak* left after the LP. Beware *low pressure* headache after LP and don't confuse it with persisting symptoms! In contrast to high-pressure headache symptoms are relieved by lying down and worsened by sitting up.

- Short-term symptomatic treatment with acetazolamide. Monitor electrolytes.
- In chronic symptomatic cases consider lumbo- or ventriculoperitoneal shunting. (VP shunting technically harder than in hydrocephalus as ventricles not enlarged; however, LP shunts have a high failure rate over time).
- Surgical optic nerve fenestration to protect optic nerves against ischaemia.
- Unambiguous counselling regarding need for long-term monitoring of visual fields.

Hydrocephalus

Physiology

- Cerebrospinal fluid (CSF) is produced by modified ependymal cells in the choroid plexus within the lateral ventricles.
- Having exited the ventricular system via the foramina of Luschka and the midline foramen of Magendie, bulk flow continues through the cerebromedullary cistern down the spinal cord and over the cerebral hemispheres.
- CSF returns to the vascular system passing through arachnoid granulations into dural venous sinuses; there is probably extracranial spinal venous reabsorption as well.
- Total CSF volume above 2 yrs approximately 150 mL, of which the ventricular system comprises ~35 mL.
- CSF production ~30 mL/hour.
  - i.e. complete CSF turnover occurs every few hours at most.

Blood–brain barrier

- Cerebral blood capillaries unique in having endothelial cells joined by tight junctions which are the physical basis of the blood–brain barrier (BBB).
- BBB excludes all water-soluble molecules with molecular weight >500 Daltons. Lipid soluble molecules (oxygen, carbon dioxide, ethanol, steroid hormones) penetrate BBB readily.
- Specific transporters exist to allow and regulate entry of important hydrophilic molecules including glucose and amino acids.
- At certain sites e.g. circumventricular organs, capillaries are fenestrated normally and neurons can 'sample' circulating blood.
- Inflammation of meninges disrupts the BBB and may enhance antibiotic penetration into the brain.
- Blood-CSF barrier anatomically distinct and composed of choroid plexus and arachnoid membrane.
- No major barrier between CSF and brain extracellular space so drugs introduced intrathecally bypass the BBB.

Definitions and variants

- *Hydrocephalus*: increase in volume of CSF spaces in the brain particularly the ventricles (ventriculomegaly) associated with ↑ICP and associated signs and symptoms.
- *Ventriculomegaly*: radiological appearance of ↑ventricular volume not necessarily implying ↑pressure (e.g. could be due to parenchymal atrophy).
- *Obstructive (non-communicating) hydrocephalus*: obstruction to CSF flow in the ventricular system before reaching the subarachnoid space.
- *Communicating hydrocephalus*: ↓absorption of CSF from arachnoid villi and subarachnoid spaces; or ↑CSF production (choroid plexus papillomas).
- *External hydrocephalus*: enlarged subarachnoid spaces, e.g. around the frontal lobes, without ventricular dilation. May be a normal variant in infancy: see Figure 3.3 in Chapter 3 p. 163.

- *Normal pressure hydrocephalus:* ventricular dilatation, no parenchymal atrophy and normal CSF pressure with chronic symptoms (classically gait disturbance, cognitive deterioration, and incontinence in the elderly). Not known to occur in children.

Aetiology and associated conditions

Congenital causes of obstructive hydrocephalus
- *Aqueduct stenosis:* (level of obstruction confirmed by enlarged lateral and third ventricles in presence small fourth ventricle ± MRI CSF flow studies). X-linked aqueduct stenosis due to mutations in *L1CAM* accounts for 5% hydrocephalus in ♂'s (also have adducted thumbs).
- *4th ventricle foraminal stenosis:* genetically determined stenosis at the foramina of Luschka and Magendie.
- *Dandy–Walker syndrome:* developmental cystic dilatation of the 4th ventricle with vermis hypoplasia.
- Combined incidence of congenital variants: 5–8 per 10 000 births.
- Congenital aetiologies may still cause adult presentations when the hydrocephalus decompensates.

Developmental disorders featuring ventriculomegaly/hydrocephalus
- Neural tube defects: particularly myelomeningocoele and encephalocoele.
- Achondroplasia.
- Syndromic craniosynostosis: 40% of Crouzon, Pfeiffer, Apert syndromes.
- Myotonic dystrophy.
- Neurofibromatosis type 1, Hurler, Down syndromes.
- Hemimegalencephaly (ventriculomegaly may mimic obstructive hydrocephalus).
- Macrocephaly and ventriculomegaly sometimes seen in idiopathic autism.
- There may be associated brain (agenesis of corpus callosum, septo-optic dysplasia) or non-neurological lesions (cardiac lesions in Down syndrome).

Acquired causes of obstructive hydrocephalus
- Intraventricular haemorrhage: 80% of premature babies with grade 3 and grade 4 haemorrhage develop progressive ventricular dilatation. Can also cause communicating hydrocephalus.
- Tumours and cysts: e.g. subependymal giant cell astrocytomas in tuberous sclerosis, colloid cyst of the 3rd ventricle; arachnoid cysts; ependymomas (including spinal ependymomas).
- Vascular malformations, e.g. AVM, vein of Galen aneurysm.
- Other: parenchymal oedema, ventricular scarring after toxoplasmosis, tuberculoma, trauma.

Communicating hydrocephalus
- Post-meningitis: e.g. pneumococcus, tuberculosis, fungi.
- Intracranial haemorrhage: subarachnoid, subdural, neonatal intraventricular haemorrhage, trauma.

- Foramen magnum and skull base lesions: Chiari malformations (type II more than type I), myelomeningocoele, craniosynostosis.
- Cerebral venous sinus thrombosis.
- Leptomeningeal tumour.

Antenatally detected hydrocephalus

There has been a reduction in the incidence of congenital hydrocephalus due to termination after foetal detection of gross ventriculomegaly and/or myelomeningocoele at routine antenatal screening.

Actions
- Detailed scan to identify further anomalies (spine, heart, urological).
- Foetal MRI to assess cerebral architecture is increasingly available.
- Amniocentesis offered for foetal karyotype (e.g. trisomy 21) or aCGH.
- TORCH screen (e.g. toxoplasmosis).
- Parental counselling by specialist foetal management group including a neurosurgeon (see Ventriculomegaly in Chapter 5 ➋ p. 539).
- Neonatal team notified if pregnancy continues.
- Monitoring for progression or resolution of ventriculomegaly *in utero*.
- After birth: neonatal examination, neurosurgical follow-up as required.

Outcome
See Ventriculomegaly in Chapter 5 ➋ p. 539.

Symptoms and signs of hydrocephalus

Hydrocephalus may present with acute or chronic symptoms of ↑ICP if it 'decompensates'; or asymptomatically, e.g. as macrocephaly picked up on routine surveillance (arrested hydrocephalus).

Early infancy
- Accelerated head growth; OFC crossing the centiles (may also be seen with benign external hydrocephalus); >1 cm per week in neonates.
- Bulging fontanelle (even when upright and settled).
- Cranial sutures widened.
- Prominent scalp veins.
- Sun-setting eyes.
- Parinaud syndrome (limited upgaze, ± convergence nystagmus).
- Irritability, poor feeding.
- Impaired development including abnormal visual behaviour.

Later childhood
- Macrocephaly, may be an isolated finding in arrested hydrocephalus.
- Headache.
- Vomiting.
- Lethargy and somnolence.
- Visual disturbance (check visual acuity and fields).
- Papilloedema is not reliable: often absent in acute decompensation.

> ❶ Check for bradycardia and elevated blood pressure: if present, urgent management of ↑ICP required. The absence of this combination does not preclude ↑pressure.

Investigations

- *Cranial ultrasound*: in neonates and infants with open fontanelle, for monitoring progressive ventricular dilatation after IVH and response to treatment.
- *CT scan*: useful for emergency evaluation of possible ↑pressure (e.g. need for immediate neurosurgical intervention). Outside emergency contexts MRI is preferred. CT findings may include hypodensity of periventricular brain tissue (trans-ependymal CSF flow); enlargement of temporal horns of lateral ventricles; barrel-shaped third ventricle; obliteration of basal cisterns and cortical sulci effaced.
- *MRI*: ↑periventricular T2 signal suggests ↑pressure (trans-ependymal CSF flow). Information contributed in addition to CT includes identifying aqueduct stenosis (CSF flow studies) and parenchymal lesions.
- *Genetic investigation*.

Treatments

Progressive ventricular dilatation in neonates

See Management of established ventricular dilation in Chapter 5
p. 568
- Diuretics (furosemide, acetazolamide).
- Repeated ventricular taps and lumbar puncture.
- Other methods: intraventricular fibrinolysis.
- 20–30% of those with grade 3 or 4 IVH needing repeated CSF removal eventually require a shunt.

Shunts

- Ventriculoperitoneal shunts: a proximal catheter in the lateral or 4th ventricle, a distal catheter in the peritoneal cavity. A long length of tube can be placed in the hope of avoiding re-operation between infancy and adulthood, although shunts placed in the neonatal period often fail (typically at about 5–6 yrs age) due to displacement of either the proximal or more commonly the distal catheter tip with growth.
- A selection of valve types is available with either fixed or externally adjustable ('programmable') valve opening pressures. The reservoir may be separate from the shunt-valve system.
- Ventriculo-atrial shunts are now out of favour due to need for re-operation with child's growth, and higher morbidity and mortality (renal failure, infection).

Endoscopic 3rd ventriculostomy

- For obstructive hydrocephalus particularly due to aqueduct stenosis.
- Typically not possible in the presence of Chiari malformation due to distortion of the third ventricle, and not effective in post-haemorrhagic hydrocephalus.
- Main advantage is avoidance of over-drainage symptoms and reduced risk of infection.
- A hole in the base of the 3rd ventricle creates a connection to the subarachnoid space of the basal cisterns.
- 70% success rate: any failures usually occur in the first 2–3 months. Less successful in youngest infants. Infective complications occur in 2%.

- Ventricular size reduces less after ventriculostomy than after shunt placement: imaging less useful in evaluating possible failure.
- Very rarely, there is late (fatal) rupture of the basilar artery traumatized at ventriculostomy.

Monitoring for sequelae

Shunt complications

See Shunt complications in Chapter 5 p. 570.

Epilepsy

- Incidence 1 in 3 by 10 yrs post-shunt.
- Underlying aetiology is a significant predictor: TORCH, post-meningitis, parenchymal injury in neonates all cause epilepsy independent of ventriculomegaly.
- Subacute/chronic shunt dysfunction can occasionally present with worsening seizures: urgent neurosurgical referral is required if there is status epilepticus.

Headaches

Under-drainage (ICP high)

- Typical high-pressure symptoms.
- Inadequate pressure relief from shunt.
- Decompensating hydrocephalus in non-shunted child.
- Chiari malformation (consider if occipital headache; CT may miss the lesion).

Over-drainage (ICP low)

- Typically, over-drainage produces a picture the reverse of a high-pressure headache: the headache is worse standing up and relieved by lying down (although this is not an entirely sensitive or specific finding).
- MRI may show tonsillar descent.

Slit-ventricle syndrome

- Post-shunt episodic headaches, vomiting.
- Investigation confirms collapsed ventricles in the presence of raised, or fluctuating high and low ICP.
- Diagnosis: ambulatory ICP monitoring. Baseline ICP in the upright position is usually –ve.

'Shunt migraine'

- May be very resistant to pharmacological therapy: consider referral to the pain management team and psychological interventions.

Other chronic problems

- General cognition and specific deficits (see below).
- Fine motor and coordination: tremor, clumsiness.
- Gross motor: cerebral palsy, spasticity (evolving upper motor neuron signs may suggest decompensating hydrocephalus).
- Endocrine disorders: precocious puberty.
- Vision: colour vision deficits, visual scotoma, and field defects, strabismus.

Cognitive disability

The typical cognitive profile seen in children with hydrocephalus (also very characteristic of children with spina bifida) includes good expressive language but weaker comprehension and impaired frontal lobe skills. The former leads to overestimation of cognitive abilities and under-recognition of the latter resulting in 'cocktail party syndrome': ability in overlearned 'small-talk' but with limited intuitive and empathetic understanding of what is being said. Specific deficits: attention, short-term memory, reasoning, sequencing actions, mathematics (subcortical information processing deficits). Personal insight into difficulties often limited: some parallels with the cognitive issues after ABI (see Prognosis [in ABI section] in this chapter ➲ p. 222).

Prognosis

5% mortality overall: shunt blockage remains a significant cause.

Spina bifida and related disorders

Developmental spinal disorders in which contents of the vertebral canal protrude through defects in the vertebrae. The spinal level of the lesion is a major determinant of morbidity.

The classic variants are:

- *Meningocoele*: meninges and CSF in the lesion.
- *Myelomeningocoele*: cord elements within lesion.
- *Lipomyelomeningocoele*: myelomeningocoele with intra/extra-dural lipoma in continuity with subcutaneous fat.

The lesion may be covered with skin or open to the environment. The opening may be subtle (dermal sinus tract) or large (rachischisis), the latter associated with significant morbidity and mortality.

- *Spina bifida occulta*: implies a developmental vertebral anomaly without overt spinal cord lesion. Generally not included in epidemiological studies of spina bifida, but may share latter's aetiology.

Associated conditions

Abnormal development of the spinal cord and ectopic elements

- *Lipoma*: dorsal spinal cord only, or a more extensive *transitional* lesion as in lipomyelomeningocoele.
- *Fatty filum terminale*: lipoma restricted to filum.
  - Common: may be thickened and associated with other dysraphism.
- *Dermoid cysts*: may grow in size, or rupture. Often associated with sinus tract.
- *Neurenteric cysts*: may emerge ventrally into the abdominal or thoracic cavities.
  - Often associated with vertebral abnormalities.
- *Diastematomyelia*: 'splitting' of the cord within the canal usually by a bony or fibrocartilaginous spur.
- *Diplomyelia*: duplicated spinal cord, each with its own dural sheath.
- *Syringomyelia*: often associated with Chiari II malformations: see Chiari malformations in this chapter ➔ p. 359.
- Low spinal cord termination: the cord may terminate at L4/5.

Other malformations outside the spinal cord

- 80% of children with myelomeningocoele have hydrocephalus.
- Chiari malformation (mainly type II).
- Vertebral anomalies (e.g. Klippel-Feil syndrome, sacral dysgenesis).
- Anorectal anomalies.
- Urogenital and renal anomalies.
- Cardiac anomalies.
- Associated malformations may form a recognized syndrome, e.g. VATER, Currarino triad (sacral, anal, and urological anomalies).

Aetiology and risk factors

CNS development from the embryonic neural tube involves coordinated activation of gene networks in nascent CNS cells and neighbouring tissue. Environmental insults interact with maternal and embryonic gene mutations and polymorphisms to cause neural tube defects (NTD).

Environmental factors
- Folic acid deficiency in diet.
- ASMs (sodium valproate, phenytoin, carbamazepine, polytherapy).
- Retinoins.
- Maternal diabetes.

Genetic factors
- Folate-dependent metabolic pathway gene polymorphisms (e.g. *PCMT1*, *MTI IFR*, methionine synthase, and methionine synthase reductase).
- Folate-independent pathways (lipomyelomeningocoeles are folate resistant).
- Syndromes (e.g. 22q11 microdeletion), X-linked and autosomal dominant Mendelian disorders (e.g. Currarino triad due to *MNX1*). May show intrafamilial variation in severity. Sporadic cases described.
- Recurrence risk in non-syndromic NTD: 5% risk for sibling of proband, 0.7% with pre-conceptional folate supplementation.

Incidence
- Marked geographical variation in incidence. The dramatic reduction in incidence over recent decades has now stabilized.
- Foetal incidence of NTD 17 per 10,000 pregnancies; live birth incidence 5–7 per 10 000 live births. The disparity is due to termination of pregnancy and *in utero* deaths, particularly of severe lesions.

Antenatal detection
- ↑maternal serum AFP and acetylcholinesterase.
- Anomaly scan at 20 weeks may show ventriculomegaly, posterior vertebral arch defects or talipes.
- ~15% of spina bifida not detected antenatally (poor visualization due to foetal position).

Assessment of the child with spina bifida
As with other complex neurodisability, a multidisciplinary approach to assessment and management is essential with early involvement of neurosurgeon, renal or urological specialist and spinal orthopaedic surgeons.

Neonatal period and early infancy
The child may present antenatally or with an unexpected lesion after birth:
- Open lesion.
- Large midline lipoma, preventing supine positioning, and cares.
- Asymmetrical natal cleft.
- Dermal sinus above the natal cleft.
  - Distinguish from benign sacral dimple in coccygeal region: latter typically in the midline, just above natal cleft, without associated hair or haemangioma.
  - If in doubt ultrasound valuable to 6 months of age; MRI thereafter.
- Midline nevus e.g. hair patch (a subtle dermal sinus may also be present).
- Kyphosis or scoliosis.
- Talipes (may be asymmetrical).

Identify the following on examination:
- Anatomical level of the lesion (MRI spine).
- Neurological level is often higher than the anatomical level and is a significant predictor of future disability. Assess muscle bulk, spontaneous anti-gravity movements, spinal reflexes, abnormal spread of reflexes, and sacral sensation.
- Associated CNS malformations.
- Bone or joint deformities, e.g. congenital hip dislocation (20%). kyphosis, and talipes. Refer to specialist orthopaedic teams.
- Dermal sinus tract. Leads to risk of CNS infection. Often associated with underlying spinal malformation. Referral to neurosurgeon.
- Non-neurological anomalies (e.g. check anus, heart).
- Bowel dysfunction. Assess anal tone. Neurogenic constipation often present (also effects of concurrent anorectal anomalies).
- Bladder dysfunction: often-incomplete bladder emptying against outflow resistance, leading to secondary reflux nephropathy. Check for a good urinary stream—urgent urological referral if not seen.

❶ Refer all children for urodynamic studies

Monitoring for later sequelae

Periodically reassess the child for sequelae that may evolve over time:
- Hydrocephalus requiring VP shunt:
  - Required in 80% of myelomeningocoele. Uncommon in other variants.
- Chiari malformation and syringomyelia:
  - Progressive occipital headaches, squint, bulbar signs, upper limb dysaesthesia. Neurosurgical referral for posterior fossa decompression if present.
- Cord tethering syndrome:
  - Back pain, mixed upper motor neuron (spasticity) and lower motor neuron signs (clawing of feet, going 'off feet'), enlarging area of sensory disturbance, incontinence.
  - May occur many years after apparently successful primary surgical repair due to rapid linear growth.
  - Urgent MRI spine if suspected and referral to neurosurgeon, though intervention may not be necessary.
- Urinary dysfunction:
  - Overflow and urge incontinence, bladder dyssynergia, UTI, risk of silent renal damage.

❶ Ensure regular renal/urology team follow-up.

- Management with continence advice, regular catheterizations, medication (pro- or anti-cholinergics) and surgical procedures (intravesical botulinum toxin and resineferatoxin injections; vesicostomy; bladder augmentation and bladder neck procedures).
- Bowel dysfunction:

- Constipation with overflow soiling; faecal impaction may worsen urinary dysfunction.
- Managed with continence advice, diet, laxatives, and enemas. Refer to paediatric surgeons.
- Conduit procedures for anterograde colonic washouts may be required.
- Progressive bone and joint deformities:
  - Kyphoscoliosis (20–40%), pathological fractures, hip dislocation, foot problems.
  - Secondary cardio-respiratory, seating, and ambulation issues. Treatments include bracing, rigid orthoses, spasticity management, physiotherapy, and surgery.
- Bone health. Multifactorial reductions in bone strength with tendency to distal femur fracture (25%) and pain.
- Upper limb manipulation problems and truncal imbalance. Occupational therapist will assist with assessment and management.
- Muscular symptoms e.g. fatigue and pain. Often seen in ambulant children. Not necessarily related to anatomical defect.
- Cognition, vision, and hearing deficits, particularly in context of shunted hydrocephalus: see Cognitive disability [in Hydrocephalus section] in this chapter ➲ p. 354.
- Nutrition. Inadequate nutrition or obesity.
- Trophic skin lesions. Poor healing, pressure ulcers on pelvic ischia and feet.
- Psychosocial issues. Puberty and sex education, self-image problems, educational and occupational exclusion.
- Latex allergy. 15% sensitized. Potentially life-threatening anaphylaxis. Manage by latex avoidance during hospitalizations. Refer to allergy expert.
- Tumours. Teratoma and benign dermoid cysts may present late with paraparesis.

Prognosis

See also Spina bifida and myelomeningocele in Chapter 5 ➲ p. 542.

Ambulation

Neurological level of lesion is main predictor of future need for mobility aids and ambulatory ability. Cognitive ability, perceptual disturbance, coordination, spasticity, and bone deformities may impose further limits.

- L5 strength (ankle dorsiflexion) predicts community ambulation: outdoors walking and independent transfers. Ankle orthoses and foot care only.
- L3–4 strength (knee extension) predicts household ambulation: standing for transfers, walking short distances with hip-knee-ankle-foot orthoses, rigid gait orthoses, and wheelchair for longer distances.
- T6–L2 (trunk stability and hip flexion) predicts non-functional ambulation: therapeutic weight bearing with orthoses. Wheelchair indoors for mobility.
- Ambulation may deteriorate in later childhood.

Cognition
Most children with myelomeningocoele do not have overt learning disability. Mean IQ shows downward shift (~90). Performance IQ typically <verbal IQ. Recurrent VP shunt infections predict lower IQ.

Mortality and morbidity
↑risk of death in infancy with high spinal lesions, open lesions, and multiple malformations.
    Causes of ↑mortality:
- Decompensated hydrocephalus.
- VP shunt infection.
- Renal failure.
- Peri-operative (particularly scoliosis surgery).

Most children can expect to survive well into adulthood.
- 30% of adults continue to require daily additional help.
- Quality of life affected by sequelae and functional limitations rather than level of lesion *per se*.

Chiari malformations

Chiari I
The result of a small posterior fossa: contents may be displaced downward with cerebellar tonsils descending below foramen magnum. Fourth ventricle is in normal position; odontoid retroverted. If CSF flow at skull base affected can result in secondary syrinx.
- Large displacement (tonsils >10 mm below foramen magnum) nearly always symptomatic: occipital headache with ICP features (worsened by cough, straining); cerebellar symptoms; downbeat nystagmus; tongue wasting, dysphagia; stridor; limb paraesthesiae and loss of pain secondary to syrinx but preserved joint position sense; central sleep apnoea. May present with paroxysmal, acute persistent, or chronic progressive pictures. Requires surgical posterior fossa decompression.
- Incidental asymptomatic Chiari I malformations are a relatively common finding on MRI. Minor degrees of descent (<5 mm) should be managed conservatively if asymptomatic. Tonsillar descent in young children may resolve spontaneously with posterior fossa growth. See Descent of cerebellar tonsils in Chapter 2 ⊃ p. 76.
- Possibly symptomatic. Not always clear if symptoms e.g. headache that led to detection of Chiari are related. Typically, tonsillar descent 5–10 mm. Potential iatrogenic harm from inappropriate operative correction of Chiari. MRI studies of CSF flow may help clarify whether descent is significant. If a child is experiencing headaches ICP monitoring may be indicated.
- Similar appearances (sometimes associated with low pressure headache) can be seen due to CSF over-drainage after LP.

Chiari II
- = 'Arnold-Chiari malformation'.
- In addition to tonsillar descent the pons is 'under-segmented' and the pons and fourth ventricle are abnormally low. The association with spina bifida is directly causative: the higher the spinal lesion the more

severe the Chiari malformation. Isolated posterior fossa decompression is rarely indicated.

Chiari III
- Rare, with additional feature of herniation of posterior fossa contents through posterior meningocoele.

Infection of the CNS

Meningitis

- Inflammation of the meninges, particularly the arachnoid and pia mater.
- Infective and non-infective causes.
  - Bacterial infection usually associated with a polymorphonuclear response in the subarachnoid space.
  - Viral, tuberculous, and fungal infection cause a lymphocytic response (see Table 4.6).

All cases of meningitis are notifiable in the UK.

Meningitis can be divided into acute (developing over hours to days) and chronic (days to weeks) forms.

Acute bacterial meningitis

Incidence and aetiology

- Epidemiology changing because of immunization patterns.
- Host factors are important (e.g. immunocompromised individuals).
- *Neisseria meningitidis* (meningococcus). Gram –ve diplococcus; most common form of bacterial meningitis in the UK; mostly group B, shifting to group C. Vaccines available for serogroups A, C, W, Y, and B. Winter epidemics. Characterized by purpuric rash, septicaemia (mortality 5–20%).
- *Streptococcus pneumoniae* (pneumococcus). Mortality 20%. Gram + ve diplococcus; infants receive 13 valent conjugate vaccine as part of immunization programme in UK.
- Group B *streptococcus, E.coli, Listeria, Klebsiella* in neonates.
- *Haemophilus influenzae* type b (HiB). Gram –ve pleomorphic coccus; affects neonates and young children. Mortality <5%. Rare in countries where vaccine is given in infancy. Encapsulated *haemophilus* types a-f can rarely cause meningitis.
- Rarely *Streptococcus pyogenes* and *Staphylococcus aureus*.

Pathogenesis

- 95% of bacterial meningitides originate from blood-borne dissemination; 5% from local spread (e.g. mastoiditis, skull trauma: particularly *pneumococcus*).

Table 4.6 CSF finding in meningitis

	Appearance	Cells	Cell count	Protein	Glucose
Bacterial	Turbid	Polymorphs	100–1000+	<1.5 g/dL	<50% plasma
Viral	Clear	Mononuclear	50–1000	<1 g/dL	>50% plasma
TB	Fibrinous	Mononuclear	100–500	1–5 g/dL	<50% plasma
Fungal	Clear	Mononuclear	100+	<1 g/dL	>50% plasma

- Bacteria from the circulation probably enter CSF across choroid plexus and capillaries. Once in the CSF, an area of impaired host defence, they multiply. This generates an immune response and an inflammatory cascade killing the bacteria, but also causing brain injury.
- Additional mechanisms:
  - direct toxic effect of agents released by bacteria or the immune system;
  - hypotension or vasculitis resulting in thrombosis and infarction;
  - development of vasogenic and cytotoxic oedema resulting in ↑ICP and diminished perfusion;
  - development of collections, ventriculitis, or abscess formation.

Clinical features
- Symptoms:
  - triad of fever, headache, and neck stiffness;
  - may be associated photophobia and myalgia.
- Signs:
  - meningism (Brudzinski and Kernig signs);
  - ↓consciousness;
  - petechial/purpuric rash only seen in meningococcus;
  - seizures (30%), cranial nerve signs (15%), other focal neurology (10%);
  - septicaemic shock (particularly with meningococcus).
- In young and ex-premature infants and in the immunocompromised, symptoms and signs may be less specific and more subtle, and a high index of suspicion is needed.

Investigations
If meningitis is suspected, LP is essential to make definitive diagnosis. Failure to LP can result in unnecessary prolonged treatment, particularly with antiviral therapy. If meningococcal infection is suspected, or the child is extremely ill and meningitis is suspected, start antibiotic & supportive treatment prior to investigation.
- Blood:
  - FBC and differential;
  - blood culture;
  - CRP, U&E, glucose; consider ESR, PCR for bacterial DNA, rapid antigen screen (RAS);
  - Interferon gamma test (with Mantoux) if TBM suspected.
- CSF:
  - LP unless focal neurological signs including signs of herniation, or reduced level of consciousness: see Examine for signs of herniation in Chapter 6 ⊃ p. 614.
  - LP is unnecessary in unequivocal systemic meningococcaemia (purpuric rash, shock, etc.).
  - Measure opening pressure and send for culture and sensitivities, protein, glucose, lactate.
  - PCR for bacterial DNA, herpes simplex virus, varicella zoster virus, enterovirus, RAS, consider viral culture, and if TB is suspected PCR for *M. tuberculosis*. Ziehl–Neelsen for acid-fast bacilli and TB culture if

TBM, although yield low as large quantities CSF required (minimum 5 mL).
- Sputum (induced if necessary) or if unavailable, gastric washings if TB suspected.
- Radiology. If consciousness is reduced and/or there are focal neurological signs, CT/MRI to exclude cerebritis, encephalitis, venous sinus thrombosis, vasculitic infarct, sub-dural empyema/abscess or ventriculitis. Contrast studies may show meningeal enhancement in any meningitis.
- CXR/sinus X-ray if clinically indicated (particularly if TB suspected).
- Measure occipitofrontal circumference (OFC) daily in infants.

Treatment
Antibiotics
Choice depends on the age of the child and local epidemiology, resistance patterns, and microbiological advice.
- Typical regime based on a third-generation cephalosporin (cefotaxime or ceftriaxone).
- In neonates, consider adding ampicillin (*Listeria*) and an aminoglycoside for Gram –ve cover.
- Once the pathogen is identified from initial blood cultures or CSF, treatment can be tailored to known sensitivities.
- The prevalence of penicillin-resistant pneumococci is rising; these can also be resistant to cephalosporins and carbapenems as they all act on penicillin-binding proteins. The drug of choice then is combination therapy with vancomycin (high dose).
- Duration of treatment is 7–10 days. Pneumococcus and HiB can continue to spike temperatures for 7–10 days: consider imaging of the head for effusion/empyema or local abscess formation.
- Consider repeat LP or CSF tap via the fontanelle if not improving.

Steroids
Controversial. Steroids have been shown to decrease the CSF inflammatory response, decrease ICP, and reduce mortality and the severity of both acute and long-term neurological and auditory complications. However, the effect seems to be pathogen-specific, with most benefit seen with HiB (now rare because of vaccination). Adverse effects of high-dose steroids have been reported and the anti-inflammatory effect in theory may decrease CSF penetration of certain antibiotics and delay sterilization of the CSF.
   If given, they should:
- Ideally be administered before the first antibiotic dose at a dose of 0.6 mg/kg/day dexamethasone in four divided doses for 2–4 days.
- Not be used in neonatal meningitis.
- Benefits probably greatest for HiB and *S. pneumoniae*.

Contacts
- For children >1 month (ideally started within 24 h).

  - For HiB: rifampicin 20 mg/kg/dose (max 600 mg) once daily for 4 days
  - For meningococcus: under 1 year rifampicin 5 mg/kg/dose; over 1 year 10mg/kg/dose (max 600 mg). Both twice daily for 2 days.

Fluid management
Do not assume hyponatraemia indicates SIADH (see Hyponatraemia in a neuro-intensive care setting in Chapter 5 ⊋ p. 581). Fluid restriction may further compromise cerebral circulation, so before restricting fluids check plasma and urinary sodium and osmolality, and urine output.

Complications (depends on severity of disease)
- *Acute*: cerebritis or encephalitis, effusions, and empyema (low threshold for neurosurgical referral where collections develop); seizures, ventriculitis leading to hydrocephalus, abscess, venous sinus thrombosis, infarct due to vasculitis.
- *Chronic*: hearing or visual impairment, learning difficulties, epilepsy, spasticity; as well as more subtle cognitive and behavioural changes.

Chronic bacterial meningitis
- Bacteria: *M. tuberculosis, Borrelia burgdorferii*, syphilis, nocardia.
- Fungal: cryptococcus, histoplasmosis, and coccidiomycosis.
- Also consider non-infectious collagen vascular disease: see Inflammatory disease of the CNS in this chapter ⊋ p. 391.

Tuberculous meningitis (TBM)
Incidence and aetiology
- Caused by *M. tuberculosis* or occasionally *M. bovis*.
- Incidence in the UK is low but increasing. In high incidence countries, TBM is often the most common form of bacterial meningitis.
- Extrapulmonary TB is more common in children, particularly in the under 5 years age group.
- BCG is of contentious efficacy, but studies seem to imply protection against the severer forms of TB in the developed world.

Pathogenesis
- Primary infection occurs when the tubercle bacillus is inhaled into the lungs and taken up by alveolar macrophages. In most cases, this primary infection passes unnoticed, with only the development of a +ve tuberculin skin test to indicate that infection has taken place.
- In other individuals the mycobacteria continue to replicate after primary infection, overcome host immunity and disease develops either as localized pulmonary disease or as a disseminated form of TB such as miliary TB or TBM.
- Very young children and HIV-infected people are particularly prone to progressive primary TB and dissemination, suggesting that the competence of the host immune system plays an important role in containment of infection.

Clinical features
Non-specific prodromal features develop over days to weeks.
 Staging is useful in predicting prognosis. MRC grading:
- *Grade 1*: non-specific fever, malaise, loss of weight, headaches.
- *Grade 2*: confusion, focal neurological signs, e.g. cranial nerve palsies, seizures.
- *Grade 3*: coma, hemiplegia, or paraplegia.

Investigations
- *Blood*: FBC, U&E, blood culture, CRP and ESR, interferon gamma test.
- *Mantoux*: may be non-reactive, although up to 60% +ve.
- *Sputum* (post induced cough if necessary) or gastric washings × 3 for acid-fast bacilli.
- CSF protein elevated, low glucose with predominant lymphocytosis; can be completely acellular in Grade 1. Sensitivity of PCR for acid-fast bacilli (AFB) is low: 20–40% in adults. Sensitivity of CSF culture is also low in children (<10%) because of small numbers of organisms in a small volume of CSF (higher in adults where HIV-related TB is more typical). Rapid antigen test available.
- *Radiology*: CXR: 50–90% have a primary focus on CXR.
- CT/MRI with contrast: triad of meningeal enhancement (particularly in basal cisterns), hydrocephalus, and infarction (secondary to vasculitis).

Diagnosis is often difficult to confirm initially and needs to be based on clinical suspicion. Even if LP is −ve, in view of the progressive disease course, do not delay treatment.

Treatment
Controversial: no consensus on number of drugs or duration. Typical UK regime: four drugs (isoniazid, rifampicin, pyrazinamide, ethambutol) for 2 months and then two drugs (isoniazid, rifampicin) for a further 10 months. Ethionamide causes fewer ocular problems and crosses the BBB better, but is not easily available in the UK. Prednisolone, again controversial, is added in high doses for the first month (2–4 mg/kg), and then tailed off. Acetazolamide or ventriculoperitoneal shunting may be used for hydrocephalus (usually communicating).

Mortality
Mortality is 10–50% depending on stage of presentation; neurological morbidity (particularly visual impairment) is common.

Contacts
- Screening and chemoprophylaxis for contacts is essential.
- Notifiable disease.

Viral ('aseptic') meningitis
Common. Clinical features include headache, fever, and neck stiffness following a prodromal flu-like illness. Children do not look 'toxic' and drowsiness is uncommon. Look for other features that may give a clue to the aetiology.

CSF findings
White cell count can be 10–1000 but usually <300 × 10⁶/L. Usually lymphocytes but may have neutrophils in the first 48 h of illness. Protein is normal or mildly ↑to 0.5–1 g/L. Glucose is normal but may be low in mumps & CMV.

Differential diagnosis
- Other infections: partially treated bacterial meningitis, brucellosis, *Listeria monocytogenes, Mycoplasma pneumoniae*, leptospirosis, Lyme disease, syphilis, rickettsial infections, TBM, fungal meningitis, parasitic infections.

- Non-infectious causes of CSF inflammation including collagen vascular and autoimmune disease, lymphoma, and some drugs: see also Recurrent aseptic meningitis in this chapter ➲ p. 381.

Treatment is supportive. Prognosis: usually full recovery within 2 weeks. May have fatigue and malaise for longer.

Causative agents
Enteroviruses
Responsible for 85% of cases. Include echovirus, Coxsackie, poliovirus. All cause diffuse rashes with or without more specific features:
- *Echovirus*: conjunctivitis, myopathy.
- *Coxsackie*: hand, foot, and mouth disease, myocarditis, pericarditis, pleurisy.
- *Polio*: isolated meningitis or meningitis before onset of typical paralysis.

Mumps
Parotitis, orchitis, pancreatitis with elevated amylase and lipase (extraneural manifestations occur in 50% cases).

Other herpes viruses
- *HSV type 1 and 2*: usually no cold sores or genital herpes present. Either a direct infection or reactivation of the virus.
- *Varicella zoster* (VZV): may have typical chicken pox rash with fluid-filled blisters.
- *Epstein–Barr* (EBV): pharyngitis, lymphadenopathy, splenomegaly, atypical peripheral lymphocytes, may have abnormal LFTs.
- *Cytomegalovirus* (CMV): may have abnormal LFTs and retinitis.

Measles
Confluent rash, lymphadenopathy, conjunctivitis, pneumonia.

Adenovirus
Conjunctivitis, respiratory infection, vomiting, and diarrhoea.

Lymphocytic choriomeningitis
Orchitis, myocarditis, parotitis, alopecia. May have had contact with rodents.

Viral (meningo-) encephalitis
Uncommon. Clinical features include fever, headache, and encephalopathy. May have focal neurological signs and seizures. May have insidious onset with abnormal behaviour/memory problems that can be mistaken for psychiatric illness.
- A direct viral cause attributed in approximately 50% cases, most commonly HSV, enterovirus, and varicella.
- Para/post-infectious encephalitis following recent systemic viral illness (e.g. ADEM) is other main type of encephalitis.

▶ It seems likely that a significant proportion of past 'presumed viral' encephalitis cases where no pathogen was identified were unrecognized cases of autoimmune encephalitis, e.g. anti-NMDA receptor disease: see Autoimmune encephalopathy in this chapter ➲ p. 391.

Causes

HSV-1 and -2 are the most commonly diagnosed causes in Western countries, but globally Japanese encephalitis virus and rabies are more important.

HSV-1 and -2

- Most common causes of viral meningoencephalitis in the UK.
- Beyond the neonatal period, most cases are due to HSV1.
- One-third primary infection, two-thirds reactivation.
- In neonates, HSV-2 infection can be blood-borne, causing multiorgan infection and diffuse encephalitis, and subsequent diffuse encephalomalacia.

Herpes zoster encephalitis

- Can occur during acute infection or due to later reactivation.
- The presence of a rash is unreliable: prognosis is poorer in those without a rash.
- After chicken pox, virus lies dormant in ganglia along entire neuraxis.
- Encephalitis is due to small or large-vessel vasculitis.
  - The former is usually in the immuno*competent* and typically leads to arterial stroke (see Focal cerebral arteriopathy in this chapter ➋ p. 508): mean onset is 7 weeks after the initial illness (up to 6 months).
  - Large-vessel encephalitis usually occurs in the immuno*suppressed*: zoster infection occurred weeks to months earlier, followed by chronic progressive encephalitis. MRI reveals large and small ischaemic haemorrhagic infarcts of grey and white matter.

HHV6

- The cause of roseola infantum—can occasionally be associated with meningoencephalitis.

Parechovirus

- Typically, young infants. May have respiratory and gastrointestinal features. Very destructive. CSF frequently acellular.

Enteroviruses

- Epidemics are common in the Asia-Pacific region.

Arboviruses

- Require an infected mosquito bite: Japanese encephalitis virus (S or SE Asia), West Nile virus (most continents except N. Europe).

HIV and HIV-associated progressive encephalopathy.

- Encephalitis may be part of the seroconversion illness. HIV-associated progressive encephalopathy (HPE) is a child-specific AIDS-defining illness affecting about half of untreated children. HPE is much less common (a few percent) in children on highly active antiretroviral therapy (HAART). HAART can arrest HPE progression.

- Features are of developmental stagnation and later neurological and general cognitive regression with pyramidal signs, hypokinesis, and evolving dysphagia and feeding difficulties. In older children, deteriorating school performance, social withdrawal, and emotional lability are seen.

CSF findings

Similar to that of viral meningitis although the protein count may be up to 6 g/L. May be normal if LP is performed in the first 48 h of illness. PCR for viral DNA/RNA is possible for many viral infections but may be –ve if LP <48 h or >14 days after onset of illness. Viral isolation is sometimes possible. Measure IgM for specific viruses in the CSF. Discuss with the clinical virologist.

MRI findings

- HSV-1 and -2: most commonly cause signal abnormality (often with haemorrhage) in temporal lobes, insular cortex, frontal lobes, and thalami. Neonates: widespread signal abnormality: hypointense on T1, and hyperintense on T2. DWI is more sensitive. Cerebellum may also be involved. May have meningeal enhancement after gadolinium. Midline shift may be present if significant cerebral oedema is present.

▶ Appearances may be atypical.

- VZV: multiple abnormal signal in grey and white matter representing vasculitis and infarction.
- Enteroviruses: may have abnormal signal isolated to brainstem or thalami.
- Arboviruses: may have abnormal signal in the basal ganglia and thalami.
- Parechovirus: often extensive destructive white matter change (in infant brain).

EEG abnormalities

Diffuse slowing of the background, focal abnormalities, and later periodic lateralizing epileptic discharges (PLEDS) may be present; however, EEG is not sensitive or specific and cannot be relied upon to establish or exclude diagnosis.

Brain biopsy

Not used routinely. Consider if diagnosis is unclear and findings will change management, e.g. if considering micro-abscesses from an embolic source, TB, or fungal/parasitic infection or a non-infectious immune-mediated encephalitis.

Treatment

- Proven *HSV-1 and -2*: IV aciclovir for 21 days. Monitor renal function. If relapse occurs, re-treat and consider prophylaxis with oral aciclovir or valaciclovir for 90 days.
- *CMV*: ganciclovir and foscarnet combination therapy. Discuss with clinical virologist.

- Treat seizures, ↑ICP and other complications with supportive measures. Use of steroids is controversial. Consider using 3 to 5-day pulse of methylprednisolone or dexamethasone in severe cases with ↑ICP. Consider surgical decompression in cases where ↑ICP is refractory to medical treatment.
- Secondary anti-NMDA receptor-mediated encephalitis (see Autoimmune encephalopathy in this chapter ➲ p. 391) is responsible for the late neurological deterioration (with recurrence of encephalopathy and often a movement disorder) sometimes seen 2 to 3 weeks after proven HSV encephalitis. Treatment is with immunomodulation: see Autoimmune encephalopathy in this chapter ➲ p. 391.

Prognosis
Depends on the cause and severity of the illness at presentation. Mortality is improved by 40% in HSV-1 and -2 encephalitis if aciclovir is given promptly.

Influenza A & B
Neurological manifestations rare but more common in children than adults.
- Post-infectious encephalitis (including ADEM).
- Encephalopathy including Acute Necrotizing Encephalitis (ANE) which can be associated with a familial/isolated *RANBP2* mutation.
- Other neuroradiological phenotypes e.g, Mild encephalopathy with a reversible splenial lesion (MERS), featuring a precisely midline area of restricted diffusion ± T2 signal change in the splenium of the corpus callosum, also sometimes referred to as Cytotoxic Lesion of the Corpus Callosum (CLOCC).
- Some evidence Influenza A (H1N1) more neurotropic.

Diagnosis: PCR respiratory secretions; CSF may show mild pleocytosis, CSF PCR usually −ve.

Treatment: oseltamivir has no effect on neurological complications. Supportive treatment for complications e.g. seizures, ↑ICP.

Consider corticosteroids (high-dose ADEM regime) if very unwell and Tocilizumab (interleukin-6 blockade) in ANE.

Worse outcome in children with pre-existing neurological disorders.

SARS-CoV-2
CNS manifestations of COVID-19 much less common than in adults but include:
- Post-infectious encephalitis (including ADEM), other demyelinating disorders often associated with +ve MOG antibodies e.g. optic neuritis and myelitis;
- Encephalopathy including ANE, MERS and stroke (haemorrhagic and ischaemic).
- The Kawasaki-like systemic post-COVID inflammatory syndrome known as Paediatric Inflammatory Multisystem Syndrome temporally associated with SARS-CoV-2 (PIMS-TS) in UK and Multisystem Inflammatory Syndrome in Children associated with COVID (MISC-C) in North American literature.

- Can include encephalopathy (often with behavioural change/ hallucinations and sometimes with MERS appearances on imaging), and status epilepticus as part of systemic illness. There are probably multiple mechanisms but neuroimmune is the most frequently identified.

Diagnosis: PCR respiratory secretions for SARS-CoV-2. CSF may show mild pleocytosis, CSF PCR usually –ve.

Treatment: Supportive treatment for complications e.g. seizures, ↑ICP. Consider corticosteroids (high-dose ADEM regime) if very unwell or for specific demyelinating phenotypes and tocilizumab in ANE. Other treatments depend on the specific syndrome.

Determinants of outcome are not fully understood, but neurological sequelae are likely for many.

Other rare causes of infectious encephalitis

Viral causes are found in approximately 50% cases of encephalitis. Increasingly suspected that most 'presumed viral' encephalitides (where no pathogen can be identified) are autoimmune: see Autoimmune encephalopathy in this chapter ➔ p. 391.

Consider the following if no viral cause is found especially if there is an appropriate travel history or if the child is immunocompromised.

- *Bacterial*: TB, *Mycoplasma pneumonia* (usually para/post-infectious); *Listeria monocytogenes* (common in transplant patients); *Borrelia burgdorferii*; Leptospirosis; Brucellosis; *Legionella*; *Tropheryma whipplei* (Whipple disease); *Nocardia actinomyces*; *Treponema pallidum*; *Salmonella typhi*; other causes of pyogenic meningitis/abscess especially if septicaemia and micro-abscesses are possible.
- *Rickettsial*: (rash usually present). *Rickettsia rickettsii* (Rocky Mountain spotted fever); *Rickettsia typhi* (endemic typhus); *Rickettsia prowazekii* (epidemic typhus); *Coxiella burnetti* (Q fever); Ehrlichiosis (*Ehrlichia chaffeensis*—human monocytic ehrlichiosis).
- *Fungal:* Cryptococcus (common in transplant recipients); Aspergillosis (common in transplant recipients); Candidiasis; Histoplasmosis; North American blastomycosis.
- *Parasitic:* human African trypanosomiasis (sleeping sickness); cerebral malaria; *Toxoplasma gondii*; *Echinococcus granulosus*; Schistosomiasis.

Source data from A Chaudhuri, P G E Kennedy, Diagnosis and treatment of viral encephalitis, Postgraduate Medical Journal, Volume 78, Issue 924, October 2002, Pages 575–583, https://doi.org/10.1136/pmj.78.924.575

Acute post-infectious cerebellitis

- Most commonly described after varicella infection: also enterovirus, EBV, mumps, and measles.
- More common in younger children (2–7 yrs of age).
- Abrupt onset ataxia and behavioural disturbance within 5–14 days of the chicken pox rash (occasionally can be pre-eruptive).
- Symptoms are worst at onset or within 1–2 weeks then improve over 4–8 weeks, with full recovery for the majority.
- Management is supportive. Antivirals are not routinely given.

- Neuroimaging is only recommended in an atypical presentation or course (progressive deterioration, waxing and waning, altered sensorium (risk of hydrocephalus), diminished reflexes).
- Differential includes Miller–Fisher syndrome: see Miller–Fisher syndrome in this chapter ⊃ p. 436.

Anterior horn cell infection

Poliovirus

Poliovirus is an enterovirus causing biphasic febrile illness with initial prodrome then further fever with acute onset asymmetrical progressive flaccid paralysis of one or more limbs. Signs of aseptic meningitis with severe neck and back pain are common. No sensory involvement. Paralysis may also be bulbar and may also have autonomic involvement.

Peak incidence was in the 1950s. Since introduction of WHO global eradication programme cases have declined by 99% but outbreaks have occurred in some low-income countries in recent years; caused by a mixture of wild virus and mutated live vaccine strains (active monitoring for virus in wastewater in many countries).

- *Investigations*: isolate poliovirus from stool.
- *Treatment*: supportive.
- *Prognosis*: mortality 10%. Weakness continues to improve up to a year from onset of illness. Children may develop later onset of weakness >30 yrs after initial illness—post-polio syndrome.

Enterovirus 71

Causes outbreaks of hand, foot, and mouth disease in the Asia-Pacific region. Young children present with fever, rash on the soles and palms, and oral ulcers. May develop shock and pulmonary oedema. May develop polio-like neurological manifestations from infection of the anterior horn cells.

Enterovirus D68

Enterovirus D68 appears to be responsible for recent outbreaks of acute flaccid myelitis (AFM).

Japanese encephalitis virus (JEV), West Nile virus (WNV), Tick borne encephalitis virus (TBEV), Dengue & Chikungunya virus

These are arbo ('arthropod-borne') viruses requiring a bite from an infected mosquito or tick. Encephalitis linked to these viruses are linked to the geographical location of transmission. Children are more likely to be symptomatic with JEV. Those infected with the flaviviruses JEV, WNV, and TBEV may develop polio-like neurological manifestations with or without meningitis or encephalitis. There are vaccines available for JEV and TBEV, but no specific treatments are available.

Paralytic rabies

Differential diagnosis: Guillain–Barré syndrome (classical AIDP, or AMAN), tick paralysis (toxic venom), diphtheritic polyneuropathy, botulism, enterovirus, or flavivirus polio-like paralysis.

Focal CNS infection

See Table 4.7.

Table 4.7 Causes of focal CNS infection

	Bacterial	Parasitic	Fungal
Immunocompetent	Mycobacterium; Staphylococcus; Streptococcus; Fusobacterium	Neurocysticercosis; Echinococcus; Amoebiasis; Paragonimiasis; Sparganosis; Schistosomiasis; Malaria	Histoplasmosis; Blastomycosis; Coccidiomycosis; Aspergillosis
Immunocompromised	Pseudomonas; Nocardia	Toxoplasmosis	Candidiasis; Cryptococcus; Rhizopus

Cerebral abscess

Brain abscesses can be caused by bacteria, fungi, or parasites, with the most common causal organisms being Staphylococcus, Streptococcus, and Haemophilus. Anaerobes such as bacteroides, Streptococcus milleri, and Fusobacterium are also commonly found. Infection commonly follows haematogenous spread from a distant focus; these abscesses frequently form at the grey–white matter junction. Direct extension can occur from the ears or sinuses, or abscesses can develop following trauma or meningitis. Congenital cyanotic heart disease is a major predisposing factor.

Clinical features

Symptoms depend on the size and location, but generally present with fever, signs, and symptoms of ↑ICP and focal neurological deficits.
▶ Children may look deceptively well!

Investigations

- Imaging: MRI or CT with contrast shows ring-enhancing lesions with surrounding oedema (may be multiple). DWI restricted diffusion (low signal on ADC).
- LP is contraindicated.
- Bloods: blood culture (frequently –ve); CRP, ESR, WBC (to monitor treatment).
- Cardiac echo to look for vegetations (embolic source).

Treatment

5–6 weeks of broad-spectrum IV antibiotics such as a third-generation cephalosporin with anaerobic cover (metronidazole) is recommended. Antibiotic treatment alone is often insufficient, and surgical drainage needs to be considered. Aspiration and/or excision relieve pressure and enable a microbiological diagnosis. Steroid use is controversial and is mainly used for mass effect. Radiological resolution is frequently slow, with a ring lesion persisting for weeks to months.

Complications
40% of children have neurological sequelae, with 25–30% developing seizures.

Protozoan and parasitic infections

Cerebral malaria
- Responsible for over a million deaths annually, the majority in children.
- Mechanism of coma unknown.
  - Reduced cerebral perfusion (secondary to ↑ICP, increased plasma viscosity, and systemic hypotension), severe anaemia, hypoglycaemia, seizures, and the local release of cytokines may all be contributory factors.
- Strict case definition: unrousable coma which persists >60 min after a seizure; asexual *Plasmodium falciparum* forms on blood film and exclusion of other causes of encephalopathy.
- In practice, any child with a history of travel to an endemic area, presenting with fever, seizures, or a diminished level of consciousness, needs to have malaria excluded. In children the time from onset of fever to coma is typically around 48 h.

Investigations
- Thick and thin smear for diagnosis and parasite count.
- Send multiple samples to avoid false –ve results.
- Blood glucose, venous pH, electrolytes (renal failure), FBC (anaemia).
- LP once consciousness is improving to exclude bacterial meningitis.
- EEG if there is concern re subclinical status.
- CT or MRI if there is concern re diagnosis.
- MR venogram to exclude venous sinus thrombosis if focal neurological signs.

Treatment
- Supportive treatment with oxygen, fluids for shock, blood for anaemia, and benzodiazepines for seizures.
- Specific treatment depends on type of parasite and area where acquired (to consider drug resistance). Parenteral quinine is usually the drug of choice, as chloroquine resistance is high (converting to oral quinine when improved: total 1 week treatment). Other possible treatments include quinidine, artemisinin derivatives, or sulphadoxine/pyrimethamine.
- Seek advice from Infectious Diseases team.

Complications
Mortality is high at around 20%, but in those that survive, the majority (~80%) have a normal outcome unless venous infarction occurs.

Neurocysticercosis
- Results from ingestion of infected pork and the encysted form of *Taenia solium* comes to rest in the brain parenchyma.
- The most common parasitic infection of CNS.
- The leading cause of late-onset epilepsy in developing countries.

Clinical presentation
- The majority of infections are asymptomatic, with symptoms starting when the cysticerci start to die.
- 90% of children present with seizures, focal or general, with 20% in status. 10% present with symptoms and signs of ↑ICP.
- Occasionally cysticercotic encephalitis can occur when numerous degenerating lesions invoke an acute inflammatory reaction.

Diagnosis
- *Blood:* FBC (occasional eosinophilia), neurocysticercosis ELISA (frequently +ve in at risk individuals as this is an endemic disease, thus not specific).
- *CSF:* normal, or occasionally mild pleocytosis and protein elevation. ELISA for neurocysticercosis on CSF more specific.
- *CT:* ring-enhancing lesion with oedema, frequently multiple.
  - A single lesion may pose diagnostic dilemma as it is difficult radiologically to exclude tuberculoma. MRI may show scolex.

Treatment
- Need for drug treatment is controversial but recent trials seem to indicate better outcome with treatment.
- Albendazole at 15 mg/kg/day 8 hourly for 8 days.
- Steroids only if there are multiple lesions or cysticercotic encephalitis.
- Symptomatic treatment with ASM is required in most patients.
- Some may need neurosurgical intervention.
- Re-image at 6 weeks to 3 months to confirm resolution.

Echinococcosis
- Caused by *E. granulosus* or *multilocularis*.
- Prevalent in temperate areas/sheep-grazing areas.
- Hepatic and pulmonary infection common: CNS involvement in only 1–2% (mainly children 5–10 yrs old).
- Symptoms and signs are of a space-occupying lesion with ↑ICP.
- Treatment with albendazole ±steroids. Surgical resection is occasionally required after drug treatment for large lesions.

Amoebiasis
- Amoebic infections of the CNS produce either meningoencephalitis (*Enteramoeba naegleria* and *acanthamoeba*) or cerebral abscess (*E. histolytica*).
- Transmission following either ingestion of contaminated water, or nasal inhalation. Cases present with fever, and signs of either ↑ICP or meningoencephalitis.
- Treatment with amphotericin B, miconazole, or rifampicin.

Mycotic infections of the CNS
- Produces either meningitis or abscesses, mainly in the immunocompromised host: see CNS infection of the immunocompromised host in this chapter ⟳ p. 377.
- The main organisms are *Candida albicans* and *Cryptococcus*.

CNS candidiasis
- Occurs mainly in susceptible neonates and infants.
- The course can be subacute, and detection can be difficult. CSF findings are variable.
- Radiology: micro-abscesses, thrombi, or haemorrhages.
- Treatment is with amphotericin B (ideally liposomal).

Cryptococcosis
- Causes a granulomatous arachnoiditis presenting with headache, disturbance of consciousness, or focal neurological signs.
- CSF is abnormal (see Table 4.6) and Indian ink staining is +ve in 60% of cases. Cryptococcal antigen is +ve in 98%.
- Treatment is with amphotericin B and 5-fluorocytosine.

Slow-viral and prion infections
Subacute sclerosing panencephalitis (SSPE)
- A late neurological presentation of previous measles caused by the host response to persistent measles virus in the brain.
- Very rare, although an increase is anticipated with documented falls in MMR vaccine uptake and measles outbreaks.
- Age at presentation 5 to 15 yrs. Primary infection is usually at <4 yrs.
- ♂: ♀ 2:1.
- Neurological regression with insidious onset over weeks to months.
  - Behavioural changes and decline in school performance.
  - Later tremors, myoclonus, seizures (often drop attacks), visual loss secondary to chorioretinitis or cortical blindness, chorea, pyramidal signs, cerebellar ataxia.
  - Rapid motor deterioration, develop abnormal posturing, autonomic dysfunction, and become comatose.
  - Neuropathological features follow an occipitofrontal and cephalocaudal progression which accounts for symptom progression.

Diagnosis
- CSF is usually acellular. May have elevated protein. Glucose is normal. Anti-measles IgG in CSF and plasma and unmatched oligoclonal bands.
- EEG is very characteristic: bilateral, synchronous, symmetrical periodic delta wave complexes present from early stages with electrodecremental periods following the complexes. The background becomes increasingly slower with disease progression.
- MRI abnormalities: changes present early in disease progression. Hyperdensities on T2-weighted images are seen in the periventricular frontal, temporal, and occipital white matter. Approximately 50% of children will have ↑signals on T2-weighted images in the basal ganglia and thalamus. Generalized cerebral atrophy and ventricular dilatation occur with disease progression.

Treatment
No established treatment. There are reports from open trials that combinations of antiviral drugs (ribavirin, inosiplex, and interferon α) may be worth considering. Some need intraventricular route.

Prognosis
Most children die within 3 yrs of diagnosis usually from pneumonia, UTI, pressure sores, etc. Approximately 10% will live longer, rarely up to 10 yrs.

Variant Creutzfeld–Jakob disease (vCJD)
- A *prion* disease: the infectious agent is the converted form of a normally occurring, host-produced protein encoded on chromosome 20.
- Variant CJD (vCJD) is the only form of CJD presenting in the paediatric age range and is thought to be due to transmission from cattle by eating infected meat or between humans via blood transfusion. First reported in 1996 in the UK and seems to have peaked in 2000, it seems now thankfully to have become extremely rare again, but ongoing vigilance is warranted.

Clinical features
Early symptoms are psychiatric (withdrawal, depression, and anxiety) followed by a decline in school performance and painful paraesthesias in the limbs. After approximately 6 months, ataxia and involuntary movements (dystonic, choreiform, and myoclonic) develop. There is progressive neurological decline with dysphasia, dementia, dysphoria, rigidity, hyperreflexia, and primitive reflexes. Death occurs less than 3 yrs from the onset of symptoms (mean 14 months).

Investigations
Changes on DWI and ↑T2 signal in the posterior thalamus (pulvinar) is characteristic in established cases. EEG is non-specific (unlike adult sporadic CJD). CSF: neuronal protein 14-3-3 +ve in 50% of cases of vCJD. Consider a brain biopsy.

▶ EEG, LP, and brain biopsy require specific stringent infection control precautions if vCJD is suspected.

Treatment
Supportive only at present. Discuss suspected cases with National CJD surveillance unit in Edinburgh. Useful website: ℘ www.cjd.ed.ac.uk.

Lyme disease
- Multisystem disease caused by the spirochete *Borrelia burgdorferii*.
- Vectors are infected deer *Ixodes* ticks.
- Common in North America and parts of Europe (including UK).
- The incubation period is 7–30 days.

Clinical features
- Most commonly affected organ systems are the skin, nervous system, joints, and heart.
- Expanding 'bull's eye' erythematous rash (erythema chronicum migrans).

- Flu-like symptoms, myositis, hepatitis, arthralgias, and rare cardiac conduction abnormalities.
- Approximately 15% develop nervous system involvement that typically consists of all or part of the triad of lymphocytic meningitis, cranial neuritis, and painful radiculitis. Cranial nerves most typically involved are the 7th nerves bilaterally.

Described neurological presentations
Peripheral
- Mononeuropathy multiplex.
- Cranial neuropathy (usually bilateral 7th nerve).
- Radiculopathy.
- Brachial plexopathy.
- Lumbosacral plexopathy.
- Diffuse polyneuropathy.
- Motor neuropathy.
- Guillain–Barré like picture (not demyelinating).

Central nervous system
- Infection in subarachnoid space.
- Radiculitis.
- Cranial neuropathy.
- Meningitis.

Parenchymal infection
- Encephalitis ('multiple sclerosis-like' variant): very rare.
- Myelopathy.

Diagnosis
- Exposure plus serology testing of serum and CSF.
- Confirm with Western blot test of the child's serum against *B burgdorferi* antigens.
- May get a false +ve result with syphilis infection. Culture is difficult. PCR is not routine: the spirochaete concentrates in collagen-rich connective tissues and the blood/CSF borne stage is brief.

Treatment
With CNS involvement, IV ceftriaxone (for total 21 days; can switch to oral doxiciclone for latter part of treatment course in older children). Meningitis often resolves spontaneously. No evidence for use of steroids.

Prognosis
Usually very good.

CNS infection of the immunocompromised host
This presents diagnostic challenges due to unusual pathogens, atypical insidious, and non-specific presentations. There are management challenges due to difficulty in eradicating some organisms and severe long-term consequences. Typical 'teaching hospital' contexts include:
- Prematurity (naïve immune system).
- Congenital immunodeficiency (DiGeorge, Bruton, common variable immunodeficiency, severe combined immunodeficiency, etc.).

- Iatrogenic acquired immunocompromise through steroid treatment of chronic inflammatory conditions, treatment of malignancy, or use of immunosuppression in oncology, immunology, or bone marrow transplant settings.
- Infective immunodeficiency due to HIV/AIDS (the CNS is second most commonly affected site: see HIV and HIV-associated progressive encephalopathy in this chapter p. 367).
- After splenectomy, including the progressive 'auto-splenectomy' of children with sickle cell disease.

The type of organisms that pose a risk depend on the cause and precise nature of the immunodeficiency.

Deficient B cell function
Meningitis caused by encapsulated bacterial pathogens.

Deficient T-cell or macrophage function
CNS infections caused by intracellular organisms.
- Fungi (*Aspergillus*).
- Bacteria (*Nocardia*).
- Viruses (HSV, JC, CMV, HHV-6).
- Protozoa (*Toxoplasma gondii*).
- Unusual bacterial meningitis organisms: *Listeria* or *Cryptococcus*.

Organisms
Bacterial
- Encapsulated organisms.
- Gram +ve and −ve.
- *Mycobacterium*.

Viral
- Herpes.
- HSV1/CMV/Varicella/HHV-6.
- Enteroviruses.

Fungal
- *Candida*.
- *Cryptococcus neoformans*.
- *Aspergillus*.

Parasitic
- *Toxoplasma gondii*.

Presentation
Often there is a non-specific neurological presentation (encephalopathy, seizures, focal neurological signs). The question is often whether this is this infection or a complication of treatment?
- 'Radiological presentation': (the incidental finding of an intracerebral mass lesion particularly in the context of T-cell deficiency). Consider TB, lymphoma, toxoplasmosis.

Toxoplasmosis (reactivation)
- Subacute or acute presentation with confusion and headache, ± fever and malaise.
- Meningeal signs are rare.
- Focal neurological signs are present in 60%.
- Seizures.
- Focal motor deficits and cranial nerve palsies.
  - sensory abnormalities;
  - cerebellar signs;
  - movement disorders;
  - neuropsychiatric symptoms.
- Antibodies are detectable in serum but are not useful in following the course of the illness.
- MRI brain: multiple ring-enhancing lesions ± oedema reflecting multifocal necrotizing encephalitis.
- Frontal, parietal, basal ganglia, cerebellum, grey and white matter.

Treatment
- Combination therapy with sulphadiazine, pyrimethamine with folinic acid (clindamycin can be substituted for sulphadiazine).
- Ineffective against the tissue cyst form.
- Must continue as maintenance therapy.
- Prophylaxis in HIV-1 +ve children with CD4 <100.

Aspergillus fumigatus infection
- Mass lesions or cerebral infarcts; meningitis is rare.
- MRI brain.
- CSF PCR, antibody, antigen (galactomannan) or culture.
- Biopsy.

Treatment
- Voriconazole.
- Liposomal amphotericin B in neonates.

Cryptococcal infection
- Inhalation of encapsulated fungus; avoids phagocytosis.
- Basilar chronic meningitis.
- Micro-abscesses in the basal ganglia (cryptococcomas).
- Focal neurological signs or seizures in 10%; ↑ICP in 50% (mechanism unknown).

Diagnosis
- CSF protein elevated, glucose low; WCC<20. India ink stain (sensitivity 75–80%).
- Cryptococcal capsular antigen in the blood (99%) or CSF.
- CSF PCR.

Treatment
- Induction: 2 weeks:
  - intravenous amphotericin B and 5-flucytosine.
- Consolidation: 8 weeks/CSF culture –ve:
  - fluconazole.
  - relapse occurs in 25–60% of HIV-1 children.
- Maintenance therapy:
  - fluconazole.
  - Granulocyte–Macrophage Colony–Stimulating Factor in high-risk patients.

JC virus

JC virus is common. 70–90% of adults are infected. Primary infection is asymptomatic. The virus remains latent in the kidney, CNS lymphocytes. Immunosuppression permits reactivation and mutation to pathogenic virus which causes progressive multifocal leukoencephalopathy (PML).

▶ PML has been reported in connection with use of natalizumab (humanized monoclonal antibody against α 4-integrin used in treatment of multiple sclerosis and Crohn disease) and rituximab.
- Focal neurological deficits.
- Progressive dementia.
- Coma and death are common over a period of 4–6 months.
- Fever and headache are *absent*.
- MRI shows multifocal white matter lesions without mass effect or enhancement.
- CSF PCR for JC virus DNA has high sensitivity and specificity. Quantitation is useful prognostically.
- Brain biopsy with immunohistology (definitive).

Treatment
- Cidofovir is unproven.
  - Some trials are supportive in children with HIV-1.
  - Poor response in non-HIV-1 children.
- Mefloquine.
- Reversing immunosuppression.
- HAART in HIV-1.

CMV encephalitis
- Children with T-cell counts <50.
  - SCID/HIV-1/bone marrow transplant/solid organ transplant.
- Extra-CNS sites (retina, adrenals, gastrointestinal tract).

Features
- Subacute dementia and focal neurological signs.
- Microglial nodules found diffusely in the grey matter.
- Ventriculo-encephalitis.
- Delirium.
- Ventriculomegaly.
- Cranial nerve deficits.

Diagnosis
- *CSF*: pleocytosis, hypoglycorrhachia, elevated protein.
- PCR DNA (PPV 92%, NPV 95%):
  - Quantitative PCR is useful prognostically.
- Areas of ↑signal on T2 MRI.

Treatment
- Induction: ganciclovir ± foscarnet; cidofovir?
- Maintenance: ganciclovir.

HHV-6 encephalitis
There are two variants A and B: type A is more neurotropic. Seen in solid organ and bone marrow transplant recipients due to reactivation or re-infection. Causes encephalitis. There may be interactions between herpes-viruses: HHV-6 may exacerbate CMV encephalitis. Possible cofactor in HIV disease? Detection of HHV-6 in CSF by multiplex PCR in the immunocompetent is often a false +ve representing viral chromosome integration or reactivation. Seek ID advice.
- *Treatment*: ganciclovir, foscarnet, cidofovir.

Varicella zoster CNS infection
Seen in T-cell deficiency, primary immunodeficiency, HIV-1 infection, and in the context of high-dose steroid use.
- Myelitis, ventriculitis, meningitis.
- Large and small-vessel encephalitis:
  - stroke (large vessel);
  - chronic progressive encephalitis (small vessel).
- *Diagnosis*: PCR VZV DNA.
- *Treatment*: high-dose IV aciclovir for 21 days. If vasculitis thought to be significant, consider prednisolone 2 mg/kg/day for 3–5 days (Gilden *N Engl J Med* 2000; 342:635).

Recurrent aseptic meningitis

Mollaret disease
Recurrent self-limiting episodes of aseptic meningitis lasting 2–4 days. Rare in children. Assumed to have an infectious cause: may be associated with HSV type 1 and 2. Monocyte cells with characteristic 'footprint nuclei' are present in CSF. They also have an elevated CSF IgG level.
- *Differential diagnosis*: collagen vascular diseases, sarcoidosis, lymphoma, complement factor 1 deficiency, meningeal carcinomatosis, structural causes, e.g. CNS tumours, midline fistula between skin and dura, or epidermoid cyst, toxic drug reactions: NSAIDs, IVIG, some chemotherapy agents, some antibiotics, e.g. penicillin, cephalosporins, trimethoprim.

Congenital infection

The CNS of the neonate can be infected antenatally, during delivery, or in the early postnatal weeks. The most important agents are those in the TORCH group (Toxoplasmosis, 'Others' (syphilis and HIV), Rubella, CMV and herpes simplex); however, other agents are important including VZV, Lymphocytic Choriomeningits Virus (LCMV), enteroviruses, and Zika virus.

Damage results from direct teratogenic effects (disruption of CNS development), tissue destruction due to inflammation, or a combination of the two.

Infection before 20 weeks' gestation may be suspected but difficult to prove as the fetus cannot produce specific antibodies in early pregnancy. Testing saved antenatal & postnatal maternal blood may be helpful. All the agents can cause an asymptomatic infection.

CMV infection

The most common and potentially serious congenital infection. Primary maternal infection in the first or second trimester (which is often asymptomatic) will result in foetal infection in 60% of pregnancies. 10% of these are symptomatic at birth.

Clinical features
CNS abnormalities include:
- Meningoencephalitis, with parenchymal damage in the germinal matrix, periventricular white matter, and cortex. Atrophy occurs later.
- Calcifications: periventricular, cortical, or both.
- Microcephaly.
- Ventriculomegaly.
- Neuronal migration disturbances—all types seen.
- Cerebellar hypoplasia.
- Hearing loss.

Systemic features include:
- Intrauterine growth retardation; premature delivery.
- Chorioretinitis.
- Hepatosplenomegaly, jaundice, anaemia, thrombocytopaenia, petechiae, ecchymoses.
- Inguinal hernias.
- Pneumonitis.

Infection is usually persistent (50% still have virus in the urine aged 5 yrs) and may cause progressive damage, particularly sensorineural hearing loss, and retinitis.

Investigations
- CSF demonstrates pleocytosis (typically <100, mainly lymphocytes) and ↑protein (usually <1.5 g/dL).
- CT is abnormal in 80%, demonstrating calcification and major cortical and white matter abnormalities.
- MRI is more sensitive and may indicate neuronal migration abnormalities.
- 60% have abnormal brainstem auditory evoked responses at birth (may manifest later so follow-up studies are important).

Diagnosis
- Discuss with infectious diseases colleagues.
- Demonstration of CMV seropositivity (or CMV excretion in urine) in an older child with neurological impairments does not establish a causal role for CMV. Infection in later postnatal life is commonly asymptomatic and seropositivity is very likely to be coincidental.
- The retained Guthrie (neonatal screening blood spot) sample is invaluable in retrospectively establishing timing of infection.
- Virus culture from urine.
- PCR for CMV DNA in urine, serum, CSF, cord blood, Guthrie card.
- Presence of IgM in foetal serum or persistence of foetal IgG in an older infant. Compare titres with maternal results.

Outcome
Depends on severity of CNS involvement but 95% with symptomatic CNS infection at birth will have major neurological sequelae.

Treatment
- Symptomatic: treatment of seizures, tone abnormalities, etc.
- Specific: ganciclovir or valganciclovir reduce progression of hearing deficits and improve neurodevelopmental outcomes. Discuss with virologist.

Toxoplasmosis

Acquired transplacentally after primary infection in the mother. Risk factors include contact with cat litter or faeces and eating undercooked meat.
- Maternal infection in first or second trimester results in foetal infection in 25% of whom 50% will be symptomatic.
- Maternal infection in third trimester results in foetal infection in 65% however large majority will be asymptomatic.
- Treatment of the mother reduces transmission risk and improves outcome but maternal infection is often asymptomatic.

Clinical features
Similar systemic features to CMV infection although IUGR and prematurity are less common. May have these features without any neurological syndrome at birth but develop neurological abnormalities later. CNS abnormalities are seen in two-thirds of cases and include:
- Meningoencephalitis—multifocal, diffuse, necrotizing, and granulomatous.
- Hydranencephaly or porencephaly.
- Hydrocephalus secondary to obstruction of aqueduct.
- Intracranial calcification.
- Microcephaly—secondary to loss of brain tissue.
- Hearing loss.

Investigations
- CSF demonstrates pleocytosis (typically <100) and protein (usually >2 g/dL).
- Ultrasound & CT may reveal basal ganglia & periventricular calcification.
- MRI helps define abnormalities.

Diagnosis
- Discuss with paediatric infectious disease colleagues.
- Presence of foetal IgM is most useful test. Compare IgG titres with maternal results.
- Confirm with PCR for Toxoplasma DNA in blood and or CSF.

Treatment
- *Symptomatic*: treatment of seizures, tone abnormalities, etc.
- *Specific*: pyrimethamine and sulfadiazine (with folinic acid supplementation) for 1 year. Consider steroids if CSF protein >1 g/dL. Discuss with infectious diseases colleagues.

Prognosis
Even those with asymptomatic infection may have problems identified later including learning difficulties, hearing impairment, and retinitis. For those with symptomatic infection, the neurological outcome depends on the severity and location of brain damage. If treated, approximately 25% will have motor deficits and an IQ of <70. 90% will have a retinopathy.

Rubella

Incidence is low in UK due to high levels of vaccination. Foetal infection is acquired transplacentally after primary (usually asymptomatic) infection in the mother. The frequency & severity of infection are greater the earlier in gestation it occurs. Ocular and cardiac defects only occur in the 1st trimester. Infection later than 4 months' gestation is usually asymptomatic.

Clinical features
Similar systemic features to CMV & toxoplasmosis infections. In addition, cardiac (peripheral pulmonary stenosis, PDA, and myocardial necrosis) occur in up to 20%. Ocular abnormalities include 'salt and pepper' retinopathy, cataracts (pearly and central), and microphthalmia. Dermal erythropoiesis causes 'blueberry muffin' syndrome. Bony radiolucencies may be seen on x-rays of long bones.

CNS abnormalities include:
- Meningoencephalitis: multifocal necrotizing, diffuse, perivascular infiltrates.
- Full anterior fontanelle.
- Lethargy, hypotonia, and irritability.
- Opisthotonos and retrocollis.
- Progressive microcephaly due to impaired cell replication.
- Impaired myelination.
- Hearing loss—inflammation of cochlea (may be difficult to detect at birth).

Investigations
- CSF: pleocytosis (typically <100 mainly monocytes) and protein (usually <1.5 g/dL).
- USS and CT may show focal calcification in basal ganglia.
- MRI helps define focal lesions (usually in white matter) and demonstrate impaired myelination.

Diagnosis
- Discuss with paediatric infectious disease colleagues.
- Isolate virus from urine, throat, or rectal swab, or CSF.
- Presence of foetal IgM. Persistence of IgG in older infant. Compare titres to maternal results.

Treatment
Symptomatic only as above. No specific treatments are available.

Outcome
90% symptomatic infants will have sequelae including motor deficits, microcephaly, cognitive impairment, behavioural problems, and hearing loss.

Herpes simplex

Fetus usually infected during delivery: rarely postnatal infection from close contacts (usually HSV1). 50%–75% type 2 and remainder type 1. Asymptomatic infection common is in the mother but unusual in the infant. Premature infants more frequently affected. Foetal scalp electrodes are a risk factor.

Clinical features
Damage caused by inflammation and destruction. Features shared by other TORCH infections. Severe cases have multiorgan involvement: predilection for reticulo-endothelial system (anaemic, jaundice, bleeding). Specific features include vesicular mucocutaneous lesions (often over the site of viral entry), conjunctivitis, and keratitis. If infection is localized (without visceral involvement), symptom onset is later (2nd or 3rd week of life).
   CNS abnormalities include:
- Meningoencephalitis: multifocal, severe, and diffuse.
- Seizures/coma.
- Bulging fontanelle.

Investigations
- CSF pleocytosis (<100 usually lymphocytes), RBCs, and protein (<1.5 g/dL). Glucose may be low.
- CT and USS may identify parenchymal abnormalities.
- MRI helps define focal lesions with DWI useful for identifying early changes.
- EEG: Periodic lateralized epileptiform activity may be seen and is associated with a poor prognosis.

Diagnosis
- Discuss with paediatric infectious disease colleagues.
- Examination of vesicular fluid/skin scrapings:
  - histology: multinucleated giant cells or intranuclear inclusions;
  - electron microscopy: viral particles identified.
- Viral isolation from throat, stool, urine, CSF (viral culture media swabs needed).
- PCR of CSF, early samples may be –ve. Consider repeat LP.
- Serology less useful as IgM response may be delayed.
- Elevated liver enzymes suggest disseminated disease.
- Refer mother to sexual health clinic for testing.

Treatment
- Aciclovir (see Aciclovir in Chapter 7 ➋ p. 650) for 21 days.
- Supportive treatment.

Outcome
Mortality is highest for those with disseminated infection (30–60%). Lower in those with isolated CNS disease (15%). High levels of morbidity in survivors from both groups.

Syphilis
- Incidence remains low in the UK but is rising.
- Consider if risk factors exist such as intravenous drug abuse or maternal HIV infection.
- Transplacental infection usually occurs in the 2nd or 3rd trimester (due to a protective effect in the early placenta).
- Maternal spirochetaemia can occur in the primary, secondary, or early latency stages of her disease. Outcome is worse if infection occurs in the primary or secondary stages.
- The spirochetes infect many organs.

Systemic features
Features are not usually present until the infant is at least 2 weeks old. Similar systemic features to other TORCH infections but skin and mucocutaneous lesions are common with a predilection for the face, oral, and anogenital regions. Liver enzymes are ↑. Abnormalities in long bones x-ray in ~65% of symptomatic newborn.

Neurological signs are usually absent but signs of a subacute meningitis maybe present with a CSF pleocytosis (usually less than 50) and a mildly elevated protein (<1 g/dL). Cranial nerve palsies (VII, III, IV, and VI), a bulging fontanelle, or hydrocephalus may be present.

Investigations
Combination of tests usually needed including:
- Dark field microscopic examinations of placenta, skin, mucocutaneous lesions, nasal discharge, umbilical cord.
- Serology, VDRL test in serum or CSF (can get false +ves).
- IgM Fluorescence Treponema antibody-absorbed (FTA-ABS) assay (more specific).
- PCR for *Pallidum* DNA in serum or CSF.

Treatment
Penicillin G for 14 days. If the mother has been treated in pregnancy, treatment of the infant may not be necessary.

Outcome
Prognosis depends on severity of damage before treatment is started. Neurological sequelae are rare if treated promptly.

Enteroviruses
Maternal infection with coxsachie viruses A or B or echovirus just prior to or during delivery can cause an aseptic meningitis or meningoencephalitis.

Abnormal signal may be seen in the cerebral white matter on MRI. Infections are more common in summer or autumn.

Diagnosis
- PCR for enterovirus RNA in CSF.
- Viral isolation from urine, throat, rectal swabs, and CSF.

Outcome
Generally good.

Varicella

Two syndromes exist. Both are rare.

Congenital varicella syndrome
- Infection in first 20 weeks of pregnancy.
- CNS features include meningoencephalitis, myelitis, dorsal root ganglionopathies, denervation, and hypoplasia of muscle, cutaneous scars in a dermatome distribution, chorioretinitis, microphthalmia, cataracts, optic atrophy, Horner syndrome. Mortality 30%.

Perinatal varicella
- Due to maternal chickenpox infection within 7 days of (before or after) delivery.
- Multiorgan infection similar to herpes simplex with necrosis of the brain parenchyma.
- Diagnosis is by viral isolation from lesions or IgM in serum.
- Treatment: VZIG within 48–96 h birth. Consider additional prophylactic aciclovir IV 10 mg/kg tds for 10 days, if mother developed chickenpox within -4 to + 2 days of delivery.

Diagnosis
- CSF analysis at birth is usually normal.
- IgM in serum.
- PCR for varicella DNA in serum and CSF.

Outcome
- Depends on the degree of damage to CNS/PNS.
- It is unclear if immune globulin or aciclovir administered to the mother gives any protection to the fetus; however, outcome of the perinatal form can be improved by giving VZIG to affected neonate.

Lymphocytic choriomeningitis virus (LCMV)

Uncommon but possibly under diagnosed.
- Exposure to rodents needed (virus stable in murine urine and faeces).
- Foetal infection requires maternal infection in 1st or 2nd trimester.
- CNS features similar to other TORCH infections including neuronal migration defects, microcephaly, and periventricular calcifications. All cases have chorioretinitis.
- Higher rate of spontaneous abortion.
- Diagnosis serological: PCR not available.
- No specific treatment is available.

Zika virus

- Zika is a flavivirus transmitted by mosquitos. Epidemic causing infection in early pregnancy in Brazil caused public health emergency in 2016; 10-fold increase in microcephaly recorded.

Diagnosis
- CSF PCR, serum IgM.
- Exposure can cause congenital abnormalities including microcephaly (with overriding sutures) caused by parenchymal hypoplasia/atrophy or abnormal cortical development, subcortical/cerebellar calcification, ventriculomegaly, ophthalmic (macular scars/retinal/optic nerve abnormalities) and osteoskeletal abnormalities (arthrogryposis/hip dysplasia).

Treatment
- No specific treatment is available.

Outcome
- Miscarriage, still birth, Children surviving develop a severe cerebral palsy phenotype.

'Pseudo-TORCH' syndromes

Aicardi–Goutières syndrome is the best known example of a range of genetically determined disorders of regulation of inflammation causing pictures closely resembling congenital infection including CSF pleocytosis ± intracerebral calcification. See 'Autoinflammatory' conditions in this chapter ➔ p. 401.

Consequences of congenital HIV infection

Children with congenital HIV are increasingly surviving into adulthood due to antiretroviral treatments (ART). HIV is a neurotropic virus and neurological manifestations are common. Presentations depend on:
- Age of the child.
- Level of immunosuppression as reflected in CD4 count:
  - opportunistic infection more likely if <200 cells/mL.
- Viral load.
- Access, adherence, and resistance to ART medication.

HIV-related syndromes of CNS
- Meningitis:
  - *Acute*: all bacterial causes more likely including *Listeria*;
  - *Chronic*: Fungal e.g. *Candida*, TB, *Cryptococcus, Nocardia*.
- Encephalitis.
- HSV, VZV, CMV.
- JC virus causing progressive multifocal leukoencephalopathy (PML). See JC virus in this chapter ➔ p. 380.
- Space-occupying lesions:
  - *Infection-related*: all bacterial abscesses more common; infective granulomas due to TB, *Toxoplasma, Aspergillus*; JC virus (PML).
  - *Neoplasia*: primary CNS lymphoma (may be associated with EBV), glioma.

HIV-related syndromes of PNS
- Polyradiculitis due to CMV or VZV.
  - neuropathic pain localized to one or more dermatomes.
- Myelitis due to HIV.
- Peripheral neuropathies:
  - HIV sensory neuropathy;
  - shingles (VZV);
  - Guillain–Barré syndrome (more common in adults as part of seroconversion illness);
  - ART complications.
- Myositis: HIV, CMV, ART complications.

Stroke-like syndromes and dementia
- *Vascular*: Embolic or secondary to venous thrombosis, VZV vasculitis, cerebral aneurysms, moyamoya syndrome.
- *Infection*: HIV dementia, JC (PML).

Static encephalopathy
- Developmental impairment (occasionally regression) with microcephaly.
- Cerebral palsy syndromes particularly spastic diplegia.

History and examination
HIV infection may have already been diagnosed but should be considered if no diagnosis or cause has been identified for children with neurological disorders in the above list, particularly if the course is unusual, if the child has other illnesses suggestive of HIV (lymphadenopathy, weight loss, oral ulcers, parotid gland swelling, haematological abnormalities, elevated immunoglobulin levels, etc.) or if parental risk factors exist.

Antenatal screening is routine in the UK and many countries but patients can opt out or have inadequate antenatal care. Occasionally asymptomatic abnormalities are detected on neonatal USS, e.g. basal ganglia calcification or an infarct.

Investigations
- Establish HIV status with parental consent.
- If +ve consider investigations depending on the neurological presentation:

CNS infection or space-occupying lesion
- Liaise with infectious diseases colleagues before taking samples. Consider CSF PCR for TB, toxoplasma, CMV, JC, HSV, VZV, EBV.
- Send blood for cultures, cryptococcal antigen.
- Store serum sample for serology.
- Check HIV viral load in plasma and CSF.
- Fundoscopy for retinitis in CMV.
- Consider brain biopsy if diagnosis still unclear or no improvement after specific treatment(s).
- Cranial imaging findings depend on neurological syndrome but may reveal basal ganglia calcification or cerebral atrophy as well as other abnormalities.

PNS picture

- Send CSF for PCR for CMV, VZV, HSV. Check HIV viral load in plasma & CSF.
- Nerve conduction studies/EMG.

Stroke-like syndrome or dementia

- Send CSF for PCR for VZV.
- Liaise with neurosurgical colleagues if an aneurysm or moyamoya is suspected (formal angiography may be needed).

Static encephalopathy

- Cranial imaging.

Treatment

Liaise closely with infectious diseases colleagues:

- TB: see Tuberculous meningitis in this chapter ➲ p. 364.
- *Toxoplasma*: pyrimethamine (with folinic acid) and sulphadiazine.
- CMV: ganciclovir ± foscarnet.
- *Cryptococcus*: manage ↑ICP, amphotericin B and fluconazole: see Cryptococcosis in this chapter ➲ p. 375.
- *Aspergillus*: amphotericin.
- PML: see JC virus in this chapter ➲ p. 380.
- Neurosurgical referral as required for treatable vascular disorders, brain abscesses, complications of CNS infections causing ↑ICP, consideration of brain biopsy.
- Child development team referral.

Inflammatory disease of the CNS

CNS manifestations and/or complications are recognized in many auto-immune diseases. For discussion of CNS complications of *known systemic* autoimmune disease including juvenile idiopathic (rheumatoid) arthritis (JIA), and Kawasaki disease see Rheumatology consults in Chapter 5 → p. 604. For diseases with prominent renal involvement (Henoch Schönlein purpura, haemolytic–uraemic syndrome) see Renal consults in Chapter 5 → p. 597.

This section addresses *primary* CNS neuroinflammation. This possibility should be considered particularly in the context of:

- New-onset encephalopathy of unidentified cause, particularly if associated with a movement disorder and/or psychiatric features and sleep disturbance.
- New-onset movement disorder of unidentified cause.
- Focal deficits including cranial nerve signs or mononeuritis multiplex.
- Very rarely, isolated new-onset aggressive epilepsy in school-age children.

The differential diagnosis of neuroinflammatory disease will include other causes of psychosis and acute confusional state (see Agitation and confusion in Chapter 3 → p. 114). Important differentials include infectious encephalitis, glioma, and lymphomatous infiltration.

We can conveniently distinguish *autoimmune* disorders due to dysregulation of the adaptive (specific) immune system and *autoinflammatory* disorders due to dysregulation of the innate (general) immune response.

Autoimmune encephalopathy

Autoimmune encephalopathies typically present in previously well young people. Onset of neurological deficits is abrupt, although a prodrome of subtle cognitive or behavioural changes may be reported.

Detectable serum and/or CSF antibodies may be present, directed against ion channels, receptors, and synaptic proteins. Although the antigenic targets are generally expressed throughout the CNS, the clinical syndrome may reflect a more focused target. Exclusion of active CNS infection is essential.

Clinical presentation

Neuropsychiatric features are common and reflect dysfunction of the hippocampus (short-term memory loss), the wider limbic system (confusion, seizures, psychosis) and/or brainstem (central hypoventilation), producing a 'limbic encephalitis' phenotype. (Some of these features help distinguish autoimmune from viral aetiologies):

- Altered level of consciousness.
- Amnesia.
- Cognitive impairment (developmental regression in younger child).
- Confusion.
- Expressive dysphasia/ mutism.
- Focal neurologic deficits.
- Seizures.
- Psychiatric features.

- Movement disorder.
- Autonomic instability.
- Sleep disturbance (e.g. insomnia).

Investigation
- Blood tests: FBC, ESR, CRP, ferritin, serum lactate, TSH, free-thyroxine, and thyroid antibodies; serologic testing for infectious causes.
- MRI is unremarkable in the majority.
- CSF: opening pressure, cell count, lactate, culture, and PCR for virus. CSF may show some evidence of inflammation such as oligoclonal bands (see Table 2.4. Interpretation of oligoclonal band findings in Chapter 2 ➋ p. 99).
- EEG shows encephalopathic change (see Fig. 4.7).
- Investigation for underlying malignancy in appropriate contexts (e.g. ovarian imaging in ♀s over the age of 12yr).

CNS autoantibodies
- Pathogenic mechanisms vary between autoantibodies. The detected antibody may not always be directly responsible for the clinical phenotype (i.e. may be an epiphenomenon).
  - Antibodies targeting cell surface antigens are more probably pathogenic than those targeting intracellular antigens.
- Different antibody-detection techniques vary in sensitivity and specificity.
- A partial list of antibodies implicated in neuroimmune disorders to date is listed in Table 4.8 in this chapter ➋ p. 396).
- Many adult neurological paraneoplastic syndromes are due to antibodies reacting with *intracellular* antigens (e.g. anti-Hu): these do not respond well to treatment. In contrast, conditions related to *cell surface* antigens respond more favourably to immunomodulatory therapy.

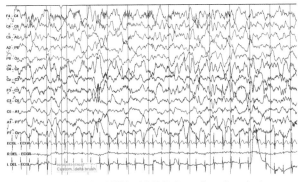

Fig. 4.7 Extreme 'delta brush' EEG in NMDAR disease (frontally predominant runs of rhythmic beta superimposed on generalized delta).

▶▶The most frequent antibodies detected in children with autoimmune encephalitis are NMDAR-Ab and MOG-Ab. These should be tested in all patients with suspected autoimmune encephalitis (in serum and CSF).

N-Methyl D-Aspartate Receptor (NMDAR)-Ab

- Antibodies should be tested in the serum and CSF (the latter is more sensitive).
- Presentation typically an encephalopathic syndrome with prominent psychiatric symptoms, a movement disorder, and seizures.
- The movement disorder is characteristically complex, with chorea in almost all causes, plus other hyperkinetic movements (most commonly complex stereotypies/repetitive movements).
- About 40% under the age of 18yr.
- Typically severe: 75% admitted to ICU.
- NMDAR was originally reported as a paraneoplastic syndrome in young adult ♀s with ovarian teratoma.
  - Abdominal and pelvic imaging (MRI or US) should be performed in all cases (with additional chest MRI for neuroblastoma in under 5 s) although association with malignancy less frequent in children.
- Brain MRI frequently normal despite severe illness ('clinical radiologic paradox').
- EEG is encephalopathic in the majority, with generalized rhythmic delta activity with or without epileptic discharges. Extreme 'delta brush' is a continuous EEG pattern initially thought specific to NMDAR-Ab encephalitis but now known to also be a feature of other severe encephalopathies (Fig. 4.7).
- Recovery is slow (up to 18 months) and in reverse order of symptom presentation (last symptom to develop is the first to resolve).
- Relapses (in ~12%) are often less severe than initial presentation.
- Complete recovery in 75%.
- Milder or partial phenotypes of NMDAR can occur either at initial presentation or at relapse: these episodes are also immunotherapy responsive.
  - Fewer than 1% of NMDAR cases have a single symptom: the clinical relevance of a low +ve titre should be questioned in those presenting with *isolated* psychiatric symptoms, seizures, or movement disorder.
- There is some correlation between antibody titres and clinical state but the utility of monitoring antibodies levels during disease course is not clear. High titres in both the serum and CSF may persist despite clinical recovery.
- Previously –ve antibody titres rising again in association with recurrent symptoms suggests relapse.

Treatment

No high-quality trial evidence, but consensus guidelines are available:
- Immediate first-line immunotherapy with intravenous methylprednisolone (IVMP), followed by IVIG in more severe patients.

Maintenance of first-line therapy (monthly IVIG or IVMP or oral steroids) for several months is recommended.
- Increasing trend to *very early rituximab use* which appears to shorten duration (effect depends on falling CD20 cell count which typically takes 2–3 weeks hence early use).
- Cyclophosphamide, and escalation to tocilizumab, if improvement is not clear or sustained.
- In very encephalopathic patients, risk–benefit of PLEX needs to be considered (risk of dysautonomia) and usually entails ICU stay where secondary morbidity is common.
- Further rituximab or mycophenolate mofetil (MMF) generally given if symptoms persist or if maintenance immunotherapy over a prolonged course is required.
- Symptomatic treatment with long-acting benzodiazepines, anticonvulsants, and clonidine can be beneficial.
- Antipsychotic-related adverse effects are common, but these medications are frequently also required.

NMDAR antibodies in Herpes encephalitis

NMDAR antibodies have been identified in 50% of children with clinical relapse in the weeks after HSV encephalitis. Typically there is:
- No evidence of ongoing active HSV infection in CSF.
- New movement disorder.
- Subtle cognitive decline (more common in older children).
- White matter change on MRI (often bilateral).
- Good response to immunotherapy.

Caution is required when in giving steroids in view of possible viral reactivation, but worsening of reported cases with steroid treatment is yet to be reported.

Anti-MOG antibody encephalitis

As well as the more typical acute demyelination syndrome associated with MOG antibody disease (MOGAD, see Paediatric MOGAD in this chapter ➔ p. 270) an encephalitic picture with prominent seizures is increasingly recognized as 'the other important identifiable paediatric autoimmune encephalitis' (~7% all cases). Clinically it resembles a 'viral meningitis'. It has characteristic MRI changes in ribbon-like distributions along the cortex showing hyperintensity on FLAIR. For investigation and treatment see Paediatric MOGAD in this chapter ➔ p. 270.

Limbic encephalitis and other seronegative autoimmune encephalopathies
- Although these phenotypes were initially reported in association with neuronal antibodies, around 50% patients are antibody –ve by currently available methods.
- Presentation with polysymptomatic encephalopathy with seizures, psychiatric features, and movement disorder.
- EEG encephalopathic.
- Phenotype is typically less severe but long-term outcome worse with higher rate of cognitive difficulties and epilepsy compared to 'antibody +ve' autoimmune encephalitis.

- 'Seronegative' patients may nonetheless respond to immunotherapies.
- Increasing role of rituximab as first-line treatment in this group (provided other diagnosis such as explosive onset epilepsies have been excluded).

Hashimoto encephalitis

- Sometimes referred to as steroid responsive encephalopathy associated with autoantibodies to thyroperoxidase (STREAT).
- Acute encephalopathy (often with seizures), responding to steroids and immunomodulation, often developing in children with recently identified hypothyroidism (although some children may be euthyroid).
- Anti-thyroid peroxidase (ATPO) antibodies are typically present , but are also commonly found in neurologically asymptomatic hypothyroid individuals.

Paraneoplastic syndromes in children

Opsoclonus-myoclonus ('dancing eyes and dancing feet') syndrome

- Affects infants and young children.
- Characterized by complex eye and limb movement disorder.
  - Opsoclonus (sometimes known as 'saccadomania') is a condition of uncontrolled, frequent, conjugate, saccadic eye movements often occurring in flurries.
  - Although the syndrome is named for this feature, it is often fleeting and subtle—the most striking feature is often extreme irritability.
  - Small amplitude limb myoclonus and true ataxia are also present to varying extents.
- Strongly associated with neuroblastoma and appears to be a paraneoplastic autoimmune phenomenon. Although post-infectious opsoclonus-myoclonus (OMS) is described, some suggest that in apparent neuroblastoma –ve cases the tumour has simply regressed.
- Although the oncological prognosis is usually good, the neurodevelopmental outlook can be poor unless aggressive immunosuppression is instituted.
- Mainstay of treatment is immunomodulation with corticosteroids (e.g. monthly dexamethasone pulses) and cyclophosphamide or rituximab. IVIG and plasmapheresis are also reported as being effective.
- Investigation:
  - spot and 24 h urine collection for catecholamines (may be –ve);
  - MIBG (iodine-131-meta-iodobenzylguanidine) scintigraphy can help localize a neuroblastoma (requires blockade of MIBG uptake into thyroid with potassium iodide for several days before and after injection);
  - MRI ± surgical biopsy confirm tumour presence.

Anti-Hu neuropathy

- Well-described in adults: occasionally presents before 18.
- Paraneoplastic relationship to neuroblastoma with opsoclonus-myoclonus recognized.
- The neuropathy is often purely sensory and associated with cerebellitis, limbic encephalitis, autonomic dysfunction, and/or brainstem encephalitis.

Table 4.8 Described autoimmune syndromes

Targeted antigen	Main phenotypes in adults	Phenotypes in children	Disease course
NMDA receptor	Characteristic autoimmune encephalopathy.	Similar phenotypes to adults. 40% of patients are children	Prolonged course. 75% admitted to ICU. Full recovery in 75%; relapse in 12%. Associated with ovarian teratoma.
	HSV encephalitis neurological relapse (children >adults).		Good respond to immunotherapy
Myelin Oligodendrocyte Glycoprotein	NMOSD, cortical encephalitis	ON, TM, ADEM, cortical encephalitis Encephalopathy with seizures (normal MRI, typically ↑CSF WCC)	Monophasic or relapsing; persistence of antibodies associated with relapsing disease.
Anti-aquaporin 4	ADS: NMOSD	NMOSD	Immunotherapy responsive, relapsing. Worsening symptoms with MS drugs.
GFAP	Meningoencephalitis with CSF lymphocytosis and ↑protein	As adults: characteristic MRI appearances ('freckling' of pons with halo around aqueduct)	Immunotherapy responsive. Typically monophasic.
LGI1	Limbic encephalitis	Very small numbers of reported paediatric cases for all these Very small numbers of reported paediatric cases for all these	Often monophasic. Good response to immunotherapy. Memory problem may persist beyond the acute event.
CASPR2	Peripheral nerve hyperexcitability		Chronic disease. Symptomatic treatment.
	PERM, 'stiff-person' syndrome		Immunotherapy responsive.

GABA$_B$	Encephalitis with prominent seizures.	Some response to immunotherapy. Associated with small cell lung cancer.
GABA$_A$	Encephalopathy with refractory seizures and status epilepticus.	Extensive cortical and subcortical MRI abnormalities. Positive TPO and GAD65 antibodies Long-term outcome is poor.
DPPX	Cognitive dysfunction, psychiatric features, resting tremor, and myoclonus PERM	Immunotherapy responsive (aggressive). Associated with diarrheal illness.
mGluR1	Cerebellar ataxia +/- Hodgkin's Lymphoma	
mGluR5	Limbic encephalitis	Improvement with tumour resection. Immunotherapy responsive.
AMPA receptor	Limbic encephalitis.	Frequently relapse. Associated with multiple tumours. Response to immunotherapy.
GAD	Stiff-person syndrome	Usually chronic disorders.

For abbreviations see text and Symbols and abbreviations list (p. xix).

Autoimmune CNS vasculopathies

- CNS vasculitis may occur as an isolated phenomenon of unknown cause (primary CNS vasculitis) or be associated with an identifiable systemic condition. The size, distribution, and degree of stenosis of affected vessels correlates with the neurologic manifestations.
- The most common CNS vasculitis in children is Systemic Lupus Erythematosis (SLE).
  - Occurs much less frequently in adults with SLE.
  - Patients may present with encephalopathy and/or seizures, headaches, or focal neurological deficits secondary to infarction.
  - Investigations include MRI and MRA, CSF analysis including oligoclonal bands and EEG if history of encephalopathy/behaviour change or seizures.
- Even in patients with known systemic autoimmune disease it is important to exclude non-vasculitic causes for neurological symptoms such as:
  - Infection in immunocompromised patient.
  - Hypertensive encephalopathy (due to renal disease or steroid use).
  - Uraemia.
- Management of CNS vasculitis is typically in conjunction with rheumatologist using a combination of steroids and steroid-sparing alternatives.

Sydenham chorea

This is regarded as a major neurological manifestation of rheumatic fever (i.e. by definition, preceded by group A β-haemolytic streptococcal infection). As with other post-streptococcal diseases, it had been very rare but has become more common again in recent years. Chorea is often a late feature, so clear history and/or evidence of the preceding infection is often absent.

Clinical features
- Insidious onset over weeks.
- Emotional lability often very prominent.
- Fidgety or clumsy involuntary movements: mostly myoclonic or semi-purposeful proximally with more complex distal movements (e.g. chorea of outstretched hands).
- Classically described features of motor *impersistence* including:
  - 'Jack in the box tongue' (inability to maintain protrusion).
  - 'Milkmaid's grip' (inability to maintain a grasp of the examiner's fingers resulting in rhythmic gripping).
- Also:
  - 'Spoon hands' (wrist flexion, hyperextension of the metacarpophalangeal joints, finger straightening, and thumb abduction).
  - 'Hung up' tendon reflexes (slow relaxation).
  - Hippus (slow rhythmic constriction and dilation of pupil).
- Prominent facial, tongue, and bulbar involvement.
- Speech is often dysarthric and/or 'explosive'.

- May be strikingly *asymmetrical* particularly at the outset.
- Writing, dressing, and feeding difficulty due to poor coordination.

Typically, spontaneous recovery is seen over 3 months. Rarely a paralytic chorea develops with extreme hypotonia and immobility (chorea mollis).

Investigations
- MRI: usually normal, but a transient ↑T2 signal in the head of caudate and putamen may be observed.
- Elevated ASOT and anti-DNAase B in supportive clinical context.
- Check copper and caeruloplasmin, TFTs, ANA and antiphospholipid antibodies (lupus anticoagulant, anticardiolipin) to exclude alternative diagnoses.
- Echocardiogram to look for evidence of cardiac involvement; it may show the characteristic pattern of mitral regurgitation.

Treatment
May be left untreated. If debilitating, consider:
- Levetiracetam, carbamazepine, sodium valproate (see Contraception and reproductive health in this chapter ⊃ p. 320) .
- Tetrabenazine, pimozide, or haloperidol.
- Rheumatic fever prevention with long-term antibiotic prophylaxis.
- The role of immunomodulation (IVIG, steroids or MMF) is unproven although has been used with increasing numbers of anecdotal +ve reports.

Cardiological aspects
- All children should be evaluated for rheumatic cardiac valve disease and if found should commence anti-streptococcal penicillin prophylaxis.
- Regimes and duration are controversial but should be continued at least until adulthood. Regimes include daily oral penicillin V (risk of poor long-term compliance) or particularly in developing countries monthly IM benzathine penicillin.

PANS (paediatric acute neuropsychiatric syndrome) and PANDAS (paediatric autoimmune neuropsychiatric disorders associated with streptococcus)

Controversial!
- Original descriptions in 1990s of acute onset OCD and/or tic disorders apparently related to infection with Group A Streptococcus (GAS) with subsequent relapsing/remitting course.
  - Dubbed PANDAS with hypothesized mechanism analogous to Sydenham Chorea (cross-reactivity of immune response against presumed basal ganglia targets) however this has not been consistently demonstrated, and large cohort studies have failed to demonstrate temporal relationship with exposure to GAS.
- In response to acknowledged limited experimental evidence for PANDAS hypothesis proponents proposed a broader PANS (Paediatric Acute Neuropsychiatric Syndrome) hypothesis expanded to implicate other and as yet unidentified infectious triggers in a wide variety of acute onset neuropsychiatric presentations.

- Proponents stress the agreed need for thorough evaluation of children with psychiatric presentations for potential infectious/autoimmune encephalitic processes.
- Sceptics concerned about over-emphasis on posited inflammatory mechanisms over genetic, metabolic, neurodevelopmental (e.g. unrecognized ASD) and functional causes; with consequent demands for immunomodulatory treatment with real risks and likely placebo effects.
- Postulated involvement of as yet unidentified viruses and/or pathogenic mechanisms with no proposed biomarkers makes it difficult to exclude clinically or research scientifically.
- Periodic exacerbations of symptoms are well recognized in children and young people with (presumed non-inflammatory) chronic OCD and/or tic disorders.

The role for immunomodulation in PANS/PANDAS presentations remains unproven, though there is consensus on the importance of symptomatic treatment of psychiatric symptoms which may often be highly disabling.

Rasmussen encephalitis

Rare condition presenting with new-onset, increasingly continuous, and aggressive epilepsy, often *epilepsia partialis continua* (EPC).
- Onset typically between 5 and 15 years.
- Untreated, disease follows slow but inexorably progressive course with development of increasingly fixed focal motor (hemiplegia) and cognitive (e.g. aphasia) deficits, with intractable epilepsy.
- Clinical course mirrored by MRI evidence of slowly progressive, confluent, and uni-hemispheric inflammatory process, progressing eventually to unilateral atrophy.
- Histology shows a T-cell mediated inflammatory process.
- Some cases appear to have been triggered by minor head trauma.
- An autoimmune mechanism is presumed, but the autoantigen has not as yet been identified. Why disease should remain uni-hemispheric is unclear.
- Immunomodulatory treatment is an important option in the early stage of the disease.
  - First-line treatment with oral or IV steroids associated with IVIG.
  - Second-line therapy: azathioprine, rituximab, or adalimumab. Natalizumab, MMF, and anakinra show promise.
- Functional hemispherotomy usually required to provide adequate seizure control and may improve cognitive outcome if performed early, but with inevitable morbidity of a dense hemiparesis, and ipsilateral hemianopia.

'Autoinflammatory' conditions

Growing recognition of conditions where inflammatory processes have been activated without evidence of infection or specific adaptive immune responses (either humoral or cellular), hence 'autoinflammatory' rather than 'autoimmune'. Many of these are due to mutations of inflammation regulation genes resulting in amplification of one of four components of the innate immune response:

- Interleukin 1 (e.g. Chronic infantile neurological cutaneous and articular (CINCA) syndrome).
- Type 1 interferon (e.g. Aicardi–Goutières syndrome).
- NF-κB (nuclear factor kappa-light-chain-enhancer of activated B cells).
- Macrophages (e.g. Haemophagocytic lymphohistiocytosis (HLH)).

Interferonopathies

A family of conditions due to mutations in at least 7 different genes causing nucleic acid accumulation, interferon up-regulation, and an inappropriate activation of the innate immune system. Their clinical pictures differ significantly but they share the same 'interferonopathy signature' and interferon expression patterns in CSF are readily examined by specialist laboratories.

Neonatal form (Aicardi–Goutières Syndrome (AGS))

The originally described neonatal-onset form (AGS1 commonly due to mutations in *TREX1*) gives a picture extremely reminiscent of congenital infection ('pseudo-TORCH' syndrome) with encephalopathy, hepatosplenomegaly, abnormal LFTs, cerebral calcification on CT, and CSF pleocytosis. Epilepsy, acquired microcephaly, and severe neurodisability develop with time.

Infant-onset forms

Later-onset variants are most frequently due to *RNASEH2B* (AGS2) gene mutations. After a period of weeks to months of normal development the child develops encephalopathy with regression, declining OFC, and recurrent sterile pyrexias. Progression usually stops after a period of several months.

Later-onset forms

Other AGS subtypes show SLE-like features including chilblains, autoantibodies, and polygammaglobulinaemia. The subtype due to *SAMHD1* mutations (AGS5) features a large-vessel cerebral arteriopathy: children are at risk of catastrophic intracerebral haemorrhage.

Investigations

- CSF is initially abnormal but *becomes normal with time* (risking false −ves if performed late).
  - Findings include pleocytosis (typically ~20 cells but always <100) and elevated CSF interferon-α and neopterins.
- Radiological features comprise:
  - Intracerebral calcification of variable extent and distribution but most commonly affecting basal ganglia and deep white matter.
  - Can develop after several months (i.e. *false −ves* if done too early); may be missed on MRI.

- White matter changes—periventricular distribution.
- Atrophy—global with time including brainstem and cerebellum.

Management
- Janus Kinase 1 (JAK1) inhibitors (e.g. baricitinib) recommended for mongenic interferonopathies in children >2 years of age, with evidence to suggest a slowing of disease progression.

Haemophagocytic lymphohistiocytosis (HLH)

- Traditionally thought of as a systemic inflammatory condition, characterized by cytokine storm and multiorgan dysfunction.
- More recently isolated CNS presentations have been reported with no signs of systemic inflammation on initial presentation.
- Aetiology may be a primary genetic condition (familial haemophagocytic lymphohistiocytosis (fHLH)) or secondary to trigger such as infection, autoimmune disease, or malignancy.
- Current diagnostic criteria of systemic HLH require at least five of eight cardinal features:
  - Fever,
  - Splenomegaly,
  - Bicytopenia (i.e. low counts of at least two of RBC, WBC or platelets),
  - Hypertriglyceridemia and/or hypofibrinogenemia,
  - Haemophagocytosis,
  - Low/absent natural killer (NK)-cell-activity,
  - Hyperferritinemia,
  - High-soluble interleukin-2-receptor levels.
- Elevated CSF protein and prominent contrast enhancement on MRI are suggestive.
- Clinico-radiological discordance may be seen where extensive neuroimaging abnormalities are out of proportion to mild clinical signs and symptoms.

▶▶HLH should be considered in any presentation suggestive of atypical chronic or recurrent CNS inflammation. One historic clinical-radiological entity known as Chronic lymphocytic inflammation with pontine perivascular enhancement responsive to steroids (CLIPPERS) should be treated with particular suspicion. CLIPPERS comprises signs and symptoms referrable to the brainstem plus enhancing lesions in brainstem (especially pons) and sometimes supratentorial structures on MRI showing marked steroid responsiveness. Consider immunological and/or genetic testing for fHLH even in the absence of systemic inflammation.

- Mechanisms of CNS-restricted neuroinflammation are not fully understood but may relate to functional defects in T lymphocyte and NK cell cytotoxicity causing impaired antigen clearance.
- Steroids and chemotherapies (e.g. etoposide) are used to limit the hyperinflammatory state (after ruling out malignancy).

- Intrathecal steroid and methotrexate for patients with CNS involvement.
- Haematopoietic stem cell transplantation (HSCT) is the mainstay of treatment for fHLH, with unfortunately a high rate of treatment failure and morbidity and mortality.

Sarcoidosis

- Multisystem granulomatous inflammatory process.
- Recessive (loss of function) mutations in *NOD2* give rise to Early Onset Sarcoid (EOS).
- NOD2 is also a susceptibility gene in Crohn disease and Blau syndrome (a rare AD granulomatous disease).
- Common sites of involvement outside the CNS include the chest, joints, uveitis, testes, and kidney.
- Neurological manifestations are protean.
  - Sterile meningitis (visible on MRI with contrast) causing multiple cranial neuropathies and/or peripheral mononeuritis multiplex.
  - Diffuse CNS infiltrative disease particularly of the hypothalamus and pituitary.
  - Myelopathy.
  - Peripheral neuropathy.
- ↑serum (and CSF) ACE levels supportive, but not specific.
- Tissue diagnosis: demonstration of non-caseating granulomatous process, with exclusion of mycobacterial infection. Kveim test discontinued because of infection risk.
- *NOD2* gene testing.

Treatment is steroids ± azathioprine, MMF, or cyclophosphamide.

Mitochondrial disease

A heterogeneous group of diseases caused by failure of mitochondrial oxidative metabolism, with symptoms and biochemical defects therefore most evident in highly metabolically active organs (muscle, heart and brain) with large numbers of mitochondria. While characteristic histochemical changes such as cytochrome *c* oxidase (COX) deficient fibres and ragged-red fibres are often evident in muscle biopsies, the advent of panels and whole exome sequencing (WES) (see 'Molecular genetics', Chapter 2 ⊃ p. 81) has led to a marked decrease in the number of muscle biopsies being performed.

Suspicion of mitochondrial dysfunction may be prompted by various combinations of exercise intolerance, proximal weakness, axial hypotonia, dysphagia, hypopnea, refractory seizures, encephalopathy, delay in acquiring (or regression of) neurodevelopmental skills, unusual combinations of organ involvement (e.g. bone marrow + pancreas), elevated blood, or CSF lactate and suggestive neuroradiological findings.

The next diagnostic step is usually a genetic screen involving a large gene panel of known nuclear-encoded mitochondrial genes and separate sequencing of mitochondrial DNA (mtDNA), as current next-generation techniques do not examine mtDNA (see 'Molecular genetics', Chapter 2 ⊃ p. 81). If these results are −ve, or if other aetiologies are being considered, then this may be followed by triome whole exome (WES) or whole genome sequencing (WGS). Respiratory chain activity may be measured directly in skin fibroblasts or muscle biopsy to assess *in vivo* the functional relevance of novel or uncertain genetic findings.

As with many genetic conditions a given clinical phenotype may be caused by many mutations, in either nuclear or mitochondrial genomes; and conversely a single genotype can give rise to several distinct phenotypes.

Mitochondrial genetics

The sometimes marked genotypic/phenotypic variation has several causes:.

Two inheritance systems
- Mitochondrial DNA (mtDNA) is inherited maternally (the zygote is thought to recognize 'paternal' mitochondria from sperm shortly after fertilization and to destroy them by ubiquitination) but the *large majority* of mitochondrial proteins are in fact coded for by genes in the cell nucleus (with standard Mendelian, not maternal inheritance).
  - mtDNA codes for 13 polypeptides and 24 structural RNA molecules. The 13 polypeptides are key constituents of the multimeric respiratory chain complexes I, III, IV, and V, with only complex II being entirely encoded in the nuclear genome.
  - These polypeptides account for only a small fraction of the entire mitochondrial proteome of more than 1800 proteins, almost all of which are imported into mitochondria.
- Thus, a single phenotype (e.g. chronic progressive external ophthalmoplegia, CPEO) may be sporadic, autosomal dominant, autosomal recessive, or maternally inherited.
- It is suggested that mtDNA encoded defects give milder disease than nuclear-encoded DNA defects: they tend to present later and be

associated with better life expectancy. However, in many cases this is probably just a reflection of the proportion of mutated mtDNA present (heteroplasmy; see next)—higher levels generally being associated with earlier onset of more severe disease.

Heteroplasmy and mosaicism
- There are many hundreds of mitochondria present in a single myocyte and each mitochondrion contains approximately 10–15 copies of mtDNA. However, the mitochondria in one cell are genetically heterogeneous, and a dual population of wild-type and mutated mtDNA may co-exist (heteroplasmy) while remaining clinically silent. Only if the proportion of mutated mtDNA exceeds a tissue-dependent 'threshold', will disease ensue.
- Disease manifestations typically reflect the function of tissues highly dependent on oxidative metabolism including brain, muscle (skeletal and cardiac), kidney (tubules), liver, gut, and pancreas (endocrine and exocrine).
- Mitochondria are randomly segregated into daughter cells during meiosis, and this may result in a skewed distribution of mutated mtDNA among a cell population. When this process occurs during foetal organogenesis, some tissues inherit high levels of mutant mtDNA while levels may be considerably lower in others. For reasons which aren't entirely clear some pathogenic mtDNA variants are also 'lost' from rapidly dividing tissues; this can be problematic when testing blood DNA from older children for large-scale single deletions and specific point variants (m.3243A>G).

Greater frequency of point mutations and poorer repair mechanisms
- Estimates suggest that the carrier frequency for pathogenic mtDNA variants is 1 in 200 of the UK population, though most of these carriers will have extremely low heteroplasmy and not be at risk of developing disease. Approximately 1 in 5000 adults develop mitochondrial disease as a consequence of either mtDNA or nuclear DNA variants.

Clinical presentations

Mitochondrial disease can present at all ages but there is a bimodal distribution with a peak in early infancy and a second broader peak in late teenage to early 30s though cases may present even later. Multiple, apparently unrelated organs can be affected typically including combinations among muscle, heart, eyes, brain (including hearing, seizures, extrapyramidal syndromes), liver, blood, and pancreas. Some combinations have been defined as 'syndromes' although even these can be incomplete or overlap.

Myopathy
The single most common feature: typically proximal and may include the face and exercise-related features such as myalgia and rhabdomyolysis.

Eye movements
Ptosis and/or external ophthalmoplegia (i.e. inability of either eye to abduct) are very characteristic changes in adults but less often observed in

children. Typically these are slowly progressive: the main differential in practice is myasthenia.

Eye involvement

Retinal pigmentation, cataracts, or optic atrophy are seen. (see Leber hereditary optic neuropathy (LHON) this chapter p. 409).

CNS involvement

CNS manifestations can be protean, and relatively non-specific, including pyramidal and extrapyramidal syndromes (dystonia), seizures (epilepsia partialis continua), migraine, and stroke-like episodes.

- MRI can be correspondingly non-specific but highly symmetrical changes can be an indicator of metabolic processes (rather than injury by extrinsic processes).
- Symmetric high T2 signal of the basal ganglia and brainstem is effectively the radiological counterpart of Leigh syndrome (historically defined pathologically) and is particularly suggestive of mitochondrial disease (although there are alternative causes).
- Calcification of the basal ganglia (CT imaging) is seen in MELAS (see below) as well as a number of other 'metabolic' disorders. Areas of infarction associated with mitochondrial stroke-like episodes tend to occur in the parieto-occipital regions and often do not conform to a single vascular territory.
- Diffuse symmetrical white matter changes are associated with a number of pathogenic nuclear DNA variants (*SURF1, NDUFS1, TYMP, DARS2* and *ISCA2*) and much less frequently, pathogenic mtDNA variants (large-scale single deletions, m.8344A>G).
- MR spectroscopy allows estimation of lactate contents of a 'region of interest' but in most circumstances probably adds little to CSF lactate estimation.

Sensorineural deafness

Particularly if acquired and symmetrical. A combination of deafness and diabetes (or family history of such combinations) is very suggestive. Deafness usually found in conjunction with other features of mitochondrial disease constituting part of a clinical syndrome and a common consequence of specific mutations in mtDNA (*MTTL1, MTTS1* and single large-scale deletions) and nuclear genes (*RRM2B, RMND1, SERAC1,* and *SUCLA2*).

Cardiac involvement

Unexplained hypertrophic or dilated cardiomyopathy may require transplantation, but the appropriateness of this option should be considered carefully in the presence of multisystem disease. Right bundle branch block and Wolff-Parkinson-White (WPW) syndrome may be symptomatic and require drug treatment or implanted pacemaker.

Renal disease

Tubular dysfunction (Fanconi syndrome) with mutations in *RRM2B*; cystic dysplasia (*RMND1* mutations) or focal segmental glomerulosclerosis (m.3243A>G). Transplantation may be an option though again should be considered carefully in the setting of multisystem disease.

Pancreatic disease

Exocrine pancreas dysfunction (resulting in fat malabsorption and steator-rhoea) in Pearson's Marrow-Pancreas Syndrome due to a large-scale single deletion or rearrangement of mtDNA, or endocrine dysfunction causing diabetes mellitus.

Liver disease

Hepatocerebral mtDNA depletion syndromes cause profound encephalop-athy and liver failure: when associated with seizures and later a movement disorder, suspect Alpers-Huttenlocher Syndrome (see Alpers-Huttenlocher syndrome/progressive neuronal degeneration of childhood (PNDC) this chapter ➍ p. 409) and investigate for mutations in *POLG1*. Neonatal liver failure with lactic acidaemia may be due to mutations in *TRMU* and asso-ciated with a good prognosis if the patient can be supported through the liver failure.

Haematological disease

Sideroblastic anaemia or pancytopaenia have been associated with Pearson's Syndrome, resulting from large-scale single deletions or rearrangements of mtDNA, and MLASA (Myopathy, Lactic Acidosis and Sideroblastic Anaemia) as a consequence of mutations in *PUS1* or *YARS2*.

Suspecting mitochondrial disease

Clues

- Presence of a recognized syndrome, including partial and overlapping forms.
- Multiorgan involvement of combinations of the above systems.
- Short stature.
- A history of stepwise neurological or neurodevelopmental deteriorations with variable, often incomplete, recovery between deteriorations.
- Any suggestion of disturbed respiratory drive (e.g. unexplained hypoventilation).
- High CSF protein (in the absence of CNS inflammation) suggests CNS necrosis.
  - Kearns–Sayre syndrome should be considered especially if concomitant CSF folate deficiency.
- High blood lactate, but more specifically high CSF lactate.
  - A mitochondrial basis for a clinical picture with prominent CNS involvement is unlikely if CSF lactate is normal (though CSF lactate may be normal in a predominantly peripheral, e.g. myopathic mitochondrial disease).
  - Recent status epilepticus, severe shock or asphyxia and meningitis are the main non-mitochondrial causes of high CSF lactate.

Investigation

- This should be directed by specialist advice guided by phenotype. It will often include serum and CSF lactate, urine organic acids (to detect 3 methylglutaconic aciduria), neuroimaging (MRI) and (rarely, nowadays) muscle biopsy.

- Levels of mutated mtDNA may be low or absent in blood and mtDNA pathogenic variants are not reliably detected using some methods of WES. In contrast, nuclear gene mutations are readily identified on DNA extracted from blood. WES or WGS are particularly useful in genetically heterogenous conditions such as Leigh syndrome (>75 genes currently known).
- Also important to screen for large-scale rearrangements and mtDNA depletion using other techniques such as long-range, real-time, or digital PCR in relevant tissue such as muscle.
- Multiomic approaches involving a combined assessment of genomic, proteomic, transcriptomic and metabolomic data is likely to help resolve the 30–40% of cases of suspected childhood mitochondrial disease who remain without a diagnosis despite the application of next-generation sequencing.

Muscle histochemistry

Characteristically ragged-red fibres (irregular reddish patches around the circumference of fibres visible on Gomori trichrome stain) representing accumulations or proliferations of abnormal mitochondria, though these are rarely seen in children younger than 5 years. Several important mitochondrial diseases, particularly those involving complex I and complex V, are not associated with histochemical changes on muscle biopsy; and some other non-mitochondrial primary myopathies, and even normal ageing, can also cause occasional ragged-red or cytochrome c oxidase (COX) deficient fibres. Electron microscopy may be helpful in demonstrating mitochondrial ultrastructural abnormalities.

Recognized syndromes

Leigh and Alpers-Huttenlocher syndromes are probably the most common mitochondrial syndromes in paediatric neurological practice: MELAS and MERRF are rare in children. The infantile-onset coenzyme Q_{10} (CoQ_{10}) biosynthetic defect is exceptionally rare but treatable.

Leigh syndrome

The most frequent clinical presentation of mitochondrial disease in childhood. Involvement of the brainstem and basal ganglia structures: originally defined pathologically but now essentially a radiological diagnosis. Clinically heterogeneous: often an early onset, aggressive picture of brainstem involvement (including eye movement and respiratory abnormalities, 'sighing respiration') plus a motor disorder (pyramidal & extrapyramidal). Stepwise deterioration is characteristic: occasionally a long period of stability can cause a child to be misdiagnosed as having 'cerebral palsy' before the ultimately progressive nature of the process declares itself.

A much rarer, dominantly inherited condition (autosomal dominant acute necrotizing encephalopathy, ADANE) has similar clinical features of acute deteriorations with intercurrent illness and superficially similar radiology. Its importance lies in identifying pre-symptomatic first-degree relatives who can benefit from immunization and prophylactic antibiotics to reduce risk of acute deterioration. The radiological discriminators include *involvement of the external capsule* in ADANE, which is relatively atypical for Leigh. Another Leigh-like syndrome, caused by recessive *SERAC1* mutations,

MEGDEL, is associated with urinary excretion of 3 MEthylGlutaconic acid, Deafness, Encephalopathy, and Leigh-like neuroimaging.

Alpers-Huttenlocher Syndrome/progressive neuronal degeneration of childhood (PNDC)

(See also Progressive neuronal degeneration of childhood in this chapter ➔ p. 409). Typically, present either in the toddler age group with a very characteristic picture of refractory status epilepticus (often *epilepsia partialis continua*, EPC) sometimes progressing after weeks or months to develop deranged liver function; or in adolescence with very aggressive new-onset epilepsy and EPC. In those children in whom a metabolic basis has been confirmed, nearly all have been mitochondrial with most due to mutations in *POLG1* though recently this phenotype has also been associated with mutations in the mitochondrial tRNA synthetase genes *FARS2*, *NARS2*, and *PARS2*.

Leber hereditary optic neuropathy (LHON)

Relatively painless (c.f. optic neuritis) onset of permanent visual failure occurs in late adolescence/early adulthood. This progresses over several weeks typically sequentially (one eye then the other) associated with swelling of the optic nerve head in the acute phase. Family history is found in >50% of cases. An early onset global dystonia is a rare phenotype associated with two of the primary LHON mtDNA variants (m.14484T>C and m.11778G>A).

Kearns–Sayre syndrome and chronic progressive external ophthalmoplegia

Chronic progressive external ophthalmoplegia (CPEO) is rare in children. Slowly progressive weakness of ocular muscles occurring over months or years sometimes with proximal limb weakness is very suggestive.

* Kearns–Sayre syndrome (KSS) is a more severe picture characterized by the onset of CPEO, cardiac involvement (arrhythmia or cardiomyopathy) and pigmentary retinopathy before the age of 20 yrs. Frequent additional features include proximal myopathy, ataxia, heart block (may be asymptomatic at presentation but important to detect), deafness, endocrinopathy (adrenal, thyroid, pancreas), renal tubular dysfunction, CSF folate deficiency, and extensive, sometimes cystic, white matter abnormalities.

Mitochondrial myopathy, encephalopathy, lactic acidosis, and stroke-like episodes (MELAS)

Stroke-like episodes occur (acute onset of any focal neurological syndrome) with focal acute inflammatory ischaemic changes on MRI that are not confined to a single vascular territory. Associated short stature, sensorineural hearing loss and gastrointestinal dysmotility (may present acutely as intestinal pseudo-obstruction often in conjunction with a stroke-like episode). Screen for cardiomyopathy and arrhythmias. Treat as focal epilepsy (acute EEG will usually locate focus corresponding to radiological and clinical lesion) with high-dose levetiracetam and clobazam and escalate treatment regime quickly if no response. No conclusive evidence for use of L-Arginine in acute treatment or prophylaxis of stroke-like episodes.

Myoclonic epilepsy with ragged-red fibres (MERRF)
This is a progressive myoclonic epilepsy (see Progressive myoclonus epilepsies this chapter ➲ p. 302) with typical onset in later childhood comprising seizures (multiple seizure types but including by definition myoclonic seizures), ataxia, myopathy (with ragged-red fibres), optic atrophy, headache, deafness, and progressive neurological deterioration with cognitive decline. Multiple lipomata in some individuals (Ekbom's Syndrome).

Infantile-onset coenzyme Q_{10} (CoQ_{10}) biosynthetic defects .
Recessive mutations identified in 9 genes to date. Incidence less than 1:100,000. Suspect in steroid resistant nephrotic syndrome without mutations in Nephrin or Podocin, especially in those also presenting with deafness or other CNS manifestations. Also suspect in those with clinical features of mitochondrial encephalomyopathies (especially when there is reduced activity of complex I+III and II+III), those with unexplained ataxia, those presenting with subacute exercise intolerance and weakness, or with signs of lipid accumulation in muscle, and those with chromosomal rearrangements involving chromosome 9q34. Treat with high-dose CoQ_{10} while investigation results pending.

A useful resource for parents and professionals for advice on case management is to be found at Wellcome Centre for Mitochondrial Research website: ℘ www.newcastle-mitochondria.com.

Movement disorders

Disorders in which there is excess of involuntary movement, or a paucity of voluntary or automatic movement. The speed and accuracy of movements are often disturbed. Often associated with abnormalities of tone, either hypo- or hypertonicity or a combination of the two affecting different body regions (e.g. low tone truncally and hypertonicity peripherally). Ataxia refers to the inability to produce smoothly coordinated movements.

Conditions predominated by dystonia

Transient idiopathic dystonia of infants
- Onset usually before 5mths and affects a single upper limb and trunk and to lesser degree the lower limb, causing a hemidystonia.
- Persists in sleep but attenuated.
- Abolished when infant moves purposefully.
- Resolves with no sequelae at around 12 mths.
- Familial cases have been reported, suggesting a possible genetic basis.
- One of the *transient benign paroxysmal movement disorders in infancy* which spontaneously resolve without consequences (See 'Non-Epileptic Phenomena' in this chapter ➋ p. 324).

Dyskinetic cerebral palsy
- Cerebral palsy predominated by dystonia, usually with elements of choreoathetosis.
- Accounts for 10–15% of cerebral palsy cases, but many children with spastic CP also experience intrusive dystonia.
- May result from acute, sustained, profound hypoxia-ischaemia (>10 min) in term infants, following pre-term delivery, or as a consequence of bilirubin-induced neurological dysfunction (BIND, kernicterus).
  - The latter can result from haemolytic disease of the newborn (in developing countries), ABO incompatibility in developed settings (particularly with early discharge), G6PD deficiency, or hyperbilirubinaemia in sick pre-term babies.
  - MRI of the brain frequently demonstrates basal ganglia or thalamic changes, but also may demonstrate white matter changes or, in some cases, no abnormalities.

Torticollis
- Torticollis and head tilt may result from a number of conditions (see Box 4.6). Look for associated signs such as orofacial dystonia, long tract signs, neck injury, or signs of ↑intracranial pressure.
- Episodic torticollis that is not fixed may be due to tics, paroxysmal dyskinesia (see Paroxysmal dyskinesias in this chapter ➋ p. 327), spasmus nutans (see Spasmus nutans in this chapter ➋ p. 136) or benign paroxysmal torticollis (see Benign paroxysmal torticollis in this chapter ➋ p. 325).

Isolated genetic dystonia (formerly Primary dystonia)
Group of monogenic disorders in which dystonia (±tremor) is the only neurological abnormality, and in which there are no neuroimaging abnormalities. Important causes include DYT-TOR1A, DYT-THAP1, DYT-KMT2B,

Box 4.6 Causes of torticollis
Cervical cord tumours, syrinx, and cervicomedullary junction malformations
Posterior fossa tumours
Diplopia
Sandifer syndrome
Spasmus nutans
Sternocleidomastoid injury and 'tumour'
Juvenile idiopathic arthritis
Dystonia
Tics
Benign paroxysmal torticollis of infancy
Paroxysmal dyskinesias

and DYT-GTPCH1. In all cases, dystonia disappears in sleep. Generally, these conditions are very responsive to deep-brain stimulation.

DYT-TOR1A dystonia (also known as Idiopathic Torsion Dystonia, Early Onset Generalized Dystonia)
- Important childhood cause of isolated dystonia.
- Autosomal dominant trait with reduced penetrance associated with mutations in the torsin A gene.
- Age of onset typically <15 yrs and starts as dystonia in one limb and often only in specific postures, frequently leading to misdiagnosis of a functional neurological disorder.
- Typically signs initially appear at the ankle resulting in abnormal foot posture and gait.
- Progresses over 5–10 yrs to become generalized involving the trunk and contralateral limbs. Then usually plateaus but results in significant deformity and contractures.

DYT-THAP1
- Focal, segmental, or generalized dystonia, with usually predominant craniocervical involvement.
- Typically later onset than DYT-TOR1A (mean age 19 years).
- Higher penetrance than DYT-TOR1A.

DYT-KMT2B
- Emerging important, possibly commonest, cause of childhood-onset generalized dystonia.
- Onset usually initially in lower limbs, ascending to craniocervical involvement, and prominent dysphonia.
- Variable other signs include developmental delay, microcephaly, intellectual disability, facial dysmorphism.

DYT-GTPCH1
- aka *GTPCH1* deficiency, Segawa Syndrome.

- Important form of Dopa-Responsive Dystonia (see Neurotransmitter Disorders in this chapter ⊃ p. 488).

Myoclonus-dystonia syndrome
- Autosomal dominant (AD) disorder with imprinting effects (only symptomatic if transmitted from father); onset before age 10.
- Majority due to mutations in the *SGCE* gene (DYT-SGCE), with mutations in the *KCTD17* more recently described.
- Mild dystonia usually affects proximal arm muscles and neck associated with stimulus-sensitive myoclonic jerks of proximal muscles.
- Psychiatric co-morbidity is commonly seen, particularly obsessive-compulsive disorder.
- Characteristically sensitive to alcohol (older members of the pedigree have usually identified this!).
- Myoclonus may also response to zonisamide. Beneficial responses to deep-brain stimulation are generally reported.

Mohr–Tranebjaerg syndrome
- Rare X-linked primary dystonia with profound sensorineural hearing loss.
- Deafness is early with development of dystonia in later childhood. Developmental impairment and long tract signs are also present.
- Caused by either mutation in *TIMM8A* gene or a contiguous gene deletion syndrome at Xq22.

Symptomatic and acquired dystonia
See Table 4.9 for causes of symptomatic dystonia.

Table 4.9 Causes of symptomatic dystonia

Metabolic/Genetic	Glutaric aciduria type 1
	Methylmalonic acidaemia
	Propionic acidaemia
	Lesch–Nyhan
	GM1 and GM2 gangliosidosis
	Homocystinuria
	Galactosaemia
	Niemann–Pick type C
	Mucopolysaccharidoses
	Sulphite oxidase deficiency
	Biotinidase deficiency
	Creatine deficiency
	HypoPTH
	Hartnup disease
	Tyrosinosis
	Vitamin E deficiency
	Pyruvate dehydrogenase deficiency

(Continued)

Table 4.9   (Contd.)

	Aromatic l-amino acid decarboxylase (AADC) deficiency
	Tyrosine hydroxylase deficiency
	Dopamine transporter deficiency syndrome
	5'phosphate oxidase (PNPO) deficiency
	Mitochondrial disorders
	Crigler-Najjar
	Bilirubin-induced neurological dysfunction (BIND)
	Guanidinoacetate methyltransferase (GAMT) deficiency
	Neurodegeneration due to cerebral folate transport deficiency (*FOLR1* mutations)
	Non-ketotic hyperglycinaemia
	Menkes disease
	L-2-hydroxyglutaric aciduria
	Thiamine transporter (*THTR2*) mutations (biotin responsive basal ganglia disease)
	GLUT1DS
	ATP1A3 mutations
Neurodegenerative	Ataxia telangiectasia
	Juvenile Huntington disease
	Metachromatic leukodystrophy
	Wilson disease
	Krabbe
	NBIA
	Neuronal ceroid lipofuscinosis
	Neuroaxonal dystrophy
	Rett syndrome
	Olivocerebellar atrophy
	Spinocerebellar ataxias
	Infantile bilateral striatal necrosis
	Pelizaeus–Merzbacher
	Neuroacanthocytosis
Drugs/Toxins	Phenothiazines
	Haloperidol
	Mitochondrial disease
	Metoclopramide
Others	Ischaemia or infection leading to striatal necrosis, basal ganglia infarction or porencephaly (often hemidystonia)
	Alternating hemiplegia of childhood
	HIV infection
	Basal ganglia neoplasm
	Vascular malformations

Treatment of dystonia
- Identify and treat potential triggers for dystonia, particularly any causes of pain such as constipation, GORD etc in a susceptible child (e.g. a child with cerebral palsy).
- Side effects are common with medications, consider risk/benefits when initiating.
- Clear goals for intervention should be established, with a time-line over which to measure improvement. The goal of interventions is not to reduce dystonia *per se* — there must be functional benefit to the child and/or carers through reduction of dystonia.
- Commonly used medications include trihexyphenidyl (dose ↑slowly to minimize unwanted effects), oral baclofen, and benzodiazepines.
- Gabapentin and clonidine may also be of benefit.
- For all children with idiopathic dystonia a trial of L-DOPA given in conjunction with a peripheral DOPA decarboxylase inhibitor should be considered: see Levodopa in Chapter 7 ➲ p. 682.
- Botulinum toxin A injections are increasingly used in the treatment of focal dystonias. There is an important role for physiotherapy to prevent contractures in prolonged or fixed dystonias.
- Episodes of severe generalized dystonia ('status dystonicus') can be difficult to treat: see Status dystonicus in Chapter 6 ➲ p. 682.
- Complex cases should be referred for consideration of neurosurgical interventions such as intrathecal baclofen or deep-brain stimulation.

Diseases associated with hypokinetic rigid syndrome

These frequently co-exist with dystonia. Some conditions causing a hypokinetic rigid syndrome in adults may present with dystonia in children.

Autoimmune disease
See Autoimmune encephalopathy in this chapter ➲ p. 391.

Juvenile Huntington disease
See Juvenile Huntington disease in this chapter ➲ p. 480.

Wilson disease
See Wilson disease in this chapter ➲ p. 480.

Neurodegeneration with brain iron accumulation
See Neurodegeneration with brain iron accumulation in this chapter ➲ p. 478.

Neuronal intranuclear inclusion disease
Rare heterogenous group of slowly progressive disorders with Parkinsonism, behavioural, and cognitive regression, progressive ophthalmoplegia, ataxia, intestinal pseudo-obstruction, and frequent oculogyric crises. Diagnosis is by demonstration of eosinophilic neuronal nuclear inclusions on rectal biopsy.

Primary dystonia–parkinsonism syndromes
Extremely rare conditions that include X-linked Parkinsonism and auto-somal dominant rapid-onset dystonia–Parkinsonism that may appear within 24 h. Treatment with L-DOPA and anti-Parkinsonian drugs is of limited use.

Niemann–Pick type C
See Niemann–Pick type C in this chapter ➜ p. 479.

Mitochondrial cytopathies
See Mitochondrial disease in this chapter ➜ p. 404.

Juvenile GM2 gangliosidosis (see Table 4.20)

Subacute sclerosing panencephalitis
See SSPE in this chapter ➜ p. 375.

Primary Parkinsonism and Parkinson disease
(Juvenile idiopathic Parkinsonism and early onset Parkinson's disease).
- Development of Parkinsonism before the age of 20 usually with preserved intellect.
- Heterogeneous group with different patterns of inheritance.
- *Dystonia of the feet is an early feature* in early onset Parkinson's disease: tremor and depression are less common than in the adult form.
- Main differentials are juvenile Huntington disease, Wilson disease, DOPA-responsive dystonia, and secondary causes of Parkinsonism.

All share good initial response to L-DOPA followed by fluctuating response and hyperkinetic movements. Many cases are variants of DOPA-responsive dystonia: see Neurotransmitter Disorders in this chapter ➜ p. 488.

Secondary Parkinsonism
- Due to hydrocephalus (especially aqueduct stenosis): improved by shunting.
- Central pontine myelinolysis.
- Drugs and poisons (mercury, manganese, carbon monoxide, methanol, risperidone, olanzapine, amphotericin B, cytosine-arabinoside).
- Infections (post-encephalitis, mycoplasma, influenza, PML).
- Basal ganglia neoplasm.

Symptomatic treatment of hypokinetic rigid syndrome
- Bradykinesia and rigidity respond better than tremor to dopamine agonists. Initially a trial of L-DOPA should be given in association with a peripheral decarboxylase inhibitor (benserazide or carbidopa). Entacapone may increase the bioavailability and duration of action.
- Common side effects include nausea, vomiting, orthostasis, and chorea.
- Experience of D2 agonists, such as bromocriptine, pergolide, apomorphine, pramipexole, ropinirole, and cabergoline in children is limited.
- Anticholinergic agents may also be used when L-DOPA is ineffective. Trihexyphenidyl is probably the most widely used paediatric anticholinergic agent.

Diseases associated with tremor

Physiological
- Often enhanced to clinically detectable levels by anxiety, excitement, caffeine, fatigue, or stress.

Essential
- Not a specific aetiological diagnosis, but rather a tremor syndrome with bilateral upper limb action tremor (often involving other body parts), present for at least 3 years, without evidence of other neurological signs.
- Autosomal dominant in many families, although tremor may be absent in first-degree relatives.
- Usually appears after school entry.
- Diagnosis is clinical and based on the finding of persistent fine (8–10 Hz) postural and action tremor of over 3 yr duration in the absence of other neurodevelopmental abnormalities, systemic disease, or drugs.
- May interfere with writing, is usually limited to the hands, but the jaw and neck may be affected. Exacerbated by stress and fatigue and relieved by alcohol. Treatment is not usually required, but first line is low-dose propranolol. Topiramate and levetiracetam may have some efficacy.

Jittering
- A high frequency, low amplitude tremor affecting limbs and the chin seen in nearly 50 % of all newborn infants during excitement and crying.
- Essentially a stimulus-sensitive clonus, it usually disappears in the neonatal period. It may also be a manifestation of hypoglycaemia, hypocalcaemia, drug withdrawal, or hypoxic–ischaemic injury.

Spasmus nutans
- A slow head tremor (2–4 Hz) seen in infants often with monocular horizontal nystagmus.
- Rarely seen after age 3 yrs.
- Has a benign course but needs to be differentiated from congenital nystagmus and MRI is necessary to rule out optic gliomas.

Secondary tremor

Endocrine
Hyperthyroidism; hypocalcaemia; hypoglycaemia; uraemia; vitamin B12 deficiency; Kwashiorkor.

Drugs and toxins
Salbutamol; sodium valproate; carbamazepine; L-DOPA; iron; neuroleptics; tricyclics; lithium; thyroid hormone; theophylline, caffeine; corticosteroids; calcium channel blockers; antihelminthics ('worm wobbles').

Metabolic
Hepatic and renal encephalopathy; Wilson disease; PKU; Lesch–Nyhan; NCL.

Neuromuscular
Spinal muscular atrophy; chronic polyneuropathy (Roussy–Levy syndrome); AIDP.

Structural
Hydrocephalus ('bobble head doll' syndrome); subdural haematoma.

Other
Opsoclonus-myoclonus (see Opsoclonus-myoclonus in this chapter ➲ p. 395); ataxia telangiectasia; Pelizaeus–Merzbacher; foetal alcohol syndrome; psychogenic.

Diseases associated with myoclonus

Physiological
A significant number of children have myoclonus without evidence of other neurological impairment, especially in sleep. This may comprise single myoclonic jerks at the onset of sleep or subtle erratic jerking of the hands, face, or legs in REM sleep. Rarely, physiological myoclonus can occur in wakefulness particularly after exertion, when fatigued or after a sudden sensory stimulus.

Benign neonatal sleep myoclonus; benign myoclonus of early infancy
See Benign neonatal sleep myoclonus in this chapter ➲ p. 324.

Essential
A sporadic or AD condition causing chronic focal, segmental, or generalized myoclonus. It begins in the teenage or young adult years and predominantly affects proximal and facial muscles. It tends to co-exist with essential tremor in families. The remainder of the neurological exam is normal, and the course is static. Treatment with clonazepam if required.

Hyperekplexia
See Hyperekplexia in this chapter ➲ p. 325.

Myoclonic epilepsies
- Early infantile developmental and epileptic encephalopathy.
- Juvenile myoclonic epilepsy.
- Myoclonic epilepsy in infancy.
- Dravet syndrome.
- Epilepsy with myoclonic–astatic seizures.
- Lennox–Gastaut syndrome.
- Angelman syndrome.
- Progressive myoclonic epilepsy syndromes: see The progressive myoclonus epilepsies in this chapter ➲ p. 302.

Infectious
- Subacute sclerosing panencephalitis.
- HSV.
- vCJD.

Inflammatory
- Opsoclonus-myoclonus (see Opsoclonus-myoclonus in this chapter ➲ p. 395).

Drugs and toxins
- Bismuth.
- Heavy metals.

- L-DOPA.
- Carbamazepine.
- Tricyclics.

Others

- Renal failure.
- Hepatic failure.
- Dialysis syndrome.
- Spinal trauma.
- Spinal tumour.

Lance–Adams syndrome

Action myoclonus following hypoxic injury, usually occurring during the recovery phase. May be associated with pseudobulbar palsy and cerebellar findings. Myoclonus may be unremitting and interfere with rehabilitation. Treatment is difficult—valproate (see Contraception and reproductive health in this chapter ➔ p. 320), primidone, propranolol, benzodiazepines, baclofen, piracetam, and levetiracetam have been used.

Diseases associated with chorea

Primary

Benign hereditary chorea

- Dominant condition linked to 14q and to mutations in *TITF1*.
- Movement disorder may include dystonia, tics, and myoclonus.
- Mutations in *TITF1* can result in a full brain-lung-thyroid syndrome.
- Onset before 5 years often with delay in walking, clumsiness, and frequent falling. Chorea affects mainly the trunk and proximal limbs. The disorder is static following a period of evolution, not paroxysmal, and not associated with impairment of cognition or intelligence. It may remit spontaneously.
- The chorea rarely impairs functioning and may respond to ASMs such as phenytoin, carbamazepine, as well as haloperidol or clonazepam.

GNAO1-related encephalopathy

- Initially described as cause of early onset epileptic encephalopathy, now recognized as genetic cause of early onset chorea (often <1 year), +/– seizures.
- Patients often experience frequent exacerbations of chorea which can result in PICU admission ('choreic storm').
- Some benefits reported with tetrabenazine use but increasing evidence to suggest early role of deep-brain stimulation to terminate choreic storm, and potentially reduce risk of further crises.

ADCY5-related dyskinesia

- Spectrum of hyperkinetic movement disorders, with prominent chorea, and variable degrees of myoclonus, athetosis, and/or dystonia.
- Paroxysmal exacerbation observed, often as child begins falling off to sleep.
- May also present with truncal hypotonia and intellectual disability.

- Gene expressed in medium spiny neurons of the striatum along with *PDE10*, regulating cAMP and cGMP levels.
  - Positive improvements reported in some children with use of caffeine, particular in terms of reduction of paroxysmal chorea.

PDE10
- Gene expressed in medium spiny neurons of the striatum along with *ADCY5*, regulating cAMP and cGMP levels.
- Homozygous missense mutations in the GAF-A domain of the gene present with early onset chorea, intellectual disability, truncal hypotonia, and normal imaging.
- Heterozygous mutations in the GAF-B domain present with juvenile-onset movement disorder, with bilateral striatal changes on MRI.

Secondary
See Table 4.10.

Table 4.10 Causes of chorea

Metabolic	Glutaric aciduria type 1; galactosaemia; Lesch–Nyhan; Wilson disease; B12 deficiency; hypocalcaemia; hypoparathyroidism; hyponatraemia; hypoglycaemia; hypomagnesaemia; Addison disease; porphyria; hyperthyroidism; GAMT, propionic and methylmalonic acidaemia, *FOLR* mutations, NKH, homocystinurias, L-2-hydroxyglutaric aciduria, sulfite oxidase deficiency, NPC,
Genetic	*NKX2-1* mutations; *ADCY5* mutations; Ataxia telangectasia; Canavan disease; Huntington disease; NBIA; NCL; Pelizaeus–Merzbacher disease; Fahr disease; neuroacanthocytosis; Friedreich ataxia; DRPLA; pontocerebellar hypoplasia type 2; Machado-Joseph disease; incontinentia pigmenti; abetalipoproteinaemia; PDE10 mutations
Infectious/autoimmune	Echovirus; HIV; EBV; HSV; borreliosis
	Sydenham chorea; SLE; Behcet; pregnancy (chorea gravidarum); anti-NMDAR encephalitis
Drugs/toxins	Oestrogen and OCP; L-DOPA; phenytoin; lithium; Ritalin; carbon monoxide; methanol; manganese; toluene; phenothiazines; ethosuximide; amphetamines; neuroleptic withdrawal syndrome
Vascular	Cyanotic heart disease; stroke; post-anoxia; post cardiopulmonary bypass; moyamoya; polycythaemia rubra vera
Others	Congenital malformations; HIE; post cardiac-bypass

Sydenham chorea
See Sydenham chorea in this chapter ➲ p. 398.

Anti-NMDAR autoimmune Encephalitis
See Anti-NMDAR autoimmune Encephalitis in this chapter ➲ p. 393.

Cardiopulmonary bypass ('post-pump' chorea)
- Chorea develops in 1–5 % of children with cyanotic heart disease usually with systemic pulmonary collateral circulations after cardiopulmonary bypass especially if accompanied by circulatory arrest or deep hypothermia.
- Onset typically ~2 weeks after surgery.
- May be mild and resolve.
- In some, it can be profound and unremitting, accompanied by hypotonia, orofacial dyskinesias, and pseudobulbar palsy.
- Refractory to drug treatment but sedatives are used to provide comfort. MRI and EEG are usually normal. In persistent chorea, the MRI after some months may show diffuse cerebral atrophy.

Tic disorders and Tourette syndrome

Tourette's Syndrome (DSM-V criteria)
- Multiple motor and one or more vocal tics have occurred at some time, although not necessarily concurrently (only 8% have coprolalia).
- The tics may wax and wane in frequency but have persisted >1 year since first onset.
- Onset is before age 18 yrs (typical onset 4–7, median 5 y).
- The disturbance is not attributable to the physiological effects of a substance (e.g. cocaine) or another medical condition (e.g. Huntington's disease, postviral encephalitis).

Diagnosis
- Clinical history and careful observation.
- No role for laboratory investigations or imaging other than to exclude conditions that may mimic tics.
- Psychiatric co-morbidites are common:
  - obsessive-compulsive disorder (OCD);
  - may have cognitive tics (mental rituals), e.g. reversing words in head while reading;
  - attention-deficit hyperactivity disorder;
  - trichotillomania;
  - ↑rates of learning difficulties and conduct disorder, though most will have neither;
  - ↑frequency of sleep disturbance especially somnambulism, night terrors, and enuresis;
  - Quality of life relates more to comorbidities than severity of tic disorder *per se*.
- Be aware of the existence of functional tics (see Functional Symptoms in this chapter ➲ p. 336).
- EEG is discouraged due to the high incidence of non-specific abnormalities.

- A number of medications may induce tics especially stimulants such as methylphenidate and dexamfetamine; and cannabis use.

Treatment
- Most children with tics do not require medication (do not 'treat the parent', or the teacher).
- CBT is used with success in older children.
- Distraction approaches:
  - 'Fidget toys' e.g. Rubik cube;
  - Make tic practically difficult e.g. breathe through mouth to block sniffing;
- Medical options:
  - clonidine particularly in children also with ADHD symptoms;
  - pimozide (obtain baseline ECG);
  - risperidone, aripiprazole, quetiapine, mirtazapine (anecdotal evidence of effectiveness only).
- Treatment of comorbidities is as important:
  - clomipramine for OCD symptoms;
  - selective serotonin reuptake inhibitor (SSRIs; e.g. fluoxetine) if anxiety is predominant, but caution should be used in prescribing to adolescents;
  - tricyclics especially nortryptiline are useful in management of tics associated with anxiety or ADHD symptoms;
  - Although they are known to induce tics, stimulants can be used to treat ADHD in children with tics safely; non-stimulant medication choices such as atomoxetine are increasingly used.

Prognosis
- 50–60% tic disorders resolve and 20–25% markedly improve in later adolescence. 20% persist into adulthood.
- Initial severity, and meeting threshold for Tourette, do not imply worse prognosis.

Childhood-onset disorders with bilateral basal ganglia changes

Disorders cluster into 4 major groups on the basis of MRI changes, shown in Table 4.11.

Alternating hemiplegia of childhood

Rare neurodevelopmental disorder, affecting ~1:100,000 children.
- Onset of symptoms before 18 months of age.
- Repeat episodes of hemiplegia which may affect either side of the body (often have a clear environmental trigger).
- Quadriplegia occurring as an isolated symptom, or as part of an initially hemiplegic episode.
- Relief of symptoms following sleep.
- Additional paroxysmal attacks which may include dystonia, tonic episodes, abnormal eye movements, and/or autonomic dysfunction.
- Evidence of developmental delay or neurological abnormalities including choreoathetosis, ataxia, or cognitive disability.
- Cannot be attributed to another cause.

Table 4.11 Patterns of MRI changes in bilateral basal ganglia disorders

MRI changes	Disorders
Bilateral putaminal T_2-weighted hyperintensities	*ADAR*, MEGDEL, ANE, Myelinolysis, cerebral palsy, propionic acidemia, *SLC19A3*, Complex I deficiency, Complex IV deficiency, Complex V deficiency, GA1, infectious encephalitis, Wilson's disease
T_2-weighted hyperintensities or ↑susceptibility in bilateral globus pallidus	BPAN, Cockayne Syndrome Fucosidosis, Gangliosidoses, Huntington's disease, PLAN, kernicterus, Methylmalonic Acidaemia, MPAN, PDH deficiency, SSADH, *TUBB4A*, Kearns–Sayre
T_2-weighted hyperintensities in the globus pallidus, brainstem, and cerebellum with diffusion restriction	Krabbe disease, Vigabatrin toxicity
T_1-weighted hyperintensities in the basal ganglia	*SLC39A14*

Adapted from Mohammad et al 'Magnetic resonance imaging pattern recognition in childhood bilateral basal ganglia disoders' Brain Communications 26;2(2)

- Most commonly due to mutations in *ATP1A3*, with more recent description of mutations in *RHOBT2*.

Episodes of hemiplegia often have clear environmental triggers, recognition, and avoidance of which are important aspects of management. These may include:
- Stress and excitement.
- Exercise.
- Sleep disturbance.
- Intercurrent illness.

Flunarizine, and less commonly acetazolamide, may reduce event frequency.

Ataxias

- For acute ataxias, see Acute post-infectious cerebellitis in this chapter ➲ p. 370 and Miller–Fisher syndrome in this chapter ➲ p. 436.
- For episodic ataxias, see Episodic ataxia 1 in this chapter ➲ p. 326.

Congenital, non-progressive ataxias with no initial symptom-free period
If imaging suggests unilateral or very asymmetric cerebellar involvement, it is probably an acquired (e.g. vascular) insult. Otherwise, identify the pattern of cerebellar involvement:
- Pontocerebellar hypoplasia or hypoplasia of cerebellar hemispheres.
- Vermian agenesis/dysgenesis.
- Cerebellar atrophy due to cerebellar cortical or white matter degeneration.

Syndromes with pontocerebellar hypoplasia
- At least now 17 causal genes for pontocerebellar hypoplasia (PCH) now described—types 1 and 2 most common.
- *Pontocerebellar hypoplasia type 1 (PCH1).*
  - Autosomal recessive.
  - Resembles severe type 1 SMA with addition of with pontocerebellar hypoplasia on MRI.
  - Around 50% of cases attributable to mutations in the *EXOSC3* gene, with several other genes also implicated.
- *Pontocerebellar hypoplasia type 2 (PCH2).*
  - Autosomal recessive.
  - Failure of cerebellar growth in late prenatal life.
  - Severe feeding difficulties in the neonatal period evolving into a picture of severe generalized impairment with prominent movement disorder (chorea and dyskinesia).
  - Again, pontocerebellar hypoplasia seen on MRI.
  - Linked most frequently to mutations in the *TSEN54* gene.
- Other syndromes associated with pontocerebellar hypoplasia:
  - congenital disorders of glycosylation (also known as carbohydrate deficient glycoprotein) syndromes: congenital disorder of glycosylation (CDG) I and III;
  - progressive encephalopathy with oedema (PEHO) syndrome (progressive encephalopathy with peripheral oedema, hypsarrhythmia, and optic atrophy).

Syndromes with vermian agenesis/dysgenesis
- *Joubert syndrome*: characteristic large face, prominent early breathing pattern irregularities worse when awake than asleep, + /− retinal, renal, and hepatic involvements. MRI shows the pathognomonic 'molar tooth' sign due to absent cerebellar vermis. Genetically heterogeneous.
- *COACH syndrome*: acronym for cerebellar vermis hypo- or aplasia, oligophrenia (i.e. learning disability), congenital ataxia, ocular colobomata, and hepatic fibrosis.

Non-progressive pan-cerebellar atrophy
- Chromosomal (trisomy 18, 21); extreme prematurity; congenital CMV.

Progressive pan-cerebellar atrophy
- Metabolic causes (isolated congenital ataxia is a rare presentation): pyruvate decarboxylase, mitochondrial, glutaric aciduria type 1, L-2-hydroxy glutaric aciduria (specific MRI appearances with white matter signal change in the U-fibres at the base of the sulci); succinic semi-aldehyde dehydrogenase (SSADH) deficiency; Hartnup (if intermittent).
- Phenytoin, radiation, other drugs.
- Others: see Al-Maawali *et al.* J. Child Neurol 2012 27(9):1121.

Slowly progressive ataxia (over months to years) with initial symptom-free period

Friedreich ataxia

Friedreich ataxia is an important and relatively common cause of progressive ataxia.

- By far the most common *recessively* inherited ataxia.
  - If there is a clear dominant family history then consider one of the other spinocerebellar ataxias.
- Typical presentation is between 5 and 20 yrs of age with increasing ataxia affecting gait, and prominent early dysarthria.
- Combination of spinocerebellar degeneration and peripheral neuropathy resulting in the characteristic combination of upgoing plantar responses (+ ve Babinski) with markedly reduced or absent ankle and knee reflexes (there are very few other paediatric causes of this combination of signs!).
- Cardiac involvement, pes cavus, and scoliosis occasionally pre-date onset of the full neurological picture. IDDM in 10%.
- There are rare forms with preserved reflexes, and other conditions (ataxia with oculomotor apraxia, several types) that give the cerebellar picture but without the Babinski response.
- Diagnosis confirmed genetically: expansion of an intronic triplet repeat sequence in the *FXN* gene leading to reduced transcription of frataxin.
- A number of new therapies (omaveloxolone, others) on the horizon.

In practice the most common alternative diagnostic consideration of pes cavus and areflexia is HMSN1/CMT1A, but in this condition a parent should be at least mildly affected (sometimes just an asymptomatic areflexia) and there will be no Babinski response. See Inherited neuropathies in this chapter ➲ p. 404.

▶▶ If the clinical picture resembles Friedreich but *FXN* genetic testing is normal it is vital to check vitamin E levels to identify the *treatable* mimic ataxia with vitamin E deficiency (AVED). See Ataxia with vitamin E deficiency in this chapter ➲ p. 530.

- In toddlers consider DNA repair disorders of which ataxia telangiectasia is the commonest. See Ataxia telangiectasia in this chapter ➲ p. 468.
  - oculomotor apraxia is a characteristic early feature: children cannot initiate saccades to switch gaze to another target and instead initiate eye movement with a head turn in a characteristic manner;
  - dystonia/choreoathetosis is often as prominent as cerebellar signs;
  - telangiectasias are first seen behind the pinnae and on the conjunctivae;
  - occasionally, ataxia is very early onset and appears quasi-congenital.

- Also consider Cockayne syndrome (usually with peripheral neuropathy), xeroderma pigmentosum (with photosensitivity) and ataxia with oculomotor apraxia (AOA1).

Spinocerebellar ataxias

Of the many remaining genetically determined causes of progressive ataxias nearly all are: (i) extraordinarily rare and (ii) dominantly inherited with high penetrance so that a family history will be informative. These are the spinocerebellar ataxias (SCAs). To date 41 distinct genetic causes have been identified, many due to triplet repeats. They are all slowly progressive and are associated with cerebellar atrophy but have varying associated features (see Table 4.12). Symptom overlap makes genetic testing essential. Identifiable SCA mutations account for only 60% of all dominant hereditary ataxias. When the gene is test normal consider a neurological examination for family members who are concerned they may have symptoms of ataxia.

Late-onset cerebellar ataxias

A heterogeneous group of neurodegenerative disorders that may be hereditary or sporadic, the latter symptomatic or idiopathic. Diagnosis is important for prognosis, genetic counselling, and possible therapeutic implications.

Notes to Figure 4.8:

- Six types of episodic ataxia.
- Toxic causes: alcohol, drugs, ASMs, benzodiazepines, antineoplastics, heavy metals (mercury, lead), chemicals (solvents, pesticides).

Table 4.12 SCAs capable of paediatric presentation

Type	Perecentage of all dominant ataxias	Average decade of onset (range)	Average duration before death (range)	Additional features
SCA1	10%	4th (2nd–7th)	15 (10–29)	Retained reflexes
SCA2	15–20%	3rd–4th (2nd–8th)	10 (1–30)	Slow eye movements
SCA3	20–50%	4th (2nd–8th)	10 (1–20)	Muscle weakness and atropy
SCA5	Rare	3rd–4th	Decades	Sensory loss
DRPLA	3%	4th (1st–7th)		Ataxia, choreoathetosis, myoclonic epilepsy, learning difficulties, dementia and mental illness

- Endocrine: hypothyroidism.
- Malabsorption: coeliac disease (gluten ataxia), vitamin deficiency.
- Miscellaneous: paraneoplastic syndromes, demyelinating disorders.
- Inflammatory: Whipple disease, parainfectious/immune-mediated ataxia.

Investigations to consider (see Table 4.13).

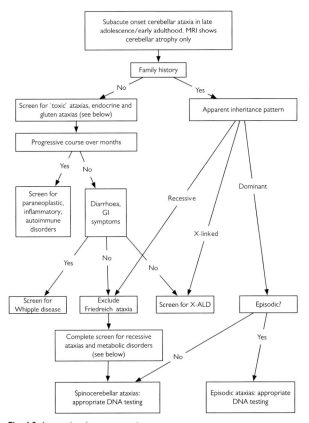

Fig. 4.8 Approach to late-onset ataxias.

Reproduced with permission from Brusse E, Maat-Kievit JA, and Van Swieten JC. Diagnosis and management of early- and onset- cerebellar ataxia. *Clinical Genetics*, Volume 71, Issue 1, pp. 12–24, Copyright © 2006 Blackwell Munksgaard.

Table 4.13 Possible investigations in progressive ataxia

Urine organic acids, plasma AAs, ammonia	MSUD, methylmalonic & propionic acids, urea cycle disorders
Biotinidase	Biotinidase deficiency
Plasma/CSF glucose ratios; specific enzyme assay	GLUT1DS, CDG deficiency
Vitamin E	Ataxia with vitamin E deficiency
Acanthocytes	Chorea-acanthocytosis, abetalipoproteinaemia
Cholesterol, triglycerides, LDLs, VLDLs	Abetalipoproteinaemia
Lactate, pyruvate, mtDNA deletions, muscle biopsy	Mitochondrial disease
Immunoglobulins, α-fetoprotein, leukocyte irradiation	Ataxia telangiectasia
Gene panel	Ataxia-oculomotor apraxia (AOA 1 and 2)
Bile alcohols	Cerebrotendinous xanthomatosis
Plasma: phytanic acid; copper, caeruloplasmin	Refsum; Wilson, acaeruloplasminaemia
β-hexosaminidase	GM2 gangliosidosis (hexosaminidase deficiency)
β-galactosidase	GM1 gangliosidosis
Arylsulfatase-A	Metachromatic leukodystrophy
β-galactocerebrosidase	Krabbe
Neuraminidase	Sialidosis
Skin biopsy; molecular genetic analysis	Niemann–Pick type C

Neuromuscular conditions

Neuromuscular conditions are disorders of the 'motor unit' comprising the anterior horn cell, peripheral nerve, neuromuscular junction, and muscle. In the past two decades enormous progress has been made elucidating the underlying genetic and cellular protein basis of many neuromuscular disorders. Many clinically defined entities are genetically heterogeneous and mutations in some genes can cause multiple clinical phenotypes.

Common presentations of neuromuscular disease

- Floppy infant: hypotonic *and* weak.
  - Ventilator dependent neonate requiring minimal ventilation but failing extubation.
  - Recurrent apnoea.
  - Arthrogryposis.
  - Feeding difficulties.
- Delayed motor development in the face of normal cognitive development (although ♂'s with Duchenne muscular dystrophy may present with global developmental delay, or speech delay with achievement of early motor milestones).
- Poor gait: slow or unable to run, falls, difficulty with steps.
- Toe-walking.
- Foot deformity.
- Episodic weakness.
- Pain on or after exercise.
- Abnormal biochemistry: ↑CK, ↑ALT.

▶▶ ALT is not liver specific but is also present in muscle. If you have no explanation for 'abnormal LFTs' check CK!

Investigation of NMD

Creatine (phospho)kinase

- Reflects muscle *destruction,* so is *normal* in many neuromuscular disorders where muscle fibres remain intact including congenital myopathies, myasthenic syndromes, SMA (may be mildy ↑in SMA type III).
- Muscular dystrophy usually >7x ULN.
- Normal or mildly ↑in neuropathies.
- Also ↑in:
  - Metabolic myopathy.
  - Inflammatory myopathy/myositis.
  - ♀ Duchenne/Becker carrier.
  - Hypothyroidism.
  - Malignant hyperthermia.
  - Status dystonicus.
  - Infective myositis.
  - Excessive exercise.
  - After EMG, IM injection, or other muscle trauma.

Electrophysiology
See Electromyography in Chapter 2 p. 96.

Muscle biopsy
See Muscle biopsy in Chapter 2 p. 104.

Genetic studies
There are a few conditions in which DNA analysis is the initial investigation of choice, these include:
• SMA.
• Myotonic dystrophy.
• Facioscapulohumeral dystrophy.
• Duchenne/Becker muscular dystrophy.
• SMARD.

In other conditions the clinical phenotype and results of muscle biopsy and/or neurophysiology guide genetic testing.

Metabolic tests
• Lactate: mitochondrial disease.
• Carnitine/acyl carnitine profile: fatty acid oxidation defects.
• Forearm ischaemic lactate test: glycogen storage disease.
• If history unclear, consider a graded exercise test to identify metabolic myopathies and/or periodic paralyses:
  • Cannulate.
  • baseline CK, lactate, K^+.
  • vigorous aerobic exercise for 20 min if possible.
  • bloods repeated at 10, 30, 60, and 120 min.
• Paired CSF/plasma glucose if GLUT1DS suspected.

Imaging
• Muscle ultrasound, MRI:
  • patterns of muscle involvement/sparing can be distinctive (especially STIR sequence) and may help diagnosis.
• Brain MRI:
  • congenital muscular dystrophies due to glycosylation defects of α-dystroglycan may be associated with cortical dysplasia or white matter abnormality.

A small but growing number of neuromuscular diseases (SMA, Pompe, some genotypes of Duchenne) have specific therapies. although this is still uncommon.

Neuropathies

▶▶These are a group of conditions caused by dysfunction of one or more peripheral nerves, typically causing weakness with or without sensory and other symptoms (see Table 4.14). The commonest causes are the hereditary neuropathies.

Hereditary neuropathies

- Typically present in the first or second decade with slowly progressive, and predominantly distal wasting; weakness; hypo- or areflexia; variable sensory involvement; and often pes cavus.
- The most common form of genetic neuropathy is Charcot-Marie-Tooth disease (CMT), also referred to as hereditary motor and sensory neuropathy (HMSN), in which both motor and sensory peripheral nerves are affected.
- CMT is divided into demyelinating (CMT1) and axonal forms (CMT2) which can be distinguished by Motor Conduction Velocity (MCV) (see Nerve Conduction Studies in Chapter 2 ➋ p. 95); with MCVs ≪38 m/s in CMT1 and ≫38 m/s in CMT2. Intermediate CMTs with borderline MCVs (25–45 m/s) are also seen.
- The other subtypes are Hereditary Sensory and Autonomic Neuropathy (HSAN) and Hereditary Motor Neuropathy (HMN) in which only sensory or motor nerves are affected respectively.

Classification of the hereditary neuropathies is complex, due to a lack of simple relationships between phenotypes and genotypes: one gene can cause multiple clinical pictures and vice versa, thus multigene (sometimes 'virtual') neuropathy panels are playing an increasing role (but only *after* exclusion of the common *PMP22* duplication/deletion) (see Table 4.15).

Charcot-Marie-Tooth disease (CMT; also known as hereditary sensorimotor neuropathies)

- Presentation can range from infancy to 40y but is usually school age.
- Slowly progressive course.
- Very early presentations can occur with hypotonia and delayed motor milestones.
- Often present with toe-walking, clumsiness, and falls.
  - Inability to walk on heels is an early sign.
- Distal weakness and wasting, affecting feet first, then hand muscles, and proximal weakness.
- Initial peroneal muscular atrophy, later spreading to calves.
- Foot deformity: pes cavus (or pes planus), ankle inversion, high arch, hammer toes.
- Areflexia.
- Mild distal sensory loss.
- Enlargement of peripheral nerves in 25%.
- Postural tremor in 25%.
- Spinal deformities.
- Intrafamilial variation is common.
- Only ~60% patients with clinical diagnosis of CMT have a confirmed genetic diagnosis.
  - *PMP22*, *GJB1*, *MPZ*, and *MFN2* are the commonest identified genes.

Table 4.14 Causes of neuropathies

Hereditary neuropathies	Acquired neuropathies
CMT/HMSN	**Polyneuropathies**
Demyelinating	*Inflammatory*
CMT1 (AD)	GBS
CMT4 (AR)	CIDP
Axonal	Vasculitis
CMT 2 (AD or AR)	Infection
Demyelinating or axonal	• HIV
CMTX (X-linked dominant, X-linked recessive)	• Lyme
	• Leprosy
Intermediate	*Metabolic*
CMTI (AD or AR)	Vitamin deficiency (B1, B2, B6, B12, E)
HMN	
AD or AR	Diabetes
HSAN	Hypoglycaemia
AD or AR	Uraemia
HNPP	Porphyria
AD	Hypothyroidism
Neuropathy associated with other disorders	Acromegaly
	Hypervitaminosis
Metachromatic leukodystrophy	*Toxic*
Krabbe disease	Arsenic, lead, mercury, thallium, vincristine, isoniazid
Abetalipoproteinaemia	Critical illness neuropathy
Refsum disease	*Paraproteinaemia*
Amyloid neuropathy	Multiple myeloma
X -linked Adrenoleucodystrophy	Waldenstrom cryoglobulinaemia
Friedreich ataxia	*Connective tissue disorders*
	Polyarteritis nodosa
	Wegener granulomatosis
	Sjögren syndrome
	SLE
	Rheumatoid arthritis
	Scleroderma
	Eeosinophilic granulomatosis with polyangiitis
	Mononeuropathy
	Traumatic
	Inflammatory

CMT1
- Pathology reflects *demyelination*: motor conduction velocities (NCVs) are markedly reduced ≪ 35 m/s.
- Autosomal dominant.

CMT2
- Pathology is *axonal*: NCVs are normal/near normal (>45 m/s) but CMAP amplitudes are reduced.
- Autosomal dominant or recessive.

CMTI (Intermediate)
- NCVs 35–45 m/s.
- Autosomal dominant or recessive.

X-linked CMT
- Mild to moderate CMT phenotype with ♂s more severely affected.
- Consider in pedigrees with no ♂-to-♂ transmission.
- NCVs are intermediate range (30–40 m/s in ♂s and 30 m/s to normal in ♀s).

CMT3
- Previously known as Dejerine-Sottas disease or congenital hypomyelinating neuropathy: use of these terms is now discouraged.
- Severe early onset—congenital or infancy.
- CSF protein may be ↑.
- De novo, AD mutations in *PMP22*, *MPZ*, *EGR*.

CMT 4
- Demyelinating pattern (reduced NCVs).
- Usually, early onset and severe.
- Autosomal recessive.

Children with CMT1A may develop very severe neuropathy after vincristine treatment: children developing post-vincristine neuropathy should have *PMP22* status checked and if +ve no further vincristine given.

Hereditary neuropathy with liability to pressure palsies (HNPP)
- *PMP22* deletion.
- Autosomal dominant.
- Onset <20 yrs.
- Recurrent episodes of mononeuropathy (simplex or multiplex) related to trauma or prolonged compression (especially peroneal nerve at fibular head, ulnar nerve at elbow, radial nerve in humeral groove, median nerve in carpal tunnel).
- Recovery over days to weeks: can be incomplete.
- Neurophysiology: slowing of motor and sensory nerve conduction in affected and unaffected nerves.
- May also present with a mild CMT phenotype.

Hereditary motor neuropathies (HMN)
- Previously referred to as distal SMA.
- Variable inheritance.

Table 4.15 Genotype–phenotype relationships in inherited neuropathies

Gene	Clinical phenotype(s)
PMP22	Duplication: typical CMT1A
	Point mutation: CMT1 (early onset and congenital phenotypes); HNPP
	Deletion: HNPP
MPZ	CMT1 (early onset and congenital phenotypes)
	CMT2I (adult-onset CMT2)
	CMT2J (CMT2 with hearing loss and pupillary abnormalities)
	CMTDIB (CMTI with cataracts, ophthalmoplegia, ptosis)
ERG2	CMT1 (early onset and congenital phenotypes)
	CMT3, CMT4E
MFN2	CMT2, optic atrophy
GARS	CMT2
	HMN5A: hand wasting predominant
GDAP1	CMT2K (late-onset CMT2)
	CMT4E (early onset severe phenotype with vocal cord and diaphragmatic paralysis)
	CMTRIA
SH3TC2	CMT4C (severe CMT1, scoliosis, cytoplasmic inclusions)
DNM2	Intermediate CMT or CMT2
	Cataracts, ophthalmoplegia, ptosis
GJB1	CMTX1: ♂s CMT1; ♀s CMT2
	May have episodes of encephalopathy and white matter change on MRI scan
	Split hand weakness (median>ulnar)
AIFM1	CMTX4 (Cowchock syndrome): CMT2 with infantile-onset, developmental delay, deafness, learning difficulties
MORC2	CMT2Z (early onset with neuropathy, cerebellar atrophy, learning difficulties)
	Childhood-onset CMT2
IGHMBP2	SMARD1, HMN6
	Childhood-onset CMT2
SLC5A7	HMN7A (vocal cord palsy)
DYNC1H1	HMN (congenital contractures, lower-limb predominant, pyramidal signs, cortical migration defects, learning difficulties)

Abbreviations: CMTRI- CMT intermediate recessive; CMTDI- CMT intermediate dominant; HMN- Hereditary motor neuropathy.

- Early onset: most <10 yrs with foot deformity or gait abnormality.
- Purely motor involvement.
- Usually lower-limb predominance (weakness and muscle wasting).
- Very slow progression.
- Nerve conduction studies: SNAPs preserved, normal NCVs. EMG: denervation.

Hereditary sensory and autonomic neuropathies (HSAN)
- Present with insensitivity to pain, silent foot ulceration, burns, and other injuries including amputations; eventual destructive arthropathy with Charcot joints. Muscle weakness and wasting can be present.
- Pain sensation is conveyed by small myelinated and unmyelinated fibres so nerve conduction studies — which predominantly reflect the function of the fastest, large myelinated fibres — *may be normal.*
- Some associated with sensorineural hearing loss.
- *Type 1*: AD inheritance. Genes include *SPTLC1 SPTLC2*, *ATL1*, and *DNMT1*.
- *Type 2*: autosomal recessive (AR). Early onset sensory neuropathy affecting all modalities of sensation. Genes include *WNK1*, *FAM134B*, and *KIF1A*.
- *Type 3* (Riley–Day syndrome): AR. Predominantly seen in Ashkenazi Jews due to *IKBKAP* mutations. Autonomic symptoms predominate, but sensory and motor signs are present. Absent fungiform papillae.
- *Type 4*: AR. *NTRK1* mutations. Congenital insensitivity to pain, anhidrosis (recurrent fever) and learning difficulty.
- *SCN9A mutations*. see Inherited Neuropathic Pain Syndromes below, this chapter ➲ p. 435.

Neuropathy in multisystem neurodegenerative disease
Neuropathy is common in many neurodegenerative and metabolic conditions and may go unrecognized because of other more prominent symptoms. Rarely neuropathy may be the presenting feature, for example in metachromatic leukodystrophy.

Brown–Vialetto–van Laere syndrome
(See also Vitamin B2 (riboflavin) in this chapter ➲ p. 523).
- Autosomal recessive disorder due to defect in the riboflavin transporter encoded by *SLC52A2* and *SLC52A3*.
- Presentation in infancy to childhood, rarely in adults.
- Presentation can be acute and resemble Guillain–Barré syndrome.
- Multiple cranial neuropathies, particularly bulbar and auditory but facial and optic nerves may also be involved.
- Sensorimotor axonal neuropathy, sensory ataxia, limb weakness.
- Prominent respiratory involvement with diaphragmatic weakness.
- Plasma acylcarnitines and urine organic acids can be suggestive (multiple acyl-CoA dehydrogenation defect).
- Good response to high-dose riboflavin.

Inherited neuropathic pain syndromes
SCN9A gene related AD causing three distinct syndromes:
- *Erythromelalgia*. Childhood-onset recurrent episodes of bilateral intense, burning pain, redness, warmth, and occasionally swelling. Feet most affected but can affect hands, legs, arms, face, and/or ears may be involved. Treatment is with cooling extremities with fan (avoid prolonged immersion in cold water due to skin breakdown risk). Carbamazepine can be considered. Avoid triggers (warmth, standing, spicy food).

- *Paroxysmal extreme pain syndrome.* Infantile-onset autonomic features including skin flushing, harlequin (patchy or asymmetric) colour change, limb stiffening. Attacks precipitated by opening bowels (rectal pain), crying, eating (submandibular pain), cold wind. Treatment: carbamazepine, stool softeners.
- *Small fibre neuropathy.* Adult-onset, glove, and stocking neuropathic pain, autonomic manifestations such as dry eyes, mouth, orthostatic hypotension, palpitations, bowel, or bladder disturbance.

Acquired neuropathies

Guillain–Barré syndrome (GBS)
- Incidence 1–2/100 000.
- The most common cause is acute inflammatory demyelinating polyneuropathy (AIDP), and the term AIDP is often used synonymously with GBS.
- Variants resulting in a similar clinical picture include acute motor axonal neuropathy (AMAN), acute motor and sensory axonal neuropathy with prominent sensory features (AMSAN) and Miller–Fisher syndrome (ophthalmoplegia, ataxia, areflexia).
- The mechanism is an immunological cross-reactivity secondary to a prodromal illness within the previous 4 weeks, typically an URTI or gastroenteritis. Implicated organisms include mycoplasma, CMV, EBV, vaccinia, variola, campylobacter, VZV, measles, mumps, hepatitis A and B, rubella, influenza A and B, coxsackie, echovirus, and SARS-CoV2.
  - *Campylobacter jejuni* is particularly associated with the AMAN variant and a more severe course.

For initial diagnosis (Box 4.7) and for management see Guillain–Barré syndrome in Chapter 6 p. 640

Miller–Fisher syndrome
- Variant of Guillain–Barré syndrome.

Box 4.7 GBS diagnostic criteria

Required
- Progressive motor weakness of more than one limb.
  - Degree of weakness can vary from minimal to complete flaccid paralysis.
- ↓or absent deep tendon reflexes in weak limbs.
- Monophasic course with time between onset and nadir 12 h–28 d.

Supportive
- Relative symmetry.
- Mild sensory involvement.
- Cranial nerve involvement.
- Autonomic dysfunction.
- CSF: elevated protein after first week; CSF leucocyte count <50.
- Nerve conduction abnormalities consistent with one of the GBS subtypes.
- Absence of other cause, e.g. porphyria, diphtheria, toxins.

- Triad of ataxia, ophthalmoplegia, and areflexia.
- Altered sensorium or abnormal EEG incompatible with Miller–Fisher and suggests brainstem encephalitis.

Other rare subtypes of GBS
- Generalized selective sensory involvement giving peripheral sensory-ataxic syndrome (due to impaired proprioception) without weakness. NCVs axonal or demyelinating.
- Pharyngeal–cervical variant with intact eye movements (cf. Miller–Fisher). NCVs axonal or demyelinating.
- Acute idiopathic autonomic involvement (NCVs normal).

Chronic inflammatory demyelinating polyneuropathy (CIDP)
▶▶ CMT is often an important differential. The following are useful pointers to CIDP rather than CMT:
- Absence of family history.
- Insidious or subacute onset.
- Cranial nerves involved.
- Hand tremor.
- Autonomic dysfunction is rare.
- CSF protein ↑in 80%.
- Electrophysiology:
  - Reduction in conduction velocity and patchy conduction block.
  - In contrast to CMT, F-responses delayed or absent.
  - Presence of nodal/para-nodal antibodies e.g. neurofascin (NF) 186/140 (NF186/140), NF155, contactin-1 (CNTN1), or contactin-associated protein-1 (CASPR1).

See Box 4.8 for diagnostic criteria

Differential diagnosis
- AIDP (see Guillain–Barré in this chapter ⊃ p. 436).
- Inherited neuropathies.

Box 4.8 Diagnostic criteria for typical CIDP
- Progressive or relapsing, symmetric, proximal and distal muscle weakness of upper and lower limbs, and sensory involvement of at least two limbs.
- Subacute course with progression over at least 8 weeks or a relapsing-remitting course.
- Absent or reduced tendon reflexes in all limbs.
- Evidence of conduction abnormalities in at least two motor nerves and two sensory nerves.
- CIDP variants:
  - Distal CIDP (distal involvement, legs>arms).
  - Multifocal CIDP (multifocal involvement, asymmetric, arms>legs).
  - Focal CIDP (single limb).
  - Motor CIDP (pure motor).
  - Sensory CIDP (pure sensory).

Much more rarely:
- MNGIE (mitochondrial neurogastrointestinal encephalomyopathy).
- Toxic/metabolic including Brown–Vialetto–van Laere (see Brown–Vialetto–van Laere syndrome in this chapter ⤳ p. 435).
- Paraneoplastic.
- Neuropathy with monoclonal gammopathy of unknown significance (MGUS).
- Infection (HIV, Lyme, leprosy, diphtheria).
- Rheumatological/vasculitic; porphyria.

Treatment
- *Steroids:* pulsed monthly regime for induction and/or maintenance; daily or alternate daily regimes.
- *IVIG:* initiated at 2 g/kg and then maintenance 1 g/kg 3–6 weekly (gradually extending interval based on clinical response).
- *Plasma exchange:* efficacious but required as often as every 4 weeks. Use as maintenance therapy limited by issues with venous access.
- *Other drugs:* Some evidence of benefit from azathioprine, cyclophosphamide, ciclosporin, mycophenolate mofetil, and rituximab.

Prognosis
- Time course may be relapsing-remitting, chronic progressive, monophasic, or have a GBS-like onset (acute onset CIDP).
- Most require chronic treatment and can have long-term morbidity.

Entrapment neuropathies

The more common entrapment neuropathies, and their scenarios.

Paucity of arm movement in a baby, following a difficult delivery involving traction of the head and/or shoulder
Erb palsy (commonest)
- Arm adducted, internally rotated, elbow extended, forearm pronated: 'waiter's tip' position.
- C5,6 upper trunk.

Klumpke paralysis
- Elbow flexed, forearm supinated, wrist extended, claw hand.
- ± associated Horner syndrome.
- C8, T1 lower trunk.

Complete brachial plexus injury
- Whole arm limp.
- Look for an associated fractured clavicle.

A child with a mucopolysaccharidosis/mucolipidosis having difficulty with fine motor tasks or loss of grip strength
Median nerve compression at the wrist, carpal tunnel syndrome:
- Can present with difficulty with pencil grip or other fine motor tasks.
- Older children can present with pain, sensory symptoms in hands (often in morning or waking them from sleep). Shaking of hands can relieve symptoms.

- Flexion of wrist for 60 s may reproduce the symptoms: Phalen test.
- Tapping over the median nerve at the wrist may induce tingling: Tinel sign.
- Many are asymptomatic so regular screening for carpal tunnel syndrome required.

A child with a fractured humerus, or a teenager after sleeping awkwardly on an arm (especially while intoxicated) presenting with wrist drop

- Radial nerve compression (in spiral groove of the humerus).
- Wrist drop with sensory loss over the lateral aspect of the dorsum of the hand between the thumb and index finger: 'Saturday night palsy'.

Foot drop following trauma to the side of the lower leg; foot drop after general anaesthesia

- Common peroneal/lateral popliteal nerve injury (around the neck of the fibula).
- Can occur iatrogenically if unrecognized compression of neck of fibula during GA.
- Foot drop with sensory loss over the lateral aspect of the leg.

Other sites

- Suprascapular nerve: spinoglenoid notch.
- Medial nerve: carpal tunnel.
- Ulnar nerve: cubital tunnel at elbow; palmar fascia and pisiform bone in hand.
- Lateral cutaneous nerve of thigh: inguinal ligament.
- Obturator nerve: obturator canal.
- Posterior tibial: tarsal tunnel, medial malleolus.

▶▶In all cases of apparent entrapment/compression peripheral mononeuropathies it is important to consider Hereditary Neuropathy with liability to Pressure Palsy (HNPP) and check for *PMP22* deletion.

Disorders of muscle

Dystrophinopathies

A number of clinical phenotypes result from mutations in the dystrophin gene: Duchenne and Becker muscular dystrophies (DMD and BMD), X-linked cardiomyopathy and a cramps/myalgia syndrome. These are now recognized as being a spectrum of Xp21 related dystrophinopathies. While DMD patients typically lose independent ambulation by 13 years, BMD ♂'s remain ambulant beyond 16 years, with those losing ambulation between 13 and 16 years considered as intermediate. The severity of the clinical phenotype depends on the amount of residual functional dystrophin.

Duchenne muscular dystrophy (DMD)
- Commonest neuromuscular condition in paediatric practice.
- Incidence 1:3 500 ♂ infants.
- 1/3 new mutations.
- Up to 10% due to gonadal mosaicism.
- Onset <5 yrs.
- Presentations include gross motor delay, gross motor difficulties, global developmental delay, or speech delay.
- Initially symmetrical proximal weakness (legs>arms) and neck flexion.
- Calf hypertrophy.
- Intellectual impairment common, affects verbal>performance IQ.
- Cardiomyopathy: annual screening from diagnosis (ACE inhibitor +/- β-blocker to be initiated around 8 years).
- Respiratory involvement, usually after loss of ambulation.
- Loss of ambulation around 9.5 yrs, historically.
- Diagnosis: Creatine kinase. DMD gene analysis. Muscle biopsy only rarely needed.

Treatment
- Steroids (prednisolone or deflazacort) slow decline in muscle function and prolong ambulation to 12–14 years. Benefits in maintaining upper limb, cardiac, and respiratory function.
  - Steroids generally started around 3–4 years.
  - Serious side effects: weight gain, osteoporosis, and fractures, cataract, slowing of height velocity, adrenal suppression, hypertension, behavioural issues, diabetes.
  - Typical regime 0.75 mg/kg (max 30 mg) prednisolone or 0.9 mg/kg (max 36 mg) deflazacort daily or intermittent (10 days on, 10 days off).
  - Check varicella status and vaccinate prior to steroids if non-immune.
  - DEXA scan at baseline and annually.
  - Spine X-ray annually for vertebral fractures.
  - BP and urine dipstick for glucose at medical review.
- Newer genetic treatments are not yet widely available and are relevant only to particular genetic subgroups:
  - Ataluren (nonsense mutation).
  - Eteplirsen (exon 51 skippable).
  - Golodirsen (exon 53 skippable).

- Casmiseren (exon 45 skippable).
- With optimal care, patients are now surviving into 30s and 40s.

Becker muscular dystrophy (BMD)
- 1:300 to 1:600 ♂s.
- Presentation like DMD, but reduced severity/later onset (5–15y).
- Slow progression, life expectancy 40 y to normal.
- Diagnosis: DMD gene test.
- Respiratory involvement only if non-ambulant.
- Cardiac: alternate year screening from diagnosis.

Atypical presentations include:
- Myalgia.
- Myoglobinuria.
- Malignant hyperthermia like reaction.
- Achilles tendon contractures.
- Cardiomyopathy.
- 'Abnormal liver function tests' (muscle isoenzymes).

Manifesting female carriers
- May present with global developmental delay/learning difficulty.
- Weakness onset usually >16 yrs, may be asymmetric.
- Isolated cardiomyopathy in about 8% DMD carriers.
- Severer DMD like phenotype rare and usually associated with chromosomal translocation.

Emery–Dreifuss muscular dystrophy (EDMD)
Clinical features
- Presentation at any age, most commonly in late childhood/early adult life.
- Early contractures before significant weakness: elbows, Achilles tendons and spinal rigidity (limited trunk and neck flexion).
- Muscle wasting and weakness in a scapulohumeroperoneal distribution.
  - scapular winging.
  - weakness biceps and triceps.
  - weakness of anterior tibial and peroneal muscles.
- High risk of cardiomyopathy with conduction defects and arrhythmias. Can be life-threatening. Most require pacing/implantable defibrillator. Annual 24 h ECG screen from 10 yrs of age. At times, cardiac conduction defects can precede muscle weakness.
- CK mildly ↑.

Genetics
Emerin and *LMNA* account for 40% of cases.
- EDMD1: X-linked, emerin.
- EDMD2: AD, Lamin A/C (*LMNA*).
- EDMD3: AR, Lamin A/C (*LMNA*).
- EDMD4: AD, *SYNE1*.
- EDMD 5: AD, *SYNE2*.
- EDMD6: X-linked, *FHL1*.
- EDMD7: AD, *TMEM43* mutations.

- Some subtypes due to *SUN1*, *SUN2*, *TTN*.

Limb girdle muscular dystrophy (LGMD)
- Heterogeneous group of muscular dystrophies presenting with childhood or adult-onset weakness with ↑CK.
- LGMD1 (10%, AD), LGMD2 (90%, AR).
- Childhood-onset similar phenotype to Duchenne and Becker with proximal >distal weakness, (waddling gait, toe-walking, scapular winging) calf hypertrophy.
- Most common childhood-onset variants:
  - sarcoglycanopathies LGMD2C (γ sarcoglycan), LGMD2D (α sarcoglycan), LGMD2E (β sarcoglycan), LGMD2F (δ sarcoglycan); LGMD2I (*FKRP*).
- Mutations in genes involved in glycosylation of α-dystroglycan may produce a LGMD phenotype as well as a congenital muscular dystrophy phenotype.

Facioscapulohumeral (FSH) dystrophy
- Autosomal dominant.
- Onset variable: usually mild, but early onset can be more progressive, ♂'s more frequently symptomatic than ♀s, intrafamilial variation.
- Facial weakness, shoulder weakness (due to poor scapular fixation) with scapular winging, proximal arm, hip girdle, ankle dorsiflexion weakness, weakness may be asymmetric.
- Severe infantile onset: 2–5% of all FSH dystrophy, facial weakness, and lumbar lordosis. Ambulation can be lost in childhood due to progressive weakness.
- Association with sensorineural deafness and Coat's disease (retinal vasculopathy) particularly with infantile and childhood onset but all ages need surveillance.
- Genetic heterogeneity:
  - FSHD1 loss of *D4Z4* DNA repeats at 4q35.
  - FSHD2 *SMCHD1* mutations, later onset, no severe infantile onset reported.

Distal myopathy
- Uncommon in childhood, mostly adult onset.
- About 25 genes recognized.
- The majority are dominantly inherited, a few are recessive, and a few may be either dominant or recessive.
- Distal weakness may involve legs only or arms and legs.
- Phenotype can resemble neuropathy or hereditary motor neuropathies—EMG helpful to differentiate (normal NCV in distal myopathies but can show myopathic changes).
- Cardiac involvement in some.

Congenital muscular dystrophies (CMDs)

A group of conditions presenting at birth or in early childhood with hypotonia, motor/global developmental delay and muscle weakness. The conditions are static or slowly progressive. CK is usually markedly ↑, and muscle biopsy shows dystrophic changes. Some are associated with disorders of myelin or neuronal migration and/or congenital eye abnormalities.

Merosin (laminin) deficiency
- Primary laminin α2 (merosin) deficiency due to mutations in *LAMA2A* gene.
- Weakness of face, trunk, and limbs usually from birth.
- Feeding and respiratory difficulties.
- CK elevated.
- Disease severity varies.
- Associated axonal neuropathy can be present.
- MRI brain: white matter changes.
- Epilepsy in 20%. Usually, normal cognition.

Collagen VI-related myopathies
These are a spectrum of myopathies due to AD or AR mutations in COL6A1, COL6A2, and COL6A3, with Ullrich CMD, Intermediate, and Bethlem myopathy as a continuous spectrum of disease.

Ullrich congenital muscular dystrophy
- Neonatal or early childhood-onset hypotonia and weakness.
- Proximal contractures.
- Distal joint laxity.
- Slowly progressive weakness and worsening contractures (shoulder, elbow, knees, and ankles).
- Respiratory insufficiency in adolescence (even if ambulant).
- Skeletal: spinal rigidity, scoliosis, torticollis.
- Skin: hyperkeratosis pilaris, keloids, and atrophic scars.

Bethlem myopathy
- Childhood onset.
- Clinical features like Ulrich but milder.
- Over time progressive flexion contractures: fingers, elbows, ankles.
- Respiratory insufficiency in adulthood.
- CK normal or slightly elevated.

CMD due to glycosylation disorders
Disorders of glycosylation of α-dystroglycan cause abnormal basal lamina formation in muscle and brain which result in varying extent of cortical lamination, muscular dystrophy, and eye problems, depending on the genetic defect. These include muscle-eye-brain disease, Walker-Warburg syndrome, and Fukuyama CMD. CK is typically ↑, and muscle biopsy shows absent α-dystroglycan. Several genes reported.

Myotonic dystrophy (DM)

Genetics
Two genes, both 'triplet-repeat' expansion disorders: severity depends on length of expansion. DM1 in particular shows *anticipation*: the repeat length expands, and disease severity increases in successive generations.
- DM1 (Steinert) CTG expansion in *DMPK* gene.
- DM2 (Proximal myotonic myopathy PROMM) CTG expansion in intron1 of *CNBP* gene.

DM1
- Severity and onset age depend on CTG expansion (larger repeats leads to earlier onset and more severe phenotype).
- >50 repeats: affected.
- >1000 repeats: congenital onset.
- Autosomal dominant.

In addition to its neuromuscular features, DM is a multisystem disorder with gut dysmotility, cataracts, gonadal failure, cardiac dysrhythmia, respiratory failure, hypersomnia, and learning disability but late-onset forms (e.g. after middle age) have minimal features (cataracts, asymptomatic myotonia).

Congenital onset
- Polyhydramnios, reduced foetal movements.
- Hypotonia, respiratory, and feeding difficulty in neonatal period which usually improves.
- Facial weakness, ptosis, talipes, arthrogryposis.
- Learning difficulties moderate to severe.
- Myotonia absent at birth and develops later in childhood.
- Motor abilities including ambulation can be achieved albeit late, followed by progressive weakness in adolescence/adult.

Childhood/Adolescence/young adult onset
- Myotonia.
- Facial weakness and ptosis.
- Limb weakness and wasting (forearms, foot dorsiflexors), neck flexion.
- Mild to moderate learning difficulties.

Cardiac conduction defects (annual ECG) and respiratory failure should be monitored for in all DM1 patients.

DM2
- Autosomal dominant.
- Onset late childhood-adult.
- Proximal muscle weakness.
- Myotonia may be asymmetric and intermittent.
- Muscle pain, variable, proximal, legs>arms, worse in cold.
- Calf hypertrophy in 50%.
- Respiratory involvement is rare and cardiac conduction defect is variably affected.

Ion channel disorders
Chloride channel CLCN1 myotonia congenita
- AD or AR.
- Onset: childhood to adult.
- Legs>face and arms.
- Myotonia and at times transient weakness, worse in cold or stress.
- Improvement in both with 'warming up'—repetitive action.
- Muscle hypertrophy.
- Treatment: mexiletine, carbamazepine, lamotrigine.

Paramyotonia congenita
- Mutations in *SCN4A* sodium channel.

- AD.
- Onset in first decade.
- Myotonia, worse with exercise and cold.
- Face, jaw, tongue and arms >legs.
- Severe subtype with neonatal/infantile onset with generalized myotonia, laryngospasm presenting as recurrent apnoea (clue is the muscle hypertrophy).
- Occasional episodic weakness (spontaneous or provoked by cold/ exercise) lasting minutes to hours.
- Treatment: keep warm, acetazolamide, mexiletine, carbamazepine, lamotrigine.

Periodic paralyses

Hyperkalaemic periodic paralysis
- Sodium channel *SCN4A*.
- AD, incomplete penetration.
- Most have ↑potassium during episodes.
- Onset in first decade.
- Paroxysmal paralysis, lasting minutes to hours.
- Weakness is usually proximal and symmetrical but may be distal and asymmetrical particularly following exercise of a muscle.
- Triggers: cold environment, rest after exercise, intercurrent illness.
- May have myotonia or muscle hypertrophy.
- Treatment: acetazolamide, potassium wasting diuretics, salbutamol(prn).

▶Increased risk of malignant hyperthermia with general anaesthesia.

Hypokalaemic periodic paralysis
- Variants due to both calcium (*CACNA1S*) and sodium (*SCN4A*) channel mutations.
- Autosomal dominant.
- Presents typically in second decade.
- Attacks of generalized paralysis, sometimes moderate weakness.
- In late night or early morning.
- Lasts hours to days.
- Trigger: muscle exercise with subsequent rest (hours later), stress, cold, carbohydrate-rich foods.
- Treatment: potassium supplements (prn or daily if frequent attacks), acetazolamide, potassium sparing diuretics, spironolactone, low sodium diet.

▶Increased risk of malignant hyperthermia with general anaesthesia.

Potassium channel KCNJ2 (Andersen Tawil Syndrome)
- AD.
- Onset first to second decade.
- Potassium usually ↓.
- Dysmorphic features; hypertelorism, mandibular and malar hypoplasia, clinodactyly, syndactyly, short stature, low set ears.

- Cardiac conduction abnormalities and ventricular tachyarrhythmia (risk of sudden death).
- Episodic weakness (milder than other PP subtypes), no myotonia.
- Treatment: acetazolamide, cardiac medication (β blockers, implanted defibrillator).

▶Increased risk of malignant hyperthermia with general anaesthesia.

Metabolic myopathies

Can present early in life as:
- Floppy infant.
- Multisystem disorder.

Or later in life with:
- Progressive muscle weakness.
- Exercise intolerance.
- Reversible weakness.
- Cramp/myalgia with exercise.
- Myoglobinuria/rhabdomyolysis.

Glycogenoses

Glycogen Storage Disease (GSD) type 2 (Pompe disease; acid maltase deficiency)

Deficiency of α1,4 glucosidase. Disease severity correlates with level of residual enzyme activity.
- Infantile form (Pompe disease).
  - Profound hypotonia and weakness.
  - Macroglossia.
  - Cardiomegaly.
  - Hepatomegaly.
  - Respiratory and feeding difficulty.
  - Death <2 yrs.
- Childhood/adolescent onset.
  - Progressive proximal weakness, onset <15years more rapid progression.
  - ↑creatine kinase.
  - Respiratory insufficiency (presenting symptom in 30%).
- Adult onset.
  - Slowly progressive muscle weakness, muscle cramps.

Enzyme replacement therapy with recombinant human α-glucosidase can stabilize disease.

GSD type 5 (McArdle disease; myophosphorylase deficiency)
- Onset usually in childhood but delayed diagnosis is common.
- Cramps and contractures with short intense exercise like sprinting.
- Second wind: improvement after continued exercise.
- Myoglobinuria, ↑CK.
- Genetics for *PYGM* gene.
- Treatment: carbohydrate loading before exercise.

Lipidoses or Fatty oxidation defects
- Typically present with intolerance of prolonged low intensity exercise such as long walks.
- In young children fever, fasting and stress can precipitate episodes.
- Myalgia, rhabdomyolysis, myoglobinuria.
- CK and acylcarnitine profile abnormal (can be normal between acute episodes).
- Skin fibroblasts analysis diagnostic.
- Treatment:
  - Frequent meals high in carbohydrates and low in long-chain fats.
  - Supplementation with slow-release carbohydrates, such as cornstarch, during illness.
  - Carbohydrate loading before exercise.

Carnitine palmitoyltransferase II (CPT2 deficiency)
- Neonatal onset (multisystem involvement).
- Infantile-onset with severe hepatocardiomuscular involvement.
- Adolescent onset with myopathic features.
- *S113L* mutation.

L-3-hydroxyacyl-CoA dehydrogenase deficiency
- Features of lipidoses.
- Cardiomyopathy.
- Pigmentary retinopathy.
- Peripheral neuropathy.
- Hypoketotic hypoglycaemia.

Mitochondrial defects of oxidative phosphorylation
(See Mitochondrial Disease in this chapter ➲ p. 404).
- Unusual to have isolated muscle involvement.
- High lactate.
- COX-deficient fibres on biopsy.
- Abnormal mitochondria on electron microscopy.

Reversible infantile respiratory chain deficiency
- Subacute onset of profound hypotonia, feeding difficulties, and lactic acidosis with or without respiratory involvement within the first months of life.
- Cytochrome oxidase (COX) –ve fibres on muscle biopsy.
- Genetic heterogeneity.

Gradual clinical improvement is the norm with persistent mild myopathic features and myalgia.

Muscle-specific phosphatidic acid phosphatase
- Onset 15 m–7 y age.
- Episodes of severe rhabdomyolysis triggered by fever, exercise, fasting, anaesthesia, or medications.
- Metabolic investigations –ve.
- Genetics for *LIPIN1*.

Congenital myopathies

Myopathies characterized by:
- Hypotonia and motor delay.
- Static or slowly progressive.
- CK normal.
- Muscle biopsy: myopathic without dystrophic changes.
- Specific appearances on histology (particularly electron microscopy) after which several of the conditions are named.
- Cardiac and respiratory involvement seen in some subtypes.

Central core disease
- Mutations in *RYR1* gene (ryanodine receptor), may be autosomal dominant or recessive.
- Muscle biopsy: central areas of derangement of sarcomeres with absence of oxidative enzyme activity, fibre type 1 predominance.
- Hypotonic from birth/infancy, delayed motor development. Can have late childhood or adult onset.
- Facial and proximal limb weakness.
- Skeletal deformities: congenital hip dislocation, scoliosis.
- Association with malignant hyperthermia.
- Cardiomyopathy and respiratory insufficiency are rare.

Minicore disease
- Genetically heterogeneous, *SEPN1* mutations recessive or sporadic; *RYR1* mutations recessive or dominant.
- Muscle biopsy: multiple small areas devoid of oxidative enzyme activity, fibre type 1 predominance.
- Hypotonia, delayed motor development.
- Variable weakness, mainly proximal and axial.
- Ophthalmoplegia in some.
- Contractures of paraspinal muscles with scoliosis.
- Early diaphragmatic involvement with respiratory insufficiency even when ambulant (*SEPN1*).

Nemaline rod myopathy
- Histologically: multiple rod-like particles derived from Z band material.
- Onset may be congenital (severe), childhood, or adult.
- Inheritance recessive or dominant.
- Congenital forms mostly due to α-actin *ACTA1*, nebulin (*NEB*), or troponin T1 (*TTN1*) mutations.
- Present with respiratory insufficiency, marked hypotonia, feeding difficulties, majority require respiratory support, may have arthrogryposis.
- Childhood-onset forms mainly *ACTA1*, NEB, α-trophomyosin (*TPM3*), or β-trophomyosin (*TPM2*) mutations.

Present with proximal weakness, often remain ambulant.
- May develop respiratory failure later.

Myotubular myopathy (centronuclear myopathy)
- Muscle biopsy: central nucleus surrounded by clear zone (resembles foetal myotubes), fibre type 1 predominance.

- Variable presentation.
- Neonatal form, X-linked, *MTM1* mutations.
- Polyhydramnios and reduced foetal movements.
- Hypotonia and weakness.
- Respiratory failure, bulbar dysfunction.
- Ptosis, ophthalmoplegia.
- Undescended testes, peliosis hepatitis with fatal haemorrhage.
- Milder forms have autosomal recessive or dominant inheritance (*DMN2*, *BIN1* mutations).

Malignant hyperthermia

Presents as:
- Generalized muscle rigidity or localized to jaw.
- Tachycardia, tachypnoea.
- Rhabdomyolysis, acidosis, hyperkalaemia, myoglobinuria, ↑CK.
- Hyperthermia occurs late.

Triggers:
- Inhalational anaesthetics (isoflurane, desflurane, enflurane, sevoflurane).
- Depolarizing muscle relaxants (succinylcholine).
- Less severe episodes may be triggered by exercise in hot conditions.

Treatment:
- PICU management of fluid balance, rhabdomyolysis, and possible renal involvement (see Status dystonicus in Chapter 5 ⮞ p. 628).

Associated with:
- *RYR1* (ryanodine receptor) mutations in 50%.
- Calcium (*CACNA1S*) and sodium (*SCN4A*) channel gene mutations in others.
- *STAC3*.

▶Anaesthetic reactions may also occur in dystrophinopathies and myotonic dystrophy. It is very important to warn patients with neuromuscular disorders of the ↑risk of anaesthetic reactions and emphasize the need for them to inform an anaesthetist of their condition prior to any procedure requiring a general anaesthetic so appropriate agents can be used.

Idiopathic Inflammatory myopathies

Juvenile idiopathic inflammatory myopathies (IIM) are a rare systemic autoimmune disorder characterized by chronic skeletal muscle inflammation of unknown causes.

Juvenile dermatomyositis
- Commoner subtype of IIM.
- 2–3 cases per million per year.
- Median age of onset 7.5y.
- ♀:♂ 5:1.
- Adult association with malignancies not seen in children.
- Systemic vasculopathy with inflammation of skin and muscle.

Presentation
- Slowly ↑ proximal weakness.
- Muscles are stiff, tender: child is *miserable*.
- Can have dysphagia.
- Heliotrope rash.
- Extensor surfaces of joints can be red, atrophic, and scaly.
- Nail bed capillary loops.
- Can have gastrointestinal involvement, arthropathy, fever, pulmonary disease, iritis.

Diagnostic criteria
- Typical 'heliotrope' purple rash on face and upper eyelids.
- Periorbital oedema.
- Gottron papules (metacarpophalangeal and proximal interphalangeal joints, extensor surfaces).
- Additional features:
  - Progressive symmetrical muscle weakness affecting proximal limb girdle and neck muscles[1].
  - ↑muscle enzymes (CK, LDH, AST, aldolase).
  - Muscle biopsy with perivascular atrophy, inflammatory infiltrates, muscle fibre necrosis.
  - EMG indicative of myopathy.
  - MRI suggestive of inflammatory myositis.
  - nailfold capillaroscopy.
  - calcinosis and dysphonia.
  - myositis-specific/-related antibodies.

Treatment
- Prednisolone.
- Other: IVIG, methotrexate, azathioprine, ciclosporin, rituximab.
- 30–70% develop subcutaneous calcinosis later in disease.

Prognosis
80% will remit without impairment. Others may be left with impairments and continuing disease.
  Poor prognostic signs:
- Skin ulceration.
- Severe gastrointestinal involvement.
- Lung involvement.
- CNS involvement.

Rarely, death from infection or cardiac involvement.

Polymyositis
- 2–8% of IIM.
- Onset generally >20 yrs.
- Neck flexor and proximal weakness.
- CK ↑50-fold.

1 Neck extensor weakness (resulting in a 'dropped head' in extreme cases) is a rare but 'hard'sign typically due (in children) to myasthenia gravis, polymyositis, dermatomyositis, chronic inflammatory demyelinating polyneuropathy, facioscapulohumeral dystrophy, myotonic dystrophy, or congenital myopathy.

- No rash (c.f. dermatomyositis).
- Overlap with collagen vascular diseases.

Infective myositis

Viral/Post viral myositis

- Common. Causes tender, aching calves or thighs (sometimes swollen).
- Associated viral illness symptoms or can be post viral.
- Elevated CK.
- Normal muscle strength and tendon reflexes.
- Viral triggers: coxsackie, influenza, EBV, CMV.
- Self-limiting (check CK in 6–8 weeks to ensure normalization).

Bacterial myositis

- Localized pain, swelling, and weakness.
- Usually due to penetrating injury.
- Treatment: antibiotics and drainage.

Parasitic myositis

- Cestodes: cysticercosis (myalgia, fever, headache, seizures).
- Nematodes: trichinosis.
- Protozoa: toxoplasmosis.

Endocrine and toxic myopathies

- Toxins and drugs can cause myalgia or myopathy. History should always include a drug history and possible exposure to toxins.
- Hypothyroidism (Semelaigne syndrome: hypothyroidism with muscle hypertrophy and short stature).

Motor neuron diseases

Spinal muscular atrophy

- Genetic testing being rapidly added to newborn screening programmes in many countries.
- Majority have homozygous deletions of exons 7 & 8 of *SMN1* gene.
- Number of copies of *SMN2*, among other factors, modifies presentation.
- Classification is clinical but there is a continuum of severity (See Table 4.16).
- Alert, normal cognition, no facial weakness.
- Pattern of weakness: proximal >distal, legs >arms.
- Absent reflexes.
- Tongue fasciculations.
- Intercostal muscles weak with diaphragmatic sparing.

Currently 3 approved treatments (Table 4.17).

Table 4.16 Spinal muscular atrophies

Type	Onset age	Higher motor skill in natural history	Life expectancy
1	<6 months	Never sit	<2 yrs without respiratory support
2	6–18 months	Sit but never walk	Adult life
3	>18 months	Independent walking	Normal
4	Adult	Independent walking	Normal

Table 4.17 SMA Treatments

Drug	Mechanism of action	Regime
Nusinersen	Antisense oligonucleotide	Intrathecal injection (4 loading doses followed by 3/year maintenance doses)
Onasemnogene Abaparvevec	Gene replacement therapy	One-time intravenous infusion
Risdiplam	*SMN2* pre-RNA splicing modifier	Once daily oral dose

SMA with respiratory distress (SMARD)

- Autosomal recessive mutations in *IGHMBP2* gene.
- Presents in infancy with motor delay and weakness, respiratory distress due to diaphragmatic weakness: elevated hemi diaphragm on CXR.
- *IGHMBP2* mutation can also present with childhood-onset neuropathy phenotype.

Pontocerebellar hypoplasia type 1 (PCH1)

Not to be confused with similarly named, but clinically unrelated PCH2 (see Syndromes with pontocerebellar hypoplasia in this chapter ➲ p. 424).

- Early onset presentation with SMA1 like phenotype but additional MRI features of hypoplasia of cerebellum and ventral pons.
- Autosomal recessive, genetic heterogeneity (*VRK1, EXOSC3, EXOSC8, LSC25A46*).
- Treatment is symptomatic.
- Poor prognosis with very limited life expectancy.

Myasthenic syndromes

These are disorders in neuromuscular transmission characterized by muscle weakness and fatigability on exercise.

Autoimmune myasthenia gravis

- ♀>♂ (4:1).
- 1–1.5 per million person-years.
- 10% present in paediatric age range.
- Antibody-mediated post-synaptic disorder.
- Autoantibodies: acetylcholine receptor (AChR) and muscle-specific kinase (MuSK).
  - AChR positivity in 2/3rd of cases, but at times standard radio-immunoassays may be –ve. Consider cell-based assay if strong clinical suspicion as greater sensitivity.

Presentation
- Insidious or acute onset (with intercurrent illness).
- Fatigable weakness on examination (attempted sustained up gaze, arms held outstretched).
- Ptosis, ophthalmoplegia, bulbar, respiratory, dysphonia, dysphagia, dyspnoea.
- Proximal >distal weakness.
- Myasthenic crisis.

Investigation
- Ice pack test for evaluation of ptosis (see Ice pack test for evaluation of possible myasthenia in Chapter 3 → p. 134).
- Antibodies (anti-AChR, anti-MuSK).
- Thyroid function and antibodies.
- Neurophysiology:
  - Repetitive nerve stimulation: decrement in compound muscle action potential.
  - Stimulated single fibre EMG: ↑jitter.
- Trial of anticholinesterases.

Treatment

Mild (ocular only, no bulbar weakness).
- Anticholinesterases. Pyridostigmine used as first line.
- Side effects due to parasympathetic effects (salivation, abdominal cramps, bradycardia) may require careful concomitant antimuscarinic use, e.g. propantheline, but there is a risk of cholinergic crisis at high doses.
- Pyridostigmine works within hours and thus effectiveness can be assessed within a couple of weeks.

Moderate
- Admission, supportive management (feeding, respiratory).
- Initiate pyridostigmine and steroids.
- Steroids: caution required as at times as they can cause an initial deterioration. Start 5 mg alternate days and ↑by 5 mg weekly until on 1–1.5 mg/kg alternate days (max 100 mg).
- Slow steroid weaning is recommended once in remission.
- Consider steroid-sparing agents when steroid dependence, steroid side effects, or poor response to steroids. Options include azathioprine, MMF, rituximab.

Severe (myasthenic crisis)
- See Myasthenic crisis in Chapter 6 ⟳ p. 645.
- ICU support for respiratory and bulbar management.
- Plasma exchange is preferred but IVIG can be considered if PLEX unavailable.
- If a first presentation, steroids can be started at maximal dose.
- Pyridostigmine usually discontinued for duration of ventilation.

Thymectomy
- Only in AChR +ve cases.
- To be considered at disease onset in all peri- and post-pubertal generalized MG. Can be considered in steroid dependent or unresponsive or pre-pubertal MG or ocular MG.
- Pre-op IVIG or plasmapheresis if symptoms still moderately severe.
- Outcome: 30% able to achieve drug free remission, 30% able to reduce level of immunosuppression.

Transient neonatal myasthenia
- Transplacental transfer of AChR subunit antibodies.
- 10–15% of myasthenic mothers.
- Hypotonia, weakness, bulbar, and respiratory insufficiency within 4 days of birth.
- Diagnosis: antibodies, response to cholinesterase inhibitors.
- Antibodies against foetal AChR only: mothers are unaffected.
infant present with arthrogryposis multiplex which may be recurrent.

▶Consider infantile botulism as a cause of myasthenia-like pictures in infants.

Lambert–Eaton myasthenic syndrome
- Autoimmune, often paraneoplastic.
- Rare in children.
- Antibodies to voltage-gated calcium channels on presynaptic nerve terminal.

Congenital myasthenic syndromes

Genetic disorders of the neuromuscular junction in which the safety margin of neuromuscular transmission is compromised.
- UK prevalence 9.2/million; most common mutations in UK are *CHRNE*, *RAPSN*, and *DOK7*.

- Notable as most are treatment responsive.
  - Responsive to anticholinesterases however note that some CMS subtypes may worsen.
- AChR and MuSK antibodies are −ve and there is no response to immunomodulation.
- Electrophysiology (See Single fibre electromyography in Chapter 2 ⊅ p. 97).

Presentation
- Birth: hypotonia, weakness (including ocular, bulbar and respiratory weakness), stridor.
- Infancy/childhood: hypotonia, fatigability, weak cry, feeding difficulties, delayed motor milestones, recurrent chest infections, episodic apnoea.
- May also present with limb girdle weakness.
- Rarely adult onset.

▶Consider congenital myasthenic syndromes in differential of apparent acute life-threatening events and severe episodic apnoea. Children may be essentially symptom-free between episodes.

Characterization
See Table 4.18 which is not exclusive but summarizes the most common types of CMS.

Medications contraindicated in all myasthenic syndromes

- Drugs directly affecting neuromuscular junction function need to be avoided or used with caution in both autoimmune and congenital myasthenia.
- Antibiotics: aminoglycosides, quinolone, tetracyclines.
- Antimalarials: chloroquine, hydroxychloroquine.
- Anaesthetic agents: succinylcholine.
- Cardiac: β-blockers, calcium channel, antiarrhythmics.
- Antipsychotics: chlorpromazine, risperidone.
- Miscellaneous: magnesium salts, botulinum toxin, penicillamine, checkpoint inhibitors.

Table 4.18 Common congenital myasthenic syndromes

	Gene defect	Inheritance	Onset	Presentation	Response to AChE inhibitor	Treatment
AChR deficiency	AChR subunit mutations, *CHRNE* most common. *CHRNGA1*, *CHRNGB1*, *CHRNGD* (cause receptor deficiency)	AR	Infancy	Weakness, ptosis, ophthalmoplegia	Improvement	AChE inhibitor, 3,4-DAP, salbutamol
Abnormal AChR clustering	*RAPSN*	AR	Variable	**Neonatal/infancy-** Reduced foetal movement, arthrogryposis, hypotonia, ptosis, feeding difficulty, episodic apnoea **Child/adult-** delayed motor development, proximal/ generalized weakness	Improvement	AChE inhibitor, 3,4-DAP, salbutamol
Abnormal AChR clustering	*DOK7*	AR	Birth– early childhood	Feeding difficulty, stridor, hypotonia, proximal/ axial weakness, respiratory issues, ptosis without ophthalmoplegia	No improvement or worse	Salbutamol, ephedrine

(Continued)

Table 4.18 (Contd.)

	Gene defect	Inheritance	Onset	Presentation	Response to AChE inhibitor	Treatment
Presynaptic CMS with episodic apnoea	CHAT, SLC5A7	AR	Neonate or infant	Hypotonia, weakness especially bulbar, respiratory problems, episodic apnoea	Improvement	AChE inhibitor
Slow channel syndrome	AChR subunit mutations, prolonged opening	AD	Variable	Selective wasting/ weakness; cervical, scapular, finger extension, ptosis with/without ophthalmoplegia	Worse	Fluoxetine, quinidine
Fast channel syndrome	AChR subunit mutations (commonest CHRNE), short channel opening	AR	Neonatal or infancy	Reduced foetal movements, generalized weakness, ptosis, ophthalmoplegia, bulbar, episodic apnoea	Improvement	AChE inhibitor, 3,4-DAP, salbutamol
Synaptic cleft	COLQ	AR	Neonatal or infancy	Feeding difficulty, hypotonia, weakness, respiratory issues, ptosis with ophthalmoplegia	Worse	Salbutamol, ephedrine

Management of neuromuscular disease

Practical and psychological support
- Family support—care co-ordinator.
- Genetic counselling.
- Access to education.
- Social worker: benefits, housing adaptations funding.
- Occupational therapy: wheelchair, equipment, and adaptations for independence.
- Palliative care.

Musculoskeletal

See also Care of the disabled child in this chapter ⊋ p. 243 although note that *spasticity* will not be an issue in this group.

Prevention of contractures
- Physiotherapy and stretching, splints.
- Encourage mobilization—splints and standing frames.
- Prevention of scoliosis: prolongation of ambulation, standing.
- Spinal surgery and other orthopaedic surgery in selected cases.

Nutrition and feeding
- Bone status, especially if on steroids: calcium, vitamin D. Bisphosphonates if vertebral fractures, recurrent fractures, or worsening bone density.
- Dietician: avoid obesity.
- Speech and language therapy assessment of swallowing: NGT or gastrostomy if swallow is unsafe.

Respiratory
Patterns
- Restrictive lung disease in muscular dystrophy (weak intercostals and diaphragm, scoliosis).
- Poor cough in SMA (weak intercostals and abdominals; poor glottis closure).
- Aspiration in SMA, severe myopathies, myotonic dystrophy (bulbar weakness, gastro-oesophageal reflux).

History
- Recurrent chest infections.
- Nocturnal hypoventilation (restless sleep, morning headache, lethargy, reduced appetite, weight loss).
- Coughing or choking during eating or drinking indicates aspiration.

Examination

▶Note that children with neuromuscular disease *cannot generate* respiratory distress!

Investigations

- FVC (lying plus sitting or standing; worse when lying indicates a weak diaphragm).
- Overnight O_2 saturations (if FVC<25% of predicted or symptomatic).
- Early morning CO_2.
- Polysomnography.

Prevention:

- Vaccinations: 23V *Pneumococcus*, influenza, Sars-Cov-2.
- Feeding assessment and advice (SALT) (see Investigations for aspiration in this chapter ➲ p. 254).
- Treatment of gastro-oesophageal reflux.
- Assisted cough (manual or mechanical).

Treatment

- Early antibiotic treatment of chest infections, antibiotic available at home, IV antibiotic if not improving.
- Assisted cough, physiotherapy.
- Non-invasive +ve pressure ventilation (NIV) for palliation, prolongation of life, better quality of life (see Long-term ventilation in Chapter 5 ➲ p. 600).
- Severe intercurrent chest infections may require ↑and/or invasive ventilation.
  - Extubation should be performed carefully under optimized circumstances (clear chest, in air, no secretions) to maximize chances of success.
- The appropriateness of such interventions should have been agreed prospectively with the family and young person concerned.

Neurocutaneous syndromes

There are several conditions in which skin abnormality is associated with neurological disorders since both skin and central nervous system originate embryologically from ectoderm.

Neurofibromatosis type I

Epidemiology

Birth frequency 1 in 2500 births; prevalence 1 in 4500. Gene (chromosome 17q11.2) codes for protein product *neurofibromin* which is found in high levels in CNS where it regulates cell growth and proliferation via RAS and mTOR (mammalian Target of Rapamycin) pathways, i.e. it has a *tumour suppressor function* (lost if mutated).

50% new mutations with no family history.

Mosaic NF1 (1:30 000) occurs when a mutation occurs in the later stages of embryo growth. May present as a mild generalized disease or more commonly as segmental NF1.

Diagnostic criteria

• Progressive condition with onset in infancy. Cutaneous features become increasingly evident through the first decade (axillary freckling appears early) but diagnosis may be missed in early years. NIH criteria updated by international consensus in 2021.

International Consensus Criteria

• Part A: The diagnostic criteria for NF1 are met in an individual who does *not* have a parent diagnosed with NF1 if two or more of the following are present.
  • six or more café au lait spots (>5 mm pre-pubertal/>15 mm post-pubertal).
  • ≥ 2 neurofibromas of any type or one plexiform neurofibroma.
  • Axillary or inguinal freckling (Crowe sign).
  • optic pathway glioma.
  • ≥2 iris hamartomas (Lisch nodules) or ≥2 choroidal abnormalities.
  • distinctive osseous lesion such as sphenoid dysplasia, or anterolateral bowing of tibia and/or fibula, or pseudoarthrosis of a long bone.
  • a heterozygous pathogenic NF1 variant with a variant allele fraction of 50% in apparently normal tissue such as white blood cells.
• Part B: A *child of* a *parent* who meets the diagnostic criteria specified in A merits a diagnosis of NF1 if ≥ 1 of the criteria in A are present.

(From Legius et al. Revised diagnostic criteria for neurofibromatosis type 1 and Legius syndrome: an international consensus recommendation. Genetics in Medicine (2021) 23:1506–1513).

Clinical features

Neurological complications account for much of the morbidity and mortality.
• CNS:
  • majority have IQ in low average range. Learning difficulties in ~60%. ADHD and ASD also common (up to 50%).
  • epilepsy 6–7% (including infantile spasms).

- cerebrovascular disease 6% (vasculopathies with stenosis and moyamoya disease; also aneurysms).
- multiple sclerosis.
- T2 hyperintensities on MRI also known as myelin vacuolation or (unhelpfully!) as unidentified bright objects (UBOs). Wax and wane and have no specific clinical implications in isolation. Common in childhood in area of basal ganglia, cerebellum, and brain stem.
- tumours: see Risk of neoplasm in this chapter ➜ p. 462.
- Peripheral nerves:
  - neurofibromas which may be subcutaneous or plexiform.
  - malignant peripheral nerve sheath tumour. Suspicion of this should elicit urgent referral to a specialist centre (red flags: persistent or nocturnal pain, rapid growth, hardening, new neurological deficit).10% life-time risk.
  - NF1 neuropathy (1% adults).
- Spinal canal:
  - neurofibromas of the spinal nerve roots;
  - spinal gliomas;
  - scoliosis (10–40%)—secondary to above lesion.
- Chiari 1 malformations.
- Aqueduct stenosis1.5%.
- Sphenoid wing dysplasia 1% (causes pulsating exophthalmos).
- Macrocephaly (45% of children have OFC >98th centile but no added clinical implications).
- Gliomas of optic nerves: see below.
- Other important complications:.
  - short stature (growth hormone deficiency);
  - hypertension (aortic coarctation, renal artery stenosis or phaeochromocytoma);
  - renal artery stenosis 2%;
  - pheochromocytoma 2%;
  - pulmonary stenosis 2%.

Risk of neoplasm

- Optic glioma (pilocytic astrocytoma): mostly chiasmic, found in up to 20% though symptomatic in <5% (↓visual acuity, visual field defect, proptosis, precocious puberty due to hypothalamus compression).
- Gliomas are usually astrocytomas of the brainstem (more common in ♀s, may cause obstructive hydrocephalus), cerebral peduncles, globus pallidus, and midbrain.
- Ependymoma, meningioma, medulloblastoma.
- The risk of malignant transformation of neurofibroma to neurofibrosarcoma is <5% in children (higher in adults). Presentation is with rapid growth of lesion and pain.
- ↑risk of Wilm tumour, rhabdomyosarcoma, leukaemia, melanoma, medullary thyroid carcinoma, and phaeochromocytoma.

Surveillance

Annual review by a paediatrician or paediatric neurologist with an interest in NF1 to monitor:

- Development and progress at school.
- Visual symptoms, VA, colour vision, and fundoscopy until age 7 yrs and then every 2 yrs until adulthood. Visual field assessment once developmentally able to co-operate.
- Increasing use of VEPs and optical coherence tomography to monitor optic pathway gliomas.
- Height and weight and pubertal assessment (precocious puberty).
- BP (consider renal artery stenosis and pheochromocytoma).
- Cardiovascular examination (pulmonary stenosis).
- Spine for scoliosis secondary to underlying plexiform spinal neurofibromas.
- Skin and other problems.
- Regular MRI is not indicated as treatment focuses on symptomatic lesions. Optic gliomas are usually indolent lesions, but some may cause local compression and require debulking and/or chemotherapy.
- Hydrocephalus is managed with ventriculoperitoneal shunting.
- Surgery is often indicated for plexiform neurofibromas that are disfiguring or painful. Neurofibromas may be paraspinal, presenting with myelopathy from cord compression and may require debulking.
- Genetic counselling for family members.

Treatment with MEK inhibitors

Selumetinib is licenced above 3 years of age for treatment of inoperative and intrusive plexiform neuromas.

NF2-related Schwannomatosis (neurofibromatosis type 2)

The hallmark of *NF2*-related schwannomatosis is the development of bilateral vestibular schwannomas which increase rapidly in size around puberty. Schwannomas of other cranial nerves, spinal nerves, and peripheral nerves also seen. Meningiomas may be both intracranial and extracranial affecting spinal and optic nerves. Others include low-grade CNS tumours and spinal ependymomas.

Epidemiology

Birth incidence 1:33 000. Prevalence 1:60 000. Autosomal dominant; chromosome 22.

Diagnostic criteria

A progressive condition with presentation typically after puberty, usually with acute hearing loss, tinnitus, vertigo due to involvement of eighth cranial nerve. Younger children present with visual deficits (juvenile posterior subcapsular lenticular opacity) or skin tumours.

A diagnosis of *NF2*-related schwannomatosis can be made when an individual has one of the following:

- Bilateral vestibular nerve schwannomas (found in 90%).
- An identical NF2 pathogenic variant in at least 2 anatomically distinct NF2-related tumours (schwannoma, meningioma, and/or ependymoma) (if the variant allele fraction in unaffected tissues

such as blood is clearly <50%, the diagnosis is mosaic NF2-related schwannomatosis).

A diagnosis can also be made in the presence of either 2 major or 1 major and 2 minor criteria as described as follows:
- Major criteria:
  - *Unilateral* vestibular schwannoma.
  - First-degree relative (other than sibling) with a confirmed diagnosis of *NF2*-related schwannomatosis.
  - ≥ 2 meningiomas (a single meningioma qualifies as a minor criterion).
  - NF2 pathogenic variant in an unaffected tissue such as blood (Note: if the variant allele fraction is clearly <50%, the diagnosis is mosaic *NF2*-related schwannomatosis).
- Minor criteria:
  - Ependymoma, meningioma (multiple meningiomas qualify as a major criteria), schwannoma (if the major criterion is unilateral vestibular schwannoma, at least one other schwannoma must be dermal in location). Can count >1 of a type, e.g. 2 distinct schwannomas would count as 2 minor criteria.
  - Juvenile subcapsular or cortical cataract, retinal hamartoma, epiretinal membrane in a person aged <40 years. Can count only once (e.g. bilateral cortical cataracts count as a single minor criterion).

Features
- Caused by a mutation in the gene coding for schwannomin on chromosome 22.
- Schwannomin is involved in the interaction between actin in the cytoskeleton and the cell membrane and suppresses tumorigenesis through contact mediated growth inhibition.
- 50% new mutation rate.
- Mosaicism (with the mutation occurring after conception and resulting two cell lineages) usually results in a less severe phenotype.
  - In mosaic individuals, the mutation may be found in too small a proportion of lymphocytes to achieve a diagnosis from genetic testing of blood.
  - In these individuals diagnosis of mosaic NF2 can only be achieved demonstrating the same mutation in two separate tumours.

New mutation for a child index case often results in a severe phenotype:
- Multi-tumour disease in early childhood (often not vestibular schwannoma related).
- Ocular presentation with proptosis and an optic nerve meningioma.
- Mononeuropathy which often affects the facial nerve and may be recurrent with poor recovery and lasting deficit.
- Amyotrophy polio-like illness with wasting of muscle groups.
- Epilepsy and focal cortical dysplasia.

Many children suffer from reduced visual acuity. Reasons include:
- Amblyopia with no obvious cause.
- 60–80% cataracts which may be posterior subcapsular lenticular opacities or cortical wedge opacities. Can present very early in life.
- Optic nerve meningiomas (again can present early).
- Extensive retinal hamartomas.

Skin:
- Features may be subtle. Present in 70% but rarely numerous.
- The commonest skin lesion is an intracutaneous plaque-like lesion, slightly raised and pigmented with hairs. Deeper subcutaneous nodules on nerves may be felt. Café au lait patches but only 1% of affected people having more than six.

Surveillance

NF2-related Schwannomatosis is a rare condition and needs specialist multi-disciplinary management. Once a tumour is present or a mutation has been found in an affected child, a brain scan needs to be done at least once a year. Spinal tumours are common but rarely need surgical treatment and 3 yearly scanning is sufficient unless there are new symptoms.

Annual hearing tests (sooner if any concerns) are essential from earliest possible age.
- Schwannomas are slowly progressive and if symptomatic may be resected or managed with stereotactic radiosurgery. Treatment may also be indicated if schwannomas are pre-symptomatic to preserve hearing.
- Genetic counselling for family members.
- Bevacizumab (monoclonal antibody that targets an isoform of VEGF that stimulates endothelial cell proliferation) is licenced for use in children in the UK with rapidly growing vestibular schwannomas with hearing impairment, meeting very strict criteria. Shown to result in shrinkage and improvement in hearing in adults. Results in children less clear.

Tuberous sclerosis complex (TSC)

Epidemiology
- 1:9000, autosomal dominant, mutations in either TSC1 on chromosome 9q34 (hamartin) or TSC2 on chromosome 16p13 (tuberin).
- Two-thirds of cases are new mutations (usually TSC2 mutations), one-third are inherited (usually TSC1 mutations), with implications for other children and family members.
- TSC2 mutation associated with more severe phenotype, although exceptions with some TSC2 mutations, and overlap of phenotype with TSC1.

Hamartin and tuberin form a complex that inhibits mTOR ('mammalian Target of Rapamycin') in early life the normal function of which is to control cell proliferation: mutations resulting in loss of function of this complex result in tumour formation in most major organs. The potential of mTOR inhibitors such as everolimus to control tuber formation is now established.

Diagnostic criteria
- Typically presents with seizures (60–90%, usually infantile spasms with onset <1 yr, 50% will be intractable), developmental impairment—especially with autistic features (25–50%).
- Learning difficulties in 45%, others have normal intellect (IQ >70, but often have specific deficits e.g. attention or memory).
- Two major or one major and two minor features must be present for the diagnosis of this condition.

Major features
- Hypomelanotic macules (>2, at least 5 mm in diameter).

  - Angiofibroma (>2) or fibrous cephalic plaque.
  - Ungual fibromas (>1).
  - Shagreen patch.
  - Multiple retinal hamartomas.
  - Multiple cortical tubers and/or radial migration lines.
  - Subependymal nodule (>1).
  - Subependymal giant cell astrocytoma (SEGA).
  - Cardiac rhabdomyoma.
  - Lymphangioleiomyomatosis.
  - Angiomyolipomas (>1).

Minor features
- Dental enamel pits (>2).

  - Sclerotic bone lesions.
  - Intraoral fibromas (>1).
  - Non-renal hamartoma.
  - Retinal achromatic patch.
  - Confetti skin lesions.
  - Multiple renal cysts.

Management
- See Table 4.19 for surveillance schedule.
- ASM therapy for seizures.

Table 4.19 Surveillance of asymptomatic patients with TSC

	Initial testing	Repeat testing
Neurodevelopmental and neuropsychiatric assessment	At diagnosis	At 0–3 yrs, 3–6 yrs, 6–9 yrs, and 12–18 yrs, and as clinically indicated
Dental assessment	At diagnosis	6 monthly
Skin examination	At diagnosis	Annual
Ophthalmology	At diagnosis	Annual
EEG	At diagnosis	As clinically indicated
ECG	At diagnosis	Every 3–5 yrs
Echocardiogram	If cardiac symptoms	If cardiac dysfunction
Renal surveillance	At diagnosis	Annual renal function. Abdominal MRI every 1–3 yrs or if concerning change on ultrasound
MRI brain	At diagnosis	Every 1–3 yrs until 25
Chest CT	In adulthood (women only)	If respiratory dysfunction

- Multidisciplinary approach for developmental problems.
- Resection of SEGA if symptomatic (±VP shunt).
  - Everolimus (mTOR inhibitor) now licenced for control of surgically unresectable SEGAs.
- Epilepsy surgery evaluation if intractable seizures.
  - May be an option if there is a single very dominant seizure focus, although more commonly epilepsy is multifocal and bihemispheric.
- Monitoring of renal function and blood pressure, monitoring of vision.
- mTOR inhibitors can be used topically for management of facial angiofibromas (off-licence).
- Monitor carefully and advice families to watch for any sudden regression in skills.
  - May represent development of hydrocephalus due to critical expansion of SEGA, or poor seizure control.
- Genetic counselling for family members.

Prognosis
- Varies with the phenotype in a particular individual.
- Major causes of death: renal disease, primary brain tumours, pulmonary lymphangioleiomyomatosis, status epilepticus, and pneumonia.

Sturge–Weber syndrome

A congenital disorder with angiomatosis of the face, eye, and meninges. Caused by post-conceptual, somatic, non-inherited mutations in the *GNAQ* gene.

Clinical features
- An ipsilateral facial port wine stain (in the distribution of the first branch of the trigeminal nerve) is present at birth.

▶ Only 15% of all children with facial port wine stain will have SWS.

- Ipsilateral leptomeningeal angioma (causing contralateral seizures ± hemiplegia, hemi-atrophy, and homonymous hemianopia).
- Progressive venous infarction of the brain underlying the leptomeningeal angioma leads to atrophy and calcification.
- Epilepsy (in 80%) starts as focal motor seizures in the first year of life; with fever sensitivity.
- Ocular vascular malformations may cause glaucoma (30%), buphthalmos, iris heterochromia, or optic atrophy.
- Hemiparesis, learning difficulties (90%), developmental impairment, dental abnormalities, and skeletal lesions.
- MRI with gadolinium demonstrates leptomeningeal enhancement, white matter abnormalities, and often unilateral hypertrophy of the choroid plexus; the vascular malformation itself may be impossible to see.
- Hydrocephalus may result from ↑venous pressure or from extensive A–V anastomosis.
- Headache is common.

Management
- Laser therapy for the port wine stain.
- Lobectomy or hemispherectomy may improve quality of life when intractable seizures are a problem——refer early as may preserve cognition.
- ASMs for seizures.
- Aspirin may reduce stroke-like episodes.
- Regular ophthalmology review to monitor glaucoma (both medical and surgical therapy may be required).
- Safe to use triptans for headache; maintain hydration.
- Psychosocial support.

Prognosis
Children with more extensive leptomeningeal involvement or bilateral disease have a worse prognosis. Early onset of intractable seizures is also associated with worse outcome and greater risk of learning disabilities.

Ataxia telangiectasia (AT)

Epidemiology
1:40 000, autosomal recessive or sporadic mutation in chromosome 11q23.3. ATM protein is absent in 85% of cases of AT and present but malfunctioning in the remaining 15%. Heterozygotes have an ↑risk of malignancy, especially breast cancer.

Clinical features
- Slowly progressive cerebellar ataxia, dystonia, and dysarthria with onset in the second year of life (precedes skin manifestations).
- Later choreoathetosis, oculomotor apraxia, nystagmus.
- Telangiectasias of the skin (ears, eyelids, cheeks, neck, antecubital and popliteal fossae), and bulbar conjunctiva.
- ↑susceptibility to bronchopulmonary infections (in ~70% due to IgA and/or IgE deficiency).
- Intelligence is preserved until late.
- Children have short stature (70%) and progeric changes (90%).
- Lymphoid tissue (tonsils, adenoids, and thymus) may be absent.
- α-fetoprotein is ↑in 95% of cases, carcinoembryonic antigen is ↑and IgA and IgE are low/absent.
- Chromosome fragility is manifest as frequent chromosome abnormalities (in 80%), especially 14:14 translocations.
- Glucose intolerance in 50% and adolescent diabetes is characterized by hyperglycaemia with infrequent glycosuria and no ketosis.
- MRI demonstrates atrophy of the cerebellum and later atrophy of the posterior columns of the spinal cord.
- If investigations for AT are –ve, consider testing for the *AOA1* (ataxia with oculomotor apraxia) gene.

Risk of neoplasm
Lymphoreticular (leukaemia, lymphoma, lymphosarcoma, Hodgkin disease), and other malignancies especially of the skin.

Management
- Control of infections with antibiotics and IVIG.

- Protection from sunlight and radiation.
- Multidisciplinary support for a progressive neurological disorder.

Prognosis

Death can occur in late childhood or early teens but many with appropriate supportive care will live well into adult life.

Von Hippel–Lindau disease

Epidemiology

1:40 000, autosomal dominant mutation in chromosome 3p25-26. The mutation leads to angiogenic neoplasms. Cysts form around these tumours and the cyst is often far greater in size than the tumour. The mass effect from the cyst is often responsible for symptoms.

Clinical features

- Usually presents in adolescence with visual symptoms or later with signs of posterior fossa mass effect.
- Although classically regarded as a neurocutaneous syndrome there is usually no skin involvement!
- Diagnostic features include:
  - retinal haemangioma/haemangioblastoma (may lead to retinal detachment if multiple);
  - CNS haemangioblastoma (especially of the cerebellum and spinal cord);
  - renal carcinoma;
  - multiple congenital cysts of the pancreas;
  - polycythaemia (from excessive erythropoietin).

Risk of neoplasm

Cerebellar haemangioblastomas are seen in around 75% of children and ultimately multiple CNS haemangioblastomas develop. Spinal cord haemangioblastomas are associated with syringomyelia in around 80%. Phaeochromocytoma, angiomas of the liver and kidney, papillary cystadenomas, and endolymphatic sac tumours all occur with greater frequency.

Management

Early detection and early surgical excision is the goal of management of symptomatic CNS haemangioblastomas. The recurrence rate is 8–15%. Radiotherapy may be used for multiple or inaccessible lesions. Regular ophthalmological examination to follow small retinal haemangioblastoma is appropriate, but if visual loss or retinal detachment occurs then this may be treated with laser photocoagulation or cryo-coagulation. Screening for phaeochromocytoma may include blood pressure monitoring and HVA and VMA assay.

Prognosis

CNS haemangioblastomas are a major cause of morbidity and are the cause of death in >50% of children with this disease. 30% of deaths are due to renal cell carcinoma.

Hereditary Haemorrhagic Telangiectasia (Osler-Weber-Rendu syndrome)

Epidemiology
- Estimated prevalence ~1: 5000.
- Autosomal dominant inheritance.
- Mutations in *ENG*, *ACVRL1*, *SMAD4*, and *GDF2* genes encoding proteins involved in vascular remodelling.
- Multiple vascular malformations develop in different organs (skin and mucous membranes, brain, lungs, and liver).

Diagnostic criteria
The diagnosis is definite with ≥3, or suspected with 2, criteria from: spontaneous recurrent epistaxis; multiple mucocutaneous telangiectasias (lips, oral cavity, nose); visceral involvement (e.g. GI telangiectasias or pulmonary, hepatic, or cerebral arteriovenous malformations); or a 1st degree relative with HHT (see Faughnan *et al* 2020. Ann. Int. Med. 2020 Dec 15;173(12):989–1001).

Clinical features
- Pulmonary AVMs can manifest as chronic hypoxemia.

Management
Refer to the Faughnan 2020 paper.

Other neurocutaneous syndromes

Hypomelanosis of Ito
An autosomal dominant condition presenting with congenital hypopigmented skin lesions (linear streaks following dermatomes or irregular whorls) in association with learning disability, seizures, motor disorder, and abnormalities of the eye (strabismus, myopia, optic nerve hypoplasia), hair, teeth, and bone.

Incontinentia pigmenti
An X-linked dominant condition affecting ♀s in >90% of cases (lethal in ♂'s). Bullous skin lesions (contain eosinophilic fluid) are found in a linear pattern on the trunk and limbs. Then verrucous lesions appear over the dorsum of the fingers from the sixth week of life. These heal, resulting in atrophic cutaneous areas. Hyperpigmented areas then appear and later gradually fade. It is associated with seizures, learning disability, and motor disorder and with abnormalities of the eye (retinal detachment, optic atrophy, papillitis, nystagmus, cataracts, and strabismus), hair (alopecia), teeth (delayed dentition, pegged teeth, and abnormal crown formation) and bone (spina bifida, hemivertebrae).

Neurocutaneous melanosis
Leptomeningeal melanosis associated with cutaneous nevi, e.g. multiple giant hairy pigmented nevi and congenital melanocytic nevi. Cutaneous giant hairy nevi usually have a 'bathing suit' or 'cape' distribution. Leptomeningeal involvement is usually brainstem, cerebral peduncles, and basilar cerebrum

and cerebellum. Hydrocephalus and learning disabilities with behaviour problems are common. CSF protein is elevated, and cytology reveals abnormal melanin-containing cells. Prognosis is poor.

Linear sebaceous nevus/epidermal nevus syndrome

A midline or near midline yellow-brown hairless plaque occurs on the face or scalp at birth or in early childhood which may become malignant. This condition is associated with CNS abnormality (unilateral lissencephaly, heterotopic grey matter and hemimegalencephaly) causing learning disability, motor disorder, and seizures, as well as eye abnormalities.

Posterior fossa malformations, haemangiomas, arterial anomalies, cardiac defects, eye abnormalities, sternal cleft and supraumbilical raphe (PHACES) syndrome

Syndrome of multiple congenital abnormalities (genetic basis unknown) that causes large facial haemangiomas (usually appearing and rapidly enlarging in early infancy).

Neurodegenerative conditions

Neurodegeneration (progressive neurological and/or cognitive decline) is caused by a heterogeneous group of conditions. Individually rare (over 600 causes described), the combined prevalence is 0.6/1000 live births.

- Combination of progressive *neurological and cognitive* decline, although either neurological or cognitive elements may predominate initially.
- Typically evolve over years after a period of normal development (this can be difficult to demonstrate if very early onset) with loss of already attained developmental skills.
- In children under 4 yrs, this may initially manifest as developmental *stagnation* before it is clear there is actual regression.
- Duration greater than 3 months.
- Evidence of generalized brain dysfunction.
- Development of abnormal neurological signs (eye signs are easily missed if not specifically looked for).
- Due to CNS dysfunction.
  - Consider non-neurological causes of apparent regression. See Non-neurodegenerative causes of apparent regression in Chapter 3 ➔ p. 183.

The most common conditions include mucopolysaccharidoses (especially type III), X-linked adrenoleukodystrophy, neuronal ceroid lipofuscinoses, mitochondrial cytopathies, metachromatic leukodystrophy, Alpers' syndrome, and GM2 gangliosidoses.

Focused investigation

- A diagnosis will be made in about 75% of cases: average time to diagnosis is 3–6 months.
- There is no general 'screen'; however, MRI and neurophysiology (EEG ± ERG and VEP) will be valuable for all. This will guide focused biochemistry, histopathology, and genetic testing.
- The clinical picture will focus differential diagnoses. See Psychomotor regression in Chapter 3 ➔ p. 183.

Importance of diagnosis

- These diseases are severe and debilitating and continue inexorably to death. Diagnosis will have enormous medical, educational, and psychosocial implications for the child and family.
- Specific diagnosis allows multidisciplinary planning, contact with condition-specific support groups and accurate and sensitive counselling regarding prognosis, inheritance, and prenatal testing.
- Until recently, diagnosis has not particularly informed therapy, however this is changing rapidly for some conditions with an increasing number of diseases amenable to specific treatments including enzyme replacement (direct or via gene therapy), substrate reduction, or bone marrow transplantation.

Most common diagnoses by age at presentation

Age at onset is one of the most useful 'handles' diagnostically. The conditions below are listed by the most typical age at onset and are discussed in more detail on subsequent pages. It is, however, *important to appreciate that many have variants*: typically, less rapidly progressing forms presenting at later ages. In these situations, the main implications of diagnosis may be for family members other than the index case.

On-line and computer-aided systems exist to help focus investigations and differential diagnoses in what can be a very confusing area.

0–2 years
- Infantile neuronal ceroid lipofuscinosis (NCL, or CLN1).
- Krabbe leukodystrophy.
- Metachromatic leukodystrophy.
- Pelizaeus–Merzbacher disease.
- Tay–Sachs: infantile.
- Infantile neuraxonal dystrophy.
- Gaucher type 2.
- Rett Syndrome.

2–5 years
- Mucopolysaccharidoses (Sanfilippo).
- Late infantile NCL (CLN2).
- Mitochondrial diseases.
- Alpers syndrome.
- Gaucher type 3.

5–12 years
- Juvenile CLN (CLN3).
- Adrenoleukodystrophy.
- Rasmussen syndrome.
- NBIA.
- Refsum disease.
- Unverricht–Lundborg disease.
- Niemann–Pick C.
- Friedreich ataxia.
- HIV dementia.

First 2 yrs of life

Rett syndrome
Rett syndrome is an important cause of regression in this age group but is not strictly a neurodegenerative condition.
- *Presentation*: initially a normal ♀ who between 6 and 18 months shows regression of speech and functional hand movements, sleep disturbance and agitation, and acquired microcephaly.
- *Clinical course*: severe cognitive impairment, stereotypical hand movements, spasticity, scoliosis, GTC seizures in the majority, non-epileptic 'vacant spells'. Respiratory rhythm disturbances including hyperventilation. See Rett syndrome in this chapter ➜ p. 473.
- *Neurophysiology*: EEG non-specific.
- *Genetics*: X-linked, predominantly ♀s; *MECP2* gene (85%). A number of other genes causing Rett-like pictures have been identified (see Rett syndrome, Rett-like syndromes, and MECP2-associated phenotypes in this chapter ➜ p. 297) for more details.

- Management:
  - symptomatic treatment of seizures, hyperventilation;
  - monitoring for scoliosis, osteoporosis;
  - periodic ECG monitoring (associated with prolongation of QT interval);
  - avoid drugs associated with prolongation of QT interval including macrolide antibiotics, haloperidol, pimozide, SSRIs.

Early infantile neuronal ceroid lipofuscinosis (CLN1)

NCLs are autosomal recessive lysosomal storage diseases, characterized by the accumulation of autofluorescent lipopigment in tissues (inclusion bodies). They are classified by age of presentation.

▶ Remember the infantile-onset form characteristically first presents with developmental impairment; the late infantile-onset form with aggressive seizures; and the juvenile-onset form with visual loss.

- *Presentation*: at end of the first year, developmental arrest, infrequent seizures, blindness, movement disorder, microcephaly.
- *Clinical course*: ↑ing irritability, hypotonia, dystonic spasms.
- *Neurophysiology*: attenuation then loss of electroretinogram (ERG) and visual evoked potentials (VEPs).
- *Histopathology*: granular inclusions in neurons on electron microscopy of skin biopsy.
- *Biochemistry*: Palmitoyl-protein thioesterase (PPT) assay: check as may not be routinely included as part of your laboratory's standard white cell enzyme (WCE) panel.
- *Genetics: CLN1* mutation analysis.

Krabbe leukodystrophy (common infantile form)

- *Presentation*: first months of life: severe irritability, spasticity, and impairment.
- *Clinical course*: regression with febrile illnesses, decerebrate by 1yr, areflexic, ↓visual awareness.
- *Neurophysiology*: ↓nerve conduction.
- *Histopathology*: needle-like inclusion bodies in macrophages and brain; demyelination on nerve biopsy; foamy histiocytes.
- *Biochemistry*: ↑CSF protein.
- *Diagnosis:* galactosylceramidase activity on WCE panel (rarely, saposin A deficiency).
- *Genetics: GALC* mutation analysis.
- *Treatment:* allogenic haematopoietic stem cell transplantation is beneficial if performed in asymptomatic symptomatic patients (typically younger siblings of index cases).

Tay–Sachs disease (classic infantile GM2 gangliosidosis)

Gangliosidoses are lysosomal storage disorders characterized by accumulation of gangliosides in neurons. Like NCLs, gangliosidoses are classified by age of presentation. This is the infantile form. ↑incidence in Ashkenazi Jewish population: screening for carrier status amongst would-be parents increasingly widespread in this community.

- *Presentation*: 4–6 months, motor weakness.
- *Clinical course*: rapidly progressive hypotonia, seizures by 6 months (massive myoclonus), blind by 1 yr, death in 4 yrs.
- *Specific features*: macular degeneration; cherry red spot; macrocephaly from year 2.
- *Neurophysiology*: EEG initially unremarkable, becomes very abnormal; VEP abolished by 18 months, ERG normal.
- *Neuroimaging*: white matter abnormalities.
- *Biochemistry*: hexosaminidase A activity on WCE.
- *Genetics*: HEXA mutation analysis.

Pelizaeus–Merzbacher disease (PMD)

Dysmyelinating disorder of the white matter. Traditionally, the classical and more severe connatal subtypes are distinguished by rate of progression, though there is considerable overlap.

- *Presentation*: onset in first year of life: nystagmus, spastic paraparesis, and movement disorder (usually dystonia).
- *Neuroimaging*: characteristic hypomyelination of cerebral white matter.
- *Genetics*: ♂'s affected (X-linked); mutation in the *PLP1* gene (75%).

Metachromatic leukodystrophy (late infantile; sulphatide lipidosis)

- *Presentation*: 18 months; regression, flaccid limb paresis, and absent reflexes (peripheral neuropathy).
- *Clinical course*: within 3–6 months hypertonia, optic atrophy, decerebrate and decorticate posture; death by 8–10 yrs.
- *Neuroimaging*: MRI shows symmetrical demyelination (typically frontal and occipital horns *but can be initially normal*).
- *Histopathology*: metachromatic sulphatides in nerves.
- *Neurophysiology*: slow nerve conduction; abnormal VEPs and somatosensory evoked potentials (SSEPs).
- *Biochemistry*: arylsulfatase A activity via WCE, ↑CSF protein.
- *Genetics*: ARSA mutation analysis.
- *Treatment*: gene therapy (atidarsagene autotemcel) approved in UK and Europe specifically for *pre-symptomatic* late infantile and *still ambulant* early juvenile forms of MLD only. Treatment comprises infusion of patients own stem cells conditioned with gene therapy.

Infantile neuroaxonal dystrophy (INAD; phospholipase associated neurodegeneration, PLAN)

Progressive degeneration of central and peripheral nervous systems.

- *Presentation*: hypotonic infant with ↓limb reflexes.
- *Clinical course*: becomes spastic, opisthotonic posturing, optic atrophy. Death by 5 yrs.
- *Histopathology*: axonal spheroids on axillary skin biopsy.
- *Neuroimaging*: MRI shows diffuse cerebellar hyperintensity and atrophy ± iron deposition in basal ganglia: INAD now regarded as a form of NBIA (see Neurodegeneration with brain iron accumulation (NBIA) in this chapter ➲ p. 478). Synonymous with PLAN (phospholipase associated neurodegeneration).

- *Neurophysiology*: EMG shows anterior horn cell disease and denervation (nerve conduction studies normal). BAERs, SSEPs, and VEPs progressively worsen (ERG is unremarkable).
- *Genetics*: PLA2G6 mutation analysis.

HIV-associated progressive encephalopathy

See HIV and HIV-associated progressive encephalopathy in this chapter ➔ p. 367.

Pre-school years (2–5 yrs)

Late infantile neuronal ceroid lipofuscinosis (CLN2)

The late infantile NCL. *Consider in all aggressive epilepsies in toddlers*: the EEG features are a useful screen.

- *Presentation*: 2–4 yrs, seizures (myoclonic and tonic–clonic).
- *Clinical course*: myoclonus is a prominent feature; motor difficulties, *progressive ataxia*. Blindness occurs late but may be preceded at times by visual inattention/lack of eye contact masquerading as autism.
- *Neurophysiology*: slow (1 Hz) photic stimulation as part of routine EEG produces large posterior spikes; VEPs and SSEPs abnormally enlarged, ERG low amplitude, eventually extinguished.
- *Histopathology*: curvilinear inclusions in white cells or neurons on electron microscopy of skin biopsy.
- *Biochemistry*: tripeptidyl amino peptidase (TPP) for the most common variety (may not be part of standard WCE panel).
- *Genetics*: CLN2 mutation analysis.
- *Treatment:* Untreated, the natural history is for death within 3–10 yrs. Enzyme replacement therapy (cerliponase alfa) is delivered intraventricularly every 2 weeks via an implanted reservoir device. It slows, but does not stop or reverse, progression (visual decline is not helped). There should be regular review to decide if treatment should continue.

Mucopolysaccharidosis type III (Sanfilippo)

Mucopolysaccharidoses (MPS) are a group of lysosomal enzyme disorders characterized by the accumulation of glycosaminoglycans (GAG). MPS III (Sanfilippo) is the most common neurodegenerative disease in childhood in the UK.

- Clinical course: triphasic; 1–5 yrs developmental impairment, 3–12 yrs behaviour disturbance (daytime aggression, hyperactive, and mood swings; night insomnia and non-epileptic paroxysms), 10–15 yrs degenerative then vegetative. Death by 15–25 yrs.
- Mild somatic MPS features: mixed deafness; hip dysplasia; diarrhoea (autonomic neuropathy due to gut deposits).
- School failure may not have been recognized at presentation although it will be identifiable on specific questioning.
- Hyperactivity is usually not helped by stimulants: nocturnal sedation can be effective.
- Biochemistry: excess urine GAG excretion (heparan sulphate), confirm by WCE.

- Enzyme replacement therapy trials to date have not shown benefits for affected children.

Mitochondrial disorders

See Mitochondrial disease in this chapter ➜ p. 404.

Progressive neuronal degeneration of childhood (PNDC); Alpers disease (PNDC with liver disease); Huttenlocher disease; infantile poliodystrophy

This name encompasses a group of diseases characterized by presentation in infancy or early childhood with neuronal degeneration and/or liver failure.

- *Presentation*: hypotonia; fail to thrive; developmental impairment; aggressive seizures, particularly characterized by resistant focal status epilepticus, e.g. of one limb (*epilepsia partialis continua*, EPC); hepatic derangement often with basal ganglia involvement.
- *Clinical course*: EPC; episodes of major status epilepticus; usually develop late hepatic failure ('Huttenlocher variant') with rapid progression to death.
- Valproate can precipitate hepatic failure and is contraindicated in suspected PNDC. Some historical cases of significant 'valproate hepatotoxicity' in young children may have been unrecognized PNDC.
- *Genetics*: familial or sporadic inheritance. Most cases appear to be due to mitochondrial defects: various mutations have been described, particularly polymerase gamma (*POLG1*) involved in mitochondrial replication.
- *Histopathology*: brain spongiosis, neuronal loss, and astrocytosis.
- *Neurophysiology*: characteristic EEG changes; abnormal flash VEPs; ERG normal.
- Can also present with a similar picture of aggressive EPC in adolescence.

Juvenile Gaucher type 3 (neuronopathic)

- *Presentation*: variable onset (infancy to adolescence); ocular motor apraxia and supranuclear gaze palsy (i.e. saccadic eye movement abnormalities but intact dolls' eye movements).
- *Clinical course*: myoclonus, ataxia, dementia. Variable prognosis.
- *Systemic problems*: bone lesions, hepatosplenomegaly, and lung involvement.
- *Biochemistry*: WCE.
- *Histopathology*: lipid-engorged Gaucher cells (deposition and storage of glucocerebroside (glucosylceramide) in tissues).
- *Neurophysiology*: changes in evoked potentials reflect disease progression; SSEPs enlarge, BAEPs deteriorate.
- *Treatment:* enzyme replacement treatment in patients with visceral symptoms, though it doesn't seem to halt neurological deterioration.

HIV-associated progressive encephalopathy

See HIV and HIV-associated progressive encephalopathy in this chapter ➜ p. 367.

School age (5–12 yrs)

Also consider more aggressive variants of diseases that typically present in adolescence.

Juvenile NCL (CLN3)

The juvenile-onset NCL, typically presenting first with visual loss.

- *Presentation*: 4–14 yrs (peak 6–10 yrs of age); subtle behaviour change; markedly ↓visual acuity (macular and retinal degeneration).
- *Clinical course*: cognitive decline, extrapyramidal and pyramidal signs; blind by 2–6 yrs; seizures occur late (absence, myoclonus of face); death in early 20s.
- *Genetics*: DNA diagnosis, homozygous deletion in the CLN3 gene.
- *Histopathology*: light microscopy shows vacuolated lymphocytes; electron microscopy shows 'fingerprint' bodies.
- *Neurophysiology*: EEG no change with photic; ERG absent early on; VEPs disappear; SSEPs ↑in amplitude.

Adrenoleukodystrophy (X-ALD)

Peroxisomal disorder; X-linked recessive (10% of ♀ carriers are symptomatic); defective ALD protein leads to demyelination.

- *Presentation*: 4–10 yrs; significant behavioural problems (withdrawal, irritability, hyperactivity).
- *Clinical course*: rapid cognitive deterioration; optic atrophy; seizures, and clinical adrenal impairment are late features. Decerebrate in 2–4 yrs.
- *Neuroimaging*: white matter abnormality, posterior to anterior progression.
- *Biochemistry*: elevated plasma very long-chain fatty acids; adrenal insufficiency.
- *Genetics*: ABCD1 mutation analysis.
- *Treatment*: 'Lorenzo's oil' improves biochemical abnormalities and may stabilize pre-clinical disease (e.g. siblings of probands with no MRI changes) but has no effect on long-term outcome in symptomatic individuals.
  - BMT is an option in selected cases with definite early MRI changes but minimal neurological signs assessed using Loess score (see Indications for haemopoietic stem cell ('bone marrow') transplant in inborn errors of metabolism in this chapter ➜ p. 483).
  - Associated adrenal insufficiency should be sought and specifically treated.
  - Gene therapy trials ongoing.

▶ Brothers and mothers of index cases should be urgently assessed for possible pre-symptomatic status.

Rasmussen syndrome

See Rasmussen encephalitis in this chapter ➜ p. 400.

Neurodegeneration with brain iron accumulation (NBIA)

An umbrella term to cover a number of disorders characterized by pallidal iron deposition, axonal spheroids, and gliosis. Includes various subtypes referred to by their genetic/enzymatic basis including pantothenate kinase-associated neurodegeneration (PKAN, formerly known as Hallervorden–Spatz disease) and phospholipase-associated neurodegeneration (PLAN), synonymous with infantile neuroaxonal dystrophy INAD, see Infantile neuroaxonal dystrophy (INAD) in this chapter ➲ p. 475.

- *Presentation*: in the first two decades of life, progressive dystonia, rigidity, and choreoathetosis with cognitive decline.
- *Supportive clinical features*: retinitis pigmentosa, optic atrophy (seizures are not prominent).
- *Clinical course*: variable rate of progression; iron chelation has not proven useful. Symptomatic benefit may be seen in some children following deep-brain stimulation.
- *Neuroimaging*: characteristic MRI appearances show basal ganglia 'eye-of-the-tiger' sign reflecting iron accumulation.
- *Genetics*: PANK2, PLAG2, and other gene mutations.
- *Neurophysiology*: VER and ERG are abnormal in 25% of cases.

Friedreich ataxia

See Slowly progressive ataxias (over months to years) with initial symptom-free period in this chapter ➲ p. 425.

Niemann–Pick type C

- *Presentation*: mid–late childhood; seizures and emerging school failure; vertical gaze palsy (particular feature: cf. horizontal eye movement disorder of Gaucher).
- *Clinical course*: heterogeneous; organomegaly, cherry red spot (50%), ataxia, dystonia. Narcolepsy and cataplexy are common features.
- *Histopathology*: foamy sea-blue histiocytes on bone marrow.
- *Biochemistry*: abnormal cholesterol studies on cultured fibroblasts (diagnosis).
- *Genetics*: NPC1 gene (not for diagnosis as majority have private mutations).
- *Treatment*: Narcolepsy may be helped by modafinil; cataplexy by tricyclics, SSRIs, or sodium oxybate. Miglustat may slow disease progression for some children.

Unverricht–Lundborg disease (ULD)

Occurs worldwide, but ↑in Scandinavia and southern Europe.

- *Presentation*: 7–16 yrs (peak 10–13), seizures (clonic, tonic–clonic, often nocturnal).
- *Clinical course*: generalized epilepsy with increasingly prominent debilitating action myoclonus, i.e. progressive myoclonic epilepsy (see The progressive myoclonus epilepsies in this chapter ➲ p. 302) and ataxia; normal cognition or subtle deficits; slowly progressive over decades, not life-limiting.
- *Genetics*: autosomal recessive; CSTB gene; deficient cystatin B, a protease inhibitor.
- *Neurophysiology*: EEG photosensitivity (90%), high amplitude SSEPs.
- *Treatment*: valproate (see Contraception and reproductive health in this chapter ➲ p. 320) for seizures; N-acetyl cysteine may be beneficial.

Leukoencephalopathy with vanishing white matter (VWM) disease
Also known as Childhood Ataxia and CNS Hypomyelination (CACH).
- *Presentation*. episodes of deterioration, including coma, following infections and minor head traumas, resulting in ↑spasticity and/ or ataxia. Variable age at onset with aggressive forms presenting in childhood and less aggressive forms later in adolescence or even early adulthood.
- *Radiology*: pathognomonic MRI changes initially showing diffusely abnormal white matter then progressing to striking cystic degeneration and disappearance of white matter and replacement with CSF.
- *Genetics*: autosomal recessive; mutations in any of the five subunits coding a transcription initiation factor eIF2B.
- Give seasonal flu vaccine and prophylactic antibiotics against respiratory or urinary infection.

Adolescence
Also consider late/milder presentations of conditions that typically present in earlier childhood.

Juvenile Huntington disease
Dominantly inherited triplet repeat disorder showing anticipation. The longer the repeat length, the earlier the presentation. Juvenile presentations are usually paternally inherited and occasionally a big expansion will result in the child presenting before the father's diagnosis has been made although a family history of progressive psychiatric or neurological symptoms is often present.
- *Presentation*: the juvenile form features rigidity, dystonia, and myoclonic and generalized seizures. This contrasts with the presentation more typical of adult-onset disease of progressive dementia with prominent psychiatric symptoms, tremor, chorea, and late seizures.
- *Diagnosis:* DNA mutation analysis but *only after specialist counselling* (because of the possible implications for the father and other at-risk/ pre-symptomatic family members). MRI may be normal early but will show progressive ventriculomegaly and caudate atrophy.

Wilson disease (hepato-lenticular degeneration)
Consider this in any unexplained neurological regression and personality change as the neurological deterioration is preventable. It is a recessively inherited defect of copper transport resulting in deposition in the brain, liver, and cornea.
- *Presentation*: extrapyramidal features predominate from adolescence, with prominent early dysarthria (hepatic presentation in younger child). Slit lamp examination of the eyes reveals Kayser–Fleischer rings (almost pathognomonic).
- *Clinical course*: penicillamine or trientine zinc chelation effectively retards disease and may partially reverse changes.
- *Biochemistry*: low plasma caeruloplasmin, low serum copper, high 24 h urinary copper. If there is any doubt, proceed to penicillamine challenge, ↑copper on liver biopsy.

- *Radiology*: low T1 and high T2 signals in lentiform nuclei, brainstem, and white matter.
- *Treatment options*: penicillamine, trientine, zinc acetate (blocks copper absorption), tetrathiomolybdate. Penicillamine has high toxicity and may *worsen* the neurological symptoms. Trientine less toxic. Once body copper accumulation has been reversed, a low-copper diet with oral zinc acetate to prevent absorption may be sufficient maintenance therapy. Seek specialist advice. Fulminant hepatic disease may require liver transplantation.

Hereditary spastic paraparesis

A heterogeneous group of conditions characterized by spastic paraparesis progressing slowly over years typically with onset in teens or twenties (but can be much earlier). X-linked, autosomal dominant, and recessive inheritance are all common. The diagnosis of the 'pure' forms (i.e. those presenting in isolation with no other neurological features) is by exclusion: evidence of slowly progressive spastic paraparesis with normal brain and spine imaging.

- Various 'complicated' forms (10% of all cases) with additional features such as optic atrophy, retinopathy, ataxia, or ichthyosis.
- Gene panels available for established causative genes (particularly dominant pedigrees) but known to be incomplete.
- Clinical features (other than inheritance pattern) generally do not permit distinction between various genetic subtypes.
- Management is supportive.

Subacute sclerosing panencephalitis (SSPE)

See SSPE in this chapter ➔ p. 375.

Lafora disease

See also the progressive myoclonus epilepsies in this chapter ➔ p. 302.

- *Presentation*: mid-adolescence, generalized tonic–clonic seizures.
- *Clinical course*: rapid course; severe myoclonus, resting and action (c.f. action only in ULD); seizures with visual features; cortical blindness; early depression; profound cognitive impairment; death in 7–10 yrs.
- *Histopathology*: Lafora inclusion bodies on axillary skin biopsy (investigation of choice for diagnosis).
- *Neurophysiology*: changes pre-date symptoms; EEG photosensitivity; giant SSEPs.
- *Genetics*: autosomal recessive, mutations in the *EPM2A* and *B* genes.

Variant Creutzfeld–Jacob disease (vCJD)

See Variant Creutzfeld–Jacob disease in this chapter ➔ p. 376.

HIV-associated progressive encephalopathy

See HIV and HIV-associated progressive encephalopathy in this chapter ➔ p. 367.

Down syndrome disintegrative disorder (DSDD)

- Also known as Down syndrome regression disorder.
- Rare but well-recognized picture of subacute loss of skills and speech in adolescence on background of (usually high functioning) Down Syndrome.
- Mechanism unclear: case reports of benefit from SSRIs and IVIG.

White cell enzymes

Deficient enzyme activity in white cells can be diagnostic of lysosomal storage diseases (Table 4.20) but first test for urine mucopolysaccharides and oligosaccharides.

Table 4.20 White cell enzymes

Group	Disease	Deficient/abnormal enzyme
Mucopolysaccharidoses	MPS I (Hurler, Scheie)	α-l-Iduronidase
	MPS II (Hunter)	Iduronate-2-sulphatase
	MPS III A (Sanfilippo)	Heparan N-sulphatase
	MPS III B (Sanfilippo)	N-Acetyl α-glucosamnidase
	MPS III C (Sanfilippo)	Acetyl-CoA: α-glucosaminide N-Acetyl-transferase
	MPS III D (Sanfilippo)	N-Acetylglucosamine 6-sulphatase
	MPS VII (Sly)	β-glucuronidase
Neuronal ceroid lipofuscinosis	NCL 1 (infantile)	Palmitoyl-protein thioesterase
	NCL 2 (classic late Infantile form)	Tripeptidyl amino peptidase I
GM$_2$ gangliosidoses	Tay–Sachs	Hexosaminidase A
	Sandhoff	Hexosaminidase A and B
Oligosaccharidoses	Fucosidois	α-fucosidase
	α-mannosidosis	α-mannosidase
	Sialidosis type I	Neuraminidase
Mucolipidoses	Mucolipidoses II (I-cell disease)	Mannose-6-phosphate phosphotransferase
Sphingolipidoses	Metachromatic leukodystrophy	Arylsulphatase A (sulphatidase)
	Krabbe leukodystrophy	Galactocerebrosidase β-galactosidase
	Niemann–Pick type A	Sphingomyelinase
	Gaucher disease	Glucocerebrosidase
	GM$_1$ gangliosidosis	β-galactosidase
	Galactosialidosis	β-galactosidase and sialidase

Indications for Haemopoietic stem cell ('bone marrow') transplant in inborn errors of metabolism

Refer to current guidelines ℅ https://bsbmtct.org/indications-sub-committee.

Supportive care for neurodegenerative conditions

Even if cure is not possible there is much we can do to help:
- Manage and talk about the parents' grief reaction as an important separate issue from the child's disease. This will help the family make some sense of their feelings and help them support each other through the grieving process and as it resolves. This process may take 3 or 4 months though the child's life may be very much longer than this. A clinical psychologist is an important member of the multidisciplinary team.
- Agree goals rather than define impairments. See Interdisciplinary working and goal setting in this chapter → p. 221.
  - How can mobility be maintained as long as possible?
  - How will feeding difficulties be overcome?
  - How will medical problems, particularly seizures, be managed?
- In the medium term as the child or young person becomes more dependent consider:
  - Involvement of a children's hospice, remembering that many hospices have outreach staff to support care in the child's home.
  - Pay attention to nutrition to maintain health, well-being, and mood.
  - Treating mood disturbance, dysphoria, or agitation. Consider SSRIs, sedation, and ultimately a morphine infusion if distress is clear.
- Always offer to meet with the family again after the child eventually dies to address unresolved issues they may have.

Late presentations of metabolic disease

These are rare presentations of rare diseases: late-onset inborn errors of metabolism (IEMs) are there to catch us out! The key is to remember to consider the possibility, if only to exclude it: if you do not think of it the diagnosis will be missed!

Diagnosis permits:
- Specific treatment.
- Prevention of metabolic decompensation.
- Accurate counselling.
- Early recognition may prevent irreversible neurological impairment.

▶ Consider a late-onset IEM particularly where there is:
- An informative family history (of course!); remember mild forms in those with partial deficiencies, e.g. organic acidaemias.
- Atypical psychiatric symptoms, particularly a striking change in behaviour or onset of psychosis.
- Subtle physical signs as part of a recognizable picture (see below).
- A late-onset cerebellar ataxia.

A particular comment on late presentations of urea cycle disorders

Presentations may be acute or chronic, and vary with age.
- Early presentations (around 12–24 months) tend to be 'hepatogastric' (i.e. gastrointestinal symptoms in association with deranged liver function) but always associated with developmental impairment.
- In the next age band (average onset 4 yrs), encephalopathy, and acute confusion predominate.
- Predominantly psychiatric presentations at a slightly later age (average onset 8 yrs).
- Deterioration with sodium valproate.
- A combination of these features is particularly suspicious!

Psychiatric presentations

Acute psychosis
- Later-onset urea cycle defects (average age at onset 8 yrs).
- Homocysteine remethylation defects.
- Porphyrias.

Chronic psychiatric symptoms in childhood or adolescence
Catatonia, visual hallucinations (aggravated by treatment)
- Homocystinurias.
- Wilson disease.
- Adrenoleukodystrophy.
- Some lysosomal storage disorders.

Mild intellectual disability, with late-onset behavioural or personality changes
- Homocystinurias.
- Cerebrotendinous xanthomatosis.

- Monoamine oxidase A deficiency.
- Succinic semi-aldehyde dehydrogenase deficiency.
- Creatine transporter deficiency.
- α and β mannosidosis.
- NPC.
- Hartnup.
- PKAN.

Early onset dementias are usually genetic rather than metabolic, e.g. Huntington where seizures predominate.

Some suggestive physical signs

Episodes of confusion, coma, or strokes
- Cobalamin C disease.
- Methylene tetrahydrofolate reductase (MTHFR) deficiency.
- Mitochondrial disorders including MELAS.
- 3-HMG CoA lyase deficiency.
- Fabry disease.
- Urea cycle defects (average age at presentation 4 yrs).
- Some leukoencephalopathies including Childhood Ataxia with CNS Hypomyelination (CACH), aka Vanishing White Matter disease (see Leukoencephalopathy with vanishing white matter (VWM) in this chapter ⊃ p. 480).
- CADASIL (cerebral autosomal dominant arteriopathy with subcortical infarcts and leukoencephalopathy).

Tremor
- Tay–Sachs disease.
- Abetalipoproteinaemia.

Polyneuropathy
- Cerebrotendinous xanthomatosis.
- MTHFR deficiency.
- Cobalamin C disease.
- Krabbe disease.
- Megalencephalic leukodystrophy with cysts.
- Respiratory chain disorders: see Mitochondrial disease in this chapter ⊃ p. 404.
- Adrenomyeloneuropathy/adrenoleukodystrophy.
- Peroxisomal biogenesis disorders.
- Polyglucosan body disease.

Proximal weakness with respiratory insufficiency
- Pompe disease.

Skin features (see Table 1.1 in Chapter 1 ⊃ p. 10)
- Xanthomata: cerebrotendinous xanthomatosis.
- Ichthyosis: Sjögren-Larsson.
- Melanoma: adrenomyeloneuropathy/adrenoleukodystrophy.
- Angiokeratoma: Fabry disease.

Visceral features
- Hepatogastric syndrome (i.e. upper GI symptoms with deranged liver function tests): early onset urea cycle defects (average age at presentation 14 months).
- Chronic diarrhoea: cerebrotendinous xanthomatosis.
- Adrenal insufficiency: adrenoleukodystrophy.
- Chronic diarrhoea, cachexia, intestinal pseudo-obstructions: MNGIE.
- Diabetes/other endocrine features: mitochondrial disorders.
- Amenorrhoea: childhood ataxia with CNS hypomyelination (CACH/ vanishing white matter).

Visual features
- Retinitis pigmentosa: cobalamin C, mitochondrial, and peroxisomal disorders, CDG, abetalipoproteinaemia, LCHAD, methylene tetrahydrofolate dehydrogenase deficiency, gyrate atrophy (ornithine aminotransferase deficiency), Vit E malabsorption (tocopherol carrier).
- Optic nerve atrophy: cobalamin C, adrenoleukodystrophy, mitochondrial disease, megalencephalic leukodystrophy with cysts, Krabbe, organic acidurias, PKU, mucolipidosis type IV, biotinidase deficiency, Pelizaeus–Merzbacher.
- Cataract: cerebrotendinous xanthomatosis, mitochondrial and peroxisomal disorders, Lowe syndrome, LPI, neutral lipid storage disease, PHARC syndrome, Tangier disease, Fabry.
- Macular dystrophy: Sjögren-Larsson, mucolipidosis type IV.
- Supranuclear gaze palsy: Niemann–Pick C (seizures, visceral involvement), Gaucher.

Hearing loss
- Mitochondrial and peroxisomal disorders.
- Brown–Vialetto–van Laere syndrome: see Vitamin B$_2$ in this chapter → p. 523.

Macrocephaly
- Glutaric aciduria type 1.
- L-2-hydroxyglutaric aciduria.
- Alexander.
- GM2 gangliosidosis.
- Canavan.

Polyneuropathy
- Cerebrotendinous xanthomatosis.
- MTHFR deficiency.
- Cobalamin C.
- Krabbe.
- Metachromatic leukodystrophy.
- Mitochondrial and peroxisomal disorders.
- Adrenomyeloneuropathy/adrenoleukodystrophy.
- Polyglucosan body disease.
- LCHAD, tyrosinaemia type 1.
- Porphyria.
- Peroxisomal disorders.
- Abetalipoproteinaemia.

Acute porphyrias

Hereditary porphyrias are a group of eight disorders of heme biosynthesis. Four of these (the 'acute hepatic porphyrias') give rise to acute attacks with neurological features including:

- *Prodrome*: minor behavioural change (anxiety, insomnia, restlessness).
- *Severe pain*: primarily abdominal but can involve back or thighs.
- *Prominent autonomic features*: nausea and vomiting; tachycardia and hypertension; diarrhoea or constipation.
- *Variable neurological features* including acute confusional state (sometimes severe), depression, or seizures.
  - Less commonly, peripheral weakness resembling Guillain–Barré syndrome.
- Attacks typically last several days to a week or more, before slowly resolving. Peripheral weakness can take longer to resolve. Pre-pubertal presentation is very rare.

Investigation in association with specialist porphyria centre:

- First line: urine porphobilinogen and 5-aminolaevulinic acid; faeces total porphyrin and plasma fluorescence emission spectroscopy (peak at 624–628 nm) to delineate the type of acute porphyria.
- All specimens must be collected in light-proof containers e.g. wrap standard universals in aluminium foil.
- Samples are likely to be false –ve between attacks and repeated testing even during attacks may be necessary if suspicion is high.
- DNA analysis and enzyme activity can subsequently be used to detect pre-symptomatic carriers.

Treatment:

- *Preventative*: avoid precipitants (list of safe and unsafe drugs; avoid alcohol, smoking, cannabis, fasting).
- *Acute specific*: repress heme synthesis with haemin, treat hyponatraemia (precipitates seizures) and maintain normoglycaemia.
- *Acute symptoms*: opiates for pain; chlorpromazine for vomiting and hallucinations; lorazepam for insomnia and anxiety.

Neurotransmitter disorders

This is a group of inborn errors of metabolism affecting synthesis, metabolism, and catabolism of neurotransmitters, their cofactors, or receptors. Neurotransmitters have wide-ranging effects: regulating neurons involved in memory and cognition, motor function, temperature, balance, and pain.

- Disorders of neurotransmission are potentially treatable causes of epileptic encephalopathies and movement disorders (complete symptom control is possible for some disorders, improved quality of life for others); untreated they can result in severe neurological dysfunction and death.
- Diagnosis is difficult and often delayed: presenting features are non-specific. Mild, moderate, and severe forms are seen, and accurate diagnosis relies upon specialized biochemical tests of CSF, urine, and plasma.

Neurotransmitters include:
- Biogenic monoamines.
  - *catecholamines*: dopamine (DA), norepinephrine, epinephrine;
  - *indoleamines*: serotonin (5-HT) and melatonin;
  - *histamine;*
  - *amino acids*: glutamate, aspartate, glycine, D-serine, gamma-aminobuytric acid (GABA).
- Acetylcholine.
- Purines (AMP, ADP, ATP).
- Neuropeptides.

In the brain, glutamate is the most prevalent *excitatory* neurotransmitter, and GABA the major *inhibitory* neurotransmitter.
There are three main categories of paediatric neurotransmitter disorders:
- Disorders of biogenic amine metabolism.
- Disorders of GABA metabolism.
- Disorders of glycine metabolism.

Disorders of biogenic amines

These are caused by the failure of synthesis of dopamine, serotonin, norepinephrine, epinephrine, or the cofactor tetrahydrobiopterin. They have characteristic CSF neurotransmitter profiles.

General characteristic features
- Epileptic encephalopathy, myoclonic epilepsy.
- Intestinal motility dysfunction, feeding difficulties.
- Developmental impairment, especially expressive speech impairment.
- Microcephaly, central hypotonia, peripheral hypertonia.
- Additional features of dopamine deficiency:
  - movement disorder (hypokinesia or dyskinesia) with diurnal variation;
  - oculogyric crises;
  - hypersalivation.
- Additional features of norepinephrine deficiency:
  - ptosis, miosis;
  - ↑secretions;

- postural hypotension.
- Additional features of serotonin deficiency:
  - disturbed temperature regulation.

Aromatic L-amino acid decarboxylase deficiency

- *Clinical features*: hypotonia; paroxysms ('spells') of limb dystonia, oro-facial dystonia, oculogyric crises, flexor spasms; myoclonic jerks; sleep disturbance; autonomic disturbance.
- *Treatment*: dopaminergic receptor agonists (no role for levodopa), MAO inhibitors, anticholinergics, pyridoxine (enzyme cofactor).
- Gene therapy available via adeno-associated virus vector injected into midbrain or putamen.

Tyrosine hydroxylase deficiency

- *Clinical features*: causes a severe infantile form of DOPA-responsive dystonia including infantile parkinsonism–dystonia, oculogyric crises, parkinsonism, tremor, ptosis, miosis, ↑oropharyngeal secretions, autonomic instability, hypotonia, toe-walking.
- *Treatment*: L-DOP-responsive, MAO inhibitors; caution: particularly sensitive to drug side effects. Earlier treatment may improve long-term developmental outcomes.

Tetrahydrobiopterin synthesis defects

- Most have ↑blood phenylalanine detected on newborn screening. BH4 synthesis and reclamation disorders have features of both dopamine and serotonin deficiency: hypotonia, dystonia, and oculogyric crises. Diagnosis is by CSF biogenic amine and pterin profile, plus phenylalanine challenge. In addition to L-DOPA, consider BH4 replacement and phenylalanine dietary restriction ('atypical phenylketonuria').

Dopamine transporter deficiency syndrome

- *Clinical features*: infantile parkinsonism, hyperkinesia, or mixed hypo-/hyperkinetic pattern; severe childhood parkinsonism, cognitive impairment, and pyramidal tract signs.
- *Diagnosis*: elevated ratio of homovanillic acid to 5-hydroxyindole acetic acid; mutations in *SLC6A3*, gene encoding DA transporter.

GTPCHI deficiency (Segawa disease)

- *Clinical features*: the most common cause of DOPA-responsive dystonia.
  - *Heterozygote* state is commoner.
  - Age of onset is usually 4–8 yrs but infant and neonatal presentations are described. Initial presentation is of insidious gait abnormality secondary to leg dystonia (L>R and usually equinovarus foot) often misdiagnosed as cerebral palsy or, in older children sometimes as a functional movement disorder.
  - The dystonia worsens through the day and improves significantly after sleep. Upper limb dystonia then appears followed by development of parkinsonism. Torticollis and truncal dystonia are uncommon. The disease plateaus in teenage years.

- Brisk tendon reflexes, striatal toe, and ankle clonus may confuse the diagnosis. Diagnosis is by DNA analysis, but a trial of L-DOPA is warranted in all suspected cases.
- Phenotypic variations with focal dystonias (e.g. writer's cramp), paroxysmal and action dystonia.
- *Homozygous deficiency* presents in infancy with more severe phenotype: will usually be identified from elevated phenylalanine levels on newborn blood spot PKU screening. More severe BH4 deficiency leads to both dopaminergic and serotinergic deficit.
- *Treatment*: L-DOPA. The response to low doses of L-DOPA is typically quick (within 72 h) and dramatic. Life-long L-DOPA treatment is required, but resistance to L-DOPA and on/off phenomena are extremely rare. 5-hydroxytryptophan supplementation generally also needed with homozygous deficiency.

Others
- 6-pyruvoyltetrahydropterin synthase deficiency.
- Sepiapterin reductase deficiency.
- Tetrahydrobiopterin reclamation defects.
- Dihydropteridine reductase deficiency.
- Dopamine β -hydroxylase deficiency.
- Monoamine oxidase deficiency.

Disorders of GABA metabolism

Characteristic features
- Developmental impairment, hypotonia.
- Ataxia.
- Seizures.

Succinic semi-aldehyde dehydrogenase deficiency
- *Clinical features*: developmental impairment, hypotonia, ↓reflexes, epilepsy, non-progressive ataxia, behavioural problems, hyperactivity; rarely psychosis, myopathy, autism. Abnormal basal ganglia signal on MRI brain.
- *Diagnosis*: urine organic acids (massive ↑gamma-hydroxybutyrate (GHB) in infancy, lessens with age), plasma enzymes, CSF ↑GHB and modest elevation in GABA.
- *Treatment*: no established treatment. Reports of usefulness of vigabatrin (irreversible inhibitor of GABA transaminase); lamotrigine (inhibits release of the major GABA precursor glutamate); SSRIs and methylphenidate for behavioural problems.

GABA transaminase deficiency
- *Clinical features*: progressive epileptic encephalopathy, developmental impairment, hypotonia, macrosomia. No established treatment.

Disorders of glycine metabolism
- Non-ketotic hyperglycinaemia: see Non-ketotic hyperglycinaemia in Chapter 5 ➋ p. 555.

Secondary disorders of neurotransmitters

Non-specific, and often relatively minor abnormalities in CSF amine neurotransmitter metabolites and pterin species can be seen as a secondary phenomenon in an enormous range of neurological disorders including: mitochondrial disease, Rett syndrome, epileptic encephalopathies, pontocerebellar hypoplasias, hypoxic–ischaemic encephalopathy, leukodystrophies, neuropsychiatric disorders, dystonias, neuromuscular disorders, cerebral palsy, autistic spectrum disorder, and non-specific developmental delay.

Investigation

While the clinical features of neurotransmitter disorders can be protean, the usual presentations of infantile parkinsonism–dystonia and early childhood dystonia are distinctive. Disorders of biogenic amines should also be considered in the child with a diagnosis of 'cerebral palsy' without apparent cause. Because most disorders of biogenic amines are treatable, they warrant careful investigation and a trial of L-DOPA. See Levodopa in Chapter 7 ➔ p. 682.

Key investigations
- CSF amine neurotransmitter metabolites and pterin species.

▶▶ There are very particular requirements for CSF specimens for measurement of neurotransmitters: check with specialist laboratory in advance.

- Typically samples must be collected directly into liquid nitrogen.
- Sequential (numbered) samples are required to aid interpretation.
- Significantly blood-stained samples will not be interpretable.
- Interpretation of borderline–normal values can be complex: liaise with specialist laboratory.
- Levels of CSF amine neurotransmitter metabolites and pterin species cannot distinguish between primary and secondary disorders of neurotransmission.
- Exercise depletes dopamine; rest replenishes (children typically 'rested' at time of LP particularly if under anaesthetic).
- Genetic tests for specific mutations.
- Plasma or fibroblast enzymes (aromatic amine decarboxylase, dopamine β -hydroxylase, monoamine oxidase, and dihydropteridine reductase deficiencies) on Guthrie card.
- Quantitative urine and plasma catecholamines.

Principles of treatment

- Monitor treatment response with repeat CSF neurotransmitter analysis.
- Replace amine neurotransmitters.

L-DOPA
- DOPA with a peripheral DOPA decarboxylase inhibitor, e.g. Co-careldopa: see Levodopa in Chapter 7 ➔ p. 682.

- 5-Hydroxytryptophan (up to 8 mg/kg/day).
- Other treatments to ↑DOPA:
  - Monoamine oxidase B inhibitors—selegiline;
  - Catechol-O-methyltransferase inhibitors—entacapone;
  - Dopamine receptor agonists—bromocriptine, pergolide, pramipexole, ropinirole.

Replace cofactors and precursors
- BH4 (up to 20 mg/kg/day).
- Pyridoxine (vitamin B6).

Sleep disorders

Development and sleep disorders

The amount of sleep and its architecture changes during life.

- Newborns sleep most of the day in evenly spaced periods of 1–4 h. REM makes up 50% of total.
- With development the length of individual sleep periods increases and proportion of REM decreases.
- Normal stages of sleep have developed by 6 months. During early childhood the sleep pattern approaches that seen in adults.
- The proportion of time in deep sleep continually declines with age.

20–30% of all children experience some sleep disturbance. The pattern of reported problems varies between countries. Most do not come to any medical attention.

REM sleep is prominent in early infancy thus sleep is naturally more fragmented. The toddler years are particularly sensitive to parenting: 25% of children have problems in settling and sleeping. Deep non-REM sleep is prominent in early childhood and arousal disorders are common in this age group.

Sleep-related problems present at two ages:

Toddlers

- 25% have problems of getting to sleep and/or night waking.

Adolescence

- Erratic sleep–wake patterns.
- *Delayed sleep phase syndrome*: inability to get off to sleep and great difficulty getting up in the morning.
  - Slow-wave sleep declines in adolescence but sleep requirements do not.
  - Natural delay in getting off to sleep is related to puberty and melatonin.
  - Social reasons for sleeping late.
  - Sleep deprivation leads to excessive daytime sleepiness, mood swings, and poor behaviour.

Parasomnias

Definition: Recurrent episodes of behaviour, experiences, or physiological changes that occur exclusively or predominantly during sleep.

Primary parasomnias are classified according to the stage of sleep in which they occur:

- Episodes that occur in the transition between wakefulness and sleep.
- Arousal disorders (from deep non-REM sleep).
- Parasomnias associated with REM sleep.
- Others.

Secondary parasomnias occur secondary to a physical or psychiatric disorder.

Primary parasomnias at sleep onset

- Sleep starts/hypnic jerks/ 'exploding head syndrome'.
- Hypnagogic hallucinations.

- Sleep paralysis.
- Rhythmic movement disorder: head banging, humming, or rocking to aid getting to sleep.
- Restless legs syndrome (difficulty getting to sleep because of unpleasant cramping sensations in the legs).

Primary parasomnias during light non-REM sleep
- Bruxism.
- Periodic limb movement in sleep (brief contractions lasting about 2 s in the toes, hips, and knees at intervals of about 20 s).

Primary parasomnias in deep non-REM sleep (arousal disorders)
These include confusional arousals and sleepwalking. Susceptibility often runs in families with children moving from one arousal disorder to another as they develop. Some households have different members exhibiting different arousal disorders. Shared features include:
- One episode per night, usually in the first half of the night.
- Genetic with a family history in up to 60%.
- Young age when slow-wave sleep is deep and long lasting.
- Associated with:
  - fever/intercurrent illness;
  - CNS depressant medication;
  - external or internal sleep-interrupting stimuli;
  - obstructive sleep apnoea.
- Curious combinations of seeming asleep and awake at the same time:
  - confused and disorientated;
  - remaining asleep during the episode although as the child grows older they tend to wake up at the end;
  - unresponsive to external stimuli including the parents' attempts to wake the child up;
  - little recall.
- A child may go from one arousal to another.

Confusional arousal
- Very common.
- Child does not wake up but partially arouses from deep non-REM, slow-wave sleep to a lighter stage of non-REM or REM sleep.
- The child is asleep during the episode itself but may wake immediately after.
- Usually occurs in infants and toddlers.
- Movements with moaning and groaning; progress to agitated, confused behaviour with intense crying, calling out, and thrashing around.
- The child may appear awake but is not and attempts to wake them increase agitation and prolong the episode.
- If carers manage to wake him/her, the child is often very confused and frightened.
- Lasts 5–15 min.
- If left alone the child will simply return to sleep.

Sleep walking
- Occur at 4–8 yrs of age; 17% children sporadically.

- Less dramatic than confusional arousal.
- The child walks about calmly, to their parent's bedroom, toilet, etc.
- Eyes wide open with a glassy stare.
- Automatisms, urinating in inappropriate places.
- Accidental injury is very possible.
- At later age may take the agitated form which is worsened by attempts to intervene, with an even greater risk of injury.

Night (or sleep) terrors (see Box 4.9)
- This occurs in 3% children mainly in later childhood.
- Later-onset cases tend to persist longer.
- Parents are woken by the child's piercing scream.
- The child is terrified, with eyes wide open, sweaty, vocalizing.
- May run into something or injure himself or others.
- Lasts a few minutes and then settles back to sleep.
- If the child wakes up, then a feeling of fear is reported but does not have the extended narrative of a nightmare.

Management of non-REM sleep disorders
- Reassurance and explanation to the parents.
- Regular and adequate sleep routines.
- Secure environment.
- Refrain from trying to waken the child.
- Refrain from recounting the episode in front of the child.
- Scheduled awakening with sleep walking/night terrors.
  - These events often occur at a fairly consistent time each evening. Fully waking the child 30 min ahead of the anticipated time is often effective at preventing them.
- Rarely, short-term use of benzodiazepine, e.g. diazepam.

Box 4.9 Night terrors and frontal lobe epilepsy

While the error of a false +ve diagnosis of epilepsy is probably much more common, the characteristic example of a false −ve is to label nocturnal frontal lobe seizures as night terrors (or confusional arousals). The error is understandable: frontal lobe seizures often comprise loud cries or shrieks and violent pedalling or thrashing movements of the limbs that do not conform to conventional notions of seizure phenomenology. If video is available careful observation of the onset will show tell-tale tonic posturing of the arms ± head turn. In clinic settings the main clues are:
- *Event frequency*. Frontal lobe seizures are often multiple per night. Night terrors very rarely if ever occur more than once per night.
- *Clustering*. Frontal lobe seizures will often occur multiply per night for several nights and then remit.

An overnight video is crucial in cases of uncertainty, but the *onset* of the attack must be captured to be informative. Frontal lobe seizures often have very little accompanying change on surface EEG but the events are stereotyped and very characteristic.

Primary parasomnias of REM sleep

Nightmares
- Very common.
- Occur in the latter part of the night when REM sleep is most abundant.
- The child wakes up, very frightened and will describe the nightmare in great detail. Involves the child or a loved one.
- Anxious and afraid to sleep again.

REM sleep behaviour disorder
- Initially thought to be a rare disorder of elderly men but now also recognized in adults with neurodegenerative disease (e.g. Parkinson) and narcolepsy.
- Seen in juvenile Parkinson disease and following withdrawal from antidepressant drugs and alcohol.
- Under normal conditions, pontine centres generate a physiological paralysis (atonia) in the limbs during REM sleep to prevent the 'acting out' of dreamed movement.
- Loss of this mechanism results in sometimes violent dream re-enactment.

Primary parasomnias on waking
- Hypnopompic hallucinations.
- Sleep paralysis.

Primary parasomnia with inconsistent relationship to sleep
- Sleep talking.

Secondary parasomnias
- Very high parasomnia rates are described in children with learning difficulties.
- Sleep disturbance is part of the 'behavioural phenotype' of some syndromes including William, Rett, Smith–Magenis, Angelman.
- Upper airway obstruction may contribute to sleep disturbance (a feature of many neurological conditions).
- High prevalence in autism, ADHD, and depression.
- Chiari malformations can present with sleep disorders.

Excessive daytime sleepiness (hypersomnia)

Most commonly reflect insufficiently restful, poor quality night-time sleep. Consider in particular:
- Lifestyle-related (i.e. inadequate nocturnal sleep due to use of computer screens, TV: a combination of emotional arousal and exposure to light of particular colour-temperatures).
- Delayed sleep phase syndrome (see above).
- Restless leg syndrome.
- Obstructive sleep apnoea syndrome.
- Factitious illness and over-reporting of symptoms.
- Chronic fatigue syndrome (i.e. confusing fatigue with actual sleepiness).

Narcolepsy

Can be conceptualized as an instability of the normal sleep/wake 'switch' resulting in rapid cycling between the two states, sleep–wake fragmentation, plus experience of sleep-boundary problems (hypnogogic hallucinations, sleep paralysis), i.e. intrusion of REM sleep phenomena into wakefulness.

- Total sleep hours per day are not that abnormal: the problem is *fragmentation* with both nocturnal sleep and daytime wakefulness very interrupted.
- Important, misunderstood, under-recognized, and poorly managed particularly in paediatric age range.
- Adult prevalence is comparable with multiple sclerosis and Parkinson disease.
- Adults retrospectively report symptoms back to early childhood.
- 50% start in childhood (3/10 000) with an average age of onset of 14 yrs but may be as young as 2 yrs.

Five main features
- *Excessive daytime sleepiness* is the defining symptom of narcolepsy: irresistible sleep attacks. Last min to 1 h. Naps are refreshing and occur anywhere.
  - Irresistible 'sleep attacks' most commonly during sedentary activity, e.g. in school classroom.
- *Cataplexy*: ('jelly legs') a sudden, temporary loss of muscle tone usually experienced as a very brief 'sag' rather than complete drop attack: triggered by strong emotion, particularly laughter.
  - The most specific feature, in 60–100% cases.
  - If truly absent, review diagnosis.
  - Consider Niemann–Pick type C and Coffin-Lowry syndrome as other very rare causes of cataplexy.
  - In early stage narcolepsy the emotion trigger for cataplexy attacks is less prominent.
  - Can appear for of a constant hypotonia especially with ptosis.
  - Chocolate can be a trigger!
- *Hypnagogic* (on going to sleep) or *hypnopompic* (just after awakening) *hallucinations*.
  - Typically extremely vivid and distressing.
  - Often not volunteered as so bizarre/embarrassing: have to be specifically asked after.
  - Occur in ~50%.
- *Sleep paralysis*. Waking from REM sleep without reversal of the physiological REM atonia resulting in inability to breath and fear of death: usually described as a 'crushing weight on chest'.
  - Occur in ~60% adults.
  - Very poor quality, *fragmented night-time sleep*.

▶▶ Note isolated daytime sleepiness (without other features) is most commonly due to lifestyle issues and inadequate nocturnal sleep.

Particular diagnostic considerations in children
- Sleepiness is difficult to assess and quantify: may manifest as poor behaviour and over-activity.
- Cataplexy may not be present initially or may be subtle (sagging at the knees).
- The child may conceal frightening or embarrassing aspects, particularly hallucination/sleep paralysis.
- Distinguish from delayed sleep maturation: the need for a daytime nap persisting beyond the toddler age group. In these children night-time sleep is not affected, and behaviour disturbance not expected.

▶ In young children, even if cataplexy is absent, some evidence of abnormal REM sleep should be present, e.g. abnormally vivid nightmares (even during daytime naps), hallucinatory experiences, and sleep paralysis.

Aetiology
- Narcolepsy is associated with ↓or absent levels of hypocretin in CSF. This is thought to be the result of degeneration of hypocretin-secreting neurons, likely to be the consequence of an autoimmune process. Associated with HLA-DQB1*0602 and the much less common HLA-DQA1*0102. 90% of patients with narcolepsy/cataplexy are +ve for HLA-DQB1*0602 which is therefore a sensitive but not specific association (seen in 20% normal population).

Evaluation
- Direct observation: facial expression, posture, yawning.
- History from family.
- Sleep questionnaires.
  - *Epworth Sleepiness Scale*. Score >10 implies sleep disorder. Narcolepsy scores 13–23.
  - *Maintenance of Wakefulness Test*. Assesses how long a patient can stay awake in a comfy chair sat in a quiet dark room. Norms for children are not established.
- The Multiple Sleep Latency Test (MSLT) is the classic investigation in adults. The test establishes that the sufferer repeatedly enters REM sleep (confirmed by simultaneous EEG) within a short time of being allowed to sleep.
  - May be technically challenging in children <10.
  - No normative paediatric data but results can be supportive.
- Polysomnography used mainly to eliminate other causes of excessive daytime sleepiness such as OSA (obstructive sleep apnoea).
- Levels of CSF hypocretin are significantly reduced or absent in cases of narcolepsy with cataplexy.
  - Unlike MSLT, not affected by symptomatic treatment with stimulants and not subject to age-dependent normal values.
  - The most robust way of obtaining a confident diagnosis of narcolepsy-cataplexy in children.
  - In the absence of cataplexy the value of measuring CSF hypocretin is debatable.
- In practice, HLA typing contributes little (sensitive but not specific).

Treatment
- Establish accurate diagnosis.
- Manage excessive daytime sleepiness with planned daytime naps with or without drug treatment.
- Address poor nocturnal sleep hygiene.
- First line treatment for daytime sleepiness is generally modafinil.
  - Dexamphetamine, methylphenidate are used as second line.
- Avoid known cataplexy triggers (laughter).
  - Consider symptomatic treatment in severe cases: clomipramine, venlafaxine.
- Sodium oxybate may be indicated for selected patients with combination narcolepsy and cataplexy.
  - Very expensive: in UK access limited to specialist sleep clinics.

Kleine–Levin syndrome
Excessive sleepiness occurring intermittently, with normal sleeping patterns between episodes.
- Rare.
- Usually presents in adolescent ♂'s but may also occur in ♀s.
- Usually follows a stressful period or a viral infection.
- Periods of hypersomnia (20 h/day) lasting for hours or weeks occur at intervals of weeks/months.
- During the awake periods:
  - overeating sometimes causing obesity;
  - hypersexual behaviour;
  - restlessness;
  - mood disorder;
  - mild confusional state;
  - short periods of elation/depression and sleeplessness may occur at the end of the phase before returning to normal.
- Tends to improve with time.
- May respond to lithium, fluoxetine, carbamazepine.

Stroke

- Overall incidence ~3/100 000 per year.
- Arterial ischaemic stroke ~1.6/100 000: rates in neonates higher at ~4/100 000 per year.

Definitions

- *Stroke*: focal neurological deficit lasting more than 24 h with a vascular basis.
- *Transient ischaemic attack*: focal neurological deficit lasting less than 24 h. In children, migraine is the commonest cause of transient focal neurological deficit in contrast to cerebrovascular disease in adults.
- *Stroke-like episode*: focal neurological deficit lasting more than 24 h (i.e. stroke) but not of a vascular basis. The main example is MELAS (see Mitochondrial myopathy, encephalopathy, lactic acidosis and stroke-like episodes (MELAS) in this chapter ➲ p. 409) where 'stroke' happens due to energy failure. Imaging will show radiological changes typical of infarction, but this is typically multifocal and not confined to vascular anatomical territories. Similar presentations can also be seen with Channelopathies (e.g. due to *CACNA1A* mutations).

Stroke and stroke mimics in the Emergency Department

Increasing interest in acute thrombolysis or thrombectomy for paediatric arterial ischaemic stroke (AIS) has highlighted the challenge of rapid identification of true AIS in the Emergency Department. Unfortunately, the challenge is greater because (unlike adult practice) AIS is not the primary cause of unilateral paralysis in paediatric emergency medicine: migraine, functional symptoms and idiopathic lower motor neuron facial nerve (Bell) palsies are important mimics (although upper and lower motor neuron facial palsy should not really be confused: see Facial movement abnormalities in Chapter 3 ➲ p. 137).

Being well in the week before presentation, GCS ≤ 12, inability to talk or walk, face and arm weakness are associated with ↑odds of AIS.

Presentations

- Acute onset focal neurological deficit (typically hemiparesis ± visual field defect)
  - Especially in contexts of known sickle cell disease, congenital heart defect, arteriopathy
- Seizures (particularly in the neonate).
- Headache.
- Neck pain.

Acute management

- ABC: maintain 100% saturation.
- Treat hypoglycaemia.
- Measure BP.
- If GCS <8 needs PICU input, consider neurosurgical referral as may need decompression (e.g. evacuation of haematoma) to manage ↑ICP.
- Treat seizures.
- Consult haematology urgently if known sickle cell disease.

Thrombolysis and thrombectomy

The role of emergency interventions to try to remove clot and restore perfusion in paediatric AIS is the subject of active ongoing research. Options include:

- Thrombolysis: infusing fibrinolytic agents (e.g. tissue plasminogen activator, rtPA) either intravenously or (less commonly) via endovascular intra-arterial infusion.
- Thrombectomy: mechanical retrieval of clot using endovascular devices.

The potential benefit of arterial recanalization has to be balanced against the risks of adverse effects (particularly major cerebral haemorrhage from thrombolysis, occurring in 5–10%). This balance is more favourable the earlier the intervention can be delivered. Adult trials suggest a window of up to 4 h from ictus.

> **These considerations put a premium on early radiological confirmation of AIS and rapid discussion with regional centres.**
>
> ▶ Although Diffusion Weighted Imaging (DWI) MRI sequences give the earliest indications of ischaemia, in practice access to MRI from the paediatric Emergency Department is often limited, particularly outside regional neuroscience centres.
>
> ▶ CT Angiography is the optimum initial imaging if there is any barrier to immediate MRI: although parenchymal changes of ischaemia/infarction are slow to develop on CT (may be normal <~4 h post ictus), CTA will confirm large-vessel occlusion if present, and exclude haemorrhage.
>
> Radiologists more used to suspected stroke in adults are likely to consider the primary indication for acute neuroimaging as being exclusion of haemorrhage which would contraindicate interventions such as thrombolysis and for which CT would be adequate. *Stronger evidence of AIS* is required in children, given the lower likelihood of this causing acute focal neurological deficit in comparison to migraine and other mimics, so CTA rather than CT is required.

Intravenous thrombolysis

Use of tissue plasminogen activator (tPA) in children can be considered in children with confirmed AIS where:

- There is an acute focal neurological deficit consistent with arterial ischaemia AND
- A Paediatric National Institute of Health Stroke Scale (PedNIHSS) score (Table 4.21) of ≥ 4 and ≤ 24 AND
- Treatment can be delivered within 4.5 hours of *known* onset of symptoms (this excludes stroke discovered on waking) AND
- Intracranial haemorrhage has been excluded:
  - CTA demonstrates normal brain parenchyma or minimal early ischaemic change with no haemorrhage AND partial or complete occlusion of the intracranial artery corresponding to the clinical or radiological deficit OR

- MRI and MRA showing evidence of acute ischaemia on diffusion weighted imaging plus partial or complete occlusion of the intracranial artery corresponding to clinical or radiological deficit.
  PROVIDING there are no contraindications:
- No CNS surgery, trauma, or haemorrhage in the previous 30 days.
- No systemic bleeding in previous several weeks.
- No general surgery in the last 7–10 days.
- No cardiopulmonary resuscitation or lumbar puncture in the last 7 days.
- No diagnosis of CNS tumour; uncorrectable thrombocytopenia or coagulopathy; pregnancy; or severe liver disease.

Young age (<8) is a relative contraindication because of the difficulty of achieving MR imaging without anaesthesia. Thrombolysis is not recommended below the age of 2. Begin thrombolysis irrespective of patient location at the point of AIS diagnosis when above criteria are fulfilled; this may well be in the local hospital emergency department or paediatric ward.

▶Where available, comparison of the extent of the stroked area on FLAIR and DWI sequences can be helpful: brain regions that show restricted diffusion on DWI but as yet no FLAIR signal change are (potentially reversibly) *ischaemic* without established *infarction*.

Endovascular thrombolysis/thrombectomy

- In practice currently, endovascular thrombolysis/thrombectomy will mainly be a consideration when a stroke occurs to a child who is already an inpatient in a centre with interventional neuroradiological expertise, where the likely mechanism is clear (e.g. post cardiac surgery), primary cerebral haemorrhage can be quickly excluded by CT and transfer delays to the angiography suite can be avoided, although such children are often fully anticoagulated which would be a contraindication.

Other acute management

Aspirin therapy

- 5 mg/kg of aspirin (maximum 300 mg) daily commencing within 24 h of onset of confirmed AIS in the absence of contraindications (e.g. parenchymal haemorrhage). After 14 days reduce dose of aspirin to 1 mg/kg (max 75 mg) daily.
- Delay administering aspirin for 24 hours in patients where thrombolysis has been given.
- Aspirin should not be routinely given to young people with sickle cell disease or on anticoagulation, presenting with AIS.
- Duration depends on risk factors identified.

Known cardiac disease

- In children and young people with cardiac disease presenting with AIS, make a multidisciplinary decision (including haematologists, paediatric neurologists and cardiologists) regarding the optimal antithrombotic therapy (antiplatelet versus anticoagulation) with assessment of the risk–benefit in individual cases.

Table 4.21 Pediatric NIH Stroke Severity Scale (PedNIHSS)

Domain	Operationalization		Score
1a. Level of Consciousness:		0	Alert; keenly responsive
		1	Not alert, but arousable by minor stimulation
		2	Requires repeated stimulation to attend, or strong or painful stimulation to make non-stereotyped movements
		3	Responds only with reflex motor or autonomic effects or totally unresponsive
1b. Level of consciousness questions:	Where is [familiar family member present]?' (>2 years)	0	Answers both questions correctly
		1	Answers one question correctly
		2	Answers neither question correctly
1c. Level of consciousness Commands:	Open / close your eyes', 'Touch your nose' (>2 years)	0	Performs both tasks correctly
		1	Performs one task correctly
		2	Performs neither task correctly
2. Best Gaze:	Assess horizontal eye movements	0	Normal
		1	Partial gaze palsy
		2	Forced deviation / complete gaze palsy
3. Visual:	Visual threat (2–6 years); confrontation, finger counting (>6 years)	0	No visual loss
		1	Partial hemianopia
		2	Complete hemianopia
		3	Bilateral hemianopia (including cortical blindness)
4. Facial Palsy:	Show teeth/raise eyebrows /close eyes	0	Normal symmetrical movement
		1	Minor paralysis (flattened nasolabial fold, asymmetry on smiling)
		2	Total or near total paralysis of lower face
		3	Complete paralysis of one or both sides

(Continued)

Table 4.21 (Contd.)

Domain	Operationalization		Score
5a. Motor Left Arm 5b. Motor Right Arm	Extend arm 90° (if sitting) or 45° (if supine)	0	No drift for full 10 s
		1	Drift ≤ 10 s
		2	Some effort against gravity
		3	No effort against gravity
		4	No movement
		5	Amputation
6a. Motor Left Leg 6b. Motor Right Leg	Extend leg 30°	0	No drift for full 5 s
		1	Drift ≤ 5 s
		2	Some effort against gravity
		3	No effort against gravity
		4	No movement
		5	Amputation
7. Limb Ataxia:	Reach for/kick a toy (<5 years); finger-nose/heel-shin (>5 years)	0	Absent
		1	Present in one limb
		2	Present in two limbs
8. Sensory:	Behavioural response to pin prick	0	Normal
		1	No sensory loss
		2	Mild to moderate sensory loss
		3	Severe to total sensory loss
9. Best Language:	Spontaneous speech and comprehension (2–6 years); describe a picture (>6 years)	0	Normal
		1	Mild to moderate aphasia
		2	Severe aphasia
		3	Mute, global aphasia

Reproduced from Ichord *et al.* (2011) Interrater reliability of the Pediatric National Institutes of Health Stroke Scale (PedNIHSS) in a multicenter study. *Stroke* **42**: 613–17.

Sickle Cell disease
- Aspirin *not* routinely used.
- Urgent transfusion to achieve HbS <30%, and Hb >100 g/l. This will typically require exchange transfusion.
- Interim transfusion to bring Hb >100 g/l if exchange likely to be delayed by >6h.

All other standard supportive stroke care.

Investigation

Important to identify the aetiology of paediatric AIS to inform recurrence risk and management.

Elements to consider in history
- Fever.
- Otitis media/mastoiditis/tonsillitis.
- Recent varicella infection.
- Pre-existing cardiac disease.
- Recent trauma particularly to the neck (can be quite trivial 'awkward' falls, gymnastics etc).
- Sickle cell disease.
- History/family history of stroke.
- Abrupt onset (favours haemorrhage or embolus) versus 'stuttering' onset (favours thrombosis).

Initial investigations (within hours)
- Baseline biochemistry, haematology including coagulation, HbS if appropriate, ESR, and CRP.

Other investigations
Should be tailored to suspected mechanism(s) (see Fig. 4.9).

Radiology

Identifying the primary cause of a stroke in childhood guides management, including steps to prevent the occurrence of possible further strokes. *The primary investigation is neuroimaging.*
- All children require MRI and MRA within a few days if not achieved acutely (for acute imaging see Thrombolysis and Thrombectomy above Chapter 4 ➲ p. 501).
  - If dissection is suspected (history of trauma, neck pain, headache, posterior circulation stroke, Horner syndrome implying carotid artery injury) ask for fine basal cuts and fat-saturation sequences.
- Imaging is crucial in distinguishing haemorrhage, arterial ischaemia, and venous ischaemia/infarction. Within the arterial ischaemic group, consideration of lesion location in relation to vascular territories (see Fig. 2.8 in Chapter 2 ➲ p. 65 and Fig. 4.9) is helpful in distinguishing embolic and thrombotic causes.

Relative indications for conventional angiography
Conventional four-vessel angiography is associated with ~1% risk of stroke from the procedure; however, it remains indicated in certain situations:
- *Haemorrhagic* stroke of unknown cause (to identify AVM, aneurysm).
  - Definitive endovascular treatment of any identified vascular abnormality may be possible in the same procedure.
- Some situations of MRA –ve AIS:
  - Posterior circulation AIS: MRA visualizes posterior circulation relatively poorly.
  - Clinical suspicion of vasculitis: MRA insensitive to small-vessel disease.

- Suspected dissection, although fat-saturation axial MRI views are generally very sensitive to the presence of dissection of the large vessels of the neck.

❶ The evidence base for secondary prevention measures in paediatric ischaemic stroke is limited. Refer to the RCPCH Stroke in Childhood clinical guidelines document (2017).

Embolic arterial ischaemic stroke

- Radiological patterns include Figure 4.9 B and D.
- From a distant source.
  - Left side of the heart in anatomically normal circulation.
  - Paradoxical embolus from *any* source in a child with congenital heart disease permitting right-to-left shunting *including the normal neonate* (due to foetal circulation) where emboli of placental origin are common.
  - Dissection of a major artery, commonly carotid or vertebral after often apparently trivial trauma to the head or neck creating an 'intimal tear'.

Investigations
- Discuss need for trans-oesophageal echo with cardiologists.
  - In adolescents transcranial doppler in conjunction with a 'bubblegram' (injection of vigorously-shaken saline) can provide evidence of right-to-left shunting through a patent foramen ovale.
- If carotid dissection being considered (history of recent 'minor' neck trauma) axial fat-saturation MR sequences (or CT angiography) are very useful in detecting this and superior to MRA: formal angiography rarely required.
- In practice, children showing pattern Figure 4.9 B will also need investigation for thrombotic causes.

Treatment and secondary prevention
- If embolic mechanism proven or strongly suspected, short-term anticoagulation with LMW heparin (see Heparin, low molecular weight in Chapter 7 ➋ p. 673) should be strongly considered (typically for a few months until source of emboli has resolved).
  - Where need for longer-term anticoagulation is anticipated (i.e. months to years), most often in the context of congenital heart disease, warfarin or newer anticoagulants (e.g. rivaroxaban) may be required.

Thrombotic arterial ischaemic stroke

- Stroke due to 'sticky blood'.
- Radiological patterns include Figure 4.9 B and D.
- The importance of primary thrombophilia is not as great as once thought.

Investigations
- Discuss timing and breadth of 'thrombophilia screen' with Haematology.
  - Transient abnormalities are common and may be important in post-infectious and other mechanisms of stroke.
  - Some polymorphisms (e.g. C655T *MTHFR*) frequent in general population and probably not sufficient cause.
  - Factor V Leiden (activated protein C resistance), protein C, protein S, prothrombin 20210 mutation, antithrombin III, antiphospholipid antibodies (anticardiolipin and lupus anticoagulant). Consider von Willebrand Factor antigen, factors VIII and XII.
- Consider:
  - Lactate, pyruvate, amino acids, cholesterol, triglycerides, lipoprotein A, NH_3.
  - Autoantibodies and ANCA.
  - Total homocysteine (fasted, within 5 days), B12, folate.
  - MELAS/MERRF mutations.
  - Viral serology + Lyme.
  - CSF protein, glucose, culture, lactate, pyruvate, zoster titres.
  - Urine organic acids.

Treatment and secondary prevention
- All children with radiologically proven ischaemic stroke should be commenced on low-dose aspirin pending further investigation unless the child has sickle cell disease, or radiological evidence of haemorrhage.
- If a prothrombotic state is confirmed and deemed significant (isolated and heterozygote states for some prothrombotic conditions such as factor V Leiden are of doubtful relevance: discuss with haematologist) then prolonged treatment with antiplatelet agents (low-dose aspirin and/or dipyridamole) should be considered.
- Children with sickle cell disease should receive an intensive blood transfusion regime (every 3–6 weeks) to maintain Hb between 10 and 12.5 g/dL and HbS <30%. This may be relaxed after 3 yrs to maintain HbS <50% and stopped after 2 yrs in patients who experienced stroke in the context of a precipitating illness (e.g. aplastic crisis) and whose repeat vascular imaging is normal at this time.

Vasculopathic arterial ischaemic stroke
- Stroke due to 'funny blood vessels'.
- Radiological patterns include Figure 4.9 B, C, and D. Pattern C particularly suggestive of small-vessel disease.

Large-vessel disease
- Moyamoya is a radiologically-defined syndrome, arising from large-vessel cerebrovascular disease of any cause. The term is Japanese for 'wisp of smoke' and relates to the angiographic appearances of the many tiny collaterals that open in response to large-vessel narrowing. Important causes include sickle cell disease, neurofibromatosis, Down, Noonan, and William syndromes.

- Look for evidence of extracranial arterial disease including evaluation for renal artery stenosis by angiography or renal artery Doppler (fibromuscular dysplasia).
- *ACTA2* arteriopathy with the typical bilateral ectasia of proximal carotid arteries and narrowing of distal internal carotid arteries and diffuse straightening of cerebral arteries ('twig-like' pattern), without Moyamoya.
  - A systemic disease with smooth muscle involvement, associated with aortic disease, hypotonic bladder, fixed dilated pupils, pulmonary hypertension. Request *ACTA2* mutations.

Focal cerebral arteriopathy

- Post-infectious focal cerebral arteriopathy is by far the commonest cause of Figure 4.9 'pattern C'. Post-varicella arteritis is particularly common: history of varicella in up to the last 6–8 months is likely relevant; also post-HHV6, mycoplasma, Lyme disease, etc.
- Varicella vasculitis in immunocompromised individuals.
- Systemic vasculitis may be suggested by elevated ESR in the presence of normal CRP. Primary cerebral vasculitis has protean manifestations and biopsy is often required to establish diagnosis.

Treatment and secondary prevention

- Antiplatelet therapy with aspirin.
- Treatment of underlying cause.
  - Post-infectious focal cerebral arteriopathy: the role of acute high-dose anti-inflammatory steroid therapy is being actively studied currently.

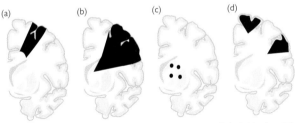

(a)   (b)   (c)   (d)

Fig. 4.9 Schematic representation of how patterns of neuroradiological involvement suggest mechanism in arterial ischaemic stroke. **A**: wedge shape infarction straddling the boundary between anterior and middle cerebral artery circulation (usually bilateral and fairly symmetrical) typical of *watershed* infarction due to hypoperfusion (e.g. period of hypotension). **B**. Wedge shaped infarction in single arterial territory (here, middle cerebral artery) implies local thrombotic *or* embolic cause. **C**. One or more small infarctions in subcortical structures implies involvement of small perforator arteries: consider small-vessel arteriopathy (especially post-infectious) as well as thrombotic conditions. **D**. Multiple wedge shaped infarctions in >1 arterial territory implies emboli from a distant source.

- In rare cases of FCA in the context of *active* chicken pox (i.e. with lesions still cropping) treat for 3 weeks with high-dose IV aciclovir.
- Aggressive transfusion programmes in sickle cell disease (see above).
- Treatment of primary vasculitides.
- Surgical vascular procedures to correct large-vessel stenoses if amenable.
  - Multiple burr-holes creation (which prompts a centripetal angiogenesis from external carotid to internal carotid circulation through each burr-hole) has largely replaced other surgical approaches to amelioration of effects of moyamoya syndrome.

Specialist and further investigations

- Flexion and extension views of the cervical spine in vertebrobasilar stroke.
- Further conventional angiograms:
  - to monitor progression of vascular disease;
  - in preoperative assessment of moyamoya.

Venous infarction

- History can be vague, and prolonged (weeks or even months).
  - Growth of thrombus can be slow.
  - Venous return temporarily compensated by collaterals.
- Radiological appearances of ischaemia in non-arterial distributions.
- CT usually suggestive of cerebral venous sinus thrombosis (CVST), confirmed by MR venography (or Doppler cranial ultrasound in neonates).
  - CVST cord sign, dense triangle sign, or empty delta sign.

Causes

Paediatric causes usually clear from clinical context:
- Sigmoid sinus thrombosis commonest form of CVST, usually associated with ipsilateral middle ear/mastoid bacterial sepsis.
- Hypercoagulable states:
  - Dehydration and/or polycythaemia in neonate.
  - Polycythaemia in congenital heart disease, sickle disease, and other haemoglobinopathies.
  - Asparaginase treatment for leukaemia.
  - Exchange transfusion in sickle cell.
- Pregnancy and use of oral contraception the most important risk factors in otherwise healthy young women.

Treatment

- Correct underlying cause.
- Systematic reviews confirm an overall benefit to formal anticoagulation.
  - Typically low molecular weight heparin.
  - Use split dosing acutely to minimize risk of haemorrhagic transformation.
  - Presence of haemorrhagic infarction not a contraindication.
  - Unfractionated heparin may be useful temporarily if neurosurgical procedures imminent (as can be rapidly reversed).
- Optimal duration of anticoagulation is unclear but repeat MRV to confirm recanalization may be helpful.
  - Where acute risk factor was identified and has been resolved, 3–6 months duration is typical.
- In severe cases with ↓consciousness, neurosurgical intervention (decompressive craniectomy) and/or endovascular procedures (clot retrieval) may be a consideration.

Cerebral haemorrhage

- For cerebral haemorrhage in the perinatal period: see Cerebral haemorrhage in the neonate in Chapter 5 ➲ p. 565.

Cerebral aneurysms

- Typically occur in the arteries of the Circle of Willis. See Figure 2.9 in Chapter 2 ➲ p. 67.
- Haemorrhage risk increases with aneurysm size.
- Because of association with Circle of Willis, aneurysms typically cause subarachnoid haemorrhage, SAH.
- SAH typically presents with very sudden onset, very severe ('ice pick') headache often followed by deteriorating consciousness. CT usually readily confirms blood in subarachnoid space: in rare cases where CT does not confirm clinical suspicions lumbar puncture should be performed.
  - LP is most sensitive 12 hours after the onset of symptoms and may be false −ve if performed <2 hours after onset of symptoms.
- Aneurysms particularly likely to be causal in SAH in an older adolescent.
- Syndromic associations of cerebral aneurysms with other conditions:
  - Coarctation of the aorta.
  - Autosomal dominant polycystic kidney disease (esp. anterior communicating artery aneurysms).
- Some aneurysms are familial (about 10% patients report a first-degree relative with SAH).
  - The role of screening for aneurysms in asymptomatic first-degree relatives of an index patient with SAH remains uncertain due to the risk–benefit ratio of surgery for an asymptomatic aneurysm.
  - It is currently suggested that screening be confined to individuals with two or more first-degree relatives with aneurysmal SAH. MRA is adequate to detect aneurysms of sufficient size (>7 mm) to warrant prophylactic surgery although the optimal timing(s) of MRA studies is uncertain (MRA at too young an age may give false −ve).
  - The presence of any symptoms or signs suggestive of SAH, or of a posterior circulation aneurysm (cranial nerve palsies or brainstem signs) clearly indicates ↑risk of haemorrhage.

Treatment

- Aim of acute treatment of SAH is to minimize risks of massive cerebral ischaemia/infarction due to delayed spasm of cerebral arteries provoked by presence of subarachnoid blood.
- So-called 3-H regime comprises induction of mild hypertensive, hyper-volaemic, and haemodiluted state, though no class I evidence. Nimodipine appears to reduce morbidity.
- Given the associations with coarctation, renal artery, and kidney disease, hypertension is an important co-morbidity. Anti-hypertensive therapy should however be delayed and very cautious until vasospasm risk period is passed.
- Treatment options include surgical clipping at open surgery, and endovascular occlusion with coils or glues. The post-operative mortality in adults who have sustained SAH is lower for coiling than clipping,

although there is some suggestion that rates of recurrence of the aneurysm may be higher.

Arteriovenous malformations

- Developmental (congenital) abnormalities of angiogenesis resulting in persistent direct large calibre connections between arterial and venous side of circulation. Haemorrhage risk related to high flow.
- A feature of several multiorgan vascular malformation syndromes e.g. Osler-Weber-Rendu, von Hippel–Lindau.
- Treatment needs to be individualized in discussion with specialist centres. Approaches are often multi-stage (e.g. sequential endovascular interventions before a definite surgical excision).
- Some AVMs will be deemed inoperable by virtue of their size and/or location, and the potential morbidity to surrounding brain tissue which may derive its blood supply from the abnormal vessels.
  - Stereotactic radiosurgery may be an option in these situations.

Cavernous haemangiomas ('cavernomas')

- Common developmental abnormality of capillary structure.
- Characteristic MRI and (usually) CT appearances due to breakdown products of blood that leak into surroundings.
- Usually not apparent on conventional or MR angiography as they are not high-flow structures.
- Catastrophic haemorrhage is rare however consideration should be given to primary surgical resection of large cavernomas.
- Tend to present with focal seizures presumed due to slow leakage of blood products into surrounding area.
- Often multiple and dominantly inherited with incomplete penetrance.
- Asymptomatic lesions are rarely treated so the clinical utility of MRI examination at regular intervals (new lesions form over time) has yet to be determined.
- Molecular genetic testing (if the family-specific mutation in *KRIT1*, *CCM2*, or *PDCD10* is known) reserved for those with a family history (two affected relatives) or where there are multiple cavernomas but no family history.
- May be associated with retinal and skin vascular malformations.

Tumours of the CNS

Epidemiology

CNS tumours (incidence 3.5/100000) are the most common solid tumours in childhood, and collectively the third largest group of childhood neoplasias after leukaemias and lymphomas. The ♂ to ♀ ratio is equal except for a ♂ predominance in medulloblastoma and germ cell tumours. The most common CNS tumours are glioma (Grades I-IV) (60%), medulloblastoma (20%) and ependymoma (10%).

Supratentorial tumours

- Supratentorial tumours predominate in *infants* (especially hypothalamic-chiasmatic-gliomas, embryonal tumours, and choroid plexus tumours).
- May be hemispheric (70%, mainly gliomas, rarely ependymomas, choroid plexus tumours, embryonal tumours, ganglioglioma) or midline (low-grade glioma, craniopharyngioma, germ cell, or pineal cell tumour).
- Suprasellar tumours: craniopharyngioma, germinoma, rarely pituitary tumours.

Infratentorial tumours

- In contrast to adults (where supratentorial tumours predominate), infratentorial tumours are at least as common in children.
- Medulloblastomas (20%), cerebellar astrocytomas (usually grade 1) (15%), ependymomas (5%), malignant gliomas (Grade III-IV) (3%), brainstem gliomas including diffuse midline gliomas (8%), other rare tumours.
- Intramedullary spinal cord tumours are rare and are usually astrocytomas (60%) or ependymomas.
- Solid metastatic tumours are rare in childhood, leukaemia being the most common metastatic CNS malignancy. Other CNS tumours (predominately medulloblastoma, ependymoma, germ cell tumours) can metastasize to elsewhere in CNS.

Presentation depends on the age of the child and the location of the tumour.

Presentations by age

- Presentations become increasingly specific and localizing with age.
- Presentations in infants typically non-specific (irritability, lethargy, vomiting, and failure to thrive, developmental regression, and increasing head size).
- Young child: more likely to have focal signs; may also have symptoms/signs of ↑ICP.
- Adolescent: localizing neurological symptoms/signs more common.

Presentations by location

Supratentorial tumour presentations

- Hemispheric gliomas.
  - seizures, focal neurological deficit, personality change.
- Optic nerve gliomas, craniopharyngiomas.
  - progressive visual field defects.

- endocrine dysfunction (short stature, hypothyroidism, and diabetes insipidus).
- behaviour and appetite changes.
- diencephalic syndrome in infants and toddlers (see 'Diencephalic Syndrome', Chapter 5 ➋ p. 547).
- symptoms/signs of ↑ICP (retrochiasmatic tumours may cause hydrocephalus).
- symptoms in younger children are often solely of ↑ICP.
- Suprasellar germ cell tumours.
  - endocrine dysfunction (diabetes insipidus and/or precocious puberty).
- Pineal tumours.
  - eye movement abnormalities (Parinaud syndrome—impaired upward gaze, dilated pupils reacting only to accommodation).
  - nystagmus (particularly rotatory).
  - symptoms/signs of ↑ICP.

Infratentorial tumour presentations

- Medulloblastomas.
  - cerebellar signs (ataxia, dysmetria), symptoms/signs of ↑ICP, neck pain +/- intermittent abnormal head postures (tonsillar herniation).
- Cerebellar astrocytomas.
  - similar presentation to medulloblastoma, slower progression.
- Ependymomas.
  - nausea and vomiting are key features due to compression of areas associated with vomiting in the brainstem.
  - symptoms/signs of ↑ICP.
- Diffuse midline glioma (mainly pons and thalami).
  - rapidly progressive cranial nerve defects, pyramidal tract signs, history less than 6 months.

Intramedullary spinal tumour presentations

- Insidious onset of symptoms (pain, paraesthesia, paresis, sensory level, sphincter disturbance, spinal deformity). Torticollis and hydrocephalus may be features. Usually spinal tumours are seen in older child, astrocytomas usually occur in upper thoracic cord and ependymomas in the cervical cord (myxopapillary ependymomas [grade 2]) usually in sacral area.

WHO tumour grading system (2021)

Predicts biological behaviour of a neoplasm which influences choice of therapies. It comprises 'malignancy scales' for a variety of neoplasms: not restricted to histological criteria. Increased reliance on molecular diagnostics to allow multi-layered diagnostic output. Grades assignments are regularly reviewed in light of long-term follow-up data.

- Grade I: low proliferative potential and possible cure following surgical resection. Example: pilocytic astrocytoma, DNET.
- Grade II: generally infiltrative and despite low-level proliferative activity may recur or progress to higher grades of malignancy. Example: astrocytomas transforming to anaplastic astrocytoma and glioblastoma.

- Grade III: histological evidence of malignancy. Example: anaplastic tumour of any cell type. Most treated with radiation and/or chemotherapy.
- Grade IV is assigned to cytologically malignant. Examples: glioblastoma, most embryonal neoplasms, and many sarcomas.

Low-grade gliomas (astrocytoma, oligodendroglioma)

30–40% all childhood CNS tumours. Despite their 'benign' reputation, morbidity is significant and death not unknown. Presentation is determined by site (see above). Posterior fossa presentation commonest.

Aetiology
- Inherited genetic conditions are responsible for 5%.
  - NF1 (gene *neurofibromin*) thought to be a tumour suppressor.
  - Tuberous sclerosis (associated with SEGA).
  - von Hippel–Lindau (associated with hemangioblastoma) .
  - Li-Fraumeni (mutation in *p53* tumour suppressor gene: more typically get medulloblastomas).
  - Gorlin syndromes (infant medulloblastoma of the SHH subgroup—*PTCH* mutation), also *SUFU* germline mutations.
  - *SMARCB1* mutation in rhabdoid tumours.
- Exposure to ionizing radiation a known risk factor.

Chiasmatic–hypothalamic gliomas
- 30% associated with neurofibromatosis type 1 (NF1): tend to be more indolent. Prognosis is worse in infants and when the tumour extends into the hypothalamus.
  - Clinical presentation may include visual field defects, strabismus, proptosis, endocrinopathies and diencephalic syndrome (see 'Diencephalic Syndrome', Chapter 5 ⊃ p. 547).
- In NF1, the tumour is observed with serial imaging, and surgical intervention is reserved for progressive or symptomatic tumours (usually only if vision is significantly impaired).
- In other children, chemotherapy and/or radiotherapy are used (radiotherapy deferred in younger children and those with NF1 and Li-Fraumeni syndrome if possible). Surgery is deferred for tumours causing mass effect or hydrocephalus.

Cerebellar astrocytomas
- *Usually pilocytic astrocytomas:* brightly enhancing, well demarcated partly cystic tumours with minimal surrounding oedema.
- Optimally managed by resection (achieved in >70%).
- Residual tumour may be observed as some will spontaneously regress. Recurrence is treated with re-operation if possible.
- A long-term perspective on disease control is required, with different strategies at different times.
- Operative complications are usually transient and related to cerebellar swelling: cerebellar signs, cerebellar mutism (see 'Cerebellar Mutism (posterior fossa syndrome)', this chapter ⊃ p. 520), 6th and 7th nerve palsies, pseudobulbar symptoms, and hemiparesis. Impaired initiation of voiding, chewing, and eye opening may also occur.

- Treatment is complete safe surgical resection (better to leave some than cause significant morbidity). Radical resection is associated with >75% 5-yr survival. Adjuvant chemotherapy or radiotherapy is reserved for evidence of disease recurrence or progression. 5 year survival in incomplete resection >60% (>80% with radiotherapy).
- Adjuvant treatment if needed is chemotherapy in younger children and radiotherapy over 8 years (because of demonstrated severe late cognitive effects of radiotherapy to immature CNS).
- Malignant transformation of non-irradiated low-grade gliomas is rare but surveillance for tumour progression or recurrence is necessary.
- Chemotherapy may have a role in the management of children with optic pathway glioma, for children with inaccessible disease and in recurrent or progressive tumours (after repeat resection) including targeted agents such as MEK inhibitors.
- Late cognitive morbidity probably relates to prolonged hydrocephalus.

High-grade gliomas (anaplastic astrocytomas, diffuse midline gliomas, glioblastoma multiforme)

Poorly circumscribed with ring-like enhancement and significant surrounding oedema with mass effect.

WHO grading system
Grade 3 or 4 and either:
- Diffuse midline Glioma, *H3K27* altered.
- Diffuse hemispheric glioma, H3 G34-mutant (*H3F3A*).
- Infant-type hemispheric glioma.

Treatment is by gross total resection where possible, radiotherapy to the tumour bed and a margin of surrounding brain and adjuvant chemotherapy. The extent of resection possible predicts long-term survival. Overexpression of *TP53* and glioblastoma multiforme are associated with poor prognosis. Targeted and chemotherapy have thus far not yielded significant survival benefit.

Five-yr survival following gross resection and adjuvant therapy is 10–20% outside infancy.

Brainstem gliomas

- Tectal tumours are usually slow-growing, and resection is indicated; however, shunting may be required for hydrocephalus.
- Other focal brainstem gliomas are less indolent but have a good prognosis with resection.
- In contrast, diffuse midline gliomas centred in the brainstem (80% of all brainstem gliomas) are inoperable with a very poor prognosis. These are usually diffuse and fibrillary in type with characteristic appearance on MRI.
- Median survival after diagnosis is 9 months despite aggressive radiotherapy and other interventions which have not as yet made a significant difference.

Medulloblastoma

The most common malignant CNS tumour.

- Usually in the midline posterior fossa. MRI shows a brightly enhancing mass with some necrotic/cystic areas, usually arising from the vermis, invading into the fourth ventricle and brainstem. Less commonly found in cerebellar hemispheres or cerebellopontine angle.
- More commonly seen in ♂'s; peak incidence is at 7 yrs of age.
- Prognosis depends on age (infants <3 years with non-desmoplastic histology have a worse prognosis), extent of resection, presence of metastases, and the presence of certain biological characteristics such as amplification of *c-myc* oncogene, large cell/anaplastic histology, and biological group. More detailed biology and subgrouping is playing an ever-increasing role in treatment stratification.
- Management comprises complete safe surgical resection, small residual disease is preferable to ↑morbidity.
- Proximity to the CSF makes seeding frequent (20 %) and staging is required with preoperative craniospinal MRI and CSF cytology.
- Craniospinal irradiation (usually over 3 years of age) is required to reduce the risk of metastases, followed by chemotherapy.
- Use of radiotherapy in under threes not commonly performed except in certain circumstances.
- 5yr survival for medulloblastoma is about 95% for favourable risk, 80% for standard risk, and up to 60% for high risk depending on biology of the tumour.

Embryonal tumours
- These tumours are often similar histologically to medulloblastomas but are biologically different with a worse prognosis. Biological characterization essential as there are a number of different entities.
- Neuroaxis staging is followed by gross total resection and further radiation and chemotherapy is dependent on the exact entity.
- Radiotherapy is deferred in younger children in favour of chemotherapy.
- Younger children (<3 yrs) have a worse prognosis although those with SHH subtype tend to do better.

Ependymoma

Can arise anywhere in the CNS from ependymal or subependymal cells; 60% occur in the posterior fossa.
- Incidence peaks at ~4years of age.
- Radiologically usually contrast-enhancing and *heterogeneous* with areas of haemorrhage, necrosis, and calcification.
- Typically midline and intraventricular.
- Initial management guided by staging MRI of brain and spine.
  - If no evidence of metastasis, then aiming for 100% resection particularly important, even at risk of neurological morbidity.
  - Image immediately post-op (still under GA) and return immediately to theatre if any residuum detected.
  - 10–30% tumours infiltrative and not fully resectable.

Not typically very chemo sensitive. Mainstay of adjuvant treatment is focal radiotherapy to tumour bed in over-3s (younger in posterior fossa disease). The role of radiotherapy in under threes is under evaluation: chemotherapy may have a role if there is residual or disseminated disease but has failed to reduce the need for radiotherapy in very young children. It may also improve survival if given post radiotherapy (usually proton beam radiotherapy) .

Overall 5-yr survival 50–60%.

Less common CNS tumours

Craniopharyngioma
- Benign tumour but locally aggressive and recurs.
- Proximity to optic pathways and pituitary make management difficult.
- Most tumours in childhood are calcified. On T2 MRI the tumour is hyperintense, lobulated, heterogeneous, and cystic with ring enhancement.
- Preoperatively children require documentation of visual fields and assessment for electrolyte abnormality and endocrinopathy. Children should have supplemental steroids before surgery and prior to treating hypothyroidism. Hydrocephalus should be controlled.
- Surgery may be required urgently in situations of acute visual deterioration or hydrocephalus, but otherwise endocrine and electrolyte abnormality should be corrected first.
- Surgery allows gross total resection of the tumour in 70–80% of cases and decompression in others. Trend is to maximal safe surgery avoiding the hypothalamus.
- Radiotherapy is of benefit if the resection is subtotal or for recurrent disease.
- Most children have panhypopituitarism, appetite and behavioural disturbance and memory dysfunction due to the tumour or its treatment.

Intracranial germ cell tumours (GCT)
- Heterogeneous, rare group of tumours comprising benign and malignant forms which can co-exist in a single tumour!
- Should be suspected in any case of midline tumour particularly at suprasellar or pineal location.
- Embryonal carcinoma and yolk sac tumours may secrete α-fetoprotein (AFP) and can infrequently spread to the lung or bone. Embryonal carcinoma and choriocarcinoma may secrete β-human chorionic gonadotrophin (β-HCG).
- AFP and β-HCG should be measured in the CSF as well as in serum and can be used to aid diagnosis (may obviate need for biopsy). Secreting tumours generally have a worse prognosis.
- Management comprises urgent CSF diversion (if required). If done by third ventriculostomy then endoscopic biopsy may be required (in AFP/β-HCG –ve cases).
- Teratomas managed by resection.
- Germinomas very radio- and chemotherapy sensitive.
- High risk of endocrine disturbance due to disruption of hypothalamo-pituitary axis: assess pre- and again postoperatively.

Choroid plexus tumours
- Papilloma or carcinoma, typically presenting with signs of ↑ICP due to overproduction of CSF and/or ventricular obstruction in the first few years of life.
- Lumbar puncture should be avoided.
- MRI demonstrates a large enhancing, highly vascular intraventricular mass.
- Benign papillomas have a 'cauliflower' like appearance with a distinct stalk.
- Management is gross total resection (±shunt insertion), which may be difficult due to tumour size, vascularity, and proximity to important structures.
- Endovascular procedures (intra-arterial embolization) may aid subsequent resection.
- Papillomas have a good prognosis if completely resected.
- Carcinomas are invasive and vascular (<50% achieve gross total resection at operation) and are prone to CSF dissemination, and chemotherapy and/or radiotherapy (if >3 yrs) may be required as adjuncts. Five-year survival rates are around 35%, with the extent of surgical resection being important for prognosis.

Neuroblastoma
Not a primary CNS tumour but included here because of important neurological presentations and complications.
- Malignant tumour of neural crest origin.
- May arise in the olfactory pathway, adrenal gland, or sympathetic nervous system.
- Most present with an abdominal mass and/or bone pain.
- Neurological presentations include Horner syndrome, spinal cord compression, ataxia and opsoclonus-myoclonus (see 'Opsoclonus-myoclonus', Chapter 4 ➘ p. 395) (2% presentations).
- Metastases to the retrobulbar area may present with proptosis or periorbital ecchymoses (raccoon eyes).
- Prognosis is related to age at diagnosis, clinical stage of disease and (in children older than 1yr) regional lymph node involvement.
- Unfavourable outcomes have been associated with elevated serum ferritin, neuron-specific enolase levels, and lactate dehydrogenase; amplification of *N-Myc* proto-oncogene and low TrkA expression.
- Low risk children are managed with gross surgical resection. Chemotherapy is used in addition to surgery in intermediate risk children. Myeloablative chemotherapy or chemoradiotherapy followed by autologous bone marrow transplantation is under investigation for the high-risk group.

Dysembryoplastic neuroepithelial tumour (DNET)
- Rare cortical tumour.
- Important cause of intractable focal epilepsy.
- Well circumscribed, usually supratentorial, more common in the temporal lobes and more common in ♂'s.

- Amenable to complete resection, no recurrence is expected, and prognosis is good.

Peripheral nerve tumours
Schwannoma, neurofibroma, perineuroma, malignant peripheral nerve sheath tumour.

Meningeal tumours
Meningioma, mesenchymal tumours (e.g. lipoma, fibrosarcoma, leiomyosarcoma, rhabdomyosarcoma), melanocytic tumours (e.g. malignant melanoma, melanomatosis).

Staging evaluation
This is required for posterior fossa medulloblastoma, ependymoma and for pineal lesions (e.g. PNET, germ cell tumour, etc.).
- Craniospinal MRI.
- CSF cytology.
- For malignant germ cell tumour: AFP and β-HCG may be ↑in both blood and CSF.

Complications of cranial irradiation
Radiation therapy should be deferred in very young children if at all possible. Chemotherapy is the adjuvant of choice in this group.
- *Acute/subacute complications*: drowsiness, nausea, and headache, lethargy, and fatigue.
- *Chronic complications*: alopecia, dental problems, hearing loss (also a complication of platinum chemotherapy), endocrine dysfunction (hypothalamus, pituitary and/or thyroid hormones), growth retardation (especially with CSI), radio-necrosis, vasculopathy (e.g. Moyamoya syndrome), neurocognitive and behaviour problems, secondary tumours (incidence of secondary tumours is perhaps as much as 5%, usually gliomas or meningiomas).

Additional management issues
- Antiseizure medication may be required to control epilepsy.
- Hydrocephalus may require shunting or placement of an external ventricular drain (EVD).
- Peritumoural oedema: treat with dexamethasone (see 'Dexamethasone', Chapter 7 ❷ p. 665).
- Endocrinopathy: hydrocortisone should be administered peri-operatively to children who have tumours in the vicinity of the hypothalamus. Injury to the pituitary stalk during surgery can mean that levels of vasopressin fluctuate postoperatively (typically a period of DI then SIADH, then DI returns).

Cerebellar mutism (posterior fossa syndrome)
A complication of posterior fossa surgery, particularly resection of midline posterior fossa tumours such as medulloblastoma (∴ more common in children than adults). It can be seen after other insults involving the cerebellum or brainstem. The syndrome onset is typically *delayed* by 24–48 h after insult.

- Features include persistent eye closure, sphincter incontinence, ↓oral intake and oromotor apraxia, truncal ataxia, emotional lability, and irritability and occasionally hypersomnolence.
- Language is particularly affected: the child typically is mute but may scream or whine. Comprehension of language is relatively preserved.
- Recovery is associated with a speech pattern described as ataxic dysarthria.
- Thought to be due to disruption of dentato-rubro-thalamo-cortical fibres.
- No known effective preventative measures.
- Diagnosis is clinical: characteristic picture in the appropriate context and absence of other causes.
- Changes on MRI have been reported but no characteristic pattern.
- Management is supportive, including active interdisciplinary rehabilitation.

Vitamin-responsive conditions

Worldwide the most common vitamin-responsive conditions are due to nutritional deficiency (childhood malnutrition or malabsorption). Although rare, these disorders are potentially treatable, and prompt diagnosis and treatment may have a marked impact on outcome.

Vitamin B$_1$ (thiamine)

- Thiamine is a water-soluble vitamin found in legumes, nuts, meat.
- Absorbed by rate-limited saturable process of active transport in the jejunum and ileum.
- Limited storage—in adults only sufficient for up to 18 days—unknown in children.
- Key role in tricarboxylic acid cycle: thiamine is *consumed by oxidative metabolism of glucose*.
  - Requirements relate to metabolic activity: ~0.5 mg/1000 kcal.

Wernicke encephalopathy

Particular vulnerability contexts:

- Catabolic conditions in critically ill patients—no storage.
- High glucose 'diet', e.g. IV dextrose saline or TPN without appropriate multivitamin supplements.
- Anorexia nervosa.
- Malignancy:
  - Consumption of thiamine by fast-growing neoplastic cells.
  - Poor dietary intake related to lack of appetite, nausea, malabsorption.
  - Specific types of chemotherapy interrupt conversion to thiamine pyrophosphate.
- Gastrointestinal disorders:
  - Recurrent vomiting.
  - Chronic diarrhoea.
  - Malabsorption.
  - Bowel failure.
- Renal failure:
  - Anorexia and vomiting.
  - Accelerated loss of thiamine during dialysis.

Diagnosis

- Difficult to diagnose and often goes undetected or under-treated.
  - First diagnosed post-mortem in over 80% of cases.

❶The serious consequences of untreated Wernicke's warrant a high index of suspicion and low threshold for treatment.

- Classic triad of *ophthalmoplegia, ataxia, and confusion*:
  - But only ~ 10% patients exhibit all three features.
  Other suggestive features:
- Papilloedema of optic discs with retinal haemorrhages.
- Unexplained lactic acidosis.

- Characteristic MRI changes:
  - 93% specificity but only 53% sensitivity.
  - Bilateral symmetrical abnormal T2 signal in: parasagittal frontal lobes, basal ganglia, thalami, hypothalamic, amygdala, around third ventricle (periaqueductal region, tectal plate), posterior medulla.
  - Cytotoxic and vasogenic oedema with haemorrhagic transformation (latter characteristic of severe hyperacute thiamine deficiency).
- Rare fulminant variant—Shoshin beriberi—characterized by cardiovascular collapse. Urgent thiamine supplementation can lead to rapid recovery while untreated it is fatal.
- Peripheral neuropathy including autonomic neuropathy.

Treatment
- Parenteral thiamine has a half-life of 96 min.
- Multiple doses required acutely to achieve adequate CNS concentration.
- High potency IV B vitamins with ascorbic acid (e.g. Pabrinex®) TDS for 3 days (500 mg thiamine TDS) followed by 500 mg IV OD for 5 days or until clinical improvement stops.
- Check adequacy of magnesium levels: magnesium a cofactor in the conversion of thiamine into thiamine pyrophosphate.

Thiamine transporter 2 deficiency (biotin responsive basal ganglia disease)
Recessive, leading to episodic encephalopathy, often triggered by febrile illness. Presents variously as confusion, seizures, external ophthalmoplegia, dysphagia, or coma. High-dose biotin with thiamine may lead to partial or complete recovery. Untreated, there may be progressive dystonia. MRI may show characteristic bilateral basal ganglia lesions. Should be considered in all cases of sudden-onset encephalopathy with thalamic and basal ganglia changes on MRI imaging.

Thiamine pyrophosphokinase deficiency (episodic ataxia, psychomotor retardation, and dystonia)
Phenotype variable. Presents in early childhood with episodes of acute encephalopathy (↑serum and CSF lactate) often triggered by infection. Leads to progressive impairment: gait disturbances, ataxia, dystonia, and spasticity. Cognitive function is usually preserved. Stabilized with oral thiamine supplementation.

Vitamin B$_2$ (riboflavin)
Brown–Vialetto–van Laere syndrome (BVVL) and Fazio–Londe disease
Two rare eponymous syndromes of sometimes rapidly progressive peripheral weakness with cranial nerve involvement characteristically including *severe sensorineural hearing loss*. They are now recognized to be allelic and both due to mutation in riboflavin transporters (commonly mutations in *SLC52A2* or *SLC52A3*). The clinical picture is significantly ameliorated by high-dose riboflavin supplementation: extent of resolution depends on prompt recognition and treatment.

▶▶ Since riboflavin is water-soluble, excreted in urine, and non-toxic, high-dose riboflavin should be instituted in any situation of possible BVVL or Fazio–Londe pending genetic confirmation.

Typical presentations include:
- A slowly progressive mixed sensory and motor peripheral neuropathy with optic nerve and (particularly) sensorineural hearing involvement (classic BVVL presentation).
- A rapidly progressing motor neuron disease-like picture with *bulbar* and *pharyngeal* involvement (classic Fazio–Londe presentation).
- A rapidly progressive Guillain–Barré-like picture with marked, progressive involvement of hearing.

Vitamin B$_6$ (pyridoxine and related compounds)

This is the cofactor for over 100 enzymes, including enzymes involved in the metabolism of neurotransmitters (GABA, glutamate), glycogenolysis, porphyrin synthesis, and transamination of amino acids.

There are three dietary forms:
- Pyridoxine (from vegetables).
- Pyridoxamine (from red meat).
- Pyridoxal 5'-phosphate (PLP, the active cofactor to which all are converted).

Pyridoxine-dependent developmental and epileptic encephalopathy (PD-DEE)
See Box 4.10.

Typical early onset group
- Prenatal seizures: mother may report abnormal foetal movements.
- Present in the first days of life in about one-third of cases: neonatal encephalopathy with irritability, hyper-alertness, and stimulus-sensitive startle; accompanied by systemic features that add to diagnostic dilemma: respiratory distress, abdominal distension, vomiting, and metabolic acidosis.
- Multiple seizure types emerge in days, ASM resistant.

Box 4.10 Diagnosis and treatment of pyridoxine-dependent DEE

Step 1. Response to vitamin
- Have full resuscitation available because of risk of collapse.
- EEG monitoring preferable.
- Pyridoxine 100 mg IV/pyridoxal phosphate 100 mg orally.
- Prompt response with cessation of seizures (within minutes).
- Side effect of cerebral depression in up to 20%: hypotonia, sedation, apnoea, akinesia, isoelectric EEG (support until recovery).

Step 2. Biochemical and genetic confirmation
- Urine AASA levels remain high even when supplemented with pyridoxine/pyridoxal (so can test even if being supplemented).
- Proceed to genetic testing if AASA levels supportive (*ALDH7A1* and *PLBP* in PD-DEE, *PNPO* in P5PD-DEE).
- Children with normal AASA levels may be non-specific pyridoxine responders, even if not strictly pyridoxine-dependent.
- In children with questionable responses to pyridoxine then withdrawal should taken place with careful observation for possible deterioration.

- May have associated structural brain abnormalities.
- Prompt response to IV pyridoxine. See Pyridoxine in Chapter 7 ➲ p. 669.

Atypical later-onset group
- No encephalopathy or structural brain abnormality.
- Seizures begin any time up to 3 yrs of age.
- First seizures may be febrile and develop into status.
- May show initial but unsustained response to conventional ASMs.
- Respond to oral pyridoxine.

Outcome: life-long treatment with oral pyridoxine and low lysine diet; likely learning difficulties, particularly language impairment; more severe motor disorder and developmental impairment if treatment is delayed. Some intellectual impairment is likely even when treated early.
   Treatment: pyridoxine 15 mg/kg/day, decrease if peripheral neuropathy.

Pyridoxal 5'-phosphate-dependent epilepsy
Clinical features similar to early onset pyridoxine-responsive seizures: commonly a history of foetal distress, intractable neonatal-onset seizures, EEG burst-suppression pattern, but no response to pyridoxine.
   Genetics: pyridoxine 5'-phosphate oxidase (PNPO) mutation.
   Treatment: pyridoxal phosphate 30–50 mg/kg/day in four doses (prompt response). Monitor LFTs.

Pyridoxine and pyridoxal-responsive seizures
There is a group of children with severe symptomatic epilepsy, often infantile spasms, who respond to vitamin B6, but in whom subsequent withdrawal is possible (i.e they are pyridoxine/pyridoxal *responsive*, but not *dependent*: pyridoxine is acting as an empiric ASM). Genetic mechanism(s) unclear.

Folinic acid-responsive seizures
Some children with confirmed *ALDH7A1* PD-DEE respond better to folinic acid than pyridoxine. The reason for the differential treatment response is unknown.

Biotin metabolism (Vitamin B₇)
Biotin is a B-group vitamin, essential for covalently binding to carboxylase enzymes (enzymes that have a central role in gluconeogenesis, amino acid metabolism, and fatty acid biosynthesis for the Kreb cycle).
   Dietary deficiency is extremely rare as dietary biotin is endogenously recycled: may occur as a complication of long-term parenteral nutrition if not supplemented.
   Inborn errors involve the enzymes needed for biotin recycling: biotinidase deficiency (which responds to biotin treatment); and *holo*-carboxylase synthase deficiency (attaches biotin to the carboxylase enzymes and does not respond to biotin treatment).

Biotinidase deficiency
- Clinical features: variable age of onset but most commonly with neurological symptoms, epilepsy (often infantile spasms) and hypotonia at 3–4 months of age (can be up to 10 yrs); ataxia in older children; dermatitis, alopecia, or conjunctivitis should raise suspicion. Later lactic acidosis, hearing, and visual loss.

- Diagnosis: plasma biotinidase level (usually <10% activity), organic aciduria (because of the effect on carboxylases). May show low CSF glucose with ↑lactate (c.f. GLUT1 deficiency).
- Treatment: biotin 5–20 mg/day orally; prompt resolution of abnormal biochemistry, skin, seizures, and ataxia; hearing and visual loss are irreversible.

Holocarboxylase synthase deficiency
Symptoms begin as a neonate. Seizures are less common (25–50%). May need higher doses: of biotin: 10–40 mg/day.

Biotin Thiamine responsive basal ganglia disease
See Thiamine transporter 2 deficiency (biotin responsive basal ganglia disease) in this chapter ➲ p. 523.

Vitamin B$_{12}$ (cobalamin)

An essential water-soluble vitamin from meat and dairy products. Deficiency may be seen in vegans and their breast-fed infants.

Inborn errors of B$_{12}$ metabolism
See Figure 4.10.
Most neurological disorders responsive to cobalamin are inborn errors of metabolism, inherited in an autosomal recessive manner and presenting with:
- *Neurology*: developmental impairment; peripheral neuropathy.
- *Haematology*: pallor; megaloblastic anaemia.
- *Gastroenterology*: anorexia, diarrhoea, and vomiting; failure to thrive (FTT); stomatitis, atrophic glossitis.

Treatment
- Hydroxycobalamin 1 mg/day IM until a response is seen. Expect to see improvement in haematological and biochemical indices, mood, and well-being within 1 week; in contrast, neurological improvement takes months to years, and indeed in the remethylation defects, progression continues.
- Then monthly to maintain hepatic stores.
- May also need betaine 100–200 mg/kg/day (an alternative methyl donor).
- Monitor treatment by plasma total homocysteine and methionine.

Acquired B$_{12}$ deficiency and subacute combined degeneration of the cord
Nitrous oxide exposure
- Nitrous oxide anaesthesia may lead to sudden neurological deterioration in situations of subclinical B$_{12}$ deficiency.
- Deterioration of spinal cord function resembling subacute combined degeneration of the cord (early paraesthesia followed in time by sensory gait ataxia) is increasingly recognized as a common complication of recreational nitrous oxide abuse. Outcome depends on prompt recognition, halting further exposure and urgent initiation of an intensive schedule of hydroxycobalamin injections.

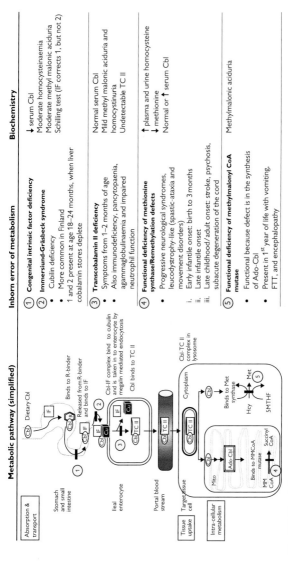

Metabolic pathway (simplified)	Inborn error of metabolism	Biochemistry
	① **Congenital intrinsic factor deficiency**	↓ serum Cbl
	② **Immerslund-Gräsbeck syndrome**	Moderate homocysteinaemia
	• Cubilin deficiency	Moderate methyl malonic aciduria
	• More common in Finland	Schilling test (IF corrects 1, but not 2)
	• 1 and 2 present at age 18–24 months, when liver cobalamin stores deplete	
	③ **Transcobalamin II deficiency**	Normal serum Cbl
	• Symptoms from 1–2 months of age	Mild methyl malonic aciduria and
	• Also immunodeficiency, pancytopaenia, agammaglobulinaemia and impaired neutrophil function	homocystinuria
		Undetectable TC II
	④ **Functional deficiency of methionine synthase/Remethylation defects**	↑ plasma and urine homocysteine
	• Progressive neurological syndromes, leucodystrophy-like (spastic-ataxia and movement disorders)	↓ methionine
	i. Early infantile onset: birth to 3 months	Normal or ↑ serum Cbl
	ii. Late infantile onset	
	iii. Late childhood/adult onset: stroke, psychosis, subacute degeneration of the cord	
	⑤ **Functional deficiency of methylmalonyl CoA mutase**	Methylmalonic aciduria
	• Functional because defect is in the synthesis of Ado-Cbl	
	• Present in 1st year of life with vomiting, FTT, and encephalopathy	

Fig. 4.10 Vitamin B$_{12}$-dependent disorders.

Others
Acquired B_{12} deficiency occurs in pernicious anaemia, an autoimmune condition resulting in destruction of the gastric parietal cells responsible for secretion of *intrinsic factor*, a glycoprotein essential for B12 absorption in the distal ileum.

- Pre-symptomatic diagnosis of B_{12} deficiency following identification of a megaloblastic anaemia is typical; however, late diagnosis can result in neurological damage.
- Many effects of B_{12} deficiency are in fact due to secondary to folate deficiency (as folate regeneration is B_{12}-dependent) and will be ameliorated by folate supplementation.
- There are, however, some specifically B_{12}-dependent processes including myelination that are not folate-responsive. This has led to debate about the wisdom of introduction of folate fortification of flour as a public-health measure to prevent neural tube defects (by ensuring adequate folate levels in women in the early days of pregnancy during neural tube formation): as folate supplementation will treat megaloblastic anaemia.

The syndrome of late neurological damage due to B_{12} deficiency comprises non-specific psychiatric features with a characteristic pattern of spinal cord involvement known as subacute combined degeneration of the cord. This resembles the findings in Friedreich ataxia (which also involves dorsal column function).

- Loss of dorsal column functions (joint position and vibration sense).
- Sensory ataxia with +ve Romberg sign (unsteadiness in standing worse on eye closure).
- Distressing paraesthesias.
- The very characteristic combination of depressed or absent deep tendon reflexes particularly at knees and ankles with upgoing plantars (positive Babinski sign), c.f. Friedreich ataxia. See Slowly progressive ataxias (over months to years) with initial symptom-free period with initial symptom-free period in this chapter ❐ p. 425.

Treatment
- As for inherited disorders of B12 metabolism.

Folate

Folates are water-soluble vitamins, essential from dietary sources (leafy vegetables, nuts, beans). The active metabolite is 5-methyltetra-hydrofolate (5-MTHF). Transport across the BBB is mediated by high affinity membrane-associated folate receptors. As folate metabolism is closely linked to B12 metabolism, clinical features are not surprisingly very similar.

Hereditary folate malabsorption
- *Biochemistry*: deficient intestinal folate absorption and deficient transport of folate into the CNS.
- *Inheritance*: autosomal recessive, but occurs mostly in ♀s.
- *Clinical features*: severe anaemia, gastrointestinal symptoms and variable neurological involvement (learning difficulties, seizures, ataxia, peripheral neuropathy).

- *Diagnosis*: megaloblastic anaemia, low serum, and red cell folate, ↑plasma homocysteine, reduced CSF 5-MTHF even after temporary correction of serum folate with 5-formylTHF injection. Mutations in *SLC46A1* identified in all cases so far.
- *Treatment*: folinic (not folic) acid (latter blocks receptor-mediated transport of 5-MTHF) initially 10–15 mg/kg once daily orally (much higher doses may be needed: dose titrated against CSF folate concentrations).
- Systemic features (anaemia etc) normalize rapidly: neurological prognosis depends on early recognition.

Cerebral folate deficiency syndrome

Three forms: an inherited genetic syndrome due to mutations in the cerebral folate receptor gene *FOLR1* (autosomal recessive); dihydrofolate reductase deficiency; and a rare infantile-onset autoimmune disorder with autoantibodies to the folate receptor blocking folate uptake into CSF.

- *Clinical features*: onset at 4–6 months of age, marked irritability, developmental impairment or regression, acquired microcephaly, cerebellar ataxia, lower-limb pyramidal tract signs, dyskinesias; later epilepsy and autism.
- *Diagnosis*: low CSF 5-MTHF but normal folate metabolism outside the central nervous system (i.e. normal serum and red cell folate, normal homocysteine levels, normal haematological indices).
- *Treatment*: folinic acid (mechanism of action uncertain).

Folinic acid-responsive seizures

- Some neonates with mutations in *ALDH7A1* (i.e. who have DEE-PDE, see Vitamin B_6 in this chapter ➋ p. 524) respond to folinic acid (and not pyridoxine or pyridoxal). Reasons for the differential treatment response are unclear.
- Treatment: folinic acid 2–5 mg/kg/day IV results in immediate cessation of seizures, then long-term 5 mg twice a day orally (increase dose with weight).

Vitamin E

- This is a generic term for a group of related compounds (tocopherols and tocotrienols). It is a fat-soluble vitamin: absorption in the gut requires bile salts. An antioxidant, particularly protecting membrane phospholipids from radical oxygen species. The CNS and retina are particularly vulnerable in vitamin E deficiency (high concentrations of susceptible fatty acids, disproportionately high oxygen supply and iron concentrations from which to generate free radicals, relative deficiency of other antioxidant systems).

▶ Particular neurological features suggesting vitamin E-responsive conditions: spinocerebellar degeneration (pyramidal tract, ataxia, polyneuropathy), and retinopathy.

- Neurological conditions responsive to vitamin E can be considered as two groups: conditions of vitamin E deficiency and conditions of ↑stress on antioxidant protection.

Conditions of vitamin E deficiency
- *Newborn and pre-term infants* have reduced serum vitamin E and are at ↑risk of oxidative stress (sudden increase in oxygen to the lung at birth). Studies have indicated that vitamin E supplementation decreases the incidence of intraventricular haemorrhage and of retinopathy of prematurity in pre-terms but may increase the risk of sepsis and necrotizing enterocolitis by impairing normal oxygen-dependent antimicrobial defences. Prophylactic vitamin E is not currently recommended, while the risk/benefit ratio remains unclear.
- *Malabsorptive conditions*: any chronic fat malabsorptive state would be expected to reduce the absorption of vitamin E.
- *Abetalipoproteinaemia*: all children have undetectable serum vitamin E. Untreated they develop ataxia, peripheral neuropathy, and retinal degeneration leading to blindness; high-dose supplementation prevents, delays progression, or reverses these neurological features (α-tocopheryl acetate 100 mg/kg/day).
- Acquired deficiency in *cholestatic liver disease*: without bile salts, vitamin E is not absorbed from the gut. Resulting ataxia and peripheral neuropathy are now rare, as all children with known cholestatic liver disease should be receiving prophylaxis with the water-soluble form of vitamin E (α-tocopheryl polyethylene glycol-1000 succinate).
- *Ataxia with vitamin E deficiency* (AVED): a familial disorder due to mutations in gene for a hepatic α-tocopherol transfer protein; severe vitamin E deficiency, but without fat malabsorption; usually presents in adolescence or adulthood with spinocerebellar degeneration and retinopathy.

▶▶ It is crucial to differentiate AVED from Friedreich ataxia, because AVED responds to vitamin E (800 mg/day).

Conditions of increased stress on antioxidant protection
There is evidence for ↑oxidative stress in Down syndrome, Friedreich ataxia, ischaemia/reperfusion injury, and the NCLs. Vitamin E, folinic acid, and antioxidant supplementation in Down syndrome has not shown benefit in terms of psychomotor development.

Chapter 5

Consultation
with other services

General principles

Consultation requests should be met with:
- A request for a clear statement of the question(s) you're being asked to address or function to be performed if you feel this is lacking (i.e. 'Why would you like us to see this patient?'). Serial involvement of subspecialty teams without clearly understood roles and responsibilities can lead to 'teaching hospital syndrome'.
- Deference and sensitivity to the relationship already built between the referring consultant and the child and family.
- Good liaison and clear agreement with the referring team on how to deliver any new information to the family and who will implement any new management plan.
- Focused discussion over specific interventions.
- Remember non-neurological colleagues may have a less experienced clinical approach; it is always best to repeat the detail of the history and carry out your own neurological examination.
- *'When all you have is a hammer, everything looks like a nail'*.
  - As a neurologist you have a responsibility to be aware of your own susceptibility to this tendency (see Synthesis in Chapter 1 ➋ pp. 49-50). Ensure the referrer appreciates the importance of considering other, non-neurological perspectives on the problem on which you were consulted.

Independent note-keeping of the contents of telephone and other 're-mote' consultations is important as you cannot check how your advice has been documented in the local clinical record.

Common referral themes will be related to specific specialist services.

Cardiology consultations

Neurological complications of cardiac disease

Neurological complications of cardiac disease typically arise either from effects of hypoperfusion (hypoxia–ischaemia) and/or embolus.

The heart
- Congenital heart disease (e.g. transposition of the great arteries; other cyanotic conditions; hypoplastic left heart syndrome), valvular disease, cardiomyopathy, and arrhythmias may result in hypoperfusion or embolus (from right-to-left shunting or arrhythmia).

Procedures
- Balloon atrial septostomy, cardiac catheterization.
- Extracorporeal membrane oxygenation (ECMO).
- Cardiopulmonary bypass and deep hypothermic circulatory arrest.

Clinical context
- Underlying conditions (e.g. genetic syndromes).
- Drugs (e.g. warfarin, ciclosporin).
- Sepsis, etc.

Stroke
- May present as cardiorespiratory instability, seizures, abnormal posturing, or headaches as well as paresis.
- Early assessment of neurological impairment and prognostication may not be possible due to systemic instability, and sedation or paralysis for ventilation. Reassess the child periodically.
- Medical instability may also delay neuroimaging and MRI may not be possible because of the prolonged study duration and/or metalwork in or near the patient.
- Brain MRI abnormalities in children with congenital heart disease may have been present *prior* to any cardiothoracic surgery!
  - Focal infarcts in 40% of Transposition of Great Artery cases due to prior atrial septostomy, cardiorespiratory depression at presentation, or perinatal events.
  - Postoperative infarcts and haemorrhages seen in 15% (micro-emboli as bypass clamps are released or from device closures; haemorrhages after ECMO and anticoagulation).

There is a high prior probability that an ischaemic stroke occurring in a cardiothoracic setting will be embolic. This is one of the few settings where in-hospital embolic stroke may occur and may allow consideration of emergency thrombolysis/thrombectomy: see Acute management [Stroke Chapter] in Chapter 4 ➔ pp. 500-4.
  - BUT consider cerebral abscess—cyanotic heart disease and endocarditis are risk factors; can have acute presentation and CT appearances resemble vascular causes (MRI will distinguish).
  - Additionally such children may well already be fully anticoagulated which would be a contraindication to thrombolysis/thrombectomy.

- Low-flow cardiac conditions, e.g. hypoplastic left heart syndrome, predispose to thrombus and embolic stroke. Requires anticoagulation and/or antiplatelet treatment.
- Paradoxical emboli from the right side of the circulation may occur in children with cyanotic heart disease (right-to-left shunting).
- Infarcts, haemorrhages, and mycotic aneurysms can be a complication of infective endocarditis.
- Central venous hypertension may predispose to cerebral vein thrombosis leading to multifocal infarcts and haemorrhages.
- Focal vascular lesions may exist on background of diffuse ischaemic brain injury which has wider neurocognitive sequelae.

Seizures

- Multiple aetiologies: stroke, diffuse hypoxic–ischaemic injury, abscess, drugs (e.g. posterior reversible encephalopathy syndrome; see Posterior reversible encephalopathy syndrome in this Chapter ➜ p. 598).
- Or related to underlying genetic syndrome, e.g. hypoplastic left heart syndrome, 22q11 deletion, Down syndrome, tuberous sclerosis.
- Distinguish from non-epileptic myoclonus, chorea, jitteriness.

Movement disorder

- 'Post-pump' chorea after bypass or ECMO: see Cardiopulmonary bypass ('post-pump chorea') in Chapter 4 ➜ p. 421.
- Myoclonus following cardiac arrest, typically interfering with voluntary movements—Lance-Adams syndrome (see Lance-Adams syndrome in Chapter 4 ➜ p. 419).
- Sydenham chorea in context of acute rheumatic fever.
- Underlying neurogenetic syndromes, e.g. Friedreich (rarely the cardiomyopathy presents before the ataxia).

Neuropathy

- Critical illness neuropathy after prolonged ventilation and intensive care: see Difficulty weaning from the ventilator in this chapter ➜ pp. 587-8.
- Compression mono-neuropathies (pressure palsies, see Entrapment neuropathies in Chapter 4 ➜ pp. 438-9) secondary to prolonged immobility.

Hypoxic–ischaemic insult

- May present with seizures, prolonged coma, or ventilation requirements.
- Hypothermia routinely provided for preoperative circulatory arrest is protective.
- Ischaemia associated with ligation of the carotid artery in ECMO.
- MRI may demonstrate diffuse injury affecting combination of white matter, basal ganglia, and cortex.
- 'Watershed' distributions of injury located particularly along the boundary between of anterior and middle (or middle and posterior) cerebral artery territories (see Fig. 2.8 Neuroanatomical sections

in Chapter 2 ➋ pp. 65-6) are particularly suggestive of subacute hypoperfusion (rather than total ischaemia).
- For assessment and prognostication following cardiac arrest: see Non-traumatic coma in this chapter ➋ pp. 585-6.

Neurodevelopmental prognosis in congenital heart disease
- Developmental scores relate more to underlying genetic syndromes (relevant in 12% of infants e.g. Down syndrome, 22q11 deletion), ApoE2 allele, and perinatal condition more than intra-operative factors.
- Hypoplastic left heart syndrome commonly associated with agenesis of corpus callosum or holoprosencephaly (10%), cortical malformations, congenital microcephaly. 60% have major disabilities.
- Neurocognitive scores in later childhood are low end of normal across multiple domains.
- May have additional focal deficits, e.g. stroke-related hemiplegia.
- Consider referral of infants with complicated in-patient course to community or developmental paediatrician.

Cardiologic aspects of neurologic and neurodevelopmental conditions

Down syndrome
- Atrial, ventricular, or atrioventricular septal defects.

Tuberous sclerosis
- Cardiac rhabdomyomas may be the presenting feature of TS, often detected on routine antenatal scan (50% turn out to have TS).
- Rhabdomyomas may cause outflow obstruction, cardiac failure, or arrhythmias in infancy but regress spontaneously by 6 yrs.

Williams syndrome
- Classically, supravalvular aortic stenosis.
- Also pulmonary stenosis, mitral valve regurgitation.
- A more generalized large-vessel arteriopathy (e.g. cranial arteries) and arterial hypertension with risk of stroke is recognized.

Noonan syndrome
- Classically, pulmonary valve stenosis, ± atrial septal defect and peripheral pulmonary artery stenosis.
- Wider arteriopathy includes moya-moya disease with risk of stroke.

Cardiomyopathies
- Barth syndrome (X-linked developmental delay, myopathy, neutropenia, low carnitine, and cardiolipins).
- Danon disease (developmental impairment, myopathy).
- CDG1a.
- Muscular dystrophies.
- Metabolic myopathies e.g. mitochondria, fatty acid oxidation, glycogenoses (Pompe).
- Friedreich ataxia.

Paroxysmal events

Discussed further elsewhere (see Funny turns (paroxysmal episodes) in Chapter 3 ➲ pp. 148-52).

❶Any paroxysmal event characterized by early pallor particularly if brought on by exertion or occurring at rest should be carefully evaluated for a primary cardiac cause.

The heart and epilepsy
- Abnormal cardiac repolarization reported in chronic epilepsy.
- Ictal and peri-ictal tachycardia common in temporal lobe seizures.
- Ictal asystole is rare but described in chronic focal epilepsy in adults, necessitating cardiac pacemaker.

Endocrinology consultations

Addison disease/adrenoleukodystrophy

A proportion of children with Addison's disease will have X-ALD (see Adrenoleukodystrophy in Chapter 4 ➲ p. 478) due to a mutation in the *ABCD1* gene. Screening is by measurement of VLCFAs.

The concern is to identify young people with X-ALD prior to onset of neurological symptoms when a bone marrow transplant (BMT) may be indicated. BMT may still be considered even with MRI changes: the presence of neurological/neuropsychological deficits increases the risk of progression following BMT. Loes' score (quantifying location and extent of CNS disease) is used to grade the condition: a score <10 is required for BMT; see Indications for haemopoetic stem cell transplant in Chapter 4 ➲ p. 483.

Growth failure

- Consider genetic disorders with growth failure including the holoprosencephaly spectrum; signs may be subtle, such as a single central incisor:
  - Correlation between the severity of the MRI, facial, endocrine, and ophthalmological features is poor.
  - MRI may fail to reveal pituitary abnormalities; but full anterior and posterior pituitary function is required as endocrine dysfunction may be life-threatening, and of late onset.
- Septo-optic dysplasia; broad phenotype, some with just isolated optic hypoplasia.
- Mitochondrial disease, e.g. Kearns-Sayre syndrome; see Clinical presentations in Chapter 4 ➲ pp. 405-7.

Hypothalamic hamartoma

- Typically associated with refractory epilepsy, including gelastic seizures, and precocious puberty.
- Cognitive and behavioural effects of poor seizure control tend to be cumulative, and early surgical remediation of epilepsy should be actively considered.
- Options include stereotactic radiosurgery and transcallosal disconnection.
- Both the immediate and late postoperative course can be complicated by anterior and posterior pituitary dysfunction.

Congenital hyperinsulinism (nesidioblastosis)

- May result in acute symptomatic seizures due to hypoglycaemia (both in the neonatal period and later) and later primary epilepsy (mechanism uncertain).
- Progress of the disorder involves pancreatic β-cell destruction by influx of calcium and eventually secondary diabetes mellitus.
- MRI may show features of hypoglycaemic damage with posterior grey and white matter damage.
- Nesidioblastosis should be considered in resistant epilepsy even with EEG features suggestive of idiopathic generalized epilepsy.

Late endocrine consequences of acquired brain injury

See Late neuro-endocrine complications of acquired brain injury in Chapter 4 ➲ p. 222.

Foetal medicine consultations

General principles

Routine screening during pregnancy includes ultrasound (USS) at 20 weeks to seek foetal anomalies. Where neurological anomalies exist on USS, *in utero* magnetic resonance imaging may be requested because it:
- Improves diagnostic accuracy by 23–29%.
- Has better diagnostic accuracy (93% for *in utero* MRI vs. 68% for USS).
- Provides useful additional information in 49% of pregnancies.
- Changes prognosis in 20%.

Paediatric neurologists are increasingly asked to counsel families on the causes and outcomes of foetal neurological anomalies. Families may decide to continue or have a termination of their pregnancy based on this information.

Features of good antenatal counselling include:
- An initial discussion about any identified anomalies and whether further tests are required.
  - Health care professionals should also point out *normal* features in the baby, such as the face, nose, hands, and not focus entirely on the anomalies.
- Rapid access to further investigations and professionals to discuss the implication of identified anomalies.
- Unrushed and uninterrupted discussions with informed professionals in comfortable rooms, with computer access to view scans and webpages of relevant charities.
- Virtual consultations may be helpful in time-sensitive situations.
- A paediatrician who is aware of the relevant history, anomalies, investigation results, and who has discussed the case with the multidisciplinary team prior to seeing the family.
- Discussions should start with asking the family what they already understand about the anomaly and what they would like to discuss.
- Explanations in lay terms.
- Diagrams of the normal anatomy and anomalies.
- An explanation of the best, worst, and most likely case scenarios based on scientific literature or, where lacking, experience.
- When discussing probability, the word 'chance' should be used rather than 'risk', and the baseline rate of developmental problems in the general population should be explained.
- Negative *and positive* framing of chance (e.g. '20 out of 100 will have developmental difficulties, but 80 out of 100 will be normal').
- Discussions on any likely resuscitation or postnatal care.
- Discussions should be neither judgemental nor pressuring and decisions on management of pregnancy respected when within the law.
- Leaflets or summaries of discussions should be provided.
- Availability of opportunities to contact the team if further questions arise.
- Emotional/psychological support should be available.

- Clear documentation of further antenatal or postnatal plans, which should be communicated to referring obstetricians and relevant paediatricians.
- Ready access to other specialities, e.g. genetics teams, when relevant.
- When a child is born and survives, follow-up with the same paediatricians should be available for continuity of care.

Ventriculomegaly

Normal ventricular size is <10 mm throughout all pregnancy. Different classifications for ventriculomegaly exist, including mild (10–12 mm or 10–15 mm); moderate (13–15 mm); severe 15 mm. These terms can be frightening to families.

Causes include:
- Normal variant.
- Cerebral atrophy from degenerative process, e.g. metabolic disease, congenital infection, infarction, genetic disease.
- Obstruction to CSF flow, e.g. aqueduct stenosis.
- Impaired CSF resorption, e.g. previous bleed or infection.
- ↑ CSF production, e.g. choroid plexus papilloma.
- Genetic disease/syndromes.

Outcomes are dependent on: size, cause, results of other investigations, and what happens throughout the rest of pregnancy. Unilateral/asymmetric ventriculomegaly probably has the same risk as bilateral ventriculomegaly.

Ventriculomegaly <15 mm
- Other structural anomalies of brain or body can be seen in 30–50% cases, of which 9% have karyotype anomalies (little data exists on aCGH or WGS).
- Congenital infection in 1.5% cases.
- 14% progress to ≥ 15 mm.
- Outcome depends on the additional anomalies found and the aetiology.

For isolated ventriculomegaly <15 mm:
- Chromosome anomalies are found in 3–5%.
- For those with no genetic anomalies, the risk of abnormal outcome is roughly the same as population rates of 2–3% for developmental impairment and 7% for specific learning issues, ADHD, ASD, attentional/concentration, motor, balance, and coordination problems.

Ventriculomegaly >15 mm
- Around 43% have other structural anomalies to the brain or body. 2% have congenital infection; 3% abnormal chromosomal anomalies.

Outcome depends on the additional anomalies found and the aetiology. For isolated ventriculomegaly >15 mm:
- 2% resolve.
- 15% improve to <15 mm.
- 12% are stillborn.
- Of survivors, 43% have normal early outcome, 18% have 'mild or moderate' developmental problems, 39% have 'severe or profound' developmental difficulties, and the VP shunt rate is 21–30%.

Agenesis of the corpus callosum (ACC)

50% are associated with other brain, body or genetic anomalies, 50% are isolated. The risk of adverse outcome in those with other anomalies depends on what they are.

Isolated ACC

Counselling of isolated ACC is very difficult because the spectrum is wide, ranging from normal outcome to early death from refractory seizures and apnoea in conditions like non-ketotic hyperglycinaemia. Often there are no clues as to where a baby's outcome will lie on the spectrum. A clear discussion of probability should be held with the family and documented in the notes.

- Anomalies on aCGH in ~10%.
- Normal outcome in 76%, but in adolescence problems with social communication, balance, and coordination, attention and concentration, and specific learning disabilities may be seen.
- 8% have severe problems (learning disabilities, motor impairment, feeding difficulties, epilepsy). Some, but not all, may die at a young age.
- Outcomes of partial and complete ACC are similar.
- Where eye anomalies are present in ♀ foetus, Aicardi syndrome should be considered.

Microcephaly

- Diagnostic definitions differ: thresholds of either 2 or 3 standard deviations (SD) below the mean.
- Obstetric reports often just report the head size as <3rd centile, so the paediatrician will need to compare to charts for gestational age and to obtain standard deviation score.
- Needs to be distinguished from abnormal head shape, such as in craniosynostosis.
- The rate of head growth and comparison to the rest of the body are important: a head size growing along the centiles and comparable to the body size is more reassuring than a head whose growth is falling off centiles.
- In the absence of other structural, genetic, or infective anomalies, a head circumference of 2–3 SD below is usually associated with good outcome, but the risk of developmental difficulties <3 SDs is likely to be high.

Macrocephaly

- Definitions include >95th centile or >2SDs above the mean in the absence of hydrocephalus.
- Familial causes should be sought by measuring the parental head size.
- Outcome data is limited to isolated cases: most are normal.
- Where other anomalies exist, genetic and metabolic causes should be considered, including Sotos syndrome, *NFIX* mutations, Neurofibromatosis, Klippel-Trenaunay syndrome, glutaric aciduria type 1, Cowden syndrome, tumours, expanding intracranial cysts, etc.

Holoprosencephaly

- A failure of the forebrain to divide into two hemispheres.
- May involve deep grey matter, olfactory bulbs, and/or optic bulbs.
- Can be divided into alobar, semi-lobar, lobar, or interhemispheric (syntelencephaly).
- The more severe the brain anomaly, the more likely to have facial anomalies like cyclopia and cleft lip and palate.
- Chromosomal anomalies are common (24–54%), especially Trisomy 13.
  - >10% have microduplications or microdeletions on aCGH.
  - 19–25% have single gene mutations.
- 20–30% live to reach 1 yr of age and survival to 11 yrs is reported, usually with relatively typical face.
  - Alobar forms usually are stillborn or die after birth and palliation planning is important for those that continue pregnancy.
- Developmental difficulties are likely, with their severity correlating to the degree of brain anomaly:
  - *alobar*: typically make little development;
  - *semi-lobar*: may take a few steps and have isolated words;
  - *lobar*: 50% walk a few steps, have mildly impaired hand function, and may speak in short phrases.
- Postnatally, diabetes insipidus and other endocrinopathies, as well as hydrocephalus, should be sought and treated.

Malformations of cortical development

The foetal brain is relatively smooth at 20 weeks and develops sulcal and gyral patterns gradually towards term. Cortical malformations may be missed on early *in utero* MRI and repeated imaging may be required where concerns exist.

- *Hemimegalencephaly*: may be associated with brainstem and cerebellar anomalies. Multiple genes are implicated, as well as tuberous sclerosis, NF1, Sturge Weber, and Klippel–Trenaunay syndromes. Developmental difficulties and epilepsy are typical.
- *Lissencephaly*: isolated or associated with other anomalies. Multiple implicated genes e.g. *DCX*, *PAFAH1B1*, *ARX*, and tubulin genes.
  - Facial anomalies, renal, cardiac anomalies, and omphalocele, consider Miller Dieker syndrome.
  - Cerebellar, basal ganglia, and brainstem involvement suggests tubulinopathies.
  - Cerebellar hypoplasia associated with *CDKL5* and *RELN* mutations.
  - CMV should be sought.
  - Developmental difficulties are likely.
- *Cobblestone malformations*: may be a sign of congenital muscular dystrophies, including dystroglycanopathies. Eye anomalies, contractures, ventriculomegaly, and kinked brainstem/bifid pons are clues. Developmental difficulties and movement problems are likely and some die before a year.
- *Polymicrogyria*: hard to diagnose antenatally. Associated with congenital infection, metabolic disease, and gene disorders. Outcome depends on site and extent of the anomaly.

- *Heterotopia*: may be band (worse outcome) or isolated nodular (better outcome). Greater degree and extent of heterotopia is associated with poorer developmental outcome and epilepsy.

Posterior fossa

Cerebellar hypoplasia

- A small cerebellum may show catch-up growth by 30–32 weeks so caution should be exercised in isolated cases.
- It can be hard to differential atrophy from hypoplasia.
- Genetic causes predominate, along with PHACES (see Posterior fossa malformations, haemangiomas, arterial anomalies, cardiac defects, eye abnormalities, sternal cleft and supraumbilical raphe (PHACES) syndrome in Chapter 4 ➲ p. 471), congenital disorders of glycosylation, CMV, foetal alcohol syndrome, and haemorrhage.
- No high-quality studies of outcome. Cognitive, motor, language, and behavioural difficulties problems are likely in bilateral cases and are also reported in unilateral cases, but rarely severe/profound.
- Unilateral cases are thought to be secondary to haemorrhage.

Dandy-Walker malformation

- Combination of cystic dilatation of fourth ventricle, hypoplastic cerebellar vermis, and elevation of tentorium.
- May be isolated or associated with other nervous system anomalies in 13–67%, and body anomalies in 9–44%.
- Developmental difficulties seen in over 63%.
- Hydrocephalus may result requiring VP shunt insertion.

Mega cisterna magna and Blakes' pouch cyst

- Enlarged cisterna magna with typical fourth ventricle, cerebellar hemispheres, and vermis.
- Risk of adverse outcome is 8–14% in small studies.
- Blake's pouch cyst represents delayed closure of the vermis and is associated with the same risk of adverse developmental outcome as the general population when isolated.

Rhombencephalosynapsis

- Abnormal fusion of the cerebellar hemispheres with degrees of vermian hypoplasia/agenesis.
- Typically genetic in origin. Outcome data is limited, but some learning, motor, and behavioural disabilities are likely.

Spina bifida and myelomeningocele

Unlike other foetal neurological conditions where the outcome is unclear, a more accurate prediction of a child's disabilities can be given for spinal lesions. For further information see Spina bifida and related disorders in Chapter 4 ➲ pp. 355-8.

Counselling is best performed by a team, including paediatric neurosurgery, paediatric neurology, neonatology, and urology.

Motor outcomes

Predicted by the anatomical level of the lesion. This can be estimated from *in utero* MRI, but clinical examination after birth may lead to revision of the functional level higher or lower (See Table 5.1).

- Walking may not be normal and can be slow, prone to trips and falls, requiring stick or frame and splints. Individuals may resort increasingly to partial or total wheelchair use in later life because of weakness, spasticity, neuropathic joints, obesity, scoliosis, or because it is faster and promotes independence.
- Upper limbs may also have reduced dexterity and coordination.

Chiari type 2 malformation

See also Chiari malformations in Chapter 4 → pp. 359-60.

- Beaked, downward displacement of the cerebellar tonsils and cerebellar vermis and fourth ventricle through the foramen magnum.
- Nearly all are associated with open myelomeningocele.
- Obstruction to CSF exit from the fourth ventricle leads to hydrocephalus.
- Rates of VP shunt insertion range 50–70%.
- Hydrocephalus and/or direct compression of the brainstem leads to swallowing/feeding difficulties, stridor, centrally mediated apnoea, and motor signs.
- 5–10% require surgical decompression.
- 1% may need tracheostomy.
- Abnormal brainstem function can be seen in absence of a Chiari 2 malformation or hydrocephalus and may be life-threatening.

Cognition

- Many families are wrongly told their child will have severe/profound learning difficulties, often with pejorative terms.
- IQ scores are in the normal/borderline range: mean IQ without hydrocephalus is ~100, with is ~80.
- 80% attend mainstream school.

Table 5.1 Rates of walking according to level of lesion

Level	% never walk	Average age of attainment in those who do walk (yr, mo)	% of those attaining walking who subsequently stop, and age (yr, mo)
Thoracic	80%	4, 6	40% (6, 9)
High lumbar	50%	5, 2	60% (6, 11)
Mid lumbar	40%	5, 0	30% (7, 0)
Low lumbar	16%	3, 10	10% (9, 1)
Sacral	0%	2, 2	N/A

Adapted from Williams EN, Broughton NS, Menelaus MB. Age-related walking in children with spina bifida. Dev Med Child Neurol 1999; 41: 446–9.

- Even with normal IQ, specific learning difficulties and attentional/concentration, memory, visuo-spatial, and executive functioning problems may exist (see Cognitive disability [in Hydrocephalus section] in Chapter 4 ➥ p. 354).
- 94% achieve high school qualification and 8–56% go on to higher education.

Bowel, bladder, and sexual function
- Most children will have bowel and bladder problems, which has a large influence on quality of life when older.
- ~75% adults use intermittent catheterization, 45% develop some continence with or without catheters.
- Intermittent catheterization will be important during early life with antibiotics and bladder relaxants until a better idea of bladder function is gained with age.
- ~50% develop bowel continence: laxatives, suppositories, digital extraction; stoma placement to permit antegrade continence enemas may be required.
- Erectile dysfunction is seen in 12–75% of men, more common with lesions around T10 and above, but responds to sildenafil or similar preparations. 55% women report dissatisfaction with sex.
- Fertility is reduced, especially in those with hydrocephalus.

Adulthood
- 23–28% marry; 52% do not form a long-term relationship.
- 24–51% have sex regularly.
- Unemployment in 44–85%, with a preponderance for part time work with reduced salary in those who are employed.
- 21–51% live independently but may need some assistance, with hydrocephalus being a risk factor.
- 85% dress themselves, 65% shop for themselves, 54% drive.
- Life satisfaction is good but reduced for: employment, friendships, self-care, relationships, physical, and mental health.

Foetal surgery
- Can be performed open or via fetoscope.
- Reduces the risk of VP shunt insertion at 12m (40% vs. 82%) and 5–10 yrs (49% vs. 85%); and rates of hindbrain herniation (64% vs. 96%) and brain stem kinking (20% vs. 48%) at 12m.
- At 5–10 yrs, prenatal surgery is associated with greater chance of independent walking, better gait, motor skills, and self-care skills. No association with improved cognition has been found.
- There is a risk of pre-term birth and maternal morbidity and mortality with surgery. Careful multidisciplinary counselling is important.

Gastroenterology consultations

Feeding difficulties in infancy

Also see Feeding in Chapter 4 ➔ p. 253.

Achieving a coordinated suck and swallow is the most demanding and complex motor task infants have to achieve and poor feeding can be the presenting feature of just about any neurological disorder in infancy. Conversely, since suck and swallow are essentially coordinated in the brainstem, even devastating supratentorial injury such as anencephaly may be surprisingly asymptomatic in the early weeks of life.

Children may be referred urgently following unexpected severity of videofluoroscopy findings, e.g. silent aspiration of thickened fluids and purees.

- Identify if oropharyngeal motor problems present, e.g. evolving cerebral palsy.
  - Drooling, history of early respiratory problems may be suggestive.
  - Worster-Drought/ congenital perisylvian syndrome (see Classic descriptions of the cerebral palsies in Chapter 4 ➔ p. 227) may show minimal generalized motor signs.
  - Children with bulbar or pseudobulbar palsy may also have gastro-oesophageal reflux disease (GORD): see Gastro-oesophageal reflux disease (GORD) and vomiting in this chapter ➔ p. 546.
- Check oropharyngeal and oesophageal structural/anatomical problems have been excluded, e.g. submucous cleft palate.
- Conditioned feeding/oral-sensory aversion with minimal motor signs is a feature of numerous neurodevelopmental disorders, e.g. extreme premature born infant, Russell–Silver, Noonan. GORD is often present.
- Profound hypotonia and marked feeding problems are characteristic of the early phase of Prader–Willi syndrome. Also consider peroxisomal disorders and congenital muscular dystrophies.
- Tongue fasciculation may suggest SMA type 1 or congenital neuropathies (early cerebral palsy typically shows milder hypotonia and better antigravity muscle strength).
- Congenital myasthenic syndromes can present with episodic dysphagia with minimal signs (ptosis, limb weakness) between episodes; see Myasthenic syndromes in Chapter 4 ➔ pp. 454-8.
- Assisted feeding via an NGT or gastrostomy tube can be necessary.

Irritability interfering with feeds can have a primary, neurological cause including:
- Krabbe disease.
- GM1 gangliosidosis.
- Leigh disease.
- NAI, cerebral injury, e.g. meningoencephalitis.

Irritability can also be secondary to malnutrition (in which case it will be eased by supplemental nasogastric feeding) due to dysphagia, which in turn may have a primary neurological basis due to an evolving motor disorder, such as dyskinetic cerebral palsy.

Other potential causes of feeding and swallowing difficulties:
- Any tone-reducing medications (e.g. benzodiazepines).

- Chiari malformation causing bulbar weakness (note CT will miss this).
- Infantile botulism. Bulbar, head and neck involvement are early with *descending* weakness (c.f. ascending in Guillain–Barré). *Absolute constipation* is a prominent feature.
- Neonatal acquired myasthenia.
- Infantile GBS (particularly pharyngeal variant).

Investigations to consider:
- MRI brain.
- aCGH and other genetic tests as indicated (e.g. 22q11 deletion, congenital myasthenia gene panel).
- LP (e.g. ↑ CSF protein in inflammatory disorders).
- EMG/NCV and specialized studies (e.g. stimulated single-fibre EMG).
- Acetylcholine receptor antibodies (MuSK antibodies typically in older children).
- Trial of pyridostigmine (may not improve and indeed may worsen some congenital myasthenia subtypes; see Congenital myasthenic syndromes in Chapter 4 ⊃ pp. 455-6).

Gastro-oesophageal reflux disease and vomiting

Acute episodes are managed symptomatically with fluid and electrolyte correction and antiemetics (lorazepam, ondansetron). There is some evidence for benefit from migraine prophylactic agents (propranolol, pizotifen).
- For management of chronic GORD in children with neurodisability; see Management [in Feeding section] in Chapter 4 ⊃ pp. 254-6.

In initial presentations or where diagnosis uncertain consider:
- Posterior fossa imaging to exclude space-occupying lesion.
- Abdominal imaging (to exclude volvulus and other causes intestinal obstruction).
- Amylase.
- Renal function.
- Ammonia (late presenting urea cycle disorders; see Late-presentation metabolic disease in Chapter 4 ⊃ pp. 484-7).
- Acid-base status.
- Plasma amino acids.
- Urine organic acids.
- Acyl carnitine profile (fatty acid oxidation disorders).
- Liver function tests.
- Urine toxicology (particularly cannabis exposure).

Sandifer syndrome

- Dyskinetic movement disorder related to severe GORD more common in children with severe neurodisability (see Management [in Feeding section] in Chapter 4 ⊃ pp. 254-5) but can also occur in neurologically intact children.
- Responds to treatment of GORD.

GI Dystonia (Feeding dystonia)

Increasingly recognized and researched late complication of severe neurodisability.

- Typically occurs in adolescents with severe CP (GMFCS IV or V, see ➔ Gross motor function in Chapter 4 pp. 245-7) who needed PEG/ fundoscopy and/or introduction of jejunal feeds in early years.
  - Constipation prominent.
- Pain behaviour, retching, vagal activation, abdominal distension and hypertonicity with temporal relationship to feeds (relationship becomes less obvious with time with more continuous symptoms).
- Diagnosis of exclusion once other causes of distress have been addressed or excluded.
  - Be wary of making diagnosis in very young child: consider metabolic disease, 'cerebral irritability', status dystonicus, complications of jejunal feeding.
- May be helped by cyproheptadine, levomepromazine, aprepitant, intrathecal baclofen, gabapentin, nabilone (off-licence).
- Typically *worsened* by anticholinergics (such as trihexyphenidyl) given in erroneous belief that the dystonia is primary.

Late intestinal failure in severe neurodisability

Increasingly recognized late complication of severe neurodisability that often follows on from GI Dystonia picture.

- Same clinical population of GMFCS V CP: often ex-premature with history of necrotizing enterocolitis (NEC).
- Picture of severe, often painful ileus associated with absolute constipation, pain behaviour, retching, abdominal distension.
- Again, worsened by anticholinergic use.
- May develop pneumatosis coli requiring colectomy or defunctioning ileostomy.
- May become total parenteral nutrition (TPN) dependent.

Cyclical vomiting ('abdominal migraine')

- Repeated bouts of vomiting lasting hours to days usually occurring at a characteristic time of day: can result in severe electrolyte imbalance. Often a family history of migraine (see Episodic Disorders that may be associated with migraine in Chapter 4 ➔ p. 343).
- Benign paroxysmal torticollis of infancy (see Episodic Disorders that may be associated with migraine in Chapter 4 ➔ p. 343) is similar with earlier onset plus torticollis and eye deviation. Both are diagnoses of exclusion (easier to be confident of diagnosis after several episodes).

Diencephalic syndrome

A child <3 yrs of age with hyperkinesis and euphoria, and striking emaciation without early gastrointestinal symptoms. Typically caused by gliomas of the 3rd ventricle.

Neurological associations of hepatocellular failure

Commonly seen following an episode of status epilepticus. Causes include:
- Hypoxic hepatic injury (commonest, with good prognosis).
- Idiopathic drug response: particularly valproate toxicity. Consider changing the ASM regime.
- Alpers disease (see Progressive neuronal degeneration of childhood (PNDC) in Chapter 4 ➲ p. 409), but probably responsible for many cases of apparent valproate-induced liver disease.

❶ Disturbed liver function is an important early presentation of Wilson disease; see Wilson disease (hepatolenticular degeneration) in Chapter 4 ➲ pp. 480-1. Hepatocellular dysfunction (typically late in the first decade of life) may pre-date development of neurological symptoms, and early chelation therapy may prevent neurological morbidity.
▶ Perform copper studies in all unexplained hepatocellular failure.

Neurological complications of prolonged TPN

- Prolonged TPN may result in trace metal deficiencies that can have neurological manifestations including myelopathy due to copper deficiency and an extrapyramidal movement disorder (with basal ganglia changes on MRI) due to excess manganese.
- Important to also consider thiamine deficiency (see Vitamin B1 (thiamine) in Chapter 4 ➲ pp. 522-3).

Neurological associations of coeliac disease, malabsorption, and inflammatory bowel disease (IBD)

- Can be associated with movement disorder thought to be caused, at least in part, by vitamin E malabsorption (also seen in other malabsorption states such as Crohn's disease).
- Antigliadin antibodies have been demonstrated in the CSF of some adults with ataxias and myoclonus ('gluten ataxia'): their coeliac disease may be subclinical.
- Neuropathy associated with coeliac disease (no single mechanism).
- IBD-associated neuropathy often subclinical, sensory.
  - Acute presentation: unilateral foot drop due to sacral nerve compression during colonoscopy.
- TNF-α antagonists may induce a chronic demyelinating neuropathy.
- Sulphasalazine-induced neuropathy.
- IBD can be a presenting feature of Niemann-Pick Type C.

Encephalopathy in gastrointestinal/liver conditions:

- Encephalopathy and seizures are common after liver transplantation, e.g. posterior reversible encephalopathy due to ciclosporin; see Posterior reversible encephalopathy syndrome in this chapter ➲ p. 598.
- Consider opportunistic infections in children on immunomodulatory treatments for IBD (e.g. natalizumab-related PML; infliximab-related

TB. See CNS infection of the immunocompromised host in
Chapter 4 ➡ pp. 377-81).
- Cerebral venous sinus thrombosis in acute IBD due to prothrombotic
state—may present without focal neurological signs.
- IBD is a recognized, and occasionally presenting, feature of Niemann-
Pick Type C.
- Sulphasalazine-related encephalopathy.
- Familial Mediterranean fever may be associated with encephalopathy,
demyelination, and seizures.

D-lactate encephalopathy

- Rare syndrome of *recurrent encephalopathy* with reduced consciousness
± ataxia (typically for hours to days) in context of *short bowel syndrome*
(e.g. ex-premature infant who required extensive intestinal resection
for NEC).
- Hallmark is biochemical evidence of:
  - metabolic acidosis with low bicarbonate.
  - high anion gap (i.e. $[Na^+] + [K^+] - [Cl^-] - [HCO_3^-] > 15$ mM).
  - but lab-reported lactate level normal or low (i.e. it appears not to be
  the missing anion).
- Solution to this paradox is that condition is caused by high levels of the
dextro enantiomer of lactate.
  - Standard lab 'lactate' assays are enzyme-based and specific for the
  'normal' L-lactate.
  - D-lactate can be assayed using D-specific enzyme, or by tandem gas
  mass spectrometry.
- D-lactate thought to be a product of gut microbiome metabolism:
  - Short ileum results in delivery of unabsorbed carbohydrate to colon
  where it is metabolized by gut flora.
- Although D-lactataemia is a reliable biomarker it is not clear that
D-lactate is responsible for the encephalopathy (infusion in healthy
volunteers doesn't reliably reproduce symptoms).
- Treatment is via dietary carbohydrate restriction; and use of non-
absorbable antibiotics and/or probiotics to alter gut flora.

Refeeding syndrome

- For neurological complications of refeeding syndrome see Central
pontine myelinolysis in this chapter ➡ p. 599.

Parenteral maintenance of antiseizure medications

A common request for advice, e.g. in the context of abdominal surgery, or
intestinal malabsorption syndromes, is for alternative maintenance regimes
for children with epilepsy taking regular ASMs.
- For routine operations (where a nil-by-mouth period is unlikely to
exceed a few hours) the risks of a single delayed dose are small, and no
special precautions are required.
- For periods of 24–48 h consider a single loading dose of IV
levetiracetam or phenytoin (particularly for children with epilepsy due
to known structural brain abnormalities) or lorazepam.

For longer periods of interruption to enteral feeding:
• Consider conversion of the existing ASM regime to the parenteral route.
• Valproate, levetiracetam, phenytoin, and phenobarbital can be given parenterally. Doses are generally unchanged although phenytoin levels should be monitored because iv administration may result in greater bioavailability; see Phenytoin in Chapter 7 ⟳ pp. 691-3.
• Carbamazepine and topiramate can be given rectally with dose adjustment: see Carbamazepine and Topiramate in Chapter 7 ⟳ pp. 659-60, pp. 704-5.
• If the existing regime is not readily adapted, consider temporary supplemental cover with IV levetiracetam or phenytoin.

Neonatal neurology

Neonatal seizures

The commonest and most specific evidence of neurological dysfunction in the newborn. Incidence is 1–5/1000 live births rising to 20–60/1000 in the very low birth weight (VLBW).

▶▶ Neonatal seizures are usually symptomatic.

Causes (in order of importance):
- Hypoxic–ischaemic encephalopathy (HIE) and stroke very much commoner than (in decreasing order):
  - intracranial haemorrhage;
  - CNS infection;
  - metabolic abnormalities;
  - malformations of cortical development;
  - inborn errors of metabolism;
  - genetic neonatal epilepsies.

Cause remains unidentified in approximately 10% (see Table 5.2 for neonatal seizure types).
- Most neonatal seizures have no clinical features to see, i.e. they are purely electrographic, and around ¾ of abnormal movements suspected to be seizures have no EEG evidence of epileptic seizures. Therefore, EEG confirmation of suspected neonatal seizures is important.
- The seizures are almost certainly *not* 'generalized tonic-clonic seizures' which are virtually unknown in the neonatal period. Look carefully at the semiology (Table 5.2).
- There is a tendency for focal *clonic* seizures to be due to acute pathology (infection, stroke) and focal *tonic* seizures to be due to 'constitutional' factors such as genetic or structural causes. Tonic seizures with apnoea is a particular feature of *KCNQ2*-developmental and epileptic encephalopathy see *KCNQ2*-DEE in Chapter 4 ➡ p. 281.

Table 5.2 Neonatal seizure types

Clonic	Focal, multifocal, bilateral asymmetric, bilateral symmetric
Tonic	Focal, bilateral asymmetric. May have eye deviation (beware generalized tonic stiffening)
Apnoea	Associated with EEG or other suspicious features
Myoclonic	Focal, multifocal, bilateral asymmetric or symmetric hiccups
Spasms	Unilateral, bilateral symmetric or asymmetric
Sequential	Variable
Automatism	Predominantly oral, may be associated with other features
Behavioural arrest	Cessation of movement and activity, often seen with other features

- Differential diagnosis includes jittering, tremor, dyskinesias, dystonia, startle responses (e.g. hyperekplexia), and sleep myoclonus: see Episodes without prominent alteration of awareness in Chapter 4 ➲ pp. 324-7.

History
- Family history (consanguinity, dominant conditions such as self-limited familial neonatal epilepsy, repeat miscarriages or infant death suggestive of metabolic conditions).
- Pregnancy (infections, drugs) including quality of foetal movements, e.g. rhythmic kicking or hiccoughing suggesting *in utero* seizures.
- Peripartum events (presentation, duration of labour, fever, or other signs of infection, mode of delivery, meconium staining of the liquor, cord pH, Apgar scores, resuscitation).
- Timing of onset of seizures.
- Description of seizure.

Examination
- Head size. Fontanelle size and shape (peroxisomal disorders).
- Dysmorphic features, rashes, neurocutaneous findings.
- Signs of metabolic abnormalities, including odour, jaundice, failure to thrive, visceral organomegaly, diarrhoea, vomiting, cataracts.
- Other signs of neurological dysfunction (including abnormalities and/or asymmetries of state, awareness, sucking and feeding, tone, eye movements, facial symmetry, movement including extraneous movements).
- Try to suppress any rhythmic movements with gentle restraint (will not be able to suppress epileptic events or benign neonatal sleep myoclonus) and attempt to stimulate/wake the baby (will terminate benign neonatal sleep myoclonus).

Investigations
Imaging
- Primary malformations of cortical development.
- Neonatal stroke.

▶ Note that some inborn errors of metabolism (e.g. non-ketotic hyperglycinaemia) are associated with structural brain abnormality (typically symmetric absence or hypoplasia of brain structures): demonstration of a structural abnormality may not be a complete explanation for the occurrence of seizures.

Neurophysiology
The gold standard for diagnosis is ictal EEG with video demonstrating electrographic seizures with a clinical correlate, however:
- The normal term and pre-term newborn EEG can have findings that are normal for maturity and are *not* indicative of an active seizure disorder. These include sharp waves, occasional spikes, slowing, δ brushes, α

bursts, and tracé discontinuó and tracé alternant patterns. Ensure your neurophysiologist is familiar with normal variants in neonatal EEG!

• Some newborn seizures may not have an EEG signature because the seizure focus is too deep to be captured by scalp electrodes.

Inter-ictal EEG may be helpful in diagnosis when it shows electrographic seizures, epileptiform features, or abnormalities of background such as low-amplitude or burst-suppression patterns.

Other investigations

Initially these should address correctable metabolic conditions and include glucose, electrolytes, Ca^{2+}, Mg^{2+}, K^+, Na^+, $HCO_3{}^-$, and NH_3.

Further investigations should be guided by the history and examination.

• Sepsis work-up including LP is usually necessary. Start broad antibiotic coverage and aciclovir until CSF cultures and HSV PCR studies are –ve.

• HIE causing significant cerebral oedema, intracranial haemorrhage, and structural anomalies can be seen on cranial ultrasound, CT, however MRI is the investigation of choice.

• In case of neonatal abstinence/withdrawal, urine toxicology is helpful.

• If an inborn error of metabolism (IEM) is suspected, initial investigations should include glucose, pH, lactate, and NH_3, and then be directed by the examination and EEG (Boxes 5.1 and 5.2).

Box 5.1 IEMs causing neonatal seizures

• Congenital hyperinsulinism (various causes)
• **Urea cycle disorders**
• Non-ketotic hyperglycinaemia
• **Pyridoxine/pyridoxal-dependent epilepsy**
• **Folinic acid-responsive seizures**
• **Biotinidase deficiency**
• Perinatal hypophosphatasia
• Adenylsuccinate lyase deficiency
• MTHFR deficiency
• D-2-Hydroxyglutaric aciduria
• Congenital disorders of glycosylation
• 3-Phosphoglycerate dehydrogenase deficiency
• GABA transaminase deficiency
• Congenital glutamine deficiency
• Glutamate transporter deficiency
• Neonatal ceroid lipofuscinosis with cathepsin deficiency
• Smith–Lemli–Opitz syndrome
• **Creatine deficiency disorders**

Conditions are ranked by (very approximate) prevalence. Conditions whose potential treatability makes them particularly important to rule out are identified in **bold**

Box 5.2 Available investigations for IEMs causing neonatal seizures

Serum
- Urgent WES/WGS
- Creatine kinase
- Lactate and pyruvate
- Ammonia
- Biotinidase
- Amino acids
- Carnitine, acylcarnitines
- Transferrin isoelectric focusing
- Copper and caeruloplasmin
- Cholesterol
- Fatty acids
- Pipecolic and phytanic acid
- Uric acid

Urine
- Alpha amino adipic semialdehyde (AASA)
- Organic acids
- Amino acids
- Acylglycines
- Sulphocysteine
- Purine and Pyrimidines
- Pipecolic acid
- Guanidinoacetate

CSF
- Glucose with paired blood glucose
- Cell count
- Lactate
- Amino acids (paired with blood for CSF: plasma glycine ratio)
- Neurotransmitters and folate metabolites

Others
- MRI and MRS (look for lactate peak, absence of creatine)
- Skin biopsy for inclusions
- Fibroblast culture
- Muscle biopsy for light and electron microscopy, electron transport chain studies

Treatment
- Correct metabolic abnormalities (glucose, calcium, sodium). Give antibiotic and antiviral treatment if sepsis is suspected.
- IV phenobarbital 20 mg/kg loading dose (may also be given orally). If no response, a further 20 mg/kg may be given in 10 mg/kg increments. There is little benefit from further dose increases once trough blood

levels of 40–60 microgms/mL have been achieved. The half-life varies from 100 to 300h in the newborn (400h in the pre-term) falling to 60h after 4 weeks. Maintenance dosing usually starts at 3–4 mg/kg/day as a daily dose.

- If no response, give phenytoin (PHT) 18 mg/kg loading dose if safe from a cardiovascular perspective. Achieving adequate plasma levels with oral PHT may be very difficult in the newborn: maintenance doses may be as high as 10 mg/kg/day.
- Levetiracetam 40 mg/kg loading dose with a further 20 mg/kg half loading dose if no response.
- Lorazepam, clonazepam, or midazolam as fourth line options until seizures are controlled. Adverse events include sedation, hypotension, and respiratory depression.

Further management

If seizures continue despite adequate therapy consider in particular:

Non-ketotic hyperglycinaemia

An autosomal recessive condition caused by deficiency in the glycine cleavage system leading to high levels of glycine in the brain and CSF with cerebral excitation but brainstem and spinal cord inhibition.

- Causes stupor, respiratory abnormalities, and hypotonia, absent sucking, characteristic hiccoughs, and refractory myoclonic seizures.
- May be mistaken for HIE but the child does not improve and there is no clear evidence of perinatal asphyxial insult.
- Diagnosis is by demonstration elevated CSF glycine and a CSF: plasma glycine ratio over 8% (normal ratio <4%).
- CSF proline < 5 microM (reported as part of same CSF amino acid profile) confirms the CSF sample is free of blood contamination and that the plasma: CSF glycine ratio is thus reliable.
- EEG usually shows a burst-suppression pattern.
- May be associated with structural brain abnormalities (e.g. agenesis of the corpus callosum) on MRI.
- Supplementation with benzoate and dextromethorphan is controversial:
  - Respiratory difficulties and early apnoeas tend to settle and child becomes extubatable, however realistic best outcome is survival into early adolescence with profound disability and little to no developmental progress.
  - Many families will opt for palliative care in the neonatal period.

Protocol for further investigation of refractory neonatal seizures of unknown cause

The importance of the individually very rare but collectively significant metabolic diseases that can present with refractory neonatal seizures lies in the ready treatability of some, and the neurodevelopmental consequences of delayed treatment. Their reliable identification requires a thorough approach, systematically applied.

Day 1
If not already performed, perform a 'metabolic' lumbar puncture to collect the following:
- Paired blood and CSF glucose.
- Paired blood and CSF amino acids.
- CSF neurotransmitters including HVA, 5-HIAA, MTHF.
- Blood homocysteine.
- Urine purine and pyrimidines.
- Urine alpha amino adipic semialdehyde (AASA).
- Transferrin isoelectric focusing.

The first priority is to exclude:

Glucose transporter-1 deficiency syndrome (GLUT1DS)
- Diagnosed by demonstration of CSF:plasma glucose ratio <40% in the absence of other causes of hypoglycorrhachia (such as systemic hypoglycaemia, meningitis).
- Confirmed by gene panel testing (*SLC2A1* mutations).
- For further details see Glucose transporter-1 deficiency (GLUT1DS) in Chapter 4 ⮞ pp. 301-2.

The second priority is to exclude:

Pyridoxine-dependent seizures
- Very rare but should be considered in all refractory neonatal seizures. Diagnose and treat by administering 100 mg B6 IV every 10 min for 200–500 mg total dose.
- Continuous EEG monitoring is desirable but not essential.
- There is a risk of apnoea during administration. EEG should normalize within 6–8h of administration if pyridoxine *dependent*.
- Urine alpha amino adipic semialdehyde (AASA) levels are diagnostic of pyridoxine- (and the closely related pyridoxal-) dependent epilepsies although results generally take several weeks to return.

For further details see Vitamin B6 in Chapter 4 ⮞ pp. 524-5.

Days 2–7
Children who are pyridoxine-*responsive* (rather than dependent) may show a delayed response, and some conditions respond to *pyridoxal phosphate* but not pyridoxine: see Vitamin B6 in Chapter 4 ⮞ pp. 524-5. Therefore it is more efficient to treat with pyridoxal phosphate if available and define the biochemical defect subsequently in more detail if a response is seen.
- Pyridoxal phosphate should be given at 10 mg/kg/day (or if not available pyridoxine is continued 100 mg per day) until urine AASA levels available.

Having obtained remaining specimens (see Box 5.2) treat with a cocktail of creatine (300 mg/kg/day), folinic acid (2.5 mg twice a day), and biotin (10 mg/day) pending remaining results.
- Biotinidase deficiency. Assay biotinidase activity in blood (associated with metabolic acidosis, skin and hair abnormalities).

- Folinic acid-responsive seizures. Diagnosed by clinical response to folinic acid: now thought to be allelic to pyridoxine-dependent epilepsy; see Vitamin B$_6$ in Chapter 4 ➲ pp. 524-5.
- Consider sending early developmental epileptic encephalopathy gene panel if an aetiology has not been identified.

Week 2

If seizures are refractory, the decision about more intensive therapy is dependent on the individual child. The options are of intravenous high-dose suppressive therapy, usually requiring continuous cardiorespiratory support and EEG monitoring; or oral ASMs (Table 5.3).

Table 5.3 ASMs in refractory neonatal seizures

High-dose suppressive IV therapy	
Phenobarbital	>30 mg/kg
Levetiracetam	40–60 mg/kg/day in 2 doses
Thiopental	10 mg/kg then 2–5 mg/kg/h
Pentobarbital	10 mg/kg then 0.5–1 mg/kg/h
Midazolam	0.2 mg/kg then 0.1–0.4 mg/kg/h
Lidocaine	2 mg/kg then 6 mg/kg/h
Valproate	20 mg/kg then 20 mg/kg/day in 2–3 doses
Oral ASMs	
Carbamazepine	15–20 mg/kg/day in 2–3 doses
Clonazepam	0.1 mg/kg/day in 2–3 doses
Levetiracetam	40–60 mg/kg/day in 2 doses
Topiramate	3–15 mg/kg/day in 2 doses
Valproate	20 mg/kg/day in 2–3 doses
Vigabatrin	50 mg/kg/day increasing to 200 mg/kg/day
Zonisamide	2.5 mg/kg/day

Discontinuation of therapy

Neonatal seizures are usually symptomatic and do not necessarily persist after an acute insult. If seizures are easy to control, the underlying aetiology resolves and the neurological examination normalizes, it is reasonable to stop ASMs early, preferably before discharge. Seizures due to cortical malformations or malignant early epilepsy syndromes will require long-term treatment (see Developmental and epileptic encephalopathies in Chapter 4 ➲ p. 277).

Outcome

This is strongly determined by aetiology. Overall 10–30% develop subsequent epilepsy but the rate is as high as 80% for malformations of cortical development and 30% for severe HIE or meningitis.

Neonatal encephalopathy

- Incidence 6 per 1000 live births.
- Associated with significant mortality (15–20%) and permanent disability (25%).
- Many causes including hypoxic–ischaemic encephalopathy (HIE), stroke, trauma, hypoglycaemia, maternal medications, and IEMs.

Hypoxic–ischaemic encephalopathy

- Incidence is 1–1.5% of live births.
- Risk factors:
  - Prematurity, IUGR/VLBW;
  - Post-maturity;
  - Abruption, cord prolapse, shoulder dystocia, breech presentation;
  - Maternal diabetes and hypertension/toxaemia in term infants.

The terms HIE and birth asphyxia should be reserved for circumstances where there is sufficient perinatal data to support the diagnosis. The term 'neonatal encephalopathy' is preferred to describe the baby who emerges with altered/reduced conscious level, limp, cyanosed, with poor heart rate or respiratory effort where *aetiology is uncertain*.

- Factors suggesting HIE include late deterioration of foetal cardiotocogram, metabolic acidosis at delivery (pH ≤7; base deficit ≥12 mM/L), Apgar score 0–6 for ≥5 min, meconium staining of liquor, and multiple organ dysfunction (renal, cardiac, hepatic, haematological, persistent pulmonary hypertension of the newborn).

Differential diagnosis
- Acute blood loss e.g. antepartum, foeto-maternal or intracranial/ abdominal haemorrhages.
- Infection.
- Inborn errors of metabolism (especially non-ketotic hyperglycinaemia).
- Intracranial haemorrhage.
- CNS malformation.
- Impediments to ventilation (e.g. pneumothorax, ascites, tracheal web).
- Cervical spinal cord injury (otherwise alert, non-encephalopathic child who cannot self-ventilate).
- Neuromuscular disease, maternal drugs including anaesthetics and cardiopulmonary disease.

Investigations
Looking for correctable metabolic disturbances, for evidence of end-organ damage and for other causes.
- FBC, glucose, Ca^{2+}, Mg^{2+}, PO_4^{2-}, pH, ammonia, lactate, urea, and electrolytes, clotting, LFTs, CK, CKMB/troponin.
- Sepsis screen (consider herpes virus).
- Consider toxicology screen for opiates, cocaine, tricyclics, SSRIs, amphetamines, barbiturates, and alcohol.
- Examination of placenta for evidence of chorioamnionitis, infarction, haemorrhage, and thrombi.
- Cranial ultrasound to rule out haemorrhage and look for evidence of oedema or infarct.

- EEG or aEEG (see Cerebral Function Monitoring in Chapter 2
  ⊃ pp. 87-91) to assess background, voltage, seizures, and for evidence
  of burst-suppression.
- The imaging modality of choice is MRI with diffusion-weighted imaging
  (DWI) although this is frequently difficult in an unstable child and may
  need to be delayed.
- It is important that neonatal MRI is reported by neuroradiologists
  familiar with the very different *normal* appearances of white matter
  in the neonate and particularly the premature infant: treat reports of
  'global white matter abnormality' with some caution.
- Areas of restricted diffusion correspond to ischaemic brain tissue and
  appear early (within an hour of insult).
  - There is potential for pseudo-normalization of diffusion 7 to 10 days
    after the insult.
- MRI will give information as to the extent of hypoxic injury, mechanism,
  and prognosis. Common patterns are:
  - *Acute profound/near total.* Typically spares cortex but cause thalamic,
    basal ganglia and brainstem injury, and dyskinetic CP.
  - *Chronic partial ('watershed') ischaemia* due to sustained hypotension
    causing loss of perfusion of border zones. Results particularly in
    parasagittal and parieto-occipital white matter loss and auditory,
    visuo-spatial, learning and language deficits. In severe cases spasticity
    and/or epilepsy may result. In pre-term infants involved cortex may
    show radiological evidence of *ulegyria* ('mushroom shaped' gyri) due
    to greater ischaemia (and thus scarring and atrophy) of cortex in the
    depth of a sulcus than on the outer convexity.
  - *Acute on chronic.* Combination of these patterns of injury, leading
    to a combination of dystonia, spasticity, learning difficulties, with or
    without epilepsy.

See MRI brain findings: diagnostic and prognostic implications in Chapter 4
⊃ pp. 234-8.

Management of HIE
- ABCs—protection of airway, maintenance of adequate respiration and
  cardiopulmonary circulation.
- Aim for normoxia and normocapnia. Avoid hypercapnia which
  may cause cerebral acidosis and cerebral 'steal phenomenon' and
  hyperperfusion. Hypocapnia may lead to ↓ CBF.
- Maintain cerebral perfusion: aim for MAP of at least 45–50 mmHg in
  term infants, 35–40 mmHg in infants 1000–2000 g and 30–35 mmHg in
  infants <1,000 g. Continuously monitor MAP ideally via arterial line.
- Prevent hyperperfusion injury by minimizing rapid boluses of colloid or
  crystalloid.
- Use inotropes as necessary to minimize need for volume expansion in
  maintenance of CPP.
- Avoid hyperviscosity by keeping haematocrit <65%.
- Avoid hypoglycaemia.
- Aim for normal serum Ca.

Therapeutic cooling for neonatal encephalopathy

72h of cooling to a core temperature of 33–34°C initiated within 6h of birth reduces death and disability at 18 months of age in:

- Infants with moderate to severe neonatal encephalopathy.
- >36 weeks' gestation.
- <6h old.
- In rare cases, neonatologists may decide hypothermia treatment is warranted outside of these recommendations.

Therapeutic hypothermia is achieved by either selective head, or total body cooling. Effective cooling is only achieved with good communication between regional neonatal intensive care and subsidiary units, supported by a multidisciplinary team experienced in neonatal intensive care, neonatal electrophysiology (such as aEEG and EEG), and neuroimaging (MRI), supervised by experienced clinicians.

    Practical considerations:

- Avoid external heat sources.
- Use cooling apparatus.
- Monitor rectal temperature.

Other measures:

- Control seizures.
- Treat cerebral oedema. Cerebral oedema can be minimized by avoiding fluid overload (consider fluid restriction) and watching for signs of SIADH and acute tubular necrosis.
- At least daily measurements of serum and urine Na and osmolarity to look for signs of SIADH or acute tubular necrosis.

Outcome

Mortality 10%; neurological sequelae in 20–40%. Indicators of poor outcome are Sarnat stage III encephalopathy (see Box 5.3), severe prolonged asphyxia, elevated ICP, early seizures, abnormal neurological signs at discharge, and markedly abnormal EEG (burst-suppression, isoelectric), and abnormal MRI.

Death by neurological criteria in neonates

Criteria for diagnosis of death by neurological criteria (DNC) in infants >37 weeks corrected gestation have been approved in the UK. (see Assessment of death by neurological criteria in this chapter ❷ pp. 583-5).

Metabolic encephalopathies

Many metabolic, toxic, infectious, and genetic abnormalities can cause neonatal encephalopathy. The placenta usually clears toxic metabolites so the onset of symptoms may be delayed by several hours or even days postpartum (cf. HIE).

    Features of metabolic neonatal encephalopathies

- Alteration in mental state: irritability, lethargy, stupor, coma.
- Seizures.
- Feeding abnormalities: poor feeding, vomiting, failure to thrive.
- Respiratory abnormalities: tachypnoea, apnoea.
- Alteration in tone: hypotonia, hypertonia.

The presentation may mimic neonatal sepsis.

Two patterns of presentation

- Apparently well newborn with a period without symptoms, who goes on to develop lethargy, poor feeding, vomiting that progresses to stupor or coma, hyper- or hypotonia, seizures, respiratory alkalosis, metabolic acidosis, and hyperammonaemia (see Figs. 5.1 and 5.2).
  - organic acidaemias such as propionic, MMA, and IVA;
  - urea cycle defects;
  - MSUD.
- Frank and early neurological syndrome with profound hypotonia, coma, seizures, and apnoea without significant acid-base disturbances or hyperammonaemia:
  - non-ketotic hyperglycinaemia;
  - molybdenum cofactor deficiency;
  - pyridoxine-dependent seizures;
  - primary lactic acidosis;
  - mitochondrial disease;
  - peroxisomal disorders.

Box 5.3 Grading of neonatal encephalopathy

Mild HIE—Sarnat Stage I
- Hyper-alert.
- Eyes wide open.
- Does not sleep.
- Irritable.
- No seizures.
- Usually lasts <24 h.

Moderate HIE—Sarnat Stage II
- Lethargy (difficult to rouse).
- Reduced tone of the extremities and/or trunk.
- Diminished brainstem reflexes (pupil/gag/suck).
- Possible clinical seizures.

Severe HIE—Sarnat Stage III
- Coma (cannot be roused).
- Weak or absent respiratory drive.
- No response to stimuli (may have spinal reflex to painful stimuli).
- Flaccid tone of the extremities and trunk (floppy).
- Diminished or absent brain stem reflexes (pupil/gag/suck).
- Diminished tendon reflexes.
- EEG severely abnormal (suppressed or flat EEG with or without seizures).

Source: data from Sarnat HB and Sarnat MS. Neonatal encephalopathy following fetal distress: a clinical and electroencephalographic study. *Archives of Neurology*, Volume 33, Issue 10, p. 696–705, Copyright © 1976 American Medical Association.

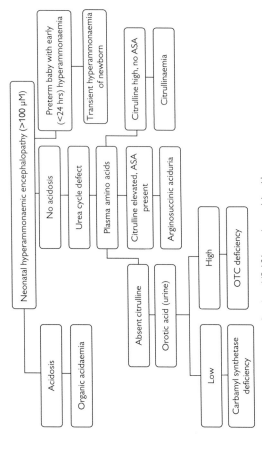

Fig. 5.1 Hyperammonaemia flowchart. NB ASA = arginosuccinic acid.

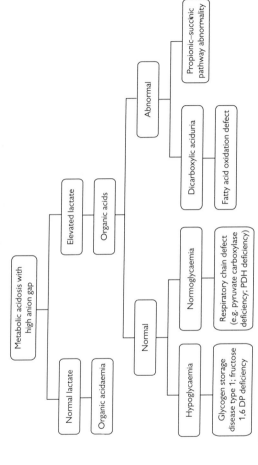

Fig. 5.2 Metabolic acidosis flowchart.

Suggestive features in peripartum history
- Absence of risk factors or clinical findings typical of HIE.
- Consanguinity, family history of multiple miscarriages or early infant death.
- Maternal acute fatty liver of pregnancy or HELLP syndrome (haemolysis, elevated liver enzyme levels, and low platelets). These complications of pregnancy are of unknown (probably heterogeneous) aetiology; however, some of the involved children later manifest fatty acid oxidation disorders.
- Oligohydramnios.
- Prolonged labour (steroid sulphatase deficiency).
- Abnormalities of foetal movement (*in utero* seizures, recurrent hiccoughs, NKH).
- Hydrops fetalis (lysosomal disorders).
- Neonatal hypoglycaemia (fatty acid oxidation disorders, glycogen storage disorders).
- Neonatal hepatic dysfunction (galactosaemia, tyrosinaemia).
- Neutropenia, thrombocytopenia.

Suggestive examination findings
- Dysmorphism: PDH deficiency, glutaric aciduria II, CDG, Zellweger, Smith–Lemli–Opitz.
- Cardiac dysfunction (mitochondrial disease, Pompe, CDG).
- Abnormal body odour (maple syrup urine disease, isovaleric aciduria, glutaric aciduria type II).
- Jaundice and hepato/splenomegaly.

Initial investigations of suspected IEM
Urgent WES/WGS is increasingly replacing traditional biochemical investigation of suspected IEM however some basic investigations will help identify broad IEM category (e.g. urea cycle disorder) and aid interpretation of WES/WGS findings:
- FBC and differential.
- Urea and electrolytes, creatine.
- Blood gas with base excess.
- Anion gap.
- Glucose.
- Lactate.
- Ammonia.
- Liver function tests.

If WGS/WES is not readily available, the following will be useful:
- plasma amino acids, uric acid, plasma carnitine, and acylcarnitine, biotinidase.
- urine ketones, reducing substances, ferric chloride reaction, organic acids with orotic acid, amino acids, sulphocysteine.
- CSF glucose, protein, cell count, lactate, amino acids, neurotransmitter, and folate metabolites.
- MRI, EEG.

Management of the newborn with a suspected metabolic encephalopathy
- Manage cardiorespiratory depression.
- Stop milk/protein feeds.
- Start 10% dextrose with electrolytes initially 3 mL/kg/h.
- Correct hypoglycaemia if present.
- Avoid over hydration if renal function is impaired.
- Monitor for cerebral oedema (fullness of anterior fontanelle); avoid hypercarbia.
- Frequent monitoring (4–6 hourly) of acid-base state and electrolytes.
- Correct metabolic acidosis with intravenous bicarbonate (may require large amounts, up to 20–40 mmol/kg of HCO_3).
- Treat hyperammonaemia if a urea cycle defect suspected with:
  - Sodium benzoate (250 mg/kg load followed by 250 mg/kg/24h infusion) or arginine 0.6 g/kg (6 mL/kg 10% arginine) over 90 min.

►► Discuss urgently with a metabolic physician if hyperammonaemia present. Urea cycle defects, MSUD, and organic acidaemias will almost certainly require haemofiltration or haemodialysis support.

- B12 1 mg IM if organic acidaemias are suspected.
- Biotin 10 mg orally daily.
- Thiamine 50 mg orally daily.
- Carnitine 25 mg/kg 6 hourly for suspected organic acidaemias or fatty acid oxidation disorders.
- Treat seizures per protocol:
  - If seizures are prominent, consider trial of pyridoxine/pyridoxal, biotin, and folinic acid; see Neonatal seizures in this chapter ➲ pp. 551-5.
- Once a diagnosis has been determined, therapy should be tailored to the underlying IEM, e.g. sodium benzoate and dextromethorphan for NKH, dietary manipulation, etc.

Cerebral haemorrhage in the neonate

Prevalence and location depend on gestational age.

Extra-axial bleeding
- Term > pre-term.
- Extradural, subdural, and subarachnoid.

Intra-axial bleeding
- Pre-term > term.
- Intraparenchymal haemorrhage—cerebral and cerebellar.
- Germinal matrix haemorrhage/intraventricular haemorrhage.

Extradural haemorrhage (EDH)
EDH is very rare in the newborn and is usually related to trauma such as skull fracture.

Subdural haemorrhage (SDH)
SDH is relatively common secondary to rupture of draining veins and sinuses due to cranial deformation and torsional forces during labour. Risk factors include non-vertex presentation, large foetal head size, primiparous

or older multiparous mother, instrumental delivery, or rapid/prolonged labour. Small clinically inconsequential SDH are common in vaginal deliveries. Most are small and resolve without treatment over the first weeks of life.
  If SDH is large, then presentation is soon after birth.
- Infratentorial haemorrhage causes brainstem compression with obtundation, respiratory abnormalities, abnormal extraocular movements, pupillary abnormalities, and nuchal rigidity.
- Supratentorial haemorrhage causes ↑ ICP, a bulging fontanelle, split sutures, and downward herniation signs. SDH over the cerebral convexities causes seizures in 50% probably due to co-existent SAH.
- A large SDH may cause systemic hypovolaemia.

Diagnosis is by CT or cranial USS. LP should be deferred if large SDH suspected. Investigate for sepsis and bleeding diathesis.
  Management:
- Supportive with treatment of seizures.
- Correct hypovolaemia and anaemia.
- Urgent neurosurgical consultation if progressive brainstem compression, opisthotonos, or tense bulging fontanelle. Surgical evacuation of the clot is warranted in the minority with a large SDH.
- Ongoing for late development of hydrocephalus and chronic subdural effusions.

▶ The occurrence of small clinically silent SDHs in otherwise well neonates is pertinent to investigation of SDH in later infancy in the context of NAI. They were noted in 8% children in one study: all had fully resolved by 4 weeks.

Subarachnoid haemorrhage (SAH)
- Primary SAH is frequent in term infants but usually clinically silent:
  - due to parturitional rupture of small leptomeningeal or bridging veins.
- Secondary SAH occurs in pre-term infants due to subarachnoid extension of an IVH or posterior fossa SDH.
- Rarely causes significant hypovolaemia.
- Usually mild alteration in mental status, irritability, and seizures. If the infant has a profoundly abnormal neurological exam, suspect either rare catastrophic large SAH (e.g. in the setting of bleeding diathesis) or HIE (in which SAH is frequently present).
- Diagnosis by CT supplemented by LP to diagnose small SAH (xanthochromic or haemorrhagic CSF).
- Treatment is supportive. Monitor occipitofrontal circumference (OFC) for development of late hydrocephalus secondary to chemical arachnoiditis.

Intraparenchymal haemorrhage (IPH)
- IPH is uncommon in term newborns but present in up to 10% of autopsied pre-term infants. Rare as a primary event: usually secondary to ruptured aneurysm or AVM, or secondary to coagulation disturbance.
- More common in a region of focal hypoxic injury (haemorrhagic transformation of arterial or venous infarction in term infants;

watershed/periventricular in pre-term). Also seen in infants on ECMO. Cerebellar IPH is more common in pre-term infants. May be primary, secondary to venous infarction or from extension of germinal matrix/ intraventricular haemorrhage.

- Cerebral IPH usually causes seizures, focal neurological signs, irritability, or obtundation. Large cerebellar IPH may be similar to posterior fossa SDH.
- CT for urgent diagnosis but should be followed with MRI with susceptibility and diffusion sequences to look for evidence of infarction, as well as MR angiography/venography.
- Management is supportive with treatment of any underlying cause (e.g. venous sinus thrombosis). A large IPH may cause obstructive hydrocephalus.
- Prognosis depends on location, size, and aetiology of IPH. A large cerebral IPH may lead to epilepsy, hemiparesis, visual, or cognitive impairment. Cerebellar IPH in term infants has a relatively good prognosis but residual cerebellar abnormalities such as tremor and ataxia may exist as well as mild cognitive and speech/language deficits. Large cerebellar IPH in the pre-term infant may lead to severe motor and cognitive deficits.

Germinal matrix/intraventricular haemorrhage (GMH/IVH)

Diagnosis is almost always made by cranial ultrasound as part of a routine NICU screening programme.

- Present in up to 20% pre-term infants <32 weeks:
  - Germinal matrix fragility is secondary to ischaemia–reperfusion (e.g. after volume infusion resulting in fluctuating CBF).
- Term IVH is usually a haemorrhage from the choroid plexus or secondary to deep venous sinus thrombosis and thalamic infarction (Table 5.4).

Table 5.4 Neonatal intraventricular haemorrhage

Grade	Description	Risk of ventricular dilation and hydrocephalus	Risk of major neurological disability
I	GMH with no or minimal IVH (<10% ventricular volume)	5%	<2%
II	IVH occupying 10–50% ventricle on parasagittal view	12%	<2%
III	IVH occupying 50% ventricular volume	75%	50%
Periventricular haemorrhagic infarction	Periventricular echo density	N/A	>90%

• Usually clinically silent but may present with a catastrophic syndrome of rapid neurological deterioration with coma, flaccid tone, tonic posturing, absence of spontaneous movements, or a subacute deterioration in alertness and spontaneous movement over hours to days.

Prevention
• Antenatal glucocorticoids.
• Any necessary infusions of colloid or hypo-osmolar fluids done slowly.
• Prevent CBF fluctuations by sedation, treatment of seizures, and gradual changes in mechanical ventilation.

Management of established ventricular dilation

• Assess speed of progression by daily OFC and clinical assessment, and weekly ultrasound.
• Determination of obstructive versus communicating hydrocephalus:
  • Perform LP aiming to remove 1–1.5 mL of CSF/kg. If little or no CSF is obtained, obstructive hydrocephalus is likely.
  • Liaise with neurosurgery for consideration of ventricular tap or placement of ventricular reservoir.
• Temporizing measures:
  • 40% of infants will show spontaneous resolution.
  • Options include serial LP, ventricular or reservoir tap, and adjunctive treatment with furosemide or acetazolamide.
• Indications for neurosurgical intervention:
  • rapid progression with deterioration in clinical status;
  • slow progression refractory to temporizing measures beyond 4 weeks.

Neonatal stroke

Up to 50% may be clinically silent in newborn period, presenting with emerging motor signs months later. Clinical evident cases present as neo-natal encephalopathy or seizures.

Causes
• Focal cerebral infarction due to embolus or thrombosis: it may be possible to distinguish on radiological patterns of involvement (See Fig. 4.9 in Chapter 4 ➜ p. 508).

Embolic stroke
• Placental via persistent foetal circulation allowing right-to-left shunting (note placental condition).
• Cardiac.

Thrombotic stroke
• Polycythaemia (4% newborns are polycythaemic).
• Venous thrombosis (suggestive radiological appearances: typically secondary to infection, dehydration, prothrombotic state, venous congestion due to heart disease).
• Primary thrombophilia; see Thrombotic arterial ischaemic stroke in Chapter 4 ➜ pp. 506-7.

Haemorrhagic stroke
- Subdural.
- Subarachnoid.
- Primary due to leptomeningeal vessel damage.
- Secondary due to extension of parenchymal or ventricular haemorrhage.
- Intraventricular/intraparenchymal.

Aneurysmal malformation of the vein of Galen

A persistent embryonic prosencephalic vein of Markowski normally present at 6–11 weeks of foetal life which drains into vein of Galen; so a misnomer! Associated rarely with dominantly inherited capillary malformation-arteriovenous malformation and *RASA1* gene mutations. Presentations:
- Cranial bruit—heard by parents!
- Developmental impairment with macrocephaly.
- High-output heart failure in the newborn from ↓ resistance and high blood flow in the lesion.
- Associated cerebral ischaemic changes: stroke or steal phenomenon with motor deficit.
- Mass effects leading to neurological impairment.
- CSF outflow obstruction and hydrocephalus.
- Haemorrhage—rare.

Management is usually by sequential endovascular embolization; however, morbidity is high and treatment should be managed by supra-regional centres with appropriate expertise.

The floppy or weak newborn

The availability of genetic therapy for SMA1 (the effectiveness of which depends crucially on timely treatment) has increased the urgency of investigation. Genetic screening for SMA1 is rapidly being incorporated into newborn screening programmes in many countries (see clinical presentations section; also see Floppy infants in Chapter 3 ➔ pp. 143-6).

Arthrogryposis

Typically affecting multiple joints relatively symmetrically (arthrogryposis multiplex congenita, AMC). Relatively common (3 per 1000).
   Indicates limited *in utero* movement which in turn may reflect:
- Primary neurological cause of weakness, either central or neuromuscular in origin. For further assessment, see Floppy infants in Chapter 3 ➔ pp. 143-6.
- Limited room for foetal movement: clear antenatal history of oligohydramnios or uterine abnormality (tends to improve in first few months postnatally).
- Orthopaedic abnormalities of joint anatomy.
- Primary muscle aplasia (amyotrophy). This is the most common cause, accounting for ~40% of AMC but a diagnosis of exclusion after assessment for primary neuromuscular disease. Scoliosis and pooling of secretions with aspiration makes a myopathy (particularly nemaline rod) likely.
- Half of those who are ventilator dependent have a developmental brain abnormality.

Neurosurgical consultations

Headache

• In a child with hydrocephalus who has had normal ICP monitoring: once raised pressure has been excluded the assessment is as for other children: primary headaches, especially migraine and tension-type headache are the most common; see Headache in Chapter 3 ⊃ pp. 165-7.

Shunt complications

In evaluation of possible shunt malfunction, a good history is at least as valuable as neuroimaging data.

Suspected blockage/fracture/other loss of function
• Up to 40% in the first year; 5–10% per year afterwards.
• 60–80% of shunts placed in infancy need revision within 10 yrs. Subsequent shunts have similar longevity.
• Symptoms are typically subacute or chronic: lethargy, headache, visual disturbance, behaviour alteration, non-specific symptoms, and occasionally seizures.
• Relationship of headaches to posture particularly helpful (raised pressure headache due to shunt blockage typically worse after period of lying down, e.g. first thing in morning, also aggravated by cough, sneeze, or straining at stool). Relationship of symptoms to recent shunt revisions also informative.
• If shunt complication is suspected, discuss this early with the child's usual neurosurgical team.

▶ CT scan and X-ray series of the shunt at local centre if the GCS is normal; otherwise defer imaging, stabilize, and arrange rapid transfer to a neurosurgical centre.
❶ Normal ventricles on CT do not exclude raised ICP!

• Consider neuroimaging data (including flow studies), ICP pressure monitoring and sampling of CSF from the shunt device (by neurosurgeons).
• A pragmatic approach is sometimes required (e.g. therapeutic trial of acetazolamide to reduce CSF production if ↑ ICP is suspected).

Over-drainage
• Lethargy. In contrast to ↑ ICP, the headache due to over-drainage ('low-pressure headache') is typically worse on *sitting or standing up*, improved by lying down.
• May occur immediately after lumbar puncture due to CSF leak.
• CT may show slit ventricles. MRI may show tonsillar descent. Ambulatory ICP monitoring may be needed for confirmation.
• If occurring immediately after lumbar puncture, then low-pressure symptoms can be managed conservatively with bed rest for a few days until the leak has closed.

- If related to recent shunt revision, then the shunt valve needs to be changed to one with a higher opening pressure.
  - Shunts with programmable valves (whose opening pressure can be adjusted remotely) are increasingly used.

Infection
- Typically due to colonization of shunt with skin flora during insertion.
- Overall incidence ~10%: 90% occur within 9 months of placement.
- Risk much higher with postoperative CSF leak.
- Drowsiness, irritability, ↑ temperature. May be difficult to differentiate from UTI. Infection screen (FBC, CRP, urgent urine microscopy).
- Most neurosurgical teams will insist on performing their own shunt taps: you do not want to be responsible for introducing infection!
- Treatment requires a period of shunt externalization (allowing the distal end of the shunt to drain into an external reservoir rather than the peritoneum), prolonged intravenous and intrathecal antibiotics, and shunt replacement once CSF indices indicate eradication of the infection.
- Antibiotic-impregnated shunts appear effective at reducing infection rates.

Other shunt complications:
- Haemorrhage, abdominal pseudo-cysts, viscus penetration, shunt migration.

Complications of intracerebral haemorrhage
- E.g. subarachnoid haemorrhage from an aneurysm or arteriovenous malformation.
- Typical contributions of the neurologist include:
  - Completing evaluation of aetiology; see Cerebral haemorrhage in Chapter 4 ➋ pp. 511-2;
  - Consideration of screening for family members; see Cerebral aneurysms in Chapter 4 ➋ pp. 511-2;
  - Seizure control;
  - Rehabilitation for acquired disability; see Interdisciplinary working and goal setting in Chapter 4 ➋ p. 221.

Sequelae of acquired brain injury
- Arrangements for the medical oversight of the early rehabilitation phase after ABI vary between centres, but clear lines of medical responsibility are important; see Medium and long-term medical management in Chapter 4 ➋ pp. 221-2.

Intracerebral sepsis
- Liaison in management of cerebral abscesses; see Focal CNS infection in Chapter 4 ➋ pp. 371-3.

Seizures in the context of neurosurgical disease
- Disordered sodium homeostasis is common:
  - Dilutional hyponatraemia: see Hyponatraemia in a neuro-intensive care setting in this chapter ➋ pp. 581-2.

- Cranial diabetes insipidus after craniopharyngioma and pituitary surgery.
- Interruption to regular intake of antiseizure medications in children with known epilepsy, e.g. due to periods of nil-by-mouth: see Parenteral maintenance of antiseizure medication in this chapter ➲ pp. 549-50.

Oncology consultations

Common reasons for consultation are management of seizures (see Seizures [in this Oncology section] in this chapter p. 575) and intrathecal methotrexate neurotoxicity. A wide range of neurological symptoms and signs can occur in the context of paediatric oncology. It is always tempting to blame the chemotherapy, but consider also:

- Metabolic derangements.
- Hypertension.
- Infection.
- Stroke.
- Disease progression with meningeal seeding of tumour.

Encephalopathy

Apply the usual clinical approach, with an open mind.

Metabolic
- Hypo- or hyperglycaemia.
- Hyperammonaemia and deranged liver function.
- Electrolyte derangements, e.g.:
  - Chemotherapy-related diarrhoea (severe mucositis);
  - Attempted correction (hypocalcaemic seizures in a child overcorrected for diarrhoeal bicarbonate loss);
  - Vincristine causing SIADH;
  - Silent GIT perforation (on steroids) and third-space losses.

Infection
- Check that antibacterial and antiviral treatments have been instituted: remember the child is likely to be immunocompromised. See Opportunistic central nervous system infections in this chapter p. 577 and CNS infection of the immunocompromised host in Chapter 4 pp. 377-81.

Drug-induced encephalopathy
Methotrexate neurotoxicity
- Relatively common complication of intrathecal *or* systemic methotrexate treatment.
- Very variable presentation:
  - mood disturbance;
  - headaches;
  - drowsiness;
  - seizures;
  - focal neurological signs.
- Cytotoxic (intracellular) oedema detectable by diffusion-weighted MR imaging is an early feature (T2 imaging may be initially normal but becomes abnormal over days).
- Dextromethorphan suggested as symptomatic treatment.

Ciclosporin neurotoxicity (see Fig. 5.3)
- A relatively common cause of encephalopathy with seizures and motor signs closely resembling (both radiologically and clinically) the posterior reversible encephalopathy syndrome (PRES) seen in hypertension; see Posterior reversible encephalopathy syndrome in this chapter p. 598.

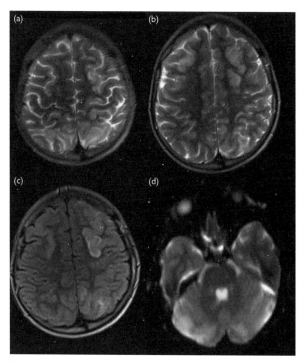

Fig. 5.3 Typical appearances of ciclosporin neurotoxicity. Note that in this case changes are relatively asymmetric and not confined to occipital cortex (c.f. posterior reversible encephalopathy syndrome, see Posterior reversible encephalopathy syndrome in this chapter ⮆ p. 598). T2 sequences top (A and B); FLAIR sequence (C) and DWI (D).

Other drug encephalopathies with white matter changes on MRI
- Amphotericin B, cytosine arabinoside, cisplatin, 5-fluorouracil (5-FU), fludaribine, ifosfamide, methotrexate, vincristine, ciclosporin, tacrolimus (FK506).
- Hypertensive encephalopathy; see Hypertensive encephalopathy in this chapter ⮆ p. 598.

Other drug encephalopathies with normal/uninformative MRI
- Aciclovir (particularly if renal function impaired).
- Cephalosporins.
- Granulocyte colony-stimulating factor.
- Ifosfamide is both directly and indirectly neurotoxic:

- causes electrolyte derangements including nephrogenic diabetes insipidus;
- non-convulsive status has been described;
- treatment of direct encephalopathy with methylene blue.
- Steroids cause mood changes and irritability as well as hypertension and intracranial hypertension.

Seizures

Causes
- Any cause of encephalopathy (see above) including antibiotics, busulfan, chlorambucil, high-dose methotrexate, vincristine (hyponatraemia).
- Non-convulsive status epilepticus particularly with cisplatin, ifosfamide.

Treatment
See Treatment of epilepsy in Chapter 4 🕭 pp. 305-16.
- Levetiracetam and phenytoin useful acutely, particularly if cause of seizures likely to be temporary.
- Standard ASM choices are appropriate in many cases.
- If hepatotoxicity present (due to chemotherapy) consider benzodiazepines.

Gait disturbance

- Disease progression may be a well-founded concern.
- Assess (see Gait abnormalities in Chapter 3 🕭 pp. 157-9) to define the *mechanism* and thus *site* of the problem more precisely:
  - Neuropathy? (mono- or polyneuropathy e.g. due to vincristine);
  - Myopathy? Loss of muscle bulk secondary to immobility or illness? Steroid myopathy?
  - Ataxia?

Paraesthesia

- Pressure palsy mononeuropathy in a debilitated child.
  - The characteristic distribution of the sensory disturbance and (if relevant) the motor deficit corresponding to the involved nerve should be sought (see Innervation of lower limb in Chapter 1 🕭 pp. 33-7).
- Peripheral neuropathy occurs with vincristine and other chemotherapy agents (see Peripheral neuropathy in this chapter 🕭 p. 576).

Stroke

- Arterial infarction is reported with certain chemotherapy combinations:
  - vinblastine, bleomycin, and cisplatin;
  - cisplatin and 5-FU;
  - carboplatin and cyclophosphamide.
- CT will rule out acute haemorrhage due to thrombocytopenia.
- Asparaginase (used in acute lymphoblastic anaemia induction) associated with dural sinus thrombosis.
  - Anticoagulate with low molecular weight heparin once secondary haemorrhage into a venous infarct has been excluded.

Headache
- Particularly related to IVIG use (may be prevented by propranolol); also ondansetron, amphotericin B.
- Intracranial hypertension with steroid use.

Cranial nerve signs
Ophthalmoplegia, ptosis
- Vincristine.

Facial palsy
- Cytosine arabinoside, ciclosporin after BMT, vincristine.

Oto-toxicity
- Carboplatin, cisplatin; cytosine arabinoside (with vestibular involvement).

Vocal cord palsy
- Vincristine (but diagnosis of exclusion: image!)

Ataxia
- Cytosine arabinoside, 5-FU.

Aseptic meningitis
- Intrathecal methotrexate.

Autonomic dysfunction
- Ileus, constipation, and bladder atony with vincristine, morphine.

Myelopathy
- Intrathecal methotrexate, cytosine arabinoside, or corticosteroids.
- Lhermitte's sign ('electric shock'-like sensations in the spine on neck flexion) may occur after cisplatin, BMT, or spinal irradiation.

Peripheral neuropathy
- Vincristine, cisplatin, cytosine arabinoside.
- Neurotoxicity with vincristine is dose-related and cumulative. A poor nutritional state may exacerbate the severity.
  - Numbness and tingling are a common early sign.
  - Muscle cramps.
  - Mild symptoms (loss of ankle reflexes, slapping gait) are common even at conventional dosages.
  - Reduction in dose of vincristine may be necessary if symptoms are severe, symptoms and signs are slowly reversible on discontinuation of the drug.

Treatment in all cases is supportive, with consideration of reduction or discontinuation of the responsible agent in conjunction with the oncology team. Check *PMP22* status (CMT1A) and if +ve consider modification of chemotherapy regimen (See Charcot-Marie-Tooth disease in Chapter 4 pp. 431-4).

Cerebellar mutism

See Cerebellar mutism (posterior fossa syndrome) in Chapter 4 ➜ pp. 520-1.

Opportunistic central nervous system infections

See also CNS infection of the immunocompromised host in Chapter 4 ➜ pp. 377-81.

Unusual infections arise due to impaired host defence as a result of:
- aggressive anticancer therapy;
- immunosuppression for organ transplantation or autoimmune disease;
- acquired immunodeficiency syndrome (HIV/AIDS).

Diagnosis can be difficult, with a wide range of possible agents including many organisms normally of low pathogenicity. Concurrent infection with more than one agent is frequent.

Manifestations of CNS infection such as headache, meningism, or fever may be mild or absent.

Survival without deficit depends on rapid diagnosis and effective therapy.

Diagnostic pointers

Clinical setting
- Children receiving chemotherapy causing marked lymphopenia (e.g. ALL, Hodgkin) and prednisolone develop a typical spectrum of CNS disease:
  - bacterial meningitis (*Haemophilus influenzae, Streptococcus pneumonii* or *Listeria monocytogenes*);
  - fungal meningitis (*Cryptococcus neoformans, Aspergillus fumigatus*);
  - Viral infections (herpes viruses and PML).
- In the context of HIV/AIDS, there is a strong association between EBV infection and the development of primary CNS lymphoma.

Time course of symptom progression
May help define the pathogen.
- Acute onset: bacterial meningitis with 'conventional' organisms.
- Subacute presentation with fever and headache: *C. neoformans, M. tuberculosis, L. monocytogenes* or herpes virus.
- Chronic progressive focal neurological picture: PML.

Pattern of clinical signs and symptoms
- Focal deficits: space-occupying lesion (toxoplasmosis, aspergillosis, PML, *Cryptococcus*, bacterial brain abscess, metastatic malignancy) or stroke (VZV vasculitis; haemorrhage secondary to thrombocytopenia).
- Spinal cord: extradural abscess, or tumour; transverse myelitis due to CMV, HSV, VZV, or parasitic infection; intrinsic infiltrative tumour.
- Radicular mononeuropathy or polyradiculopathy; HSV or CMV.

Consider data from peripheral blood count and differential, acute phase reactants, CSF cellular response (though this may be misleading), MRI, and culture of blood, CSF, nose, throat, sputum, and urine (bacteria, fungi, and viruses). Specific management requires close liaison with oncologists, microbiologists, and virologists.

Neurological complications of CAR-T therapy

T-cells that have been modified to express Chimeric Antigen Receptors ('CAR-T' cells) represent a major new class of immunotherapies rapidly establishing a role in the treatment of leukaemias and lymphomas.

- T-cells are harvested from the patient, genetically modified to express receptors making them specific to a desired target antigen (typically CD19 that identifies B-lymphocytes), multiplied *ex vivo*, and then reinfused. These target and kill cells expressing the target antigen.
- Unregulated, this cytotoxic activity causes a severe systemic 'cytokine-release' syndrome with a variable neurotoxicity (but some early reports of fatal cerebral oedema).
- Deteriorating fine motor skills (writing) and dysphasia tend to be early features.
- MRI typically normal (helpful in excluding differential diagnoses).
- Treatment is with steroids and tocilizumab.

Severe neurotoxicity becoming rarer with growing experience and prophylactic use of steroids and tocilizumab.

PICU consultations

For issues specific to cardiac ICU, see Cardiology consultations in this chapter ➲ pp. 533-5.

Coma

For acute (emergency) management of coma, see Emergency management of coma in Chapter 6 ➲ pp. 613-7.

Coma is a common medical emergency with many causes. The prevalence of each cause differs with age.

Causes of coma
Traumatic
- Accidental traumatic brain injury (TBI) or inflicted non-accidental injury (NAI).

Non-traumatic
- Hypoxia–ischaemia: cardiac/respiratory arrest, suffocation, drowning, severe hypotension.
- Infection/inflammation: meningoencephalitis, abscess, shunt infection, post-infectious ADEM, cerebellitis.
- Epilepsy: post-ictal, subtle motor status epilepticus, non-convulsive status epilepticus.
- Vascular: intracerebral haemorrhage/embolism, hypertensive encephalopathy, cerebral venous sinus thrombosis with venous infarct.
- Metabolic: hypoglycaemia, diabetic ketoacidosis (DKA), renal failure, adrenal failure, liver failure/hyperammonaemia, hyper-/hyponatraemia.
- Toxic: accidental or deliberate drug ingestion, heavy metal poisoning, e.g. lead or iron.
- Hydrocephalus: first episode (post IVH or CNS infection, tumour), or recurrence after blocked shunt.

Identification of the cause
Cause may be obvious from history. If not, consider the following:

Infectious and parainfective
- Uncommon infections: malaria, TB meningitis, or Japanese encephalitis if they have travelled previously to an endemic area or are in high-risk group. See Infection of the CNS in Chapter 4 ➲ pp. 361-81.
- ADEM: onset 1–2 weeks after viral or other infection or vaccination resulting in coma ± focal neurological signs.
- Rarely, coma can result from acute onset primary *peripheral* neuromuscular disease causing hypoventilation and hypoxia (e.g. rapidly progressing Guillain–Barré syndrome).

Trauma
- Particularly with bilateral periorbital haemorrhage, otorrhoea, or rhinorrhoea (leaking CSF will be +ve for glucose on test strip) indicating basal skull fracture.
- Non-accidental injury: retinal haemorrhages ± bulging fontanelle ± shock or pallor. The offered explanation may not be consistent with the severity of the presentation.

Metabolic/toxic
- Intoxication is a common cause of rapid-onset coma.
- Pear drops smell of ketones and tachypnoea in DKA.
- Unusual smell, decompensation after intercurrent illness (causing a catabolic state), unexplained hypoglycaemia, family history of unexplained deaths in siblings suggestive of an inherited metabolic defect.
- History of pica ± learning disability in lead encephalopathy.
- Intoxication in younger children with opportunity (e.g. access to poorly secured parental medication).

Raised intracranial pressure
- History of perinatal IVH or prematurity, previous meningitis or recent symptoms suggestive of ↑ intracranial pressure in hydrocephalus.
- Recent dehydration or family history of thrombophilia in venous sinus thrombosis.
- Child with a VP shunt.

Vasculitic
- Recent gastroenteritis in haemolytic–uraemic syndrome with CNS involvement.

Immediate investigations
See Emergency management of coma in Chapter 6 ⊃ pp. 613-7. Ensure these are complete.

Further/subsequent investigations to consider
It is not intended that this list be slavishly followed in all cases. Tailor the investigation to the clinical picture.

Blood
- Urgent WES/WGS where neurogenetic causes are being considered.
- Plasma amino acids, carnitine, and acylcarnitine.
- Haemoglobin electrophoresis.
- Serology ± PCR for other infectious causes.
- DNA for mitochondrial mutations and storage.
- Autoantibodies including ANA and dsDNA.
- ESR and CRP. An elevated ESR with a *normal* CRP can be an indication of rheumatological (e.g. vasculitic, connective tissue) pathology.
- Serum angiotensin-converting enzyme.
- Thyroid autoantibodies and function.
- Blood film for malaria.

Urine
- Sodium level.
- Porphyria screen.

LP if not contraindicated: see Immediate investigations in Chapter 6 ⊃ p. 616.
- CSF amino acids.
- Cytospin for malignant cells.

MRI
- Especially if ADEM, posterior fossa pathology or stroke is a possibility. Additional sequences such as inversion recovery, diffusion-weighted imaging, MRA, or MRV may be indicated. See Venography in Chapter 2 ➔ p. 57.

EEG
- Rarely provides direct clues to aetiology but may be useful (e.g. demonstration of marked asymmetry suggesting a focal pathology).
  - Periodic complexes in herpes encephalitis.
  - 'Delta brush' in NMDA receptor antibody encephalitis (see Fig. 4.7 in Chapter 4 ➔ p. 392).
- Exclude subtle status epilepticus.

Others
- Sputum or stool for culture and viral studies.
- Rarely, muscle or skin biopsy (fibroblast culture) for investigation of mitochondrial disorders.
- Brain biopsy: consider if the result will make a difference to management.

Hyponatraemia in a neuro-intensive care setting

Hyponatraemia occurs commonly following neurological disease (e.g. TBI, tumours, meningoencephalitis and stroke) and may indicate poor prognosis. It is particularly common after subarachnoid haemorrhage (30%).

It is an important preventable cause of secondary neurological insult, aggravating cerebral oedema, precipitating seizures, and sometimes causing irreversible white matter change (see Central pontine myelinolysis in this chapter ➔ p. 599).

Causes include:
- Syndrome of inappropriate ADH secretion (SIADH): can occur after CNS injury but *is over diagnosed and often wrongly assumed* when the true cause is either:
  - Dilutional hyponatraemia: inappropriate use of large volumes of hypotonic fluid; or
  - Cerebral salt-wasting (CSW) syndrome. The cause is unknown but appears to be primarily a natriuretic effect on the kidneys.

▶ Key to distinguishing CSW from SIADH or dilutional hyponatraemia is that CSW is associated with hypovolaemia (due to salt *and* water loss).

Evaluation of hyponatraemia
- If measured plasma osmolality is $>2 \times [\text{Na}]_{\text{plasma}}$ in the absence of uraemia, consider hyperglycaemia or mannitol as the cause of hyponatraemia.
- Blood urea is often low in SIADH (dilutional) but normal/high in CSW.
- Low output of concentrated urine in SIADH; high output of dilute urine in CSW.

In CSW there is:

- Clinical evidence of hypovolaemia: poor skin turgor, shrunken eyes, dry mucous membranes, absence of perspiration, tachycardia. Low central venous pressure (CVP <6 mmHg) and low pulmonary capillary wedge pressure if measured (PCWP <8 mmHg).
- Loss of weight on serial testing since admission (*c.f.* weight ↑ in SIADH).
- -ve water balance on input/output chart.
- -ve 24 h sodium balance (output > input over 24 h):
  - calculate input from infused fluids;
  - output (mmol per 24 h) = $[Na]_{urine}$ × urine output in 24 h;
  - sodium balance neutral in SIADH.
- Marked elevation of $[Na]_{urine}$ (variable in SIADH).
- Biochemical evidence of haemoconcentration with ↑ urea, haematocrit, potassium (not usually seen in SIADH), urate (low in SIADH).
- In complex/ambiguous cases, seek specialist (e.g. nephrology) advice.
- Some children may have SIADH first then evolve to CSW after a few days.

Management

- In dilutional hyponatraemia, correct fluid prescription.
- In SIADH, consider further fluid restriction (discuss with intensivist).

Management of CSW

- Treat the underlying neurological process especially ICP or hydrocephalus.
- Volume replacement:
  - Maintain hydration with intravenous isotonic saline (0.9% NaCl).
  - Blood products are useful if the child is anaemic.
  - Colloids may help by expanding the volume and absorbing interstitial third-space fluid.
  - Match urine loss and keep a +ve fluid balance.
- Positive sodium balance:
  - Calculate sodium deficit = $(140 - [Na]_{plasma})$ × total body water (estimate as 50–60% of ideal body weight).
  - Aim to correct at no more than 1 mM per hour with oral salt or hypertonic saline to ensure +ve sodium balance.
  - There is a risk of precipitating central pontine myelinolysis with over-rapid correction (see Central pontine myelinolysis in this chapter ➲ p. 599).
  - Consider preventing further salt loss with volume expansion using fludrocortisone (risk of hypokalaemia, fluid overload, and hypertension).
- Monitor:
  - Serum sodium, volume status (including overload with pulmonary oedema). Monitor central venous pressure or even pulmonary capillary wedge pressure.
  - Sodium and water balance.

Assessment of death by neurological criteria

The possibility that death by neurological criteria (DNC) has occurred should be considered in any deeply comatose and apnoeic child with a profound or diffuse brain insult. Common causes of insult sufficient to cause DNC in children include TBI; CNS infection; intracerebral haemorrhage; and cerebral hypoxia secondary to cardiac/respiratory arrest, drowning, smoke inhalation/carbon monoxide poisoning, or drug ingestion.

> ❶ The following discusses the UK approach to DNC: appropriate national guidelines and legislation should be followed in other jurisdictions.
> - The UK approach considers death to be 'the irreversible loss of the capacity for consciousness, combined with irreversible loss of the capacity to breathe' operationalized as 'irreversible cessation of the integrative function of the brainstem'.
> - The UK approach does not require demonstration of 'whole brain death' although this may be useful in particular circumstances (demonstration of whole brain death is *sufficient* to make a diagnosis of DNC but not *necessary*).
> - UK practice permits application of DNC testing in neonates above 37 weeks corrected age.

Diagnostic criteria for DNC
- Profound coma *of known cause* and capable in principle of causing devastating injury, with total unresponsiveness to noxious stimuli.
- A structural brain lesion sufficient to explain the clinical findings.
- Apnoea despite induced hypercapnia (see Apnoea test below).
- Absence of all reflexes subserved by the brainstem and cranial nerves (pupillary light, vestibulocular, corneal, gag, and cough reflexes).
  - Spinal reflexes, including deep tendon reflexes; and spinal myoclonus may (rarely) be preserved.
- Irreversibility.

Pre-conditions
- Body temperature >35°C.
  - Any therapeutic hypothermia must have been fully reversed.
- Metabolic and endocrine causes or contributors to coma must be excluded or reversed (e.g. waiting several drug half-lives to guarantee elimination).
- Neuromuscular blockade — if used as part of therapy — must have been demonstrably reversed by peripheral neurostimulation ('train of four') or demonstration of peripheral tendon reflexes.

Serial testing
- Two senior doctors, preferably the consultant in charge of care and another independent doctor (not a member of any transplant team), should perform testing.
- Wait 6 h from onset of the coma before initial testing.
  - Wait 24 h if the coma follows a cardiac arrest or general anaesthetic.

- Tests should be repeated in all cases to allow independent confirmation of examination findings. Timing of second test is at the discretion of medical staff but should take the family's needs into account.
  - There is no minimum interval required between the two tests: the 'irreversibility' assessment is achieved by waiting a sufficient period *before the first test*, not the interval between tests.

Cranial nerve reflex testing
Pupillary light reflexes
- Test in a dark room with a bright source. There should be absolutely no direct nor consensual response to light. Inspection with a magnifying glass may be helpful. Pupils should be average to large size: *pinpoint* pupils suggest persisting drug effects.

Corneal reflex
- Test with a cotton bud: make sure the cornea over the (coloured) iris is touched. No blink response seen.

Gag/cough reflex
- No response to pharyngeal or tracheal suction to carina via an endotracheal (ET) tube.

Vestibulo-ocular reflexes
Equivalent to oculocephalic reflex testing.
- Make sure no eardrum perforation is present.
- Elevate the head to 30° above horizontal.
- Infuse 20 mL of ice-cold water into each external auditory meatus in turn with an assistant holding the child's eyes open.
- There should be no eye movement, limb movement, or grimace.

Apnoea test
Hypercapnia is a potent stimulus to breathe. The technique of apnoeic oxygenation used is:
- Adjust ventilator settings to achieve a $PaCO_2$ of ≥ 5.3 kPa (40 mmHg).
- Use 100% FiO_2 for 10 min:
  - Pre-oxygenation will reduce the risks of the test, e.g. hypotension, cardiac arrhythmias, acidosis.
- Take baseline arterial blood gas.
- Take child off the ventilator and place a catheter at the carina with 100% O_2 at 8 L/min.
- Observe for ≥ 5 min checking oxygenation is maintained by saturation monitor.
- Ensure $PaCO_2$ levels of ≥8 kPa (60mmHg) with a rise from baseline of ≥2.7 kPa (20mmHg) and pH ≤7.3 are achieved.

Any respiratory effort including sighing signifies failure of the test.

Special circumstances
- Severe maxillofacial injury may preclude gag/cough testing.
- Severe primary injury of the upper cervical spine may affect phrenic nerve function and thus the cough reflex. *This invalidates the apnoea test.*

- In such special circumstances where clinical assessment of brainstem reflexes is necessarily incomplete, *ancillary tests* of brain function may be helpful.
  - Radionucleotide (e.g. SPECT) and/or CT angiogram demonstration of absence of cerebral and cerebellar perfusion may be used to support a diagnosis of whole brain death which as stated above is a sufficient basis for diagnosis of DNC.
  - Total absence of cerebral perfusion is unlikely in infants (with open fontanelle) and thus diagnosis of whole brain death may not be possible.
  - EEG and neurophysiological assessment of cortical electrical activity is not considered useful as metabolic/toxic suppression may give a false +ve.

Further reading: Revised UK guidance from the Association of Medical Royal Colleges (AoMRC) and Royal College of Paediatrics and Child Health (RCPCH) is expected in 2024.

Prognostication after acquired brain injury

Neurologists are often requested to assist in assessing prognosis for recovery for a child in a coma.

Traumatic injury
Predictors of mortality
- Age (mortality is high in infants and young children, lowest in mid-adolescence then rising again), but this is due largely to age-dependent patterns of mechanism and severity (e.g. inflicted head trauma in infants).
- Pupillary response (dilated non-reactive pupils persisting after initial resuscitation).
- Extracranial trauma (pelvic, chest injury).

Predictors of morbidity
- GCS motor score at 72 h:
  - M1, M2, or M3: almost invariably associated with severe disability.
  - M4, M5, or M6: good recovery or moderate disability in 75%.
  - Consider best side if function asymmetric.
- Hypoxia on admission.
- Hyperglycaemia may be an independent predictor of poor outcome.

Non-traumatic coma
Cardiopulmonary arrest
- Rare—usually in-hospital.
- Outcome is poor: ~10–30% survive to discharge from the PICU.
- Best predictor of mortality is whether consciousness was normal prior to arrest.
- Out-of-hospital arrest has extremely poor outcome: only 5% survival in better than vegetative state in one series.

Respiratory arrest (without cardiac arrest)
- 75% survival.

Near-drowning
- Outcomes after cold water immersion can be remarkably good:
  - thought to be protective effect of hypothermia;
  - intact survival reported after 60 min pulse-less immersion under ice.
- Warm water drowning (e.g. a swimming pool) is very different:
  - tends to a bimodal outcome: either vegetative or intact;
  - arterial pH, ICP, and plasma glucose predict.

Clinical assessment
- Motor response to pain is the best clinical predictor of morbidity.
- Sedation/paralysis may cause false pessimism.
- Reliably absent motor response (e.g. repeated several days apart) has 100% +ve predictive value for poor outcome.
- Radiological data may also be very informative.

Electrophysiological indicators of outcome
EEG
- Isoelectric, low-amplitude, suppression-burst, and markedly asymmetric appearances are recognized as poor prognostic signs in all age groups but +ve and –ve predictive values are uncertain.
- Normal sleep and reactive patterns suggest good outcome.
- 'Alpha coma' (coma associated with abnormally invariant and widespread α rhythms on EEG) has a poor outlook.

Evoked potentials
- Probably more useful than EEG: relatively unaffected by anaesthesia.
- Easily repeated and (lack of) change over time is particularly informative.

Brainstem auditory evoked potentials
- Largely reflect brainstem integrity: hence give similar data to clinical assessment of brainstem function.
- Reflect mortality but not morbidity.

Visual evoked potentials
- Limited value: may even be normal in vegetative state.

Cortical somatosensory evoked potentials (SSEPs)
- PPV of preserved SSEP for good outcome is 90%.
- PPV of bilaterally absent SSEPs for poor outcome is 90%.
  - Occasional false pessimism due to subdurals (can also suppress EEG amplitude).
  - Selective brainstem injury (usually radiologically evident) can interrupt SSEP transmission to an intact cortex and also cause false pessimism: therefore, interpret with care in severe traumatic injury.
  - Accuracy in neonates is less certain: false pessimism may be a risk.
- Multimodality evoked potentials (combining several data sources) may be most accurate.

Withdrawal of care decisions

Your job as consulting neurologist is to try objectively to describe future levels of neurodisability, as well as the — often considerable — width of the 'confidence interval' on that forecast.

Decisions as to whether such outcomes are 'acceptable' are highly value-laden, and family *and professional* views on these issues will be influenced by many factors. UK guidance (RCPCH) supports *consideration* of with-holding/withdrawal of intensive care on the grounds of:
• 'Futility' (delaying death with no prospect of meaningful recovery).
• 'Intolerability' (treatment is excessively burdensome).
• 'No purpose' (a judgement on future quality of life).

The only general principles that can be given here are that discussion must: (i) remain centred on the perceived interests of the child and (ii) solicit the views of all involved parties (including family, carers, and nursing staff).

Difficulty weaning from the ventilator

This is an infrequent but recurrent request for a consult from PICU, usually in the context of a child ventilated for an apparently non-neurological problem.

▶ Investigation is guided by asking whether this is a child who is not waking up, or a child who is waking but not breathing adequately. EEG may be helpful in this context. Causes of both are included below

Do not assume non-neurological causes have been excluded. Consider:

Biochemical?
• PO_4^{2-}.
• K^+ (particularly in a child with neuromuscular disease).
• Na^+.
• Malnutrition.

Drugs?
• Causing a neuropathy—vincristine.
• Causing a myopathy—steroids.
• Causing a neuromuscular blocking effect—aminoglycosides.
• Prolonged effect—thiopentone (zero order kinetics and accumulation in adipose tissue).

Cardiac or respiratory causes?
Ensure an opinion has been sought.

Secondary effect of the primary non-neurological illness/PICU setting?
• Missed high cervical cord injury.
• Missed phrenic nerve injury.
• Hypoxic–ischaemic encephalopathy—evidence for this in history, charts, imaging?
• Critical illness polyneuropathy, usually in the context of multiorgan system failure. Variable sensory-motor axonal neuropathy, myopathic changes.
• Dyskinesias (particularly choreoathetosis) associated with prolonged sedative use.

Known primary neurological illness more severe than appreciated?
- Any cerebral insult.
- Botulism—ventilatory support may be required for months.
- Guillain–Barré syndrome—particularly the acute motor axonal neuropathy (AMAN) form.
- Ongoing non-convulsive seizure activity.

Undiagnosed neurological illness revealed in the acute presentation?
Central origin
- Neurodegenerative disease.
- Inborn error of metabolism.
- Mitochondrial disease.
- Posterior fossa abnormality, e.g. Arnold Chiari.
- Brainstem pathology.
- Central hypoventilation syndrome—hypoventilation during sleep, autonomic dysfunction, pupillary abnormalities, *PHOXB* mutation analysis.

Neuromuscular origin
- Myotonic dystrophy.
- Spinal muscular atrophy with respiratory distress type 1 (SMARD1).
- Autoimmune myasthenia gravis and congenital myasthenic syndromes.

Specific investigations to consider
As well as specific tests for the above conditions:
- Tensilon test.
- Diaphragm fluoroscopy.
- Peripheral neurophysiological studies with repetitive nerve stimulation and single-fibre EMG.
- Muscle biopsy.

Abnormal movements on the ventilator

Are they seizures?
- Abnormal mouthing or chewing movements or isolated limb jerks are relatively common in ventilated children and the possibility of seizures may be queried.
- Review history:
  - evidence of significant cerebral insult?
  - medication, particularly recent changes;
  - electrolyte and biochemical status (esp. Na, Ca, Mg, glucose).
- Expert review of video may be sufficient to reach a diagnosis.
- Evidence in favour of seizures may include:
  - synchronous changes in pulse rate, blood pressure, or saturation.
- Evidence against seizure disorder includes:
  - movements relate to handling, cares, or change of position;
  - movements can be 'stilled' with gentle restraint or change of limb position (particularly in neonates).
- Differentials include:
  - post-pump and post-anoxic movement disorders; see Abnormal movements on extubation in this chapter ● p. 589.

- decerebrate posturing and status dystonicus.
- cerebral dysautonomia in severe (usually traumatic) midbrain injury; see Acute medical management of ABI in Chapter 4 ➲ pp. 219-20).

Delirium

Many aspects of the PICU environment predispose to delirium and disorientation:

- Use of sedative drugs and anaesthetics.
- Pain and use of opiate analgesia.
- Hypoxia.
- Sepsis.
- Disorienting environment (noise, absence of a circadian rhythm in levels of lighting and activity).
- Primary encephalopathy (e.g. traumatic brain injury).

For assessment investigation see Agitation and confusion in Chapter 3 ➲ pp. 114-5.

For management see Acute behavioural disturbance in Chapter 6 ➲ pp. 610-2.

Abnormal movements on extubation

Post-pump chorea.

See Cardiopulmonary bypass ('post-pump' chorea) in Chapter 4 ➲ p. 421.

Post-hypoxic movement disorders

- Lance–Adam syndrome (intention myoclonus) particularly after carbon monoxide poisoning and other severe global hypoxia (e.g. strangulation). See Lance-Adams syndrome in Chapter 4 ➲ p. 419.

Drug/sedation withdrawal

- Jittery tremors.
- Seen following withdrawal of opiates, benzodiazepines, and phenytoin.
- Treated with slow benzodiazepine taper ± clonidine.

Brief resolved unexplained events (BRUEs)

Formerly termed acute life-threatening events (ALTEs).

- A sudden, brief, and now resolved episode in an infant comprising one or more of:
  - Cyanosis or pallor.
  - Absent, ↓ or irregular breathing.
  - Marked change in tone (hyper- or hypotonia).
  - Altered level of responsiveness.
- May be recurrent.
- Rare but dramatic PICU picture with wide differential, of which primary neurological causes are relatively uncommon although BRUEs are often seen in children with neurodisability.
- Diagnosis of exclusion after appropriate history and examination.
- Criteria for lower risk include:
  - Age >60 days; or if premature born at >32 weeks and post-conceptional age now >45 weeks.
  - No previous similar events.

- No clustering.
- Duration <1 minute.
- No CPR required.
- No concerning features on history or examination.
- Investigation of low-risk BRUEs can be limited to 12-lead ECG and a brief period of oximetry.
  - In other situations consider neuroimaging, echocardiogram, EEG, and blood investigations including lactate, ammonia (see *Pediatrics.* 2016;137(5):e20160590).
- Be prepared to consider inflicted head trauma (see Non-accidental (inflicted) traumatic brain injury in Chapter 6 ⟳ p. 620). and carer-induced illness (see Factitious or induced illness in Chapter 4 ⟳ pp. 332-4).

Refractory status epilepticus

- See Treatment Algorithm in Chapter 6 ⟳ pp. 624-5 for treatment regimes.
- EEG may be used to titrate third line therapy, e.g. barbiturate coma sufficient to achieve suppression-burst for 12h before attempted withdrawal.
- Secondary complications of aggressive antiseizure therapy are common (e.g. pneumonia and intestinal ileus with thiopentone infusion).
- The aggressiveness of antiseizure treatment needs to be tailored to individual circumstances including the aetiology (if known) of the status epilepticus, response to therapy in previous episodes and prior levels of neurodisability.

Psychiatry consultations

Conduct/behaviour disorder—is it epilepsy?

This question often arises in contexts of temper outbursts or other erratic/inappropriate behaviour. A detailed history defines the nature of the events (see Funny turns: episodic events in Chapter 3 ➔ pp. 148-52). Video footage may be very useful and is certainly a higher priority than EEG.

- Are events truly paroxysmal (abrupt start and stop)?
- Are events truly stereotyped (i.e. features consistent between episodes) or are contents situational or contextual?
- Are events truly random, or do they occur in certain settings, or in the presence of particular people? Were there well-defined triggers?
  - An ABC analysis is often undertaken in children with behavioural problems, using diaries or other methods to assess the Antecedents (what was happening in the run-up to the episode of concern), the features of the Behaviour itself and the Consequences (what happened next: how others responded to the behaviour).
  - The more an ABC analysis makes sense (i.e. the behaviour is explicable on the grounds of antecedents or consequences) the less likely it is to be epilepsy.

Recourse to EEG for supportive evidence should *only* be considered after *careful reflection* if genuine diagnostic doubt persists because of the very real risk of over-interpreting non-specific findings of uncertain significance which are more likely in children being seen by psychiatry services, particularly if they have any learning difficulties.

- Psychiatrists occasionally use antiseizure drugs for 'episodic dyscontrol'. They are effective mood stabilizers: their efficacy is not evidence of epilepsy.

Previously unidentified attendant developmental coordination disorder (DCD) and/or specific learning difficulties leading to educational and other failure are a far more common cause of conduct/behaviour disturbance. Liaise with the local neurodevelopmental paediatrician and educational services.

- Define the child's educational strengths and weaknesses.
- Examination will reveal significant coordination difficulties.
- Educational liaison/remedial therapy as appropriate.

Also consider mannerisms, stereotypies, and tics.

Differential diagnosis of psychosis

Diagnostic uncertainty in the initial phases of primary psychosis is common and neurology opinions may be sought. Main differentials of primary psychiatric psychosis are:

- Behavioural problems (particularly at school) due to unrecognized learning difficulties (see School failure in Chapter 3 ➔ pp. 191-2);
- Acute confusional states (see Agitation and confusion in Chapter 3 ➔ pp. 114-5);
- Very much more rarely, primary neurodegenerative disease; see Adolescence in Chapter 4 ➔ pp. 480-1.

History

Primary psychosis (e.g. schizophrenia, schizoaffective disorder, delusional disorder) may have an acute onset, but it is more commonly preceded by a prodromal period (up to 12 months) of transient and/or attenuated psychotic symptoms, unusual behaviour, and/or social withdrawal together with falling school performance.

- Any history of an active seizure disorder?
- Is there history of substance use (e.g. alcohol, cannabis, opioids, cocaine, other stimulants, hallucinogens)? Differential diagnosis with drug-induced psychosis or co-morbidity with primary psychosis?
- Any correlation with the use of prescription drugs (e.g. Steroids, isotretinoin, anticholinergics, antidepressants, ASMs, antimalarials)?
- Family history particularly of schizophrenia and psychosis?

Symptoms

- Hallucinations?
  - *Visual* hallucination is suggestive of acute confusional state: see Agitation and confusion in Chapter 3 ⊋ pp. 114-5.
  - *Auditory* hallucination and specifically hearing 'running commentary' third-person voices talking about the patient is more typical of primary psychosis.
- Delusions (fixed or falsely held beliefs).
- Disorganized thoughts and speech.
- 'Negative symptoms' (e.g. emotional apathy, lack of drive, poverty of speech, social withdrawal, self-neglect).
- Fluctuating higher mental function.
- Cognitive impairment (e.g. working memory, verbal fluency, social cognition), usually subtle at first, often pre-date the onset of the main symptoms of psychosis.
- Is there hard evidence of true cognitive decline (i.e. actual loss of clearly previously established ability)?
- Compare 'developmental ceiling' effects: see School failure in Chapter 3 ⊋ pp. 191-2.

Examination

- The presence of motor signs (pyramidal, extrapyramidal, or cerebellar) is incompatible with a diagnosis of primary psychosis.

Assessment

- In a young child with visual and cognitive regression mistaken for 'autism' consider late infantile NCL; see Pre-school years (2–5 yrs) in Chapter 4 ⊋ pp. 476-7.
- In older children consider neurodegenerative disorders particularly:
  - Wilson disease;
  - juvenile X-linked adrenoleukodystrophy;
  - systemic lupus erythematosus and CNS vasculitides;
  - late-onset vitamin B_{12} deficiency;
  - Huntington disease;
  - vCJD, SSPE;

see Adolescence in Chapter 4 ⊋ pp. 480-1.

Acute behavioural disturbance

See Agitation and confusion in Chapter 3 pp. 114-5.

Complications of anti-psychotic drugs

Anti-psychotic drugs carry a risk of extrapyramidal syndromes including parkinsonism, acute dystonia, akathisia, tardive dyskinesia, and neuroleptic malignant syndrome. These are less likely with the newer, 'atypical' anti-psychotics.

- Parkinsonism onset typically insidious after several weeks' therapy.
- Acute dystonia is typically rapid (within a week of starting or increasing dose).
  - may last from minutes to hours.
  - most commonly involves the neck, but tongue, trunk, or limbs also seen.
- Akathisia
  - subjective sense of distress and 'inner restlessness'.
  - repetitive movements (pacing, walking on the same spot, rocking from foot to foot), standing and sitting repeatedly.
  - may be acute or delayed.
  - also seen during withdrawal of anti-psychotics.
- Tardive dyskinesia
  - usually affects mouth and face with stereotyped chewing, tongue protrusion, or lip smacking, may involve rocking or finger flexion and extension.
  - ± oculogyric crises and akathisia.
  - most often associated with neuroleptics (e.g. phenothiazines, haloperidol), atypical anti-psychotics (e.g. risperidone, olanzapine) and more rarely antiemetics (e.g. metoclopramide or prochlorperazine); also theophylline.
  - estimated incidence ~1% those taking these drugs.
  - late complication (hence 'tardive').

Management

Discontinue the drug if possible or substitute a drug less likely to cause problem.

- Parkinsonism, acute dystonia, and akathisia: consider lowering dose or switching to drug with less risk (e.g. quetiapine, clozapine), if clinical condition allows.
- Tardive dyskinesia: stop anti-psychotic if possible. If essential, switch to an agent with less risk.
- Parkinsonism and acute dystonia (including oculogyric crisis): anti-cholinergic drugs (e.g. procyclidine, benztropine).
- *Akathisia*: β-blockers; benzodiazepines also useful.
- Tardive dyskinesia: consider tetrabenazine, diazepam, clonazepam, or promethazine.

Neuroleptic malignant syndrome

May present with an altered level of consciousness or behaviour, progressing to muscle rigidity, hyperthermia, rhabdomyolysis, and autonomic dysfunction.

- Lab tests: high CK, myoglobinuria, leucocytosis.
- Withdraw the drug.
- Aggressive correction of hyperpyrexia, dehydration, and hypovolaemia in the PICU.
  - 20% mortality from respiratory failure.
- Bromocriptine may reverse the syndrome; dantrolene is helpful in achieving peripheral muscle relaxation.
- If clinically indicated, a low potency neuroleptic can be reintroduced very slowly when the individual recovers, although there is a risk of recurrence.

Neuropsychiatric liaison work

Effective liaison between neurology and psychiatry is important for children with many conditions. Examples include:
- The adolescent with dyskinetic cerebral palsy who presents with food refusal due to increasing insight into their disability.
- The child with an autistic spectrum disorder and seizures presenting with new episodes of altered awareness, odd affect, and possible auditory hallucinations.
- Rage and aggression in the context of temporal lobe epilepsy.
- Epilepsy and non-epileptic seizures.
- Acquired brain injury: see Medium and long-term medical management in Chapter 4 ⮞ pp. 221-2.
- Functional neurological symptoms. (See Functional neurological symptoms in Chapter 4 ⮞ pp. 335-9).
- Chronic fatigue or pain.

Areas of joint management

Tics and Tourette syndrome

Neurologist
- Establishing diagnosis of tics after consideration of differentials such as myoclonus or seizure disorder.
- Diagnosis of Tourette syndrome if appropriate; see Tic disorders and Tourette syndrome in Chapter 4 ⮞ pp. 447-8.
- Arranging of 12-lead ECG prior to consideration of treatment with agents that may prolong the QT interval. Check QT_c.

Psychiatrist
- Assessment and treatment of co-morbidities (OCD, ADHD).
- Advice on monitoring of medication used and its escalation.
- Advice on psychological strategies for managing tics (e.g. massed practice).

Behavioural management in difficult to control epilepsy
Children with poorly controlled seizures may have difficulties with behaviour and attention interictally. Episodic behavioural episodes may be mistaken for seizures and, for example, lead to excessive and inappropriate use of emergency seizure medication (e.g. buccal midazolam).

The role of the neurologist is to define seizure events where possible (reviewing video data); to define the extent of subclinical seizure activity and its impact on cognitive function; and to define a protocol for seizure management for psychiatry staff.

Psychotropic medications (e.g. stimulants) have the theoretical potential to lower the seizure threshold although this risk is often small in practice.

Psychiatrists may play a role in addressing some of the emotional and social effects of severe epilepsy: see Epilepsy and daily life in Chapter 4 ⮞ pp. 317-23.

Aggression, conduct disorder, and oppositional defiant disorder
Diagnostic criteria for these conditions are established, but their practical value is debated. Difficulties may occur only in the family context or in a

wider social context. The earlier the onset of conduct disorder, the worse the risk of serious offending in later life.

Described as occurring in two age groups: middle childhood/early adolescence, and adolescence. In the latter, a distinction between socialized (with preservation of peer relationships) and unsocialized (offending alone with little guilt or concern) is useful. Physical aggression is less common in adolescence: truancy becomes more common; drug taking, sexual offences and prostitution can occur, and gang fighting occurs in large cities.

Management
• Parenting skill training (e.g. Webster–Stratton for parents and children).
• Cognitive problem-solving skill training and family therapy (may be limited by learning difficulties).
• Social measures including support for housing and benefit applications.
• Very limited role for psycho-pharmacological intervention.

Consider assessment for occult learning difficulties, sensory and perceptual difficulties, and autism.

Autism and epilepsy

Epilepsy is common in children with autism (one of the strongest pieces of evidence for a neurobiological, rather than psychosocial basis for autism), and many general epilepsy management principles apply.

Autistic regression
'Setback autism'—the onset of social and communicative withdrawal *after* apparently normal acquisition of the first few words—is relatively common.
• There has been debate about the extent to which non-convulsive status epilepticus, particularly DEE-SWAS-like processes might contribute to autistic regression (by analogy with Landau–Kleffner syndrome; see (Developmental) epileptic encephalopathy with spike-and-wave activation in sleep ((D)EE-SWAS in Chapter 4 ➲ pp. 286-7).
• This hypothesis would predict some children with autism might be potentially helped by ASMs but this is controversial.
  • The incidence of epilepsy in autistic children is comparable in those with and without a clear history of regression.
  • Regression ('setback') rates are comparable in those with and without epilepsy.
  • Sleep EEG 'epileptiform' abnormalities are seen in 10% even in the absence of regression and epilepsy (19% in those with regression).
• IQ is related to the presence of regression, not the presence of the EEG abnormality.
• In practice, achieving a sleep EEG is often very challenging in children with autism and yield is low. Epileptic exacerbation of autistic symptoms appears rare; nevertheless, sleep EEG is worth considering particularly if the severity of the autistic picture appears to fluctuate.
• Autistic symptoms *do* appear particularly common in children with seizures of right temporal lobe onset.

For most children with autism and epilepsy, antiseizure therapy should be long-term even if seizure freedom has been achieved. Long-term remission (seizure freedom off medication) is probably seen in about 15%.

Renal consultations

Henoch–Schönlein purpura (anaphylactoid purpura)

An IgA-mediated autoimmune disorder affecting the joints, kidney, GIT, and skin. Neurological manifestations occur in 2–7%.

- Headaches, changes in consciousness or behaviour, seizures, hemiplegia, paraplegia, cortical blindness.
- PNS effects: polyneuropathy, mononeuropathy, and brachial plexopathy.
- Management is supportive.

Systemic lupus erythematosus (SLE)

See Autoimmune CNS vasculopathies in Chapter 4 ➜ p. 398.

Haemolytic–uraemic syndrome (HUS)

This is closely related to the pathologically indistinguishable entity of thrombotic thrombocytopenic purpura (TTP). Both cause thrombotic microangiopathy: the kidney is the major target in HUS and the brain in TTP but there is some overlap. HUS is broadly broken down into those with (D+) and without (D–) a diarrhoeal prodrome.

D+ HUS

A triad of thrombocytopenia, bloody stools, and renal failure. Associated with *E. coli* O157:H7 and *Shigella dysenteriae* infection. Typically food-borne initially though person-to-person spread a risk as it may be shed in the stool for several weeks after resolution of symptoms. Organisms produce verocytotoxins that bind to endothelial cells in the kidney.

D-HUS

Heterogeneous aetiology:

- Drugs (including ciclosporin, tacrolimus, quinine).
- Autoimmune disease including SLE.
- Neuraminidase-producing organisms including *Pneumococcus*.
- Inherited disorders of immune regulation particularly of the complement system (e.g. Complement Factor I deficiency).
- Inborn errors of metabolism (e.g. Cobalamin C deficiency) .

Children with a recurrent, familial, or neonatal course have worse outcomes. Better in those who do not require dialysis. Late mortality is as high as 25%.

Neurological features

- Neurological complications occur in 30–50%.
- Seizures, stupor, coma, hallucinations, focal deficits including extrapyramidal signs. A cerebellar syndrome with truncal ataxia and mutism has been described.
- May occur in the absence of significant renal failure or hypertension.
- Management in D+HUS is symptomatic. Neurological sequelae occur in 10–20%.
- Eculizumab therapy should be considered in D-HUS.

Hypertensive encephalopathy

Presentations
- Raised ICP syndrome with characteristic 'red flag' headache features (see Recurrent or chronic headache in Chapter 3 **⊃** pp. 166-8) and/or papilloedema.
- Focal seizures.
- New onset focal motor signs (due to haemorrhage).
- Posterior reversible encephalopathy syndrome (PRES) (see below).

Management
Liaise early with PICU/renal consultant.
- Control of seizures must be guided by blood pressure:
  - Antiseizure medications may lower blood pressure and have an impact on cerebral perfusion.
- Both cerebral and renal autoregulation are affected by hypertension.
  - Sudden drops in blood pressure are to be avoided as they increase the risk of focal infarction, particularly of the optic nerve.
- A gradual reduction in blood pressure titrated with a labetalol infusion is a recommended approach with volume boluses given as required.

Posterior reversible encephalopathy syndrome

- A relatively common cause of encephalopathy with seizures and motor signs.
- Usually occurs in children with chronic kidney disease, hypertension, autoimmune disorders (like SLE or vasculitis), or with chemotherapeutic agents.
- Non-specific: despite the name may not be strictly posterior (occipital), nor indeed fully reversible!
- Classically presents with seizures whose occipital onset are indicated by post-ictal visual loss (in otherwise alert—if terrified—child).
  - In practice, any focal neurological syndrome possible.
  - Headaches, and altered mental status are also frequent.
- Classically causes a symmetric posterior white matter signal change on MRI:
  - Distribution of signal change, however, highly variable.
  - Early diffusion-weighted imaging (DWI), will demonstrate cytotoxic oedema and intracellular swelling.
  - T2 changes may be delayed.
  - Ischaemia/infarction may enter radiological differential diagnosis: consideration of whether changes conform to an arterial territory or watershed distribution may be helpful.
- Prognosis depends on prompt recognition: usually there is near complete recovery on treatment of cause.
  - Delay in treatment may result in permanent ischaemic change.
- Treatment is supportive: treating the underlying cause, along with antihypertensive and seizure control, and withdrawal of the offending drug.
- Very similar appearances and features can be seen in ciclosporin toxicity (see Fig. 5.3 Ciclosporin neurotoxicity for typical appearances).
- Child may be of course both hypertensive and on ciclosporin!

Intracranial hypertension

- Secondary to prolonged steroid use for renal disease (e.g. nephritic syndrome).
- For investigation and management, see Idiopathic intracranial hypertension in Chapter 4 ⟳ pp. 347-8.

Rhabdomyolysis/myoglobinuria

- Rarely present primarily to the renal team although nephrological input may be required for fluid management and/or acute secondary renal failure.
- See Periodic paralyses in Chapter 4 ⟳ pp. 445-6 for investigation.

Neurological effects of uraemia

These are now rare because of early dialysis:
- Encephalopathy.
- Seizures.
- Myoclonus.
- Peripheral neuropathy:
  - Affecting two-thirds of children in chronic renal failure.
  - Distal symmetric mixed sensory-motor polyneuropathy.
  - Restless legs, burning feet sensations.
  - Rarely a fulminant course with flaccid quadriplegia.
  - Improves with dialysis and transplantation.
- Myopathy.

Neurological complications of renal transplantation

Largely the effects of chronic immunosuppression:
- Infection in an immunocompromised host: see CNS infection of the immunocompromised host in Chapter 4 ⟳ pp. 377-81.
- Ciclosporin neurotoxicity: see also Ciclosporin neurotoxicity in this chapter ⟳ p. 573.

The reason for transplant (e.g. renal dysplasia) may be associated with a risk of seizures as occurs in Bardet–Biedl syndrome. Poorly controlled seizures may warrant investigation for other causes (Laurence–Moon–Biedl syndrome has been associated with hypothalamic hamartoma).

Central pontine myelinolysis

Also known as osmotic demyelination syndrome. Rare syndrome associated with over-rapid correction of hyponatraemia. Also reported in association with end-stage renal disease and/or dialysis, liver transplantation and with over-rapid correction of chronic malnutrition states (e.g. in eating disorders, and chronic alcohol dependency in adults).
- Characteristically biphasic with initial mild to moderate encephalopathy due to hyponatraemia (seizures, confusion, visual hallucination) followed a few days later by deteriorating conscious level and in particular pseudobulbar palsy with trismus and pyramidal signs combined with a 'pseudobulbar affect' (emotional lability).
- MRI typically shows patchy pontine T2 signal change associated with restricted diffusion.
- Treatment is supportive along with addressing the underlying cause.
- Outcome better in children than reported in adult literature: intact recovery possible.

Respiratory consultations

Long-term ventilation

CNS or neuromuscular disease may lead to respiratory insufficiency. Decisions on the use of long-term ventilation must be preceded by open discussions with the child and family on the aims of treatment and quality of life issues: see Withdrawal of care decisions in this chapter ➔ p. 587. Ventilation will support respiration, and probably improve quality of life and survival.

Functional factors predisposing to ventilatory failure:

- Inspiratory failure due to poor central drive, poor coordination or weakness of diaphragm, external intercostals, or accessory muscles.
- Expiratory failure and poor cough due to poor coordination or weakness of abdominal muscles and internal intercostals.
- Bulbar paresis leading to poor swallow and secretion retention.

See also Respiratory disease in neurodisability in Chapter 4 ➔ pp. 260-3.

Nocturnal respiratory failure and support

Physiological tone reduction during REM sleep exposes diaphragmatic weakness; and/or bulbar weakness leads to obstructive sleep apnoea. Strongly suggested by daytime hypercarbia, an indication for further assessment.

Indications for nocturnal non-invasive ventilation (NIPPV):

- Night-time restlessness, frequent awakenings, or sleep-disordered breathing.
- Morning headaches.
- Daytime fatigue or hypersomnolence.
- Deterioration in schoolwork.
- $PaCO_2 > 6$ kPa (45 mmHg).
- Nocturnal oxygen saturation <88% for 5 consecutive minutes.
- Maximal inspiratory pressure <60 cm H_2O.
- Forced vital capacity <50% predicted.

Difficulties/contraindications for NIPPV:

- Poor mask tolerance.
- Bulbar involvement with secretion retention despite assisted cough.

The respiratory/long-term ventilation team will advise on mask fitting and ventilator type, usually pressure-support, bi-level type devices (BIPAP).

- A set expiratory positive airway pressure prevents airway obstruction.
- An inspiratory positive airway pressure is set together with a back-up rate for when the child does not trigger a breath.
- Set-volume type ventilators may be used to supply higher pressures when needed but cannot compensate for leaks like pressure-support devices.

Diurnal respiratory failure and support

More common in CNS disorders but use in neuromuscular disease is increasing. Often preceded by tracheostomy.
Indications:

- Diurnal hypercarbia despite adequate nocturnal ventilation.
- Dyspnoea.
- Increasing infections despite adequate cough therapy.

Disordered breathing patterns

Central apnoea

Central hypoventilation syndrome is defined as persistent alveolar hypoven-tilation and/or apnoea during sleep and impaired ventilatory responses to hypercapnia. Cessation of breathing for >20 s, ± bradycardia and cyanosis.

Generally a problem of infancy but may be seen later in childhood due to acquired brain injury, e.g. after irradiation of posterior fossa tumours.

Physiological causes

• Inefficient central control of respiration in pre-term babies (periods of regular, irregular or periodic breathing predominate), diminishing as term approaches; worse if ill.
• Temperature control (incubators).

Pathological causes

• Drugs.
• Sepsis.
• Metabolic:
  • hypoglycaemia;
  • hypocalcaemia;
  • hypo- or hypermagnesaemia.
• Intracranial haemorrhage.
• Polycythaemia with hyperviscosity.
• Necrotizing enterocolitis.
• Patent ductus arteriosus.
• Gastro-oesophageal reflux.
• Seizures.
• Neuromuscular disease.
• Encephalitis.
• Cardiopulmonary disease.
• Metabolic disease.
• Anatomical abnormalities of brainstem, including Chiari malformation.
  • usually an incidental finding but take note if posterior fossa contents 'tight'; see Chiari malformations in Chapter 4 ➜ pp. 359–60.
• Achondroplasia.
• Genetic disease:
  • Prader–Willi syndrome;
  • Riley–Day syndrome: see Hereditary sensory and autonomic neuropathies in in Chapter 4 ➜ p. 435.

Idiopathic congenital central hypoventilation syndrome

Unexplained by any of the above. Polysomnography shows hypoventila-tion predominates in non-REM sleep with absent ventilatory and arousal response to hypercapnia and hypoxia.

Seen with autonomic dysfunction: very low heart rate and respiratory rate variability, abrupt asystole, abnormal pupillary reactivity, temperature dysregulation, profuse sweating, swallowing difficulties, and/or oesophageal dysmotility.

Associations:

• Hirschprung disease (seen in 20% cases).

- Neural tumours e.g. neuroblastoma, ganglioneuroblastoma or ganglioneuroma (seen in 5–10%).
- Test for *PHOXB* gene (encodes a key transcription factor in the development of the autonomic nervous system).

Late-onset central hypoventilation syndrome

Presents following respiratory infection or anaesthesia which may trigger the need for nocturnal ventilator support. Often preceded by chronic pulmonary hypertension, right heart failure, or respiratory infections with seizures or need for mechanical ventilation. Test for *PHOXB*. Mutations show variable penetrance and environmental cofactors may provoke presentation.

Management of central hypoventilation syndromes

- Detailed history.
- Oesophageal pH monitoring.
- EEG.
- Polysomnography, as available/required:
  - When not available assemble as much data as possible from ECG/EEG/video, nursing observations.
  - In particular, what is the sequence? Bradycardia before apnoea? Reflux before apnoea? Breathing strongly against closed glottis?

Counsel parents. Consider acetazolamide, non-invasive/long-term ventilation as appropriate.

Hyperpnoea

Causes:

- ↑ ICP.
- Impending coning.
- Behavioural phenotype in a number of syndromes, including:
  - Rett, see Epilepsies with findings on genetic testing in Chapter 4 ➲ pp. 295-7;
  - Joubert, see Epilepsies with findings on genetic testing in Chapter 4 ➲ p. 424;
  - Angelman, see Symptomatic epilepsies with genetic abnormalities in Chapter 4 ➲ pp. 295-7;
  - Leigh syndrome (a number of patterns may be observed, including sighing or apnoea, see Leigh syndrome in Chapter 4 ➲ p. 408);
  - Pitt-Hopkins, see Epilepsies with findings on genetic testing in Chapter 4 ➲ pp. 295-7;
  - Learnt behaviour, often for pleasure, in children with global impairment (may enjoy inducing seizures).

Stridor

Most often in neonates or infancy. History and examination give diagnostic clues but endoscopy is usually, and imaging may be, required.

History:

- Age at onset.
- Acute or chronic.
- Character, variation, triggers, relieving or exacerbating factors.

Examination:
- Severity.
- Phase (inspiratory, expiratory, biphasic).
- General tone and posture.
- Handling secretions?
- Character of cough, cry, and voice?

Imaging:
- Lateral neck X-ray for soft tissues.
- Barium swallow: tracheo-oesophageal fistula?
- MRI.
- Possibly pH monitoring.

Stridor may be inspiratory, expiratory, or biphasic. Inspiratory stridor suggests a laryngeal obstruction, expiratory stridor implies tracheobronchial obstruction, and a biphasic stridor suggests a subglottic or glottic abnormality.

Acute stridor is almost always infective. Most neurological stridor is chronic; other causes include congenital or acquired stenosis or other compressive abnormalities, including webs, rings, aberrant vessels, etc.

Laryngomalacia
- Accounts for 75% of childhood stridor.
- Inspiratory: worse with crying or feeding.
- Better when prone.
- Consider central hypotonia or a neuromuscular disorder.
- Gastro-oesophageal reflux: remediable with treatment.

Vocal cord dysfunction
- If unilateral may give weak cry and/or biphasic stridor, improving when lying on affected side.
- Bilateral paresis may give severe respiratory distress.
- Consider:
  - syringobulbia or other ponto-medullary abnormality;
  - Chiari II abnormality;
  - recent intra-thoracic surgery;
  - congenital laryngeal nerve palsy.

Dystonia/dyskinesia of vocal cords/larynx
- Occasionally seen in older children as a focal dystonia or as part of a more generalized dystonia.
- Leads to paroxysmal dysphonia or pervasive strangulated sound to utterance.

Liaison is centred on respiratory support, chronic lung disease as a co-morbidity; see Respiratory disease in neurodisability in Chapter 4 ➔ pp. 260-3, and disordered breathing patterns.

Rheumatology consultations

CNS features of autoimmune and autoinflammatory disease

Whereas 'autoimmune' disorders typically involve cross-reactivity between a host and a target antigen, 'autoinflammatory' disorders are genetically determined disorders of the innate, general immune response.

These conditions are characterized by diffuse inflammatory changes in the connective tissue, which may involve the CNS or peripheral nervous system in isolation or as part of a systemic vasculitis. In this section, we deal primarily with CNS complications of known systemic disease. See Inflammatory disease of the CNS and 'Autoinflammatory' conditions in Chapter 4 ➔ pp. 391-400 and pp. 401-3 for discussion of CNS-first presentations of previously unrecognized autoimmune disease including:

- Sydenham chorea;
- Systemic lupus erythematosus;
- Sarcoidosis;
- Autoimmune CNS vasculopathies;
- Hashimoto encephalitis;
- Autoimmune encephalitis;
- Rasmussen encephalitis;
- Paraneoplastic syndromes;
- Haemophagocytic lymphohistiocytosis (HLH).

Henoch–Schönlein purpura (see Henoch–Schönlein purpura in this chapter ➔ p. 597) and Haemolytic–uraemic syndrome (see Haemolytic–uraemic syndrome in this chapter ➔ p. 597) are discussed elsewhere in this chapter.

Kawasaki disease

Diagnosis

Unexplained fever for >5 days and ≥4 of the 5 clinical features:

- Non-purulent bilateral conjunctivitis.
- Papulosquamous peripheral lesions.
- Erythematous trunk lesions.
- Cervical lymphadenitis, usually unilateral.
- Inflamed mucous membranes in oropharynx and respiratory tract.

Note that not all symptoms may be present simultaneously!

Thrombocytosis is common. If coronary artery aneurysms are present, the diagnosis is usually confirmed.

25% have aseptic meningitis (mononuclear CSF pleocytosis). Hemiplegia, seizures, and subdural effusions have been reported. Younger children typically show marked irritability.

Treatment

Prompt treatment with IVIG and aspirin reduces the risk of cardiovascular complications.

Steroids, infliximab, cyclosporine are treatment options in IVIG resistant patients.

Post-COVID multisystem inflammation

PIMS-TS ('paediatric inflammatory multisystem syndrome temporally associated with SARS-CoV2'), also known in North American literature as MISC-C ('multisystem inflammatory syndrome in children associated with COVID') refers to a rare Kawasaki-like multisystem inflammatory syndrome developing a few weeks after typically mild SARS-CoV2 infection.

• Presenting features are very similar to Kawasaki disease although patients typically older and coronary artery aneurysm does not appear to be typical.
• Neurological involvement in more than 30% of patients, usually with headache, seizures, confusion, drowsiness.

Treatment
• IVIG; corticosteroids; aspirin.
• Anakinra; tocilizumab.
• Supportive management of 'long COVID' symptoms (fatigue, 'brain fog').

Dermatomyositis

Although primarily a disease of muscle and skin, CNS vasculitis can occur; see Juvenile dermatomyositis in Chapter 4 pp. 449-50.

Infection in the immunocompromised host

See CNS infection in the immunocompromised host in Chapter 4 pp. 377-81.

Transition to adult services

A topic of long-overdue increased discussion and attention over the last decade.

* The move from paediatric to adult services is often a time of enormous anxiety and avoidable distress for young people and families.
* For all the inadequacies of paediatric services the reality is that their funding is relatively protected in most health systems: under-resourced adult services have had to respond to increasing numbers of 'graduates' from paediatric services with needs of ever-growing complexity. Manage expectations.
* Incompatibilities between the fundamental models of care between paediatric and adult services create enormous challenges particularly for parents:
  * paediatric services' overarching model of supporting a child *within their family* are replaced by a goal of as much independence as possible in adult living and thriving.
  * a complex package of care established over many years supporting a child with their parents may be seen by adult services as 'tying' the young person to them in ways that can only become more unsustainable with time.
  * Parental 'letting go' is a major part of the challenge.
* A longer history of medical sub-specialization in adult than paediatric medicine tends to mean adult care is divided across a greater number of teams.
* Adult services typically have much larger caseloads and expectation management e.g. around time available for discussion in clinic is important.

▶▶ The age at which young people can give and withhold consent for medical treatment varies between jurisdictions but in the UK the important concept of 'Gillick competence' recognizes that young people can demonstrate an adult understanding before the legal age at which ability to consent is universally assumed; and can give, *but not withhold* consent independently of their parents before that age (16 in the UK).

There can be no single model of transition to adult services appropriate to all young people's needs, all underlying medical conditions, and all health systems. Some principles:

* Start early. The life expectancies of children with even the severest cerebral palsies mean planning for adulthood will be needed.
* Transition is a *process*, not an event. Over a period of several years young people should be supported to develop an independent role in the management of their health needs.
  * regularly review their understanding of their health condition, its treatments, and its implications for them in adulthood (for employment, education, driving, relationships, sexuality) and help them develop this.

- ask yourself how much you are teaching and training the young person, rather than the parents.
- increasingly involve, and then favour, the young person in consultations and decision making.
- help parents to increasingly accept the role of onlooker, advocating when necessary but recognizing the appropriateness of this change.
- provide opportunities for the young person to talk to you alone, and in confidence.
- Identify the adult professionals who will take on the young person's care early and involve them in medical care during an overlap period during which the young person can get to know them.
- Special considerations arise for young people with intellectual disabilities that will limit their ability to manage their own affairs in adulthood.
  - Legal provision differs between jurisdictions, but most offer a framework for deciding to what extent and in what areas of life an adult might require a publicly appointed independent guardian to oversee their affairs and ensure their best interests and protection from exploitation.

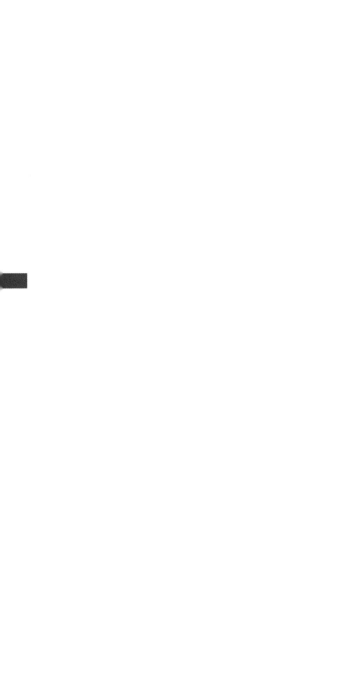

Chapter 6

Emergencies

Acute behavioural disturbance

Agitation of children and adolescents is distressing and can endanger the patient, carers, and health professionals.

Distinguish between:

- *Agitation*: uncontrolled behaviour, due to excessive motor or verbal activity, which could cause harm to self or others.
- *Delirium*: waxing and waning mental status associated with an underlying medical problem.
- *Psychosis*: aberrant thinking, perceptions, and behaviour resulting in a loss of contact with reality. Can occur as a primary psychiatric disorder or due to an underlying medical condition.

In nearly all situations, environmental, rather than pharmacological, management is to be preferred.

Environmental changes

- Reduce environmental noise (e.g. TV).
- Ensure the room is well-lit.
- Preferably use a familiar setting.
- Allow the child to mobilize to an extent consistent with safety—avoid restraint wherever possible. Consider removing hazardous items (e.g. potential missiles) from the room and allowing sleeping on a mattress on the floor.
- Reduce the number of unfamiliar bystanders to the minimum consistent with the safety of personnel.
- Have familiar caregivers present.
- Ensure any sensory impairments are minimized (find misplaced hearing aids, glasses). Satisfy basic needs (hunger, thirst).
- Establish a rapport and attempt to reassure; preferably limit the number of involved staff.
- If medication is necessary, oral medication (haloperidol or risperidone) is preferable to parenteral administration.
  - If parenteral administration is considered necessary because oral administration is not possible, intramuscular administration is usually safer and more practicable than intravenous administration in an acute situation (see Acute agitation: drug treatment, in this chapter ➔ p. 611).
  - Parenteral haloperidol can cause acute oculogyric crisis or dystonia (treat with procyclidine).

Identify and treat the cause

Delirium has many possible causes, some of which are life-threatening. It is, therefore, a medical emergency.

Causes of delirium

Morbid mnemonic! I WATCH DEATH

- Infection: extracerebral (pneumonia, UTI, sepsis, malaria) or intracerebral (meningitis, encephalitis, cerebral abscess); parainfectious including ADEM.
- Withdrawal: alcohol, benzodiazepines, opiates, and other sedatives.
- Acute metabolic: hypoglycaemia, hepatic, renal, or pulmonary insufficiency. Electrolyte imbalance. Very rarely: porphyria, late-onset metabolic disease (see Late-presentations of metabolic disease in Chapter 4 ➋ pp. 484-7).
- Trauma: head injury, burns, heatstroke.
- CNS pathology: space-occupying lesion, epilepsy (status and post-ictal states) other encephalopathies.
- Hypoxia.
- Deficiency: thiamine B_1, folate, pyridoxine B_6, B_{12}.
- Endocrine: thyroid, adrenal, hypopituitarism, or parathyroid dysfunction.
- Acute vascular: TIA; stroke; hypertensive encephalopathy; post-cardiac surgery (especially post-cardiac bypass); cardiac failure or ischaemia; subdural haemorrhage; subarachnoid haemorrhage; vasculitis, e.g. SLE; cerebral venous thrombosis; migraine.
- Toxins or drugs: prescribed (steroids, sedatives, ASMs, narcotic analgesics) or recreational. Carbon monoxide poisoning.
- Heavy metals: lead, mercury.

Drug treatment

Treat the underlying cause. Symptomatic treatment of agitation with drugs should only be used when essential and even then with care especially in children. Antipsychotics and especially benzodiazepines can aggravate delirium, exacerbate underlying causes (e.g. benzodiazepines worsening respiratory failure), and can cause significant unwanted effects, e.g. acute dystonic reactions.

> ❶ It is generally preferable to use regular rather than 'as required' dosing: as the latter implies waiting for a recurrence of the disturbed behaviour before intervening; however, this mandates *at least daily review* of the prescription in light of wanted and unwanted effects.

Benzodiazepines
- Usually preferred when delirium is associated with withdrawal from alcohol or sedatives.
- Generally *unhelpful* in post-traumatic disorientation after severe brain injury where stimulant medication (e.g. methylphenidate) can be more effective.
- May be used as an alternative or adjuvant to antipsychotics when these are ineffective or cause unacceptable side effects.
- Oral, buccal, intranasal, or intravenous lorazepam or midazolam may be given up to once every 4 h (the intranasal route can be an irritant).
- In children with delirium due to hepatic insufficiency, lorazepam is preferred to haloperidol.

- Excessive sedation or respiratory depression from benzodiazepines is reversible with flumazenil: see Flumazenil in Chapter 7 ⊃ p. 671.

Antipsychotic drugs
- Antipsychotics are the most used drugs in adults but are less popular in children because of extrapyramidal effects.
- Haloperidol is often used acutely because it has few anticholinergic side effects, minimal cardiovascular side effects, and no active metabolites. As it is a high-potency drug, it is less sedating than phenothiazines and therefore less likely to exacerbate delirium. Low-dose haloperidol is adequate for most children. In severe behavioural disturbance, haloperidol may be given intramuscularly (see Haloperidol in Chapter 7 ⊃ pp. 675-6).

Emergency management of coma

For subsequent approach to investigation after immediate stabilization of child in coma: see Coma in Chapter 5 ⊘ pp. 579-81.

Remember initial resuscitation measures: Airway, Breathing, Circulation.

Treat hypoglycaemia (if no explanation, take plasma sample before treating).

Assess Glasgow Coma Scale

- Coma level should be rapidly assessed using the age-appropriate Glasgow Coma Scale (GCS, see Table 6.1).
- If the coma score is deteriorating or <12, look for signs of ↑ ICP and examine the brainstem reflexes for signs of herniation syndromes (see Fig. 6.1) as rapid recognition and treatment of ↑ ICP can save lives.

Table 6.1 Modified Glasgow Coma Scale

	>5 yrs	<5 yrs
Eye opening		
4	Spontaneous	Same as >5 yrs
3	To voice	
2	To pain	
1	None	
Verbal		
5	Orientated	Alert; babbles, coos; words or sentences normal
4	Confused	Less than usual ability, irritable cry
3	Inappropriate words	Cries to pain
2	Incomprehensible sounds	Moans to pain
1	No response to pain	No response to pain
Motor		
6	Obeys commands	Normal spontaneous movements or in infant <9 mths, withdraws to touch
5	Localizes to supraocular pain	Same as >5 yrs
4	Withdraws from nailbed pressure	Same as >5 yrs
3	Flexion in response to nailbed pressure	Same as >5 yrs
2	Extension to supraocular pain	Same as >5 yrs
1	No response to supraocular pain	Same as >5 yrs

With permission from Morray JP, Tyler DC, Jones TK, et al: Coma scale for use in brain-injured children. *Critical Care Medicine* 12:1018-20, 1984.

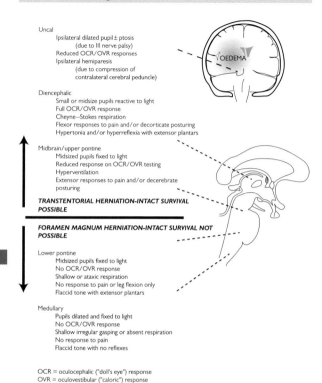

Uncal
    Ipsilateral dilated pupil ± ptosis
        (due to III nerve palsy)
    Reduced OCR/OVR responses
    Ipsilateral hemiparesis
        (due to compression of
        contralateral cerebral peduncle)

Diencephalic
    Small or midsize pupils reactive to light
    Full OCR/OVR response
    Cheyne–Stokes respiration
    Flexor responses to pain and/or decorticate posturing
    Hypertonia and/or hyperreflexia with extensor plantars

Midbrain/upper pontine
    Midsized pupils fixed to light
    Reduced response on OCR/OVR testing
    Hyperventilation
    Extensor responses to pain and/or decerebrate
    posturing

**TRANSTENTORIAL HERNIATION-INTACT SURVIVAL
POSSIBLE**

**FORAMEN MAGNUM HERNIATION-INTACT SURVIVAL NOT
POSSIBLE**

Lower pontine
    Midsized pupils fixed to light
    No OCR/OVR response
    Shallow or ataxic respiration
    No response to pain or leg flexion only
    Flaccid tone with extensor plantars

Medullary
    Pupils dilated and fixed to light
    No OCR/OVR response
    Shallow irregular gasping or absent respiration
    No response to pain
    Flaccid tone with no reflexes

OCR = oculocephalic ("doll's eye") response
OVR = oculovestibular ("caloric") response

Fig. 6.1 Herniation syndromes.

Examine for signs of herniation

Raised ICP is dangerous because:
- It reduces cerebral perfusion pressure (CPP = mean arterial pressure – intracranial pressure) which causes cerebral ischaemia.
- Differences in ICP *between* different brain compartments cause herniation syndromes that cause direct mechanical damage, ischaemia, and haemorrhage secondary to vascular distortion. Recognition requires examination of the brainstem reflexes.

❶ DON'T MISTAKE TONIC POSTURING DUE TO CONING FOR A TONIC SEIZURE: treating supposed seizures with benzodiazepines may make the situation worse as the resulting respiratory depression may cause hypercarbia, increasing cerebral blood flow, and ICP.
- Typically, *tachycardic* in convulsive status, often *bradycardic* and/or hypertensive in coning.
- History and context are typically very helpful.

Examination of brainstem reflexes

Pupil response to light

Use a bright torch. Note resting pupil size and symmetry, and briskness and symmetry of the response to light.

- Do not mistake a dilated non-reactive pupil due to an afferent pupillary defect (optic nerve involvement in fracture of the bony orbit) for third cranial nerve involvement in a herniation syndrome (the consensual response is present in the former, absent in the latter. See Pupil reactions in Chapter 1 ➔ pp. 18-9).

Oculocephalic ('doll's eye') and oculovestibular (caloric) reflexes

If cervical spinal cord injury can be confidently excluded: briskly turn the head to 90° to each side (with assistance to secure endotracheal tube), watching the eyes. The intact response is to appear as if maintaining gaze on a distant object (although it does not rely on intact vision): the eyes move relative to the head and in the opposite direction to the head movement. The abnormal response is to maintain a fixed orientation relative to the head and orbits (eyes stay looking in the direction the head is pointing).

If cervical cord injury cannot be excluded: perform the functionally equivalent oculovestibular (caloric) test. Exclude a perforated eardrum then put the head in the midline with 30° elevation. Inject 50 mL of cold water into the ear canal (collect in dish as it drains out!): observe for 1 min. Intact reflex induces tonic eye deviation toward the tested ear.

Examine fundi.

- Papilloedema in ↑ ICP (may not be present if ICP has ↑ rapidly);
- Presence of venous pulsation implies normal ICP: see Venous pulsation in Chapter 1 ➔ p. 18;
- Macular star in hypertensive encephalopathy;
- Retinal haemorrhages in NAI.

Stabilize

- If GCS is <8 or if evidence of herniation, intubate and ventilate.
- If GCS is 8–10 and evidence of herniation, give 3 mL/kg of 2.7% or 3% hypertonic saline by slow IV infusion. See Hypertonic saline in Chapter 7 ➔ pp. 702-3) or mannitol 0.25 g/kg bolus.
- Intubate and ventilate.

Intubation and ventilation of the unconscious child is likely to be justified to secure the airway and/or for the management of ↑ ICP. Borderline cases should be discussed urgently with an intensivist or anaesthetist.

- If tonic eye deviation or nystagmus, assume subtle motor status epilepticus: see Status epilepticus in Chapter 6 ➔ pp. 621-7.
- If the cause is not obvious, and the child is either <12 months age or GCS is >12, then perform LP. Treat empirically with IV 3rd generation cephalosporin plus IV aciclovir.
- If GCS <12 or deteriorating, delay LP and start IV 3rd generation cephalosporin and IV aciclovir.
- Liaise with local ICU and/or neurosurgeon and arrange transfer if necessary.
- May need urinary catheterization and arterial line.

Immediate investigations

- *Blood*: capillary glucose monitor strip and plasma glucose, alcohol level in appropriate contexts, U&E and creatinine, plasma osmolality, FBC and film, CRP, Ca^{2+}, Mg^{2+}, blood gas, ammonia, LFT, lactate, viral studies, blood cultures (if febrile), coagulation if signs of bleeding or non-blanching rash, group and save sample in context of trauma. If deliberate/accidental poisoning is a possibility, save the plasma sample.
- *Urine*: dipstick test for glucose and ketones, toxicology (notify lab of particular compounds of interest such as medications in the house a child may have had access to as this greatly aids toxicological investigation), microbiology, and osmolality. Samples for amino and organic acids. Freeze an acute sample if any suspicion of inborn error of metabolism.
- *LP if not contraindicated*: see Stabilize in this chapter ➋ p. 615. Measure opening pressure; send for cell count, Gram stain; glucose (with matching plasma sample); lactate and protein; PCR/viral antibodies for herpes simplex encephalitis ± other infectious agents. Oligoclonal bands (with matching serum sample) if ADEM is suspected. Save a sample if possible. Consider saving a cytospin sample if malignancy is a possibility.
- Brain CT/MRI (with contrast if an abscess is suspected).
- Other radiology: skull, cervical, chest, and pelvic X-rays if multiple trauma.

If an inborn error of metabolism is suspected

- Usually a neonate but occasionally a urea cycle disorder can present in later childhood with coma and hyperammonaemia.
- In any situation where a previously unidentified IEM seems possible, stop feeds (a source of protein that may further destabilize) and administer 10% dextrose to prevent tissue catabolism.
- For management of hyperammonaemia and metabolic acidosis, see NICU consults (see Neonatal encephalopathy in Chapter 5 ➋ pp. 558-69). Hyperammonaemia will almost certainly require haemodialysis or haemofiltration.

Further/subsequent investigations to consider

- See PICU consultations section (see Coma in Chapter 5 ➋ pp. 579-81).

Management of raised ICP
Basic measures
- Nurse head in midline and tilted up 30°. Keep head still. Minimal handling/suction.
- Ventilate to normocapnia. Hyperventilate/bag for brief periods only if needed to control severe ICP spikes.
- Fluid: maintain good circulating volume. Observe for SIADH or cranial diabetes insipidus. Careful fluid balance. 6 hourly U&E/osmolality.
- Consider hypertonic saline: see Hypertonic saline in Chapter 7 ➋ pp. 702-3. Hypertonic saline preferable to mannitol as latter may cause hypovolaemia as it acts as an osmotic diuretic.

- Hydrocephalus: consider VP shunt/third ventriculostomy. Discuss with a neurosurgeon.
- Seizures: treat obvious seizures as they may cause a spike in ICP.
- EEG: will be useful if subtle motor or non-convulsive status epilepticus is suspected. May be helpful in prognosis.
- Consider use of cerebral function monitor (see Cerebral function monitoring in Chapter 2 ⊃ pp. 87-91). Requires close support from neurophysiologists, including regular standard EEGs to interpret changes and ensure focal discharges is not being missed.
- Consider a brain MRI within 48 h if the diagnosis is still uncertain.
- Prophylactic barbiturates: use is controversial and not standard in the UK.
- Reducing body temperature: mild hypothermia is of confirmed value in neonatal HIE. Its role in stroke and TBI in older children remains unclear: present trial evidence would suggest no benefit or even harm. Avoid rapid rewarming.
- ICP monitoring: consider in severe head trauma or if the child remains unconscious with signs of ↑ ICP and stable BP more than 6 h after initial investigations and management (see Early neurosurgical intervention in this chapter ⊃ pp. 619-20). Contraindicated in children with low platelet count (<50×10⁹/L) and with caution in other bleeding diatheses.
- CSF drainage or surgical decompression: may be useful if elevation of ICP persists: see Early neurosurgical intervention in this chapter ⊃ pp. 619-20.

Traumatic coma

Severe TBI has a mortality of between 8% and 15% in the UK.

- Initial management should be the same as for coma: see Emergency management of coma in this Chapter ➋ pp. 613-7.
- Avoid sedative (strong opiate) analgesia until assessment has been made.
- Cervical spine immobilization is required when any of the following risk factors are present:
  - GCS <15 at any time since injury;
  - Neck pain or tenderness;
  - Focal neurological deficit;
  - Paraesthesia in the extremities;
  - Any other clinical suspicion of neck injury;
- 'Block and tape' neck immobilization preferable to poorly fitting cervical collars which can also impede cerebral venous return.
  - Only remove immobilization after neurosurgical or spinal surgical agreement: AP and lateral neck X-rays (including peg view if the child is >10 yrs) and/or MRI of the cervical spine may be required after severe trauma.
  - Preferable to avoid neck CT in young children (high radiation doses to the thyroid).
- Intubate and ventilate immediately if:
  - GCS <8.
  - Gag reflex lost.
  - Respiratory difficulties (hypoxia, hypercarbia, respiratory arrhythmia) present.
- Consider intubation and ventilation if:
  - GCS deteriorating.
  - Bilateral fractured mandible or other facio-oral injury present.
  - History of or witnessed seizures.
- Arrange CT head if:
  - GCS <13 at any time since injury or <15 at 2 h after injury.
  - Skull fracture present.
  - Any sign of basal skull fracture (haemotympanum, 'panda eyes', CSF otorrhoea, Battle's sign—blood over mastoid process).
  - History of or witnessed seizures.
  - Focal neurological deficit.
  - Persistent vomiting or severe headache.
  - Dangerous mechanism of injury, including fall from >1 m (5 steps).
  - Known coagulopathy or ↑ risk of fractures.

Abnormal CT findings

You may be the first person to look at the CT scan. Look for signs of:

- Skull fracture.
- Cerebral oedema—compression of CSF spaces, effacement of sulci, midline shift. May get a reversal sign in severe cases—white matter is hyperintense compared with grey matter.
- Haemorrhage (blood is very light grey/hyperintense):
  - Epidural: collection constrained at skull suture lines;

- Subdural: crescentic extraparenchymal collections over frontoparietal convexities. Often a compressed ipsilateral ventricle. Often bilateral. Common in infants. Consider non-accidental head injury in infants;
- Subarachnoid haemorrhage (SAH)—blood anywhere in the subarachnoid space, but most common in the posterior interhemispheric fissure or along tentorium cerebelli. Often accompanied by intraparenchymal damage;
- Intraparenchymal—homogenous hyperintense lesions within the parenchyma. May also get haemorrhagic contusions that are a mixture of oedema and haemorrhage. Contusions are often *contre-coup* injuries (on the opposite side of the head to impact, where displaced brain has struck the inner surface of skull);
- Punctate haemorrhages in cerebral white matter—indicate *traumatic axonal injury*. Seen after a rotational head injury that causes shearing at the grey/white matter border. Often associated with intraventricular haemorrhage and signs of oedema;
- Intraventricular haemorrhage—hyperintense blood seen in the ventricles.

When to get an MRI scan

- Acutely if clinical neurological deficit cannot be explained by CT findings. MRI is much more sensitive to traumatic (shearing) axonal injury which should be suspected in situations of slow recovery after severe injury with relatively 'normal' CT.
  - After the acute phase, MRI is the imaging modality of choice. Timing depends on the individual child.

When to discuss with a neurosurgeon

- Any CT scan abnormality present.
- Persisting coma or confusion despite resuscitation.
- Deterioration in GCS (especially the motor component).
- Progressive focal neurological signs.
- Seizure without full recovery.
- Definite or suspected penetrative injury.
- CSF leak.

Early neurosurgical intervention

- Evacuation of haematoma—usually necessary if a midline shift >5 mm is present or if signs of herniation syndrome are present.
- ICP monitoring—often indicated if abnormalities on CT scan are present or clinical signs of herniation. A variety of methods are used.
  - Insertion of an external ventricular drain with a pressure transducer theoretically permits CSF drainage as an additional therapeutic manoeuvre as well as ICP monitoring; however, ventricles are often already compressed and thus catheters difficult to place;
  - Alternatively, pressure transducers are placed in the subarachnoid space.
- *Decompressive craniectomy*: removal of a section of the skull vault. Indicated for severe intracranial hypertension when medical measures have failed.

- Significantly reduced mortality but perhaps at the expense of survival with very severe disability.
- Skull defect closed after several months with a synthetic plate.
- External ventricular drain—indicated if hydrocephalus is present following SAH or IVH.

Subsequent management

Liaise with ICU, neurosurgical colleagues, and therapists involved in neurorehabilitation.

- For management of ↑ ICP, see Management of raised ICP in this chapter ➔ pp. 616-7.
- *General supportive measures.*
  - Optimize nutrition.
  - Monitor for early complications of spasticity (loss of ankle dorsiflexion range): may need splinting.
  - Prevention of pressure sores.
- Observe for paroxysms of sympathetic over-activity with hypertension, fever, and hyperhidrosis as well as other brainstem signs in children with diffuse axonal injury. See Acute medical management of ABI in Chapter 4 ➔ pp. 219-20.
- Watch for hyponatraemia (see Hyponatraemia in a neuro-intensive care setting in Chapter 5 ➔ pp. 581-2).
- A VP shunt may be required if ventriculomegaly forms after clamping the EVD or if hydrocephalus develops after SAH or IVH.
- Observe for complications of direct vascular trauma including:
  - *Traumatic dissection*—usually follows neck trauma, e.g. whiplash injury. Presents with neck/head pain, stroke symptoms, and signs ± Horner's syndrome and lower cranial neuropathies. Need CT angiogram or thin-slice fat-saturated MR imaging for diagnosis;
  - *Carotid-cavernous fistula*—presents with visual problems, may have proptosis or chemosis of the eye and orbital bruits. Need CT angiogram or MRA for diagnosis.
  - *Traumatic aneurysm.*
- Tracheotomy may be necessary if prolonged ventilation is required.

For neurorehabilitation, see Interdisciplinary working and goal setting in Chapter 4 ➔ p. 221 for more details.

Non-accidental (inflicted) traumatic brain injury

The forensic evaluation of suspected non-accidental head injury is beyond the scope of this book. Your hospital should have protocols in place for the notification of concerns regarding possible inflicted (non-accidental injury) and its investigation.

From a clinical management perspective, the mechanism of injury in inflicted head trauma in infants is often repeated shaking and/or impact against a hard surface. Secondary hypoxic injury is common. The repetitive nature of the inflicted acceleration/deceleration, the severity of the forces, and the additional hypoxia can cause very aggressive cerebral oedema. Acute management of seizures can also be challenging, although this typically abates after a few days. Mortality and late morbidity rates are high.

Status epilepticus

Introduction

- Generalized convulsive status epilepticus (CSE) is defined as a continuous seizure or repeated seizures without full recovery of consciousness.
  - Duration thresholds based on when long-term morbidity is likely (for generalized CSE, animal data suggest perhaps 30 min or longer) are less pertinent than operational definitions of when intervention should occur, which for generalized CSE is usually accepted to be 5 mins.
- Outcome is aetiology and age-dependent.
  - Overall mortality is significant, up to 3%.
  - Neurological sequelae are more frequent in infants: 30% vs. 6% over 1yr of age (may reflect underlying aetiology).
- Causes of CSE include fever (febrile convulsions comprise $^1/_3$ of all CSE in childhood), epilepsy, withdrawal or change of ASMs, CNS infections, cerebral hypoxia, and metabolic disturbance.

The first steps

These steps take minutes only and can be done concomitantly with preparing to start the CSE treatment algorithm (Table 6.2 and Fig. 6.2).

Table 6.2 First steps

	Action	Comments
Airway	Open and maintain airway Give high flow oxygen	Hypoxia causes seizures and contributes to morbidity
Breathing	Support breathing	Grunting and ↑ respiratory rate are common Beware the exhausted child, the child with neuromuscular disease and respiratory depression, either central or secondary to administered drugs
Circulation	Establish IV/IO access Check blood glucose: if hypoglycaemic, draw blood for later investigation and give 5 mL/kg of dextrose 10%	If bradycardic consider possible tonic posturing due to ↑ ICP Shocked child, treat for sepsis Hypertension may be the cause of seizures
Disability	Assess conscious level, pupils, posture Check for neck-stiffness	Decorticate and decerebrate posturing can be mistaken for a tonic seizure Consider acute dystonia Consider non-epileptic attacks
Exposure	Check for rash Measure temperature	Fever (infection, ecstasy) Hypothermia (ethanol, barbiturates)

▶ Conditions that can be mistaken for status epilepticus:
• Extensor posturing due to raised ICP. Children in CSE are typically tachycardic; bradycardia should raise suspicion of raised ICP. In this setting, sedative drugs, e.g. benzodiazepines are **contraindicated** as they suppress respiration and aggravate the situation by causing hypercarbia (see Examine for signs of herniation in this chapter ➲ p. 614).
• Status dystonicus.
• Prolonged non-epileptic attack events.

Treatment algorithm

• This algorithm is useful for most children over 4 weeks of age, presenting in accident and emergency or children's wards.
• Children with an established tendency to recurrent CSE may have their own individualized treatment algorithm.
• One or both of the two first-line doses of benzodiazepine may have been given by parents, teachers or paramedics in the community prior to arrival: there is an absolute limit of *two* doses by any route before proceeding to second-line therapies.

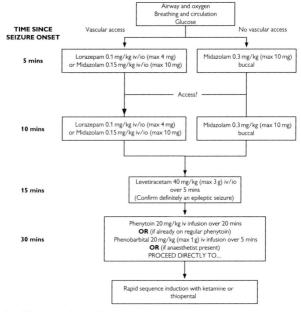

Fig. 6.2 Status epilepticus flowchart.

▶ NB: do not forget supportive medical management.
- Continue to monitor airway, breathing, and circulation.
- Maintain normoglycaemia.
- Monitor electrolytes and fluid balance.
- Treat pyrexia.
- Nasogastric tube to empty stomach contents.
- Management of ↑ ICP: see Management of raised ICP in this Chapter ➔ pp. 616-7.

Status epilepticus investigation

Need for aetiological investigation will depend on background—less pertinent for the child with known difficult epilepsy—but otherwise:
- FBC, U&Es, magnesium, calcium, phosphate, LFT, blood gas, CRP, ammonia, lactate, glucose.
- If febrile, take blood or urine cultures; consider LP.
- Consider blood and urine samples for inborn errors of metabolism, toxicology, and ASM levels (if on treatment).
- Consider the need for brain imaging once stabilized.

Practical aspects of drugs used in the CSE algorithm

Choice of first drug

There are significant international differences in the choice of first-line benzodiazepine for CSE.
- In the UK, buccal midazolam has largely replaced the use of rectal diazepam. If respiratory depression occurs, breathing may need to be supported until this wears off.
- Once IV access is established, lorazepam or midazolam are the drugs of choice. They have longer durations of action than diazepam and fewer respiratory depressant effects. A dose of lorazepam (0.05 mg/kg) or midazolam (0.15 mg/kg) may be effective for many children.

Paraldehyde

- Some 'individualized' CSE management plans will specify paraldehyde in place of parenteral benzodiazepines (less used outside UK).
- Must be diluted in an equal volume of olive oil or saline (not arachis oil because of the risk of nut allergy).
- Premixed preparations are increasingly available.
- Doses may be expressed as mL *of undiluted paraldehyde* **OR** mL *of premixed preparation* (twice the volume).
  - take particular care in correct prescribing.
- Side effects include rectal irritation and sedation.
- Paraldehyde reacts with plastic and so must be given immediately if drawn up in a plastic syringe.
- It should not be given IM (risk of sterile abscess formation).
- The use of paraldehyde should never delay the administration of 2nd line ASM. Only indicated when there are difficulties in obtaining IV/IO access.

Levetiracetam
- Intravenous levetiracetam increasingly replacing phenytoin as second line following recent trial evidence of equivalence.
- 500 mg/5 mL concentrate is diluted in 100 mL 0.9% saline and infused over 5 mins.

Phenytoin
- Phenytoin, 20 mg/kg, must be made up in 0.9% saline solution and infused slowly (over 20–30 min, max. 1 mg/kg/min) with cardiac monitoring (risk of cardiac arrhythmias).
- If the child stops seizing during the infusion, continue to infuse the full dose.
- Phenytoin is severely irritant to veins; watch carefully for signs of extravasation at the infusion site.
- If a child is already on phenytoin, consider giving a reduced load (e.g. 5 mg/kg) or consider an alternative such as phenobarbital.

Refractory convulsive status epilepticus

❗ It is very important to remember that the evidence base for the use of the following drugs and their doses in refractory status epilepticus is that of opinion, experience, and case report. Use of these drugs in status epilepticus is unlicensed. Careful attention must be paid to pharmacopoeia and administration advice. Management of these children will always be individualized in the light of underlying diagnoses, precipitants, and triggers. Seek specialist advice.

Refractory or resistant CSE may be defined as being present when two or three ASMs have failed after following the algorithm.

Manage in an intensive care setting; airway and breathing support and close monitoring of other parameters allow the use of very high doses of ASMs (Table 6.3).

Table 6.3 Possible treatment options

	Route	Dose	Note
Phenobarbital	IV	20 mg/kg/dose (max. 1 g)	Repeated doses until child stops seizing, or plasma levels >40 mg/L
Phenytoin	IV	9–20 mg/kg/dose (max. rate 1 mg/kg/min)	Repeated doses until child stops seizing, or plasma levels >20 mg/L
Midazolam	IV	0.15 mg/kg IV (max. 10 mg) or 0.3 mg/kg buccal loading dose (max 10 mg)	Loading dose followed by IV infusion starting at 2 microgms/kg/min. Increase in 4 microgms/kg/min increments every 30 min to initial max. of 20 microgms/kg/min (use of higher doses reported)

Table 6.3 (Contd.)

	Route	Dose	Note
Clonazepam	IV	50 microgms/kg/dose (max 1 mg)	Can follow with infusion of 10–60 microgms/kg/min. Troublesome secretions may limit use
Sodium valproate	IV	25 mg/kg loading dose (max 2.5 g/24 h)	25 mg/kg loading dose if not already on drug 10 mg/kg loading dose if already on drug
Levetiracetam	IV	20 mg/kg loading dose (max. 3 g)	If response, ±load again, follow with maintenance 12 hourly Accumulates if impaired renal function
Anaesthetic agents	IV and inhaled		Liaise with intensivist/anaesthetist
Thiopental	IV	5 mg/kg bolus	Infusion rate 3–5 mg/kg/h. Maintain seizure-free for 12 h (or titrate to suppression-burst on EEG) and then wean over 2–3 days Caution: hypotension, atelectasis, paralytic ileus
Ketamine	IV		Initially 0.5–2 mg/kg as slow IV injection over 1 min, followed by continuous intravenous infusion of 0.6–2.7 mg/kg/h adjusted according to response
Isoflurane and desflurane	Inhaled		Onset of action in minutes, result in burst-suppression on EEG Caution: hypotension, apnoea, atelectasis, infection, paralytic ileus
Propofol			No longer recommended, ↑ mortality compared with midazolam

There are many case reports of other drugs used with effect. If the seizure activity is highly focal, an emergency corticographically guided resection of an active seizure focus may be considered.
See also FIRES in Chapter 4 pp. 287-8.

Clustering

Either in association with an episode of CSE or as an independent event, long runs of frequent brief seizures may occur without meeting continuity criteria for status. The child should be managed in a high-dependency setting with the facility to support the airway and breathing rapidly if needed.

The intravenous drugs discussed for refractory CSE (see Table 6.3) may be considered, with awareness of the risk of respiratory depression and hypotension. Other possible treatment options are shown in Table 6.4.

Table 6.4 Other treatment options for seizure clusters

	Route	Dose	Note
Chloral hydrate	Oral	10–40 mg/kg/dose po qds for 24 h	Expect sedation
Clobazam	Oral	1–2 mg/kg/day po divided into two or three doses	Oral secretions may be limiting (as with clonazepam)
Paraldehyde	Rectal	1–3 mL/kg per dose 3–6 hourly	Sedation and rectal irritation may be limiting
Topiramate	NG	2 mg/kg/day	Rapid titration over days to 10–15 mg/kg total daily dose
Vigabatrin	Oral	50 mg/kg total daily dose	Titrate up in 10–50 mg/kg/day steps up to 150 mg/kg total daily dose

May precipitate abnormal movements |

Neonatal status epilepticus

The incidence of seizures is higher in the neonatal period than at any other time of life (2–3 per 1000 term live births rising to 10–15 per 1000 pre-terms). Most neonatal seizures are subtle, manifesting with combinations of motor, behavioural, and autonomic symptoms, making them difficult to recognize clinically. Generalized tonic–clonic seizures are exceptional.

▶ Neonatal seizures are more likely to be symptomatic, thus it is vital to look for the cause and if possible, treat it. Prognosis depends largely on this underlying cause. See Neonatal seizures in Chapter 5 ➋ pp. 551-5.

Drug treatment
There is a lack of good clinical evidence for ASM efficacy in neonatal status epilepticus and uncertainty as to the extent to which EEG evidence of seizure activity should be pursued in the absence of clinical convulsions. There are concerns from the basic science literature about possible adverse effects of ASMs on the developing brain; to be balanced against evidence of adverse effects of neonatal seizures themselves on neurodevelopmental outcome and ↑ rates of epilepsy in later life. Keep the number of ASMs used to the minimum possible (neonates quickly develop tolerance; see Table 6.5).

Table 6.5 Drugs in neonatal status epilepticus

Phenobarbital	First line
	Effective in about a third of babies
	20 mg/kg IV loading dose. A second loading dose of 20 mg/kg can be used to achieve therapeutic levels
	NB: loading doses can cause apnoea in unventilated baby
	Followed by 5 mg/kg/day in two divided doses
Levetiracetam	40 mg/kg IV loading dose. A 2nd loading dose of 20 mg/kg may be necessary
	Followed by 40 mg/kg/day iv or oral, in two divided doses
Phenytoin	Second line
	20 mg/kg IV loading dose
	Maintenance doses in neonates can be up to 10 mg/kg/24 h
	Monitor cardiac rhythm and respiratory rate
	Poor oral bioavailability. If prolonged treatment is required, switch to oral carbamazepine
Carbamazepine	10 mg/kg/day in two divided doses (first choice in suspected *KCNQ2* related epilepsy)
Midazolam	Loading dose of 150 microgms/kg followed by infusion of up to max. 300 microgms/kg/h
	Monitor respiratory depression and heart rate changes. Myoclonic jerks and dystonic posturing reported as side effects
Lidocaine	2 mg/kg then 6 mg/kg/h for 4 h; then taper over 24 h

For further details of treatment regimes, see Treatment in Chapter 5 ➔ pp. 554-5.

- Current guidelines retain phenobarbital as first-line treatment.
- Second-line options are phenytoin, levetiracetam, midazolam, or lidocaine.
- If there is a family history of epilepsy, consider phenytoin or carbamazepine as 1st line (*KCNQ2*-related epilepsy).
- Levetiracetam may be preferable to phenytoin in the context of cardiac disease.

Remember the vitamin-responsive conditions: all neonates with CSE should be empirically treated with pyridoxine, followed by a trial with pyridoxal phosphate if ineffective; and folinic acid and biotin pending further investigation. See Protocol for further investigation of refractory neonatal seizures of unknown cause in Chapter 5 ➔ pp. 555-7.

Status dystonicus

Definition

Status dystonicus (SD; also known as *dystonic storm* or *dystonic crisis*): increasingly frequent and severe episodes of generalized dystonia requiring urgent hospital admission. SD represents the severe end of a continuum of worsening dystonia. In contrast to CSE, the goal of treatment is not usually to completely stop or end dystonic spasms, but to reduce their intensity to achieve comfort and medical stability.

SD happens more commonly in children and can arise acutely in children with no past history of dystonia. A robust evidence base for treatment is lacking, but an ABCD approach is suggested:

- Address precipitants.
- Begin supportive care.
- Calibrate sedation.
- Dystonia-specific medications.

Address precipitants

A cause for SD can be found in 60–70% cases. Common causes include:

- Febrile infection.
- Pain (especially in children with background dystonia).
- Medication changes.
- Failure or interruption of deep brain stimulation (DBS) or intrathecal baclofen (ITB).

> For a child with an implanted intrathecal baclofen pump (see Surgical management of spasticity and dystonia in Chapter 4 ⊃ pp. 249–52) SD must be presumed to be due to pump or (more usually) catheter failure and resultant **acute baclofen withdrawal** until proven otherwise.

Prompt recognition and treatment of precipitants are necessary to speed up resolution of the episode.

Begin supportive care

Medical complications of SD affect many different systems. Overall mortality is around 8%.

Airway/Respiratory

- Compromise is common due to respiratory muscle spasm, vocal cord adductor spasm, aspiration, exhaustion, and use of sedative medication.

Management

- Ensure patent airway, examine chest.
- Monitor oxygen saturation, and blood gases as indicated.
- Assess the safety of oral feeding.
- Paralysis and intubation may be required.

Cardiovascular

- Tachycardia, hypertension.
- Excess sweating causing dehydration and electrolyte disturbance.

Management
- Fluid resuscitation, monitor electrolytes (↑ insensible losses through sweating and fever can rapidly lead to dehydration, and maintenance fluids may need to be ↑ by an additional 5–20% to compensate).
- Monitor vital signs, peripheral perfusion, signs of dehydration, renal function.

Gastrointestinal
- Poor oral intake, acute liver injury due to myoglobinaemia.

Management
- Early insertion NGT for fluid/feed delivery.
- Monitor LFTs:
  - note that ↑ ALT levels in isolation are more probably of muscle origin due to rhabdomyolysis than a sign of liver failure.

Renal
- *Important risk of acute kidney injury* due to dehydration and/or myoglobinaemia and ↑ CK from rhabdomyolysis.

Management
- Check for myoglobinuria (urine dipstick +ve for 'blood' in the absence of red blood cells on urine microscopy, confirmed with plasma CK and myoglobin levels).
  - Note the rise in CK is late and levels may not peak until 24–48 h after muscle damage, whereas myoglobinaemia is usually cleared within 6 h).
- Manage child on the basis of electrolyte abnormalities (usually ↑ K$^+$, PO$_4$$^{2-}$, Ca^{2+}, urate) and *not* on the basis of CK.
- Seek advice from the renal team if acute renal failure is present.
- If urine output is reasonable (>0.5 mL/kg/h):
  - High fluid input = 3 L/m^2/day (0.45% saline/2.5% dextrose);
  - Add sodium bicarbonate to fluids, aim for urine pH >7 (start with 10 mmol sodium bicarbonate/500 mL).
- If oligo- or anuric:
  - Consider fluid challenge (5–10 mL/kg), possibly with furosemide to establish urine output.
  - If unsuccessful, dialyse for severe electrolyte disturbance (CVVH should clear myoglobin reasonably well, but no real data in children).

Metabolic
- Hypoglycaemia can result from pancreatic dysfunction associated with myoglobinaemia.

Pain
- Extremely common.
- May be a trigger for episodes (vicious circle).

Management
- Identify triggers (e.g. gastro-oesophageal reflux, constipation, dental caries, mouth ulcers, hip dislocation).
- Ensure adequate analgesia.

Non-pharmacological interventions
- Many children with dystonia are much more cognitively intact than levels of impairment might lead you to predict, with the potential for considerable awareness of their situation. Psychological/emotional factors can further aggravate their underlying dystonia. This should be considered, and appropriate support provided.
- Positioning can be very helpful in aborting spasms in some children. In particular, using seating, pillows, sleep systems etc. to maintain hip flexion, and to keep the neck flexed and head in the midline position are important.
- Physiotherapy assessment may provide additional strategies to improve spasm-free periods and sleep. In some children, handling may exacerbate dystonia, and this should be minimized to necessary care.

Calibrating sedation
- Temporizing sedative strategies remain a mainstay of treatment. New-onset dystonia with acute CNS illness usually improves over time and may be managed expectantly.
- SD in the context of a chronic neurological disorder may be more difficult to manage.
- The risks of complications from severe dystonia need to be measured against the risk of unwanted effects from the high doses of sedation required (Table 6.6). Specialist advice may be required!

Consider using objective dystonia scales and serial video to assess response to treatment. Remember: the aim is to reduce dystonia and to enhance sleep, not to terminate SD abruptly or completely.

Table 6.6 Sedative medications for use in SD

Drug	Doses	Side effects to look for
Chloral hydrate	30–50 mg/kg (max 1 g/dose) TDS (can be given rectally)	Gastric irritant, rash, headache Ketonuria Eosinophilia, low WCC
Clonidine	1–3 microgms/kg/dose initially TDS, ↑ dose and/or frequency as necessary Can be given as IV infusion, initially 0.5 microgms/kg/hour, increasing in 0.5 microgms/kg/hour steps to 2 microgms/kg/hour. Higher doses may be required with expert supervision	Antihypertensive: monitor BP closely initially. Avoid sudden withdrawal
Alimemazine (Trimeprazine)	2 mg/kg/dose (max 60 mg) max BD (use with caution <6 months)	Antimuscarinic effects (urinary retention, dry mouth, GI disturbance) Extrapyramidal effects Mood change, irritability Liver dysfunction Arrhythmias

Table 6.6 (Contd.)

Drug	Doses	Side effects to look for
Diazepam oral and rectal	Rectal (PRN: can repeat dose ×1) <1 yr 2.5 mg PR 1–3 yrs 5 mg PR >3 yrs 10 mg PR Oral <1 yr 250 microgms/kg bd 1–4 yrs 2.5 mg bd 5–12 yrs 5 mg bd >12 yrs 10 mg bd	Long half-life Doses may be cumulative Drowsiness, irritability Respiratory depression Tolerance may occur
Midazolam buccal (use IV preparation if specific buccal formulation not available)	500 microgms/kg (max 10 mg) buccal or sublingual	Respiratory depression Cardiovascular depression (severe hypotension)
Midazolam IV	Slow IV injection of 100–200 microgms/kg then infusion of 30 microgms/kg/h increasing according to response	Potentiated by erythromycin and other drugs
Lorazepam IV	Used PRN 50 microgms/kg/dose (max 4 mg) Can repeat ×1 if required Max dose of 0.1 mg/kg or 8 mg in 12 h	Respiratory depression Hypotension Use with caution in liver disease

Light sedation and muscle relaxation

A number of sedatives (e.g. chloral and clonidine) and/or muscle relaxants (oral/rectal diazepam, buccal/IV midazolam, IV lorazepam) may be useful alone or in combination to provide relief from painful and exhausting spasms and allow periods of sleep. Extreme care should be taken to monitor children when using combinations of drugs with sedating properties.

Heavy sedation/muscle relaxation

• Intravenous midazolam is commonly used: it has a long half-life, allowing slow weaning. It also has a spinal interneuron blocking action, of benefit in children with dystonia.
• Intravenous clonidine is increasingly used: it causes less respiratory depression than benzodiazepines.
• Levels of sedation achieved with these drugs require close monitoring of cardiovascular and respiratory function, and this may necessitate PICU admission.

Dystonia-specific medications

A wide range of medications have been reported as potentially beneficial in SD, some outlined in Table 6.7:
- Dystonia-specific medications will likely be required for some time after an episode of SD.
- Levodopa should be considered particularly in children with idiopathic dystonia. Use for 3 months in maximal doses before discontinuing.

Table 6.7 Dystonia medications

Drug	Dose	Recognized side effect
Levodopa All doses quoted are for the levodopa component of Sinemet®	Sinemet®-62.5 (carbidopa 12.5 mg, levodopa 50 mg): start 1 mg/kg/day (below 1 yr, start at 0.25 mg/kg/day) increasing to max dose 10 mg/kg/day Once total dose of levodopa is >100 mg/day switch to Sinemet®-110 (10 mg carbidopa, 100 mg levodopa) as less carbidopa is preferable	GI upset Sleep disturbance Hypotension, arrhythmias Red urine Psychiatric manifestations Peripheral neuropathy
Trihexyphenidyl	Start 1 mg TDS (<8 yrs) or 2 mg TDS (>8 yrs). Increase total dose by 1 mg (<8 yrs) or 2 mg (>8 yrs) every 7 days until clinical effect or side effects intervene or max dose 10 mg TDS	Anticholinergic effects (urinary retention, dry mouth, dry eyes, blurred vision, GI disturbance, etc.)
Tetrabenazine	<4 yrs start 6.25 mg OD >4 yrs start 12.5 mg OD, increasing to 12.5 mg TDS Adolescent start 25 mg OD increasing to 25 mg TDS	Depression (may be severe) Risk of neuroleptic malignant syndrome with rapid escalation
Haloperidol	12.5–25 microgms/kg BD (max 10 mg/day) further increase under guidance from paediatric neurologist	Extrapyramidal signs Tardive dyskinesia
Gabapentin	Day 1: 5 mg/kg OD Day 2: 5 mg/kg BD Day 3: 5 mg/kg TDS Day 4: 10 mg/kg TDS Can be ↑ in 5 mg/kg steps to 20 mg/kg/TDS	Sedation Respiratory depression at higher doses, particularly if used with other sedatives

- Trihexyphenidyl requires a slow escalation to high dose or until unwanted effects (anticholinergic, e.g. urinary retention, blurred vision, GI upset) intervene.
  - If this occurs reduce the dose and maintain at a reduced level for a month before increasing again. This may allow greater toleration of higher doses.
- Gabapentin has a particular role when acute/chronic pain/discomfort is a driver (e.g. hip subluxation).
- More sedative medications, e.g. clonidine and benzodiazepine, may also have a long-term role, but the benefits of ongoing side effects need to be weighed against potential gains.

For all children with SD not improving within 1–2 weeks, neurosurgical interventions should be considered: intrathecal baclofen (see Surgical management of spasticity and dystonia in Chapter 4 ➋ pp. 249–52) or Deep brain stimulation. Early discussion should be initiated with specialist centres providing these interventions, particularly in children with identified causes for their dystonia known to respond well to such approaches (e.g. GNAO1-related encephalopathy).

Mimics of SD:

Mimics of SD potentially requiring specific interventions are outlined in Table 6.8

Table 6.8 Mimics of status dystonicus

Mimic	Clinical features to help distinguish from SD	Specific interventions
ITB withdrawal	Arising in child with ITB pump in situ. Confusion/delirium and seizures can occur	Urgent re-initiation of ITB therapy High-dose enteral baclofen and enteral or parenteral benzodiazepines as bridging therapy
Neuroleptic malignant syndrome	Triggered by withdrawal of dopaminergic medication, or initiation of dopamine antagonist/depletors (e.g. neuroleptics or tetrabenazine) Higher fever, rigidity, and autonomic dysfunction. Can be accompanied by rhabdomyolysis	Cessation of provoking medication Supportive care
Serotonin syndrome	Serotinergic excess most commonly due to serotinergic medications Mild symptoms include shivering and diarrhoea, more severe abnormal mental state, rigidity, fevers, and seizures	Cessation of provoking medication Supportive care
Malignant hyperthermia	Reaction to inhalational anaesthetics or depolarizing muscle relaxants Fever, rigidity, and spasms, elevated heart rate, and rhabdomyolysis	Supportive treatment with cooling Dantrolene Investigation for genetic predisposition (e.g. RYR1 mutations)

Sudden onset visual loss

The duration of visual loss is a clue to aetiology: loss for seconds in papilloedema; for minutes in transient ischaemic events (e.g. emboli) and occipital epilepsy; hours in retinal migraine; and days in optic neuritis.

⊃ Truly *monocular* visual loss (i.e. vision out of the other eye is completely normal) implies a cause *anterior to the chiasm*.

Optic neuritis
- Typical age at presentation ~7 yrs; ♀>♂.
- Preceding viral illness.
- Unilateral presentation at onset may be followed rapidly by bilateral involvement. Presents with severe loss of acuity, field defects, and central scotomata.
- Disc swelling of optic neuritis may be mistaken for papilloedema. However, in papilloedema, visual loss is late and RAPD rare.
- VEP usually abnormal (helpful in retrobulbar neuritis where no other signs may be found). VEP is normal in functional blindness.
- See Optic neuritis in Chapter 4 ⊃ pp. 266-7.

Functional visual loss
- Assessment can be challenging.
- Usually a teenage girl.
- Visual fields usually reported as markedly constricted and often 'cylindrical' (boundary of visual field a constant distance from visual axis irrespective of distance) rather than 'conical' (fixed angle from visual axis).
- Easier diagnosis when visual loss is total rather than partial.
- Helpful observations are:
  - Visual behaviour: orientated in space and able to manoeuvre without injury;
  - Pupillary responses normal;
  - Electro-diagnostic tests normal (VEP and ERG);
  - Normal nystagmus with an optokinetic drum;
  - Moving a mirror close to the face will cause the eyes to move if vision is present (refixation reflex).
- See also Functional neurological symptoms in Chapter 4 ⊃ pp. 335-9.

Retinal migraine
- A major cause of transitory monocular blindness.
- Scintillating, shimmering scotomata, abnormal perception of colour and movement, can be binocular, usually lasts less than 60 min.
- Symptoms are accompanied or followed by headache.
- Recurrences are in the same eye.

Binocular visual loss

- Progressive visual field restriction (e.g. due to a slowly expanding lesion at the optic chiasm, or a retinal dystrophy) can be surprisingly asymptomatic until it involves the macula, at which point it may present acutely. The pathology may be more longstanding than the history suggests.

The child who suddenly stops walking

The child who has lost the ability to walk should be considered a potential neurological/neurosurgical emergency and urgent imaging may be required.

▶ A seemingly more pressing acute illness may mask the fact that a child has also lost the ability to walk or mobilize. Avoid this pitfall by performing a thorough neurological assessment in any sick child.

History

The list of causes is enormous but the history will provide a starting point. Specific questions should cover:
- What can the child not do?
- What is the temporal sequence of events?
- Was there a precipitating factor?
- Are there any sensory disturbances (loss or gain)?
- Is there pain? Location and quality?
- Is there or has there been intercurrent illness?
- Is the child well or is there systemic illness?
- Is the child on any medication?
- Has there been foreign travel?
- Have there been insect bites?
- Is there a family history?
- What is the child's mood/affect?
- What does the child/family think is the cause?

▶ Always specifically ask about bladder and bowel function to identify spinal pathology.

Historical clues to aetiology may include:
- Post-ictal: Todd paresis.
- Post-migraine: hemiplegic migraine.
- Preceding trauma: cord pathology causing compression, infarction, transection; stroke due to arterial dissection.
- Recent intercurrent illness: Guillain–Barré, transverse myelitis.
- Viral encephalitis: echovirus, enterovirus, Coxsackie virus.
- Tick bite: Lyme disease.
- Semi-acute onset with bladder and or bowel involvement: spinal tumour.
- Chemotherapy: vincristine, cisplatin.
- Infant with progressive constipation, poor suck, and descending pattern of involvement: infant botulism (history of exposure to sources such as honey may not be present).
- Adolescent with a history of intravenous drug abuse: wound botulism.

Examination

▶ Establish whether this is a child who *can't* move because of weakness; or a child who *doesn't want* to walk because of pain, or fear of falling due to unsteadiness.
▶ Be persistent in cajoling and assisting the child to walk as much as possible in order to try to make this distinction.

As ever, the purpose of examination is to locate the site(s) of pathology. Acute weakness will be due to either cord, nerve root, peripheral nerve, neuromuscular junction, or muscle weakness.
- Identify the pattern of any weakness:
  - Proximal suggests myopathy.
  - Distal suggests neuropathy.
  - Symmetrical or asymmetrical?
- Are peripheral tendon reflexes present? Plantar responses?
- What is the anatomical distribution of any sensory disturbances?
  - Is it consistent with a spinal dermatomal level, or a peripheral nerve pattern? (See Table 1.6 in Chapter 1 ➋ p. 40.)
- What modalities of sensation are involved?
  - Selective loss of spinothalamic (pain and temperature) sensation with preservation of vibration and joint position sense seen in anterior spinal artery syndrome.
- Is there involvement of the sphincters?
  - Is the anal sphincter closed tight or lax?
  - Is perianal sensation intact?
  - Is the anal reflex (sphincter contraction in response to drawing point across perianal skin) preserved?

Investigation

The main urgent decision is whether this child needs an emergency MRI of the spine at appropriate level(s). This is required in any situation where examination locates the lesion to the spinal cord, as extrinsic spinal cord compression is a neurosurgical emergency with outcome depending on prompt relief of compression.

Indications for MRI if there is:
- A complaint of *back* pain (in contrast, *limb* pain is common in, and consistent with, Guillain–Barré).
- Weakness in all muscle groups below a particular spinal root level.
- History of trauma.
- A dermatomal pattern of sensory involvement (not always seen).
- Sphincter involvement typically implies intrinsic cord involvement. *Sphincter function may be preserved* in situations of external cord compression so its preservation is not necessarily reassuring. In the latter situation, there is often loss of spinothalamic sensation (temperature and pin-prick) in the perianal area.

If in doubt discuss with regional neurosurgical service urgently.

The child who can't walk and has a peripheral weakness

See Table 6.9 for causes.

Table 6.9 Causes of inability to walk and peripheral weakness

Affected region	Cause		Useful early investigations
Muscle	Myositis	Transient acute myositis/myalgia with viral illnesses	Elevated CK; viral titres
		Dermatomyositis	
	Rhabdomyolysis	Disorders of carbohydrate metabolism	Elevated CK; acyl carnitine profile when symptomatic
		Disorders of fatty acid metabolism	
	Periodic paralysis (autosomal dominant channelopathies)	Familial hypo-, hyper-, and normokalaemic periodic paralyses	K+ levels in blood; ECG
Neuromuscular junction	Autoimmune	Myasthenia gravis	Tension test; peripheral neurophysiology
	Acquired	Botulism	Peripheral neurophysiology
		Tick paralysis (North America, Dermacentor species)	
		ICU weakness (combination of neuromuscular blockade drugs, corticosteroid myopathy, and depletion of myosin; usually presenting as failure to wean from ventilator)	
Peripheral nerve	Guillain–Barré syndrome		Peripheral neurophysiology; CSF protein (late)
	Metabolic	Hypokalaemia	
		Acute intermittent porphyria	
	Toxic	Vincristine, lead, mercury, arsenic	
Anterior horn cell	Poliomyelitis		Peripheral neurophysiology

Affected region	Cause		Useful early investigations
Spinal cord	Spinal cord compression		MRI
	Epidural	Metastases (leukaemia, lymphoma, neuroblastoma)	
		Abscess	
		Haematoma (haemophilia, trauma)	
		Bony compression (Morquio syndrome, Down syndrome; fracture/dislocation of vertebrae)	
	Intradural	Neurofibroma	
	Intramedullary	Glioma	
		Ependymoma	
		Hydromyelia	
	Spinal cord transection	Trauma	MRI
	Transverse myelitis		MRI
	Vascular	Anterior spinal artery occlusion (infarction of anterior portion of cord resulting in loss of spinothalamic pain and temperature sensation, with preservation of dorsal column light touch, proprioception, and vibration due to different blood supply)	MRI
		Vascular malformations (may present with acute bleed or infarct in first two decades of life)	
	Discitis	(Rare before adulthood)	MRI
	Metabolic/toxic	Recreational nitrous oxide use	History
		Biotinidase deficiency	Biotinidase activity

Guillain–Barré syndrome

GBS is an acute immune-mediated demyelinating polyradiculoneuritis, frequently preceded by a non-specific infection, and presenting with a classic triad of *weakness, areflexia and elevated CSF protein without pleocytosis* (the latter may not be present early). (See Guillain–Barré syndrome in Chapter 4 ➔ pp. 266–7); also see Box 6.1 Practice points.

> **Box 6.1 Practice points**
> - Uncommon conditions with clinical presentations resembling Guillain–Barré syndrome include neurotropic viral infections (poliomyelitis, West Nile virus, Japanese encephalitis); botulism; and metabolic conditions including Brown–Vialetto–van Laere syndrome (presence of hearing impairment should alert you to the latter).
> - Acute flaccid myelitis due to Enterovirus D68 typically predominant upper limb involvement (c.f. polio) but can be misdiagnosed as Guillain–Barré. Cases peaks in summer and early autumn.
> - Examination should correlate with neuroanatomy or else suspect a functional cause

Presentation
- Progressive ascending motor weakness with areflexia/hyporeflexia.
- Almost half will become non-ambulant.
- Usually symmetrical.
- Not uncommonly:
  - Sensory impairment, often with distressing paraesthesiae;
  - Cranial nerve involvement;
  - Autonomic dysfunction.
- Transient sphincter dysfunction occasionally occurs.

Clinical features
- Ascending weakness starting in legs: usually symmetrical though can be quite asymmetric on occasions.
- Absent deep tendon reflexes.
- Can have bulbar and ocular involvement.
- Respiratory involvement in 50%: monitor respiratory function (no single parameter is reliable in children).
- Pain, paraesthesia. Toddlers in particular may present with predominant early symptoms of back pain rather than weakness.
- Deafness is *inconsistent* with Guillain–Barré: if present consider the vitamin-responsive Brown–Vialetto–van Laere syndrome: see Vitamin B_2 (riboflavin) in Chapter 4 ➔ pp. 523-4.
- Autonomic dysfunction (constipation, urinary retention, incontinence, excessive sweating, hypertension, arrhythmias).
- Rarely diagnostic confusion can occur if encephalopathy due to hypoxia has already occurred, masking the peripheral site of the pathology.

Investigations
CSF
- ↑ protein (after first week).
- Typically <10 white cells/mm³.

Nerve conduction studies
- Typically slow nerve conduction with conduction block.
  - Very low CMAP amplitudes on early (<1 week) EMG can be due to conduction block.
  - Only place significance on this finding (i.e. inferring it's an acute motor axonal neuropathy (AMAN) with implications for slower and poorer recovery) if present after a week.
- Distal latencies ↑ (may not be abnormal for several weeks).

Imaging
- Enhancement of nerve roots on MRI.

Others
- Serology for mycoplasma, EBV, CMV, VZV, *Borrelia*.
- Stool for *Campylobacter*, Coxsackie.
- Antiganglioside antibodies (may be helpful where there is diagnostic doubt but typically take several weeks).
  - Anti-GQ1b in Miller–Fisher variant;
  - Anti-GM1 in AMAN variant.
- Consider MRI brainstem and cord if doubtful features:
  - Clear sensory level;
  - Predominant bladder or bowel dysfunction;
  - Explosive/rapid onset.

▶Careful monitoring of bulbar, respiratory (FVC), cardiovascular, and autonomic status is vital.

Management
See Table 6.10 for complications of GBS.

Table 6.10 Complications of Guillain–Barré syndrome

Bulbar dysfunction	Dysphagia, weak cough, unable to clear secretions
Respiratory compromise	Vital capacity below 15–20 mL/kg, breathlessness on exertion; deteriorating blood gases (rising CO_2)
	Do not wait until the child becomes hypoxic or exhausted. Most deaths in childhood are due to preventable respiratory complications
Autonomic instability	Sweating, sinus tachycardia, hypertension, labile blood pressure, bradycardia, arrhythmias
	Monitor temperature, heart rate, BP, respiratory rate, vital capacity, pupils, GCS, cough, swallow, urine output

Treatment

IV immunoglobulin
- 2 g/kg divided over 3–5 days.

Indicated if: progressive deterioration at the time of presentation; non-ambulant; bulbar dysfunction; respiratory compromise.
- Accelerates the rate of recovery.
- Late treatment (3 weeks after symptom onset) is not of proven benefit.

Plasmapheresis is as effective as IVIG, but there are practical difficulties. Long-term outcome is *worsened* by steroids.

Admit to PICU if
- Rapidly progressive tetraparesis.
- Respiratory compromise.
- Bulbar dysfunction.
- Autonomic cardiovascular instability (autonomic instability is a predictor of fatal cardiac arrhythmias).

General care
- Thrombosis prophylaxis in older, larger children (stockings and low-molecular weight heparin).
- Nutrition, skin care.
- Gabapentin useful for painful dysaesthesiae (common in the recovery phase).
- Psychology.
- Rehabilitation.
- Monitor for occasional late complications of communicating hydrocephalus due to high CSF protein.

Typical clinical course
- Deterioration over 2–4 weeks (>4 weeks implies CIDP; see Chronic inflammatory demyelinating polyneuropathy in Chapter 4 ➲ pp. 437-8).
- May be severe with respiratory compromise requiring ventilation (15–20%).
- Plateau phase.
- Recovery phase:
  - Good recovery for most with significant improvement evident within about 2 weeks;
  - Morbidity, about 10% left with significant residual disability;
  - Mortality, from respiratory and autonomic dysfunction, is lower than in adults (1–8%).
- Positive prognostic factors: milder course, early start of recovery, younger age, no evidence of denervation.

Spinal cord compression

See Box 6.2

> ### Box 6.2 Key features of spinal cord dysfunction
> - Sensory level.
> - Level of motor weakness.
> - No cranial nerve involvement.
> - Urological symptoms (frequency, dribbling, retention, priapism).
> - *Breathing may be affected in high lesions*

Symptoms
- Paraesthesiae in the legs.
- Weakness (difficulty climbing stairs).
- Bladder and bowel (constipation).
- Back pain.

Early signs
- Tender over the affected area of the spine.
- Loss of pin-prick sensation in the legs.
- Loss of proprioception and vibration sense in the feet.
- Deep tendon reflexes in the legs are brisker than in the arms (or may be paradoxically reduced, particularly in thoracic lesions).
- Sweat level (↓ sweating below the lesion).
- Sensory level (more reliably examined over the back, not the abdomen).

Late signs
- Definite weakness.
- Definite hyperreflexia and extensor plantars.
- Loss of abdominal reflexes.
- Loss of anal tone.

Investigations
- All children with suspected spinal cord compression need urgent spinal imaging (MRI).
- Investigations for malignancy as appropriate.

Management
- High-dose steroids in all, dexamethasone 0.25 mg/kg IV (max. 10 mg).
- Neurosurgical referral.
- Specific treatment depends on the cause:
  - Surgical decompression;
  - Radiotherapy;
  - Spinal shock in traumatic spinal cord injury (loss of sympathetic tone to blood vessels resulting in delayed capillary refill time, hypotension, bradycardia), IV methyl prednisolone 30 mg/kg load, then continuous infusion of 5 mg/kg/h for 15 h.
- Supportive care: respiratory support; careful attention to bladder and bowel; GI stress ulcer prophylaxis; prevention of pressure sores; nutrition.

- Rehabilitation: multidisciplinary team: see Acquired spinal cord injury in Chapter 4 ➔ pp. 224-6.

Transverse myelitis

Transverse myelitis is an acute focal inflammation of the spinal cord with demyelination and swelling, most often thoracic (80%) or cervical (10%). Affected children are usually aged 5 yrs or older. (See Acute transverse myelitis in Chapter 4 ➔ pp. 267-8).

Post-infectious, autoimmune, and primary inflammatory mechanisms have been suggested; a preceding infection is noted in 60% (EBV, mumps, myco-plasma, rubella, rubeola, varicella).

Clinical course
- Abrupt or rapid onset, over 1–2 days, of the features of spinal cord dysfunction.

Early symptoms
- Paraesthesia of the legs.
- Back pain at affected segmental level.
- Fever, lethargy, malaise, myalgia.
- Later motor loss (initial spinal shock—weak and flaccid—becoming spastic and paraplegic).
- Loss of bowel and bladder function.
- Improvement usually begins after 1 week (though may not be for weeks).

Examination
- Identify the segmental level.
- Transitional zone (between affected and unaffected spine) dysaesthesia and hyperalgesia.
- Loss of sweating below the level.
- Flaccid paralysis initially (may become spastic with UMN signs as recovery proceeds).

Investigations
- MRI to exclude spinal cord compression and to confirm the lesion—moderate cord swelling, ↑ signal on T2, enhanced with gadolinium.
- CSF pleocytosis (lymphocytosis), normal or slightly ↑ protein, normal glucose.
- EMG normal (there may be some anterior horn cell dysfunction in involved segments).
- Serology for likely infections.
- Recreational nitrous oxide inhalation can cause relatively acute transverse myelitis via effects on vitamin B_{12} metabolism.

Treatment
- High-dose IV steroids.
- IV immunoglobulin and/or PLEX especially where neuromyelitis optica is a concern.
- NB: supportive care (as for spinal cord compression).
- Rehabilitation: see Acquired spinal cord injury in Chapter 4 ➔ pp. 224-6.

- Catastrophic onset (hyperacute, complete paralysis) is a poor prognostic indicator.

Myasthenia gravis

Myasthenic crisis
- Life-threatening complication of myasthenia.
- Defined as weakness severe enough to require intubation and ventilation:
  - Unable to clear secretions;
  - Ineffective cough;
  - Nasal voice;
  - Dysphagia;
  - Pneumonia with hypoxia;
  - Vital capacity below 15 mL/kg.
- May be precipitated by infection, surgery, stress, menses, under-medication.
- Occurs in 15–20% of children, most within 2 yrs of the disease.

Management
- Supportive.
- Pharyngeal suction.
- Ventilation.
- Consider plasma exchange or, in neonates, exchange transfusion.
- IV immunoglobulin.

Cholinergic crisis
- Due to overmedication with anticholinesterases.
- Diarrhoea, cramps, sweating, muscle weakness, miosis, bradycardia, salivation, fasciculation (presence often allows differentiation from a myasthenic crisis—but it can be difficult).
- Withhold anticholinesterases.
- Consider atropine.

The child unwilling to walk because of pain or unsteadiness

See Table 6.11 for causes of unwillingness to walk for factors other than weakness.

Table 6.11 Causes of unwillingness to walk due to factors other than weakness

Skin and nails	Infections, injuries	
Bones and joints	Irritable hip Perthes' disease Septic arthritis	
	Inflammatory arthritides	Henoch–Schönlein purpura
Brainstem and cerebellum	Acute cerebellar ataxia	
	Infectious and post-infectious	Varicella, measles, mumps, herpes simplex, EBV Mycoplasma Meningitis Cerebellar abscess
	Paraneoplastic	Opsoclonus-myoclonus syndrome (± neuroblastoma)
	Posterior fossa space-occupying lesion	Tumour Bleed
	Toxic	Alcohol, ASMs, sedatives, methotrexate, piperazine, lead
	Metabolic	Maple syrup urine disease Urea cycle defects (arginosuccinic aciduria) Organic acidurias Mitochondrial disorders Hartnup disease Pyruvate dehydrogenase deficiency (may be precipitated by fever or excitement) Thyroid disease
	Genetic	Episodic ataxia types 1 and 2
	Demyelination	Multiple sclerosis
	Head injury	Haematoma Vertebro-basilar occlusion
	Hydrocephalus	
	Vascular	Basilar migraine Basilar artery thrombosis/embolism Kawasaki disease

Table 6.11   (Contd.)

Basal ganglia and cortex	Movement disorder	(new-onset dystonia)
	Stroke	
	Epilepsy	Todd's paresis (post-ictal)
		Non-convulsive status epilepticus
		Alternating hemiplegia
	Vascular	Hemiplegic migraine
Eyes and ears	Vertigo	
	Labyrinthitis	
	Visual loss	
Other	Functional	
	But always take complaints of back pain seriously as it is rarely a functional symptom in childhood: consider discitis	

Acute ataxia

(See Acute ataxia in Chapter 3 ➔ p. 207).
In children, ataxia usually indicates disease involving the cerebellum (see Table 1.5 in Chapter 1 ➔ p. 29). In the child who was previously healthy, the most common causes are:
- Drug ingestion (especially aged 1–4 yrs; ask about medications in the home).
- Acute post-infectious cerebellitis.

Non-cerebellar causes of acute ataxia include
- Sensory ataxia—Guillain–Barré syndrome, Miller–Fisher variant.
- Disequilibrium in severe epilepsy (e.g. due to frequent myoclonic jerks).
- Primary brain tumours usually cause progressive ataxia, but acute ataxia may signify a bleed or acute hydrocephalus. Alternatively, the ataxia may seem of acute onset because it has only just been noticed.
- Striking ataxia, sometimes of relatively acute onset, may be the presenting feature (particularly in the preschool child) of opsoclonus-myoclonus syndrome (see Opsoclonus-myoclonus in Chapter 4 ➔ p. 395) with the eye and limb movement disorder developing later.

Investigations
Expect to find a diagnosis for most:
- CT or MRI for posterior fossa space-occupying lesion and structural lesions.
- Acute and convalescent sera for viral titres (including varicella, EBV, measles, mumps, echovirus, Coxsackie B).

Where clinical picture suggests appropriate:
- CSF for protein, cytology, and infection (if scan is normal and no cause is apparent).
- Toxicology screen.
- Amino acids, organic acids.
- Relevant investigations (see Opsoclonus-myoclonus in Chapter 4 ➔ p. 395) in suspected neuroblastoma-related opsoclonus-myoclonus.
- EEG for subtle seizure activity.

Chapter 7

Pharmacopoeia

❶ This section is intended as general guidance and is not intended to override advice contained in national or hospital formularies. The doses quoted have been obtained from a variety of sources and/or used over a number of years by experienced neurologists. At times, they may exceed recommended dosages in formularies.

The unwanted effect and contraindication data are not intended to be exhaustive. Consult more detailed sources of information before using drugs with which you are unfamiliar.

If in doubt, consult your pharmacist and other colleagues.

Young children typically require higher doses per kilogram body weight than adults. Doses are given on a per kilogram basis together with typical maximum adult doses. Per kilogram dosing typically becomes excessive in older adolescents, and doses in adolescents calculated on a per kilogram basis should be reviewed (and possibly reduced) in line with typical adult doses.

Acetazolamide

Neurological indications

Reduction of CSF production in treatment of raised ICP including neonatal post-haemorrhagic ventriculomegaly and idiopathic intracranial hypertension. Occasional adjunctive treatment of focal, generalized, and absence seizures.

Dosing

Starting doses and escalation regimen

- *Raised ICP.* PO/IV (>1 months): 8 mg/kg eight hourly, increased by increments of 24 mg/kg/day as necessary to max. 100 mg/kg/day (usual adult max. 1 g/day but some reports of up to 4 g/day).
- *Epilepsy.* PO/IV (<12 yrs): 2.5 mg/kg/day divided 2–3 times daily, increased at weekly intervals to 15 mg/kg/day, maximum 750 mg/day. PO/IV (12–18 yrs): 250 mg 2–4 times daily. (Adult max. 1000 mg/day).

Preparations

250 mg tablet, 250 mg modified-release capsule, 500 mg IV injection. Tablets can be crushed and dispersed in water.

Contraindications

Adrenocortical insufficiency, hypokalaemia, hyponatraemia, hyperchloraemic acidosis, sulphonamide hypersensitivity.

Important interactions and unwanted effects

Rash and (rarely) Stevens–Johnson syndrome. Paraesthesiae. Nephrotoxicity with concomitant NSAID use. Elevates carbamazepine concentrations. Acetazolamide potentially increases the risk of toxicity when given with valproate.

Comments

Not recommended for prolonged use. Use with caution in patients with hyperammonaemia. Monitor electrolytes: alkalosis causes hypokalaemia that may need bicarbonate or potassium supplementation. Maintain bicarbonate level >18 mmol/L.

Aciclovir

Neurological indications

Treatment of suspected or confirmed herpes simplex or varicella zoster encephalitis.

Dosing

Possible herpes encephalitis (i.e. precautionary treatment pending CSF virology)

- IV (Neonate–3 months): 20 mg/kg 8-hourly
- IV (3 months–11 yrs): 250 mg/m² 8-hourly
- IV (>12 yrs): 5 mg/kg 8-hourly

Probable or confirmed HSV encephalitis, or if immunocompromised.
- Double the dose above. Treat for 21 days.

Preparations

250 mg and 500 mg IV injection. Tablets (200 mg, 400 mg, and 800 mg), dispersible tablets (200 mg, 400 mg, and 800 mg), and liquid (200 mg in 5 mL and 400 mg in 5 mL)

Important interactions and unwanted effects

Dose must be decreased in renal impairment: risk of toxic encephalopathy. Ensure adequate hydration.

Comment

Give as IV infusion over 1 h (at all ages). The significant sodium load may be an issue in some situations.

ACTH (tetracosactide)

Neurological indications

Treatment of infantile epileptic spasms syndrome and epileptic encephalopathies. The biological preparation of ACTH is not available in the UK. Tetracosactide (tetracosactrin) is a 1 mg/mL synthetic analogue. 500 microgms Synacthen Depot® IM on alternate days has approximately the bioactivity of 40 IU of ACTH IM daily.

Dosing

- IM: 500 microgms of Synacthen Depot® into the buttock on alternate days increasing to 750 microgms on alternate days if no response after 1 week.

Discontinuation regimen
- Dose typically maintained until seizure free for 1–2 weeks then decreased to 50% dose for 2 weeks, then 25% dose for 2 weeks before stopping.
- Discuss with endocrinology whether treatment dose/duration warrants short synacthen test (assessing potential adrenal suppression) to guide withdrawal.

Preparations

- Synacthen Depot® 1 mg/mL

Contraindications

Acute systemic infection. Do not use in neonates (depot contains benzyl alcohol).

Important interactions and unwanted effects

Risk of anaphylaxis (see product literature). Hypertension and hyperglycaemia are common (monitor blood pressure and for glycosuria at least weekly). Irritability may be marked. Increased appetite and weight gain. Due to the increased risk of infection tetracosactide should not be used in the presence of active infectious or systemic disease or in the presence of a reduced immune response unless adequate disease specific therapy is being given. Sepsis can be overwhelming, and prompt medical attention should be sought at any sign of intercurrent illness. Gastrointestinal haemorrhage.

Comments

Some authorities regard ACTH as superior to oral prednisolone although the evidence for this is weak and it is typically less well tolerated.

Amitriptyline

Neurological indications

Chronic headache (including migraine and tension-type headache) and other chronic pain syndromes particularly with sleep disruption; second-line treatment of peripheral neurogenic pain (gabapentin, pregabalin are preferred).

Dosing

Starting doses
- PO (2–12 yrs): Initially 200–500 microgms/kg (max 10 mg) at night.
- PO (>12 yrs): 10 mg at night.

Maintenance doses
- PO (2–12 yrs): max 1 mg/kg BD (under specialist advice).
- PO (>12 yrs): max 50–75 mg at night.

Discontinuation regimen
- 50% of the dose for 4 weeks; 25% of the dose for 2 weeks, then stop. Avoid abrupt discontinuation. Withdrawal effects may occur within 5 days of stopping treatment; usually mild and self-limiting but in some cases can be severe.

Preparations

Tablets (10 mg, 25 mg, 50 mg); oral solution (10 mg/5 mL, 25 mg/5 mL, 50 mg/5 mL). A variety of oral solutions available with different excipients: ensure product is suitable for use in children.

Contraindications

Cardiac arrhythmias, heart block, and acute porphyria. ECG is advisable before use.

Important interactions and unwanted effects

Many interactions: check current information. Unwanted effects include confusion, fatigue, sedation, postural hypotension, syncope, and 'anticholinergic' effects (dry mouth, blurred vision, urinary retention, constipation). In the event of overdose, do not treat arrhythmias with anti-arrhythmic drugs—IV sodium bicarbonate may be used.

Comments

- Limit treatment duration to a total of 3 months. Licensed for treatment of depression over 16 in UK.
- Tricyclic antidepressants lower the seizure threshold and should be used with caution in patients with a history of convulsions.

Aspirin

Neurological indications

Stroke prophylaxis (antiplatelet agent) in specific contexts, e.g. stenotic cerebrovascular disease.

Dosing

- PO: 5 mg/kg (max 300 mg) once daily for first 14 d after confirmed arterial ischaemic stroke decreasing thereafter to 1 mg/kg (max. 75 mg) once daily.
- Dose can be titrated using an *in vitro* functional assay of inhibition of platelet function: a platelet thromboelastograph ('Platelet TEG®').

Preparations

75 mg dispersible and enteric-coated tablets. For doses <75 mg, put dispersible tablet in 15 mL of water and give the appropriate volume, discarding the remainder. Give with food or milk.

Contraindications

Severe hepatic or renal impairment, haemophilia, active peptic ulceration, and bleeding disorders.

Important interactions and unwanted effects

Not common in a low-dose regimen; however, hypersensitivity may occur.

Comments

May increase risk of hyperammonaemic encephalopathy particularly in metabolic disorders and should be suspended during acute febrile illnesses especially varicella and influenza. Alternative antiplatelet medications should be considered if aspirin use interrupted for more than a few days.

Atomoxetine

Neurological indications

Treatment of attention-deficit hyperactivity disorder (ADHD). Symptomatic treatment in narcolepsy.

Dosing

Starting doses and escalation regimen
- PO (>6 yrs body weight up to 70 kg): 500 microgms/kg/daily for 7 days. Increase at weekly intervals.
- PO (>6 yrs body weight >70 kg): 40 mg/daily for 7 days. Increase at weekly intervals.

Maintenance doses
- PO (>6 yrs): 1.2–1.8 mg/kg/day (max. 120 mg daily) as a single dose or divided into 2 doses (BD dosing may reduce unwanted effects).

Preparations

Capsules (10 mg, 18 mg, 25 mg, 40 mg, 60 mg, 80 mg). Oral solution (4 mg in 1 mL)

Contraindications

Phaeochromocytoma or history of phaeochromocytoma. Narrow-angle glaucoma.

Important interactions and unwanted effects

Atomoxetine should not be used in combination with monoamine oxidase inhibitors. Caution in concurrent use with CYP2D6 inhibitors.
Anorexia, dry mouth, nausea, drowsiness, liver failure.

Comments

- Ocular irritant: flush affected eye immediately with water and seek medical advice.
- Use with caution in cardiovascular or hepatic disease.
- Some children with ADHD have co-existing epilepsy. It has been reported that stimulants may exacerbate seizure tendencies: in our opinion, this risk is not high, and epilepsy is not a contraindication to stimulant therapy if otherwise clinically indicated.
- May take 4–6 weeks to see an effect.
- Monitor pulse and blood pressure.
- Seek medical attention in the case of unexplained nausea, vomiting, darkened urine, or jaundice.

Baclofen

Neurological indications

Treatment of spasticity and dystonia.

Dosing

Starting doses and escalation regimen
- PO (<10 yrs): 300 microgms/kg/day in 2–4 divided doses. Increase gradually.
- PO (>10 yrs): 300 microgms/kg/day in 2–4 divided doses or 5 mg TDS. Increase by this amount at weekly intervals.

Maintenance doses
- 0.75–2 mg/kg/day (max 100 mg/day).
- In the context of acute intrathecal baclofen withdrawal (e.g. failure of baclofen pump or catheter see Effects of baclofen withdrawal in Chapter 4 ⟳ p. 250) higher doses may be needed in conjunction with aggressive intravenous benzodiazepine treatment.

Discontinuation regimen
- Avoid abrupt withdrawal (see Effects of baclofen withdrawal in Chapter 4 ⟳ p. 250). Reduce to 50% for 1 week, then 25% for 1 week, then stop.

Preparations

Tablets (10 mg; may be crushed and dispersed in water). Oral solution (5 mg/5 mL).

Contraindications

Peptic ulceration.

Important interactions and unwanted effects

Lethargy, sedation, and bulbar compromise: often limit usefulness. Some oral solution contains 2 g sorbitol per 5 mL which may cause diarrhoea.

Comments

Baclofen also may be delivered as a continuous intrathecal infusion (see Intrathecal baclofen in Chapter 4 ⊃ p. 249): intrathecal doses are typically 100–1200 microgms/day.

Biotin (vitamin H)

Neurological indications

Inborn errors of metabolism: defects of biotin metabolism including biotinidase deficiency, biotin responsive basal ganglia disease, isolated carboxylase defects.

Dosing

Starting doses and escalation regime
- PO (neonates): 5 mg daily, then increase according to response (e.g. 5 mg every 2 days).
- PO (1 month to 18 yrs): 10 mg daily, then increase according to response (e.g. 5 mg every 2 days).

Maintenance doses:
- PO (neonate): 10–50 mg daily.
- PO (1 month to 18 yrs): 20–50 mg daily (up to 100 mg daily in isolated carboxylase defects).
- Biotin-thiamine responsive basal ganglia disease (see Thiamine transporter 2 deficiency (biotin responsive basal ganglia disease) in Chapter 4 ⊃ p. 523): 5–10 mg/kg/day.

Preparations

Tablets 5 mg may be crushed and mixed with food or drink. Injection 5 mg/mL.

Contraindications

None known.

Important interactions and unwanted effects

None known.

Comments

May be used pragmatically initially if a disorder of biotin metabolism suspected. Close contact with tertiary specialists in metabolic disease advised. High-dose biotin can interfere with immunoassays for T3 and T4 giving false impression of 'thyrotoxicosis'.

Botulinum toxin A

Neurological indications

Treatment of focal dystonia or localized spasticity attributable to specific muscle groups.

Dosing

❶ It is essential to be aware that the dosing units of the commonly available commercial preparations are **not equivalent** and to specify the preparation intended on the prescription.

Maximum total dose per administration
- Dysport®
- IM injection to the lower limb (>2yrs): 15 U/kg (max. 1000 U) if single limb. 30 U/kg (max 1000 U) if both limbs.
- IM injection to the upper limb (>2 yrs): 16 U/kg (max. 640 U) if single limb. 21 U/kg (max. 840 U) if both limbs.
- IM injection to upper and lower limbs (>2 yrs): 30 U/kg (max. 1000 U) per administration if injecting multiple sites (see Table 7.1).
- Typically, 30–50% of the maximum permitted dose used at first administration.

Table 7.1 Typical target doses (Dysport® units*)

	Dose	Injection sites per muscle
Biceps	3–6 U/kg	1–2
Brachioradialis	1.5–3 U/kg	1
Gastrocnemius	5–15 U/kg	2–4
Soleus	4–6 U/kg	1–2
Tibialis posterior	3–5 U/kg	1–2
Flexor carpi radialis	2–4 U/kg	1–2
Flexor carpi ulnaris	1.5–3 U/kg	1
Adductor policis	0.5–1 U/kg	1

*1 Botox® unit = approximately 2.5–4 Dysport® units. Doses should be reduced proportionately in situations of reduced muscle bulk.

Preparations

Powder is reconstituted immediately before use in 0.9% saline usually at a dilution of 100 Dysport® units/mL or 200 Botox® units/mL (higher concentration, smaller-volume injections may be useful in some contexts). Refer to product literature for further information.

Contraindications

Myasthenia. Concurrent aminoglycoside use.

Important interactions and unwanted effects

Some diffusion from injection sites typically occurs: cervical injection (typically for dystonia) may cause dysphagia and injection of hip adductors may affect continence. Effects may be potentiated by aminoglycosides. Sometimes flu-like symptoms.

Comments

Specialist use only. Target muscles are identified by clinical examination. Needle placement is guided by surface anatomy and/or ultrasound guidance. Confirmation of placement prior to administration can be achieved by observing the needle pivoting about the insertion point in the skin as the target muscle is passively extended.

Clinical effects last 8–12 weeks. All targeted muscles should be treated at a single session. Frequent administration probably increases the risk of antibody formation that limits effectiveness.

Additional indications include treatment of drooling by injection into salivary glands (in specialist centres).

Brivaracetam

Neurological indications

Generalized, absence and focal seizures.

Dosing

Starting doses and escalation regimen
- PO/IV (>2 yrs; weighing 10–49 kg) 1–2 mg/kg/day (divided in 2 doses)
- PO (>2 yrs; weighing >50 kg): 50–100 mg/day (divided in two doses)

Maintenance doses
- PO/IV (>2 yrs; weighing 10–49 kg): Up to 4 mg/kg/day, occasionally 5 mg/kg/day.
- PO (>2 yrs; weighing >50 kg) 200 mg/day divided in two doses.

Preparations

Tablet (10 mg, 25 mg, 50 mg, 75 mg, 100 mg). Oral solution (10 mg/mL) can be diluted in water or juice shortly before swallowing. IV (50 mg/5 mL)

Contraindications

Hypersensitivity to brivaracetam or other pyrrolidone derivatives

Comments

- May be less prone to causing unwanted behavioural effects than levetiracetam. Can be directly substituted (without a transition period) for levetiracetam.
- Avoid abrupt withdrawal. Reduce by a maximum of half the daily dose every week until either a dose of 1 mg/kg daily (in children weighing up to 50 kg) or 50 mg daily (in children weighing over 50 kg) is reached and given for 1 week then reduce to 20 mg daily for a final week.
- Use with caution in hepatic impairment, dosing adjustment may be required.
- Brivaracetam film-coated tablets contain lactose. Patients with rare hereditary problems of galactose intolerance, total lactase deficiency or glucose-galactose malabsorption should avoid.

Calcium and vitamin D supplements

Neurological indications

Prophylaxis of osteomalacia in the context of long-term steroid or phenytoin use.

Dosing

- Typical regimes provide ~500 mg of calcium (12 mmol Ca²⁺) and 400 units (10 mg) of cholecalciferol daily (e.g. Calcichew D3 Forte® once daily). Higher doses may be used under specialist advice.

Preparations

Various calcium/vitamin D preparations are available: individual preference and palatability may be important.

Comments

Monitor bone mineral density in long-term steroid use (e.g. >3 months).

Cannabidiol

Neurological indications

Seizure control in Dravet and Lennox–Gastaut syndrome (adjunctive treatment with clobazam) and epilepsy associated with tuberous sclerosis.

Dosing

Starting doses and escalation regimen
- PO (>2 years): 5 mg/kg/day divided in two doses for 1 week then 10 mg/kg/day divided in two doses.
- Increasing in steps of 5 mg/kg/day according to response at weekly intervals

Maintenance doses
- PO (>2 years): Usually 10–12.5 mg/kg/day divided in two doses.
- Seizures associated with Lennox–Gastaut or Dravet: max 20 mg/kg/day divided in two doses.

- Seizures associated with tuberous sclerosis (adjunctive treatment): max 25 mg/kg/day divided in two doses,

Missed dose regimen
- If more than 7 doses are missed, dose should be re-titrated to therapeutic dose.

Preparations
Oral solution (100 mg/mL) contains sesame oil

Important interactions and unwanted effects
Loss of appetite, cough, diarrhoea, drowsiness, fatigue, fever, increased risk of infection, irritability, nausea, rash, seizures, vomiting.

Comments
Specialist use only. Consider reducing concomitant clobazam doses. Food may affect absorption (give at a consistent time with respect to meals). Transaminase elevation is the commonest reason for discontinuation, particularly if also on valproate. Monitor liver function before, and 1, 3, and 6 months after starting then periodically; more frequently if also on valproate.

Discontinue if >30% seizure reduction not achieved within 6 months.

Carbamazepine

Neurological indications
Treatment of focal seizures; some paroxysmal movement disorders; neurogenic pain; empiric mood-stabilizer in psychiatric practice (including bipolar disorder). Will *worsen* primary generalized epilepsies (especially JME), tonic, atonic, and absence seizures.

Dosing
Starting doses and escalation regimen
- PO (>1 months): 5 mg/kg/day divided in 2 doses, increasing by 5 mg/kg/day every 3–7 days.

Maintenance doses
- PO (>1 months): maximum doses guided by clinical assessment of tolerance. Typically 20 mg/kg/day but occasionally fast metabolizers tolerate and may need higher doses. Maximum adult dose is typically 1.2 g/day, occasionally higher (1.6–2 g/day).

Discontinuation regimen
- 75% of the dose for 2–4 weeks; 50% of the dose for 2–4 weeks; 25% of the dose for 2–4 weeks, then stop.

Missed dose regimen
- Give next dose when due: no additional doses.

Preparations

Tablets (100 mg, 200 mg, 400 mg). Oral solution (100 mg/5 mL). Controlled-release tablet (thought to limit post-dose drug level peaks, 200 mg, 400 mg): can be halved if scored but not crushed without loss of controlled-release effect. Suppository (125 mg, 250 mg).

Contraindications

Atrio-ventricular conduction abnormalities (unless paced). History of bone marrow depression, acute porphyria.

> ⓘ Test children of Han-Chinese or Thai origin for HLA-B*1502 allele prior to treatment commencing as ↑ risk of Stevens–Johnson Syndrome. Consider testing for other south- and east-Asian ethnicities.

Important interactions and unwanted effects

- Drowsiness or unsteadiness may occur transiently on introduction or dose escalation (reduce rate of escalation) or as a dose-limiting unwanted effect at higher doses. May also occur transiently 1–2 h after dosing as blood levels peak: either fractionate dose further (e.g. into 3 divided doses) or use controlled-release preparation.
- Should be withdrawn immediately in aggravated liver dysfunction or acute liver disease.
- Occasional rash. Rare lupus-like syndrome. Rare blood dyscrasias and osteomalacia. Hyponatraemia (SIADH).
- Plasma carbamazepine levels are increased by concomitant CYP3A4 inhibitors and inducers such as macrolide antibiotics. For interactions between antiseizure medicines, see this Chapter ⟁ p. 709. Many other important interactions: see other sources.

Comments

- Rectal administration (suppository or liquid) is possible for periods of up to 1 week: dose should be increased by 25% (max. 250 mg QDS). When using oral liquid rectally—should be retained for at least 2 hours (but may have laxative effect).
- Enzyme induction will reduce effectiveness of standard oral contraception.
- Carbamazepine use in pregnancy has been associated with dose-dependent increased rates of congenital malformation. Its use in female patients should only be after informed discussion of risks (see Contraception and reproductive health in Chapter 4 ⟁ p. 320).
- Different formulations of oral preparations may vary in bioavailability. Patients being treated for epilepsy should be maintained on a specific manufacturer's product.

Carnitine (levocarnitine)

Neurological indications

Primary carnitine deficiency; carnitine-responsive metabolic disorders (e.g. mitochondrial disorders). Some authorities recommend carnitine supplementation for children on the ketogenic diet.

Dosing

- PO (all ages): Up to 200 mg/kg/day divided in 2–4 doses (usual maximum 3 g/day).
- IV (all ages): Up to 100 mg/kg/day divided in 2–4 doses. To be administered over 2–3 mins.

Preparations

Tablets (330 mg, 1 g). Capsules (250 mg, 500 mg). Oral solutions (300 mg/1 mL, 100 mg/1 mL). IV (as L-carnitine) 1 g/5 mL.

Contraindications

Use with care in diabetes.

Important interactions and unwanted effects

Nausea, vomiting (dose-dependent); abnormal body odour.

Comments

Use in many indications unlicensed. Monitor free and acyl carnitine levels.

Chloral hydrate

Neurological indications

Refractory status dystonicus, agitation, insomnia. Use in sedation for procedures now discouraged but see Acute sedation protocols in this chapter 🔂 p. 708.

Dosing

- PO: 80–240 mg/kg/day divided in 4–6 doses.

Discontinuation regimen
- 50% of the dose for 3–5 days; 25% dose for 3–5 days, then stop.

Preparations

Oral solution (143.4 mg/5 mL, 500 mg/5 mL). Mix with milk, water, or fruit juice to mask taste.

Contraindications

Use with care in respiratory disease. Avoid in severe hepatic or renal impairment, cardiac disease, gastritis, or acute porphyria.

Important interactions and unwanted effects

Gastric irritation, nausea, vomiting, sleepiness, rash.

Comments

Do not use concomitantly with triclofos (as it is a derivative of chloral). Not licensed in children for sedation. Recent revision of UK MHRA guidance limits licensed use to short term (<2 week) use only due to potential for carcinogenic effects based on animal data. Extended off-licence use is occasionally necessary in situations of severe intrusive movement disorder preventing sleep or otherwise severely affecting care and quality of life. It is recommended that written informed consent (including awareness of known carcinogenicity in animal studies) is documented.

Clobazam

Neurological indications

Anti-epileptic.

Dosing

Starting doses and escalation regimen
- PO (>1 months): 500 microgms/kg/day divided in 2 doses. Increased according to response after 5–7 days.

Maintenance doses
- PO (>1 months): 1 mg/kg/day (max. <12 yrs: 30 mg/day, 12–18 yrs: 60 mg/day) divided in two doses.

Discontinuation regimen
- 75% of the dose for 2 months; 50% of the dose for 2 months; 25% of the dose for 2 months, then stop (faster withdrawal is possible if treatment duration is short).

Preparations

Tablet (10 mg) can be crushed and dispersed in water. Oral solution (5 mg/ 5 mL, 10 mg/5 mL)

Contraindications

Ventilatory/pulmonary insufficiency, sleep apnoea syndrome; severe hepatic impairment; depression, unstable myasthenia gravis, phobic states, obsessional states.

Important interactions and unwanted effects

Sedating, particularly in combination (e.g. with phenobarbital).

Comments

Risk of withdrawal seizures if discontinued abruptly. Clobazam may in rare cases cause restlessness and muscle weakness. For interactions between antiseizure medicines, see this chapter p. 709.

Clonazepam

Neurological indications

Anti-epileptic.

Dosing

Starting doses and escalation regimen
- PO (<5 yrs): 250 microgms at night increased at weekly intervals.
- PO (5 to 11 yrs): 500 microgms at night increased at weekly intervals.
- PO (12 to 18 yrs): 1 mg at night increased at weekly intervals.

Maintenance doses
- PO (<1 yr): 0.5–1 mg/day divided in 2–4 doses.
- PO (1 to 4 yrs): 1–3 mg/day divided in 2–4 doses.
- PO (5 to 11 yrs): 3–6 mg/day divided in 2–4 doses.
- PO (12 to 18 yrs): 4–8 mg/day divided in 2–4 doses.

Discontinuation regimen
- 75% of the dose for 1 month; 50% of the dose for 1 month; 25% of the dose for 1 month, then stop.

Preparations

Tablet (500 microgms, 1 mg, 2 mg); intravenous injection; oral solution (500 microgms/5 mL, 2 mg/5 mL)

Contraindications

See Clobazam in this chapter ♦ p. 662.

Important interactions and unwanted effects

Increased salivation and airway secretions (may be temporary, worse with IV administration); sedation; irritability; behaviour disturbance.

Comments

Individual sensitivity for both wanted and unwanted effects is very variable. Intravenous preparation can be used rectally in acute situations. For interactions between antiseizure medicines, see this chapter ♦ p. 709.

Clonidine

Neurological indications

Treatment of agitation (particularly post-traumatic brain injury and opiate withdrawal e.g. after prolonged PICU stay); status dystonicus; tic disorders.

Dosing

Starting doses and escalation regimen
- PO: 1.5–3 microgms/kg/day divided in 3 doses, increased if necessary every 5–7 days.

Maintenance doses
- *Sedation.* PO: 5–25 microgms/kg/day (max. 1.2 mg/day).
- *Tic disorders.* PO: 3–10 microgms/kg/day (max. 300 microgms/day).

- *Satus dystonicus*. IV infusion 0.5 microgms/kg/hr increments every 6–12 h up to 2 microgms/kg/hr — occasionally up to 3–5 microgms/kg/hr under specialist supervision may be required, see Status dystonicus in Chapter 6 ➲ p. 628.

Discontinuation regimen
- *Tic disorders*. 75% of the dose for 2 days; 50% of the dose for 2 days; 25% of the dose for 2 days, then stop.
- Discontinuation needs to be more gradual in status dystonicus.

Preparations

Tablet (25 microgms, 100 microgms): can be crushed and dispersed in water. Oral solution: (50 microgms/5 mL). IV injection (150 microgms/mL).
Transdermal patches (2.5 mg, 5 mg, and 7.5 mg): changed weekly these deliver approximately 100, 200, and 300 microgms/day respectively. Patch location should be rotated to reduce risk of local irritation: can take 2 to 3 days to reach steady-state levels initially.

Contraindications

Porphyria. Severe bradyarrhythmia secondary to second or third-degree heart block or sick-sinus syndrome

Important interactions and unwanted effects

Antihypertensive: monitor blood pressure (particularly on induction and withdrawal). Avoid sudden withdrawal to prevent hypertensive crisis withdrawal syndrome. It may cause drowsiness, parasomnias, and nightmares.

Co-enzyme Q10 (ubiquinone)

Neurological indications

Metabolic supplementation in mitochondrial and related conditions.

Dosing

Starting doses (all ages)
- PO: 5 mg 1–2 times a day.

Maintenance doses
- PO (Neonate): Up to 200 mg/day.
- PO (>1 months): Up to 300 mg/day.

Preparations

Tablet (30 mg) and capsules (30 mg, 100 mg, 200 mg, 300 mg) can be opened and dispersed in water. Oral solution (25 mg/5 mL, 50 mg/5 mL)

Important interactions and unwanted effects

Gastro-oesophageal reflux/heartburn. Reduce dose in moderate to severe hepatic impairment. May reduce insulin requirements in people with insulin-dependent diabetes.

Comments

Take with food.

Dexamethasone

Neurological indications

Emergency and perioperative management of cerebral oedema associated with cerebral tumour. Treatment of bacterial meningitis (see discussion in Treatment [Meningitis section] in Chapter 4 ➲ p. 363).

Dosing

Cerebral tumour

Given in units of dexamethasone base:

- Child under 35 kg: 16.6 mg slow IV stat; then 3.3 mg IV/PO every 3 h for 3 days; then 3.3 mg IV/PO every 6 h for 1 day; then 1.7 mg IV/PO every 6 h for 4 days, then decrease by 0.83 mg/day daily.
- Child over 35 kg: 20.8 mg slow IV stat; then 3.3 mg IV/PO every 2 h for 3 days; then 3.3 mg IV/PO every 4 h for 1 day, then 3.3 mg IV/PO every 6 h for 4 days, then decrease by 1.7 mg/day daily.

Pneumococcal meningitis

- IV (Child 3 months to 15 yrs): 150 microgms/kg (max. Per dose 10 mg) every 6 h for 4 days starting before or with first dose of antibiotic.
- IV (Child 16–17 yrs): 10 mg every 6 h for 4 days starting before or with first dose of antibiotic. See Treatment in Chapter 4 ➲ p. 363.

Preparations

Injection (3.3 mg (as base)/mL, 3.8 mg (as base)/mL). Tablets (500 microgms, 2 mg, 4 mg) may be crushed and dispersed in water. Soluble tablet (2 mg, 4 mg, 8 mg, 10 mg, 20 mg). Oral solution (2 mg/5 mL, 10 mg/5 mL, 20 mg/5 mL).

Important interactions and unwanted effects

As for ACTH.

Comments

Well absorbed orally. Note that dosing may differ based on specific oncology protocols.

For discussion of withdrawal see Prednisolone in this chapter ➲ p. 695.

Dexamfetamine

Neurological indications

Treatment of attention-deficit hyperactivity disorder.

Dosing

Starting doses and escalation regimen

- PO (3–5 yrs): 2.5 mg/day increasing by 2.5 mg/day increments at weekly intervals typically given in an 8 am and noon regimen.
- PO (>6 yrs): 5 mg/day increasing by 5 mg/day increments at weekly intervals typically given in an 8 am and noon regimen.

Maintenance doses
- PO (3–5 yrs): Up to 20 mg daily.
- PO (>6 yrs): Up to 40 mg daily.

Doses may be given in 3–4 divided doses if necessary.

Discontinuation regimen
- 50% for 1 week then stop.

Preparations

Tablet (5 mg, 10 mg, 20 mg) can be halved. Modified-release capsules (5 mg, 10 mg, 15 mg). Oral solution: 5 mg/5 mL

Contraindications

Cardiac disease, hypertension; agitation or psychosis, anorexia, and hyper-thyroidism, porphyria, glaucoma, concomitant use of MAOIs (or use in 14 previous days).

Important interactions and unwanted effects

Anorexia. May aggravate tic disorders, agitation, or psychosis.

Comments

- Very short acting: doses typically given in morning and at lunchtime with food to limit rebound effects late in evening. Monitor weight and height as appetite suppression and growth restriction may occur during prolonged therapy (drug free period may allow catch up in growth). Monitor pulse, blood pressure, psychiatric symptoms, and growth at least every 6 months or following each dose adjustment.
- Many children with attention-deficit hyperactive disorder may have co-existing epilepsy. It has been reported that stimulants may exacerbate pre-existing seizure tendencies: in our opinion, this risk is not high and epilepsy is not a contraindication to stimulant therapy if otherwise clinically indicated.
- NOTE: Controlled Drug (CD) regulations apply in the UK.

Lisdexamfetamine is a pro-drug converted to dexamfetamine after absorption. Very similar wanted and unwanted effect profiles. 50 mg of lisdexamfetamine dimesylate $\cong$ 20 mg dexamfetamine sulphate.

Diazepam

Neurological indications

Status epilepticus (rectal route particularly useful in out-of-hospital settings but buccal midazolam is preferable), muscle spasm (e.g. after orthopaedic procedures in children with dystonic cerebral palsy), severe/dangerous sleep walking.

Dosing

- Status epilepticus:
  - IV (<12 yrs): 300–400 microgms/kg (max. per dose 10 mg), repeated after 10 min if necessary. Given over 3–5 min.

- IV (>12 yrs): 10–20 mg repeated after 10 min if necessary. To be given over 3–5 min.
- PR (neonates): 1.25 to 2.5 mg, repeated after 5–10 min if necessary.
- PR (1 months to 1 year): 5 mg repeated after 5–10 min if necessary.
- PR (2–11 yrs): 5–10 mg, repeated after 5–10 mins if necessary.
- PR (12–17 yrs): 10–20 mg, repeated after 5–10 mins if necessary.
- Muscle spasm (PO):
  - 1–11 months: 500 microgms/kg/day divided in two doses.
  - 1–5 yrs: 5 mg/day divided in two doses.
  - 5–12 yrs: 10 mg/day divided in two doses.
  - 12–18 yrs: 20 mg/day divided in 2 doses; max. 40 mg/day.
- Sleep walking:
  - PO (>12 yrs): 1–5 mg at night.

Discontinuation regimen
- Avoid prolonged use if possible. After short-term use (e.g. <2 weeks) reduce to 75% for 1 week; 50% for 1 week; then stop. After prolonged use, taper more gradually, e.g. 75% of the dose for 1 month; 50% of the dose for 1 month; 25% of the dose for 1 month; then stop.

Preparations

Tablets (2 mg, 5 mg, 10 mg); oral solution (2 mg/5 mL, 5 mg/5 mL); emulsion for intravenous injection (5 mg/mL: avoid in neonates as contains benzyl alcohol); enema (5 mg/2.5 mL, 10 mg/2.5 mL).

Contraindications

Respiratory depression and unstable myasthenia gravis

Important interactions and unwanted effects

Respiratory depression particularly in the context of IV treatment for status epilepticus. Can be late, occurring 20–30 min after injection: keep child monitored. Risks are greater (and likelihood of seizure termination poorer) with multiple, smaller doses rather than a single larger dose. Dependence/tolerance may develop.

Paradoxical aggravation of agitation may be seen if used in acute confusional states (see Acute behavioural disturbance in Chapter 6 ➲ p. 610).

Eslicarbazepine

Neurological indications

See under carbamazepine in this chapter ➲ p. 659: particularly useful in situations of partial response to carbamazepine where higher doses are being prevented by emerging unwanted effects. Will *worsen* primary generalized epilepsies (especially JME), tonic, atonic, and absence seizures.

Dosing

Starting doses and escalation regimen
- PO (6–17 yrs and <60 kg): 10 mg/kg/day as single daily dose increasing by 10 mg/kg/day every 1–2 weeks.

- PO (6–17 yrs and >60 kg): 400 mg once daily increasing after 1–2 weeks to 800 mg once daily.

Maintenance doses
- PO (6–17 yrs): 30 mg/kg/day (max. 1.2 g) as single daily dose.

Discontinuation regimen
- 75% for 2 weeks; 50% for 2 weeks; 25% for 2 weeks; then stop.

Preparations
Tablets (200 mg, 400 mg, 600 mg, 800 mg). Oral suspension (50 mg/mL).

Contraindications
Second- or third-degree heart block

Important interactions and unwanted effects
See Carbamazepine in this chapter ⊃ p. 659.

❶ Test children of Han-Chinese or Thai origin for HLA-B*1502 allele (see Carbamazepine in this chapter ⊃ p. 659).

Comments
Like oxcarbazepine (see oxcarbazepine in this chapter ⊃ p. 688) eslicarbazepine is related to carbamazepine, modified to prevent conversion to a particular metabolite responsible for many of the dose-related unwanted effects of the latter. In theory, therefore, it should be similarly efficacious and better tolerated. Once-daily dosing may be advantageous. Can be directly substituted (without a transition period) for carbamazepine.

For interactions between antiseizure medicines, see this chapter ⊃ p. 709.

Ethosuximide

Neurological indications
Treatment of absence and myoclonic seizures.

Dosing
Starting doses and escalation regimen
- PO (1 month to 5 yrs): 10 mg/kg/day (max. 250 mg/day) divided in two doses, increasing by 10 mg/kg/day increments divided in two doses at 7 to 14-day intervals.
- PO (>6 yrs): 250 mg twice daily increasing by 250 mg/day increments divided in two doses at 7 to14-day intervals.

Maintenance doses
- PO (1 months to 5 yrs): 20–40 mg/kg/day (max 1 g/day) divided in 2 doses.
- PO (>6 yrs): 500–750 mg twice daily, increased if necessary to max 2 g/day.

Preparations

Capsule (250 mg): some brands contain soya oil. Oral solution (250 mg/ 5 mL).

Contraindications

Porphyria.

Important interactions and unwanted effects

Oral solution can have an unpleasant taste. Dose-limiting effects are usually gastrointestinal (nausea, diarrhoea, anorexia ± weight loss), or dizziness. Rarely blood dyscrasias. For interactions between antiseizure medicines, see this chapter ❯ p. 709.

Comments

Counsel to seek prompt medical advice if fever, sore throat, mouth ulcers, bruising, or bleeding.

Everolimus

Neurological indications

Treatment of (unresectable) sub-ependymal giant cell astrocytoma (SEGA) associated with tuberous sclerosis complex (TSC). Adjunctive treatment of refractory seizures associated with TSC.

Dosing

Adjunctive treatment of refractory seizures associated with TSC
Treatment of SEGAs associated with TSC

- PO (1–3 yrs): 7 mg/m^2/day as a single daily dose
- PO (>3 yrs): 4.5 mg/m^2/day as single daily dose
- Dose adjusted in light of trough blood level measurements to achieve concentrations typically of 5–15 ng/mL.
- PO (<6 yrs without co-administration of CYP3A4/PgP inducer): 6 mg / m^2/day as a single daily dose
- PO (>6 yrs without co-administration of CYP3A4/PgP inducer): 5 mg / m^2/day as a single daily dose
- PO (<6 yrs with co-administration of CYP3A4/PgP inducer): 9 mg / m^2/day as a single daily dose
- PO (>6 yrs with co-administration of CYP3A4/PgP inducer): 8 mg / m^2/day as a single daily dose

Preparations

Tablets (0.25 mg, 0.75 mg, 2.5 mg, 5 mg, 10 mg); dispersible tablet (2 mg, 3 mg, 5 mg) must be dispersed in water before administration.

Important interactions and unwanted effects

Pneumonitis, stomatitis, thrombocytopenia, neutropenia.

Comments
- Specialist use only. Tablets should be swallowed whole or where not possible crushed thoroughly in 30 mL water and allowed to disperse for ~10 mins before drinking.
- CYP3A4/PgP inducers include carbamazepine, phenobarbital, phenytoin, steroids.
- Tablet and dispersible tablet doses are *not interchangeable*.
- Inhibitor of mammalian Target of Rapamycin (mTOR). Has immunosuppressive properties like tacrolimus and sirolimus: may predispose to intercurrent infection including *pneumocystis* pneumonia and aspergillosis.
- Regular monitoring of levels and full blood count required, including serum triglyceride and serum-cholesterol. Seek prompt medical advice if fever, sore throat, ulcers, bruising, or bleeding.

Fenfluramine

Neurological indications
Adjunctive treatment of seizures in Dravet syndrome.

Dosing
Starting doses and escalation regimen
- PO (2–17 yrs): 0.2 mg/kg/day divided in two doses, increasing to 0.4 mg/kg/day divided in two doses after one week with further adjustments as required every 5–7 days.

Maintenance doses
- PO (2–17 yrs): up to 0.7 mg/kg/day divided in two doses (max 26 mg/day).
- Lower doses up to 0.4 mg/kg/day (17 mg/day) with concomitant stiripentol use.

Preparations
Oral solution (2.2 mg/mL).

Contraindications
Pulmonary arterial hypertension, valvular heart disease (aortic or mitral).

Important interactions and unwanted effects
Appetite suppression, constipation, or diarrhoea.

Comments
- Specialist use only. Appetite suppression can be significant: monitor body weight.
- Significant risk of cardiac valve stenosis: echocardiogram should be performed before starting treatment, every 6 months for the first 2 years, and annually thereafter.
- Do not discontinue abruptly, the dose should be decreased gradually.

Folinic acid

Neurological indications

Pragmatic treatment for neonatal onset seizures.

Dosing

Starting dose and escalation regime

PO/IV (neonates): 10 mg/day in two divided doses This is likely to be the maintenance dose though with advice of a neurometabolic paediatrician larger doses may be tried.

Preparations

Tablets (15 mg) as calcium salt. Tablets may be crushed and dispersed in water. Solution for injection (various strengths available). Can be given IV as calcium folinate.

Contraindications

None known.

Important interactions and unwanted effects

None.

Flumazenil

Neurological indications

Reversal of severe sedation and/or respiratory depression secondary to excessive benzodiazepine use.

Dosing

- IV (all ages): 10 microgms/kg (max 200 microgms) administered over 15 seconds; repeated every min if required, followed by intravenous infusion 2–10 microgms/kg/h (max 400 microgms/h), adjusted according to response.
- Limit total dose per course of treatment to 50 microgms/kg (max 1 g) in older child.

Preparations

Solution for injection (500 microgms/5 mL).

Cautions

Nausea and vomiting common. Be aware of consequences of sudden reversal of benzodiazepine effects dependent on purpose for which they were given (recurrence of seizures, severe anxiety/panic attacks, status dystonicus, etc.). Flumazenil has a short half-life compared to benzodiazepines: excessive effects of the latter may recur if flumazenil discontinued prematurely.

Comments

Unlicensed.

Flunarizine

Neurological indications

Migraine prophylaxis, particularly familial hemiplegic migraine.

Dosing

- PO (<40 kg): 5 mg at night
- PO (>40 kg): 10 mg at night.
- Higher doses may be necessary in some patients.

Preparations

Capsule (5 mg). Tablet (5 mg) can be crushed and dispersed in water prior to administration.

Contraindications

Depression or previous episodes of serious depression, Parkinson's disease, or a family history of Parkinson's disease or liver damage.

Important interactions and unwanted effects

Weight gain, increased appetite, drowsiness, headache, low mood.

Comments

Effects on headache frequency may be delayed for several weeks. Full effect can take up to 12 weeks.

Gabapentin

Neurological indications

Neurogenic pain and dysesthesias. Adjunctive treatment of focal seizures. Adjunctive treatment of dystonia.

Dosing

Starting doses and escalation regimen

- PO (>2 yrs): 10 mg/kg/day (max. 300 mg) once daily on day 1, BD on day 2, and TDS thereafter.

Maintenance doses

- PO (>2 yrs): 30–40 mg/kg/day. Higher doses (up to 70 mg/kg/day; adult max. 4.8 g/day) have been used with benefit.

Discontinuation regimen

- 50% of the dose for 1 week then stop.

Preparations

Capsules (100 mg, 300 mg, 400 mg) can be opened but bitter taste: mask with strong tasting liquid such as undiluted fruit cordial or a teaspoon of soft food such as yoghurt. Tablets (600 mg, 800 mg). Oral solution (50 mg/mL).

Important interactions and unwanted effects

Sedation at high doses. Occasional insomnia, dizziness.

Comments

- Generally, well tolerated even at high dose although respiratory depression has been occasionally reported particularly in combination with other sedative drugs.
- Oral solution contains large amounts of artificial sweetener (acesulfame K, saccharin etc.). At high doses, sweetener intake may exceed recommended daily limits: consult product literature.
- NOTE: Controlled drug (CD) regulations apply in the UK.
- For interactions between antiseizure medicines, see this chapter ➜ p. 709.

Glycopyrronium bromide (glycopyrrolate)

Neurological indications

Reduction of oral and upper airway secretions particularly in severely disabled child.

Dosing

- PO (all ages): 120–400 microgms/kg/day divided in 3–4 doses.

Preparations

Tablet (1 mg, 2 mg) can be crushed and dispersed in water. Solution for injection (200 microgms/mL) can be given orally. Oral solution (320 microgms/mL equivalent to 400 microgms/mL of glycopyrronium bromide).

Contraindications

Urinary retention, bladder outflow obstruction. Chest infection. Angle-closure glaucoma, gastrointestinal obstruction. Severe ulcerative colitis.

Important interactions and unwanted effects

See under Trihexyphenidyl. Thicker, more viscous airway secretions may be harder to clear, aggravate atelectasis, and precipitate chest infections. Profound antimuscarinic effects may be seen. Doses should be given at consistent times with respect to food. High fat food should be avoided.

Glycopyrronium bromide tablets and oral solutions doses are not interchangeable due to differences in bioavailability. Sialanar® oral solution has approximately 25% higher bioavailability than tablets and generic oral solutions.

Heparin (low molecular weight)

Neurological indications

- Prophylaxis of deep vein thrombosis in immobile, post-pubertal adolescents in hospital settings according to local policies.
- Treatment of established venous thrombosis.
- Medium term prophylaxis (for periods of up to a few months) for risk of recurrent arterial ischaemic stroke (especially risk of embolic stroke e.g. in the case of carotid artery dissection).

- Low molecular weight heparin (LMWH) has largely replaced warfarin for this indication.
- Children at *long-term* risk of embolic stroke (e.g. due to heart valve disease) who need anticoagulation for months to years still tend to be given long-term warfarin despite its complexities, or newer oral anticoagulants such as rivaroxaban, as LMWH has to be given subcutaneously.
  - If long-term anticoagulation is planned, heparin is discontinued once an appropriate alternative anticoagulant has been established.

Several LMWHs are available but the dosage units are **not interchangeable**.

Enoxaparin
- Prophylaxis of thrombosis
  - SC (<2 months): 0.75 mg/kg/dose 12-hourly.
  - SC (>2 months): 0.5 mg/kg/dose 12-hourly (max 40 mg/day).
- Treatment of thrombotic and thromboembolic episodes
  - SC (<2 months): 1.5–2 mg/kg/dose 12-hourly.
  - SC (>2 months): 1 mg/kg/dose 12-hourly.
  - Doses adjusted as necessary in light of anti-Xa levels (see Table 7.2).

Tinzaparin
Has the advantage of once-daily dosing.
- Nevertheless, split (twice daily) dosing may be considered for first few days of therapy in some contexts (e.g. cerebral venous sinus thrombosis where haemorrhagic transformation of venous infarction is a concern)
- Prophylaxis of thrombosis
  - SC (all ages): 50 U/kg/day
- Treatment of thrombotic and thromboembolic episodes
  - SC (<2 months): 275 U/kg/day
  - SC (2–11 months): 250 U/kg/day
  - SC (1–4 yrs): 240 U/kg/day
  - SC (5–9 yrs): 200 U/kg/day
  - SC (10–18 yrs): 175 U/kg/day
- Doses adjusted as necessary in light of anti-Xa levels (see Table 7.2).

Dose adjustment for treatment of established thrombosis

Table 7.2 Target anti-Xa level (4 h post-dose) 0.5–1.0 U/mL

Anti-Xa level	Action
<0.35 U/mL	Increase dose by 25% and recheck anti-Xa after 3 doses
0.35–0.49 U/mL	Increase dose by 10% and recheck anti-Xa after 3 doses
0.5–1.0 U/mL	No change to dose. When dose steady, a weekly level check is adequate
1.1–1.5 U/mL	Decrease dose by 20% and recheck anti-Xa after 3 doses
1.6–2 U/mL	Decrease dose by 30% and recheck anti-Xa in 3 doses
>2 U/mL	Withhold dose. Re-dose only when anti-Xa level <0.5 U/mL. Decrease dose by 40% and recheck anti-Xa after 3 doses

Contraindications

Reduce dose in severe renal and hepatic involvement: unfractionated heparin may be preferable (see next).

Comments

LMWH has a longer duration of action than standard (unfractionated) heparin given by continuous infusion. Unfractionated heparin can also be rapidly reversed by giving protamine whereas protamine reversal of LMWH is incomplete. Use of unfractionated heparin may therefore be preferable in certain complex situations particularly in ICU settings (e.g. if surgery is anticipated) although it requires much closer monitoring and careful dose titration. For general uses, however, subcutaneous administration and the reduced need for monitoring of coagulation profiles are major advantages of LMWH.

Haloperidol

Neurological indications

Treatment of severe chorea and tic disorder; emergency treatment of severe aggression or violent behaviour in autism or pervasive developmental disorder.

Dosing

Starting doses and escalation regimen
- Tics and chorea.
  - PO (1–10 yrs): 25–50 microgms/kg/day divided in two doses.
  - PO (10–17 yrs): 0.5 mg twice daily or 0.16 mg three times a day.
- Acute agitation (specialist use).
  - PO (6–11 yrs): 10–30 microgms/kg PO repeated after 60 min if necessary.
  - PO (>12 yrs): 1–5 mg repeated after 60 min if necessary.
  - IM (>12 yrs): 2.5–5 mg repeated after 60 min if necessary.

Maintenance doses
- Tics and chorea.
  - PO (1–10 yrs): 50–75 microgms/kg/day (max. 10 mg/day) divided in 2–3 doses.
  - PO (10–17 yrs): 6–15 mg/day (occasionally more) divided in 2–3 doses.

Discontinuation regimen
- After long-term use: 75% for 2 weeks; 50% for 2 weeks; 25% for 2 weeks; then stop.

Preparations

Tablet (500 microgms, 1.5 mg, 5 mg, 10 mg). Oral solution (200 microgms/mL, 1 mg/mL, 2 mg/mL). Solution for injection (5 mg/mL).

Contraindications

Significant liver or renal disease. Cardiac electrophysiology disorders. Uncompensated heart failure. Uncorrected hypokalaemia.

Important interactions and unwanted effects

(See Unwanted drug effects in Chapter 5 ⊃ p. 593).

Early dyskinesia after a few doses (reversible); tardive dyskinesia (may be incompletely reversible); other extrapyramidal unwanted effects. Neuroleptic malignant syndrome (very rare).

Measure prolactin at start of therapy and at 6 months, then yearly. Baseline and periodic check of ECG recommended.

Histamine

Neurological indications

Identification of autonomic neuropathy in consideration of neuropathic causes of apparent indifference to pain.

Dosing

- Intradermal injection: 0.2–0.5 mL of 1:10 000 histamine solution (usually supplied as 1:1000 solution so needs ×10 dilution).

Comment

Lack of wheal response suggests autonomic neuropathy (i.e. significant result).

Hypertonic saline (2.7% or 3%)

Neurological indications

Treatment of acutely raised intracranial pressure.

Dosing

- IV (all ages): 3 mL/kg slow infusion over 20 min by peripheral or (preferably) large central vein. Repeat as clinically necessary: recheck plasma sodium frequently.

Comments

- Management of acutely raised ICP should be in conjunction with intensivists and/or neurosurgeons.
- 3% hypertonic saline is not routinely available as a pre-prepared fluid. Draw 36 mL out of a 500 mL bag 0.9% saline and replace with 36 mL 30% saline to make 500 mL 3% saline.
- 2.7% saline may be available as a pre-prepared fluid.
- Use the same dose irrespective of whether 2.7% or 3% saline is being used.

Hypertonic saline reduces intracellular volume by osmotic extraction of intracellular water, a similar mechanism of action to mannitol, although it has several advantages over mannitol. It tends not to cause a late rebound intracellular swelling due to intracellular accumulation (see Mannitol in this chapter ➲ p. 683); it does not cause an obligatory diuresis thus preserving circulating volume and mean arterial pressure; and treatment can be more readily monitored as the molecule responsible for osmolality change (sodium chloride) can be directly measured. Plasma sodium will typically rise by 2–3 mM after infusion of 3 mL/ kg. Discuss use in presence of baseline hypernatraemia with intensivist colleagues.

Indometacin (indomethacin)

Neurological indications
Treatment of chronic paroxysmal hemicrania and cluster headache. See Cluster headache and other trigeminal autonomic cephalgias in Chapter 4 ➲ p. 344.

Dosing
- PO (>1 months): 0.5–1 mg/kg/dose (max 12 hourly)

Preparations
Capsules (25 mg, 50 mg)

Contraindications
(As with other non-steroidal anti-inflammatories) cardiac failure, bleeding diathesis including risks for GI haemorrhage.

Important interactions and unwanted effects
(As with other non-steroidal anti-inflammatories), exacerbation of asthma, cardiac failure, GI bleeding.

Intravenous immunoglobulin (IVIG)

Neurological indications
Treatment of AIDP (Guillain–Barré) and CIDP. Treatment of autoimmune encephalitis. Considered in treatment of acute demyelinating syndromes including transverse myelitis and severe ADEM. Treatment of myasthenic crisis in myasthenia gravis.

Dosing
- All indications. Total dose 2 g/kg typically fractionated over 5 consecutive days. Standard infusion protocols start at very low dose to minimize risk of anaphylaxis and escalate over several hours: consult product leaflet.
- Monitor temperature, pulse, and respiration frequently during administration.

Preparations
Various: no evidence of differential efficacy.

Contraindications

Known anti-IgA antibodies. IgA deficiency must be excluded prior to first use.

Important interactions and unwanted effects

Fever, rash (consider continuing with antihistamine/steroid cover). More rarely anaphylaxis. As a pooled-blood product, risk in principle of transmission of infectious agents though all known pathogens screened.

Comments

Advisable to store a serum sample before administration to permit serological testing after use.

Obese patients should be dosed according to *ideal* body weight.

Ketamine

Neurological indications

Third line treatment of absence status epilepticus (See Absence status epilepticus in Chapter 4 p. 289).

Dosing

- PO (1–18 yrs): 1.5 mg/kg/day divided in two doses for up to 5 days.
- PICU protocol: continuous infusion initially 0.5–2 mg/kg as slow IV injection over 1 min, followed by continuous intravenous infusion of 0.6–2.7 mg/kg/h adjusted according to response.

Discontinuation regimen
- Oral treatment is typically maintained alongside conventional ASMs for 5 days then discontinued without weaning.

Preparations

Solution for injections (10 mg/mL, 50 mg/mL, 100 mg/mL): parenteral preparation can be given orally in fruit juice. Oral solution available.

Contraindications

- Hypertension (BP >95th centile for age and height).
- Concerns about raised intracranial pressure.
- Acute stroke/severe cardiac disease.
- Severe liver disease.

Important interactions and unwanted effects

Respiratory suppression.

Comments

For intravenous infusion, dilute to 1 mg/mL with 0.9% saline or glucose 5%. NOTE: Controlled Drug (CD) regulations apply in the UK.

Lacosamide

Neurological indications

Treatment of focal seizures; adjunctive therapy of primary generalized tonic–clonic seizures.

Dosing

Starting doses and escalation regimen
- PO (2–17 yrs and <50 kg): 1 mg/kg/day divided in two doses. Increase by 1 mg/kg/day at weekly intervals.
- PO (2–17 yrs and >50 kg): 100 mg/day divided in two doses. Increase by 100 mg/day at weekly intervals.
- In status epilepticus or seizure clusters. PO/IV (all ages, unlicensed <16 yrs): 2 mg/kg/day, to max 10 mg/kg/day if tolerated.

Maintenance doses
- PO (2–17 yrs and <50 kg): up to 10 mg/kg/day (occasionally 12 mg/kg/day under 40 kg)
- PO (2–17 yrs and >50 kg): up to 300 mg BD.

Preparations

Tablets (50 mg, 100 mg, 150 mg, 200 mg). Oral solution (10 mg/mL). Solution for intravenous infusion (200 mg/20 mL).

Important interactions and unwanted effects

Dizziness common. Risk of PR-interval prolongation: do not use in presence second- or third-degree heart block.

Comments

Intravenous formulation available: no dosing adjustment required.

For interactions between antiseizure medicines, see this chapter ➔ p. 709. Use in children under 16 yrs of age must be under specialist supervision. May *worsen* primary generalized epilepsies (especially JME), tonic, atonic, and absence seizures.

Lamotrigine

Neurological indications

Treatment of focal, generalized, and absence seizures.

Dosing

Starting doses and escalation regimen
- *Without valproate, and without enzyme-inducing drugs*:
  - PO (2–11 yrs): 300 microgms/kg/day in 1–2 divided doses, increasing after 14 days to 600 microgms/kg/day for further 14 days, then increasing in steps of up to 600 microgms/kg every 7–14 days.

- PO (>12 yrs): 25 mg once daily, increasing after 14 days to 50 mg once daily, then increasing in steps of up to 100–200 mg/day every 7–14 days in 1–2 divided doses.
- *Without valproate but with enzyme-inducing drugs*: double the above doses.
- *With valproate* (which inhibits lamotrigine degradation):
  - PO (2–11 yrs and <13 kg): 2 mg once daily on alternate days for 14 days then 300 microgms/kg once daily for further 14 days then increased in steps of up to 300 microgms/kg every 7–14 days.
  - PO (2–11 yrs and >13 kg): 150 microgms/kg once daily for 14 days then 300 microgms/kg once daily for further 14 days then increased in steps of up to 300 microgms/kg every 7–14 days.
  - PO (12–17 yrs): 25 mg once daily on alternate days for 14 days then 25 mg once daily for further 14 days then increased in steps of up to 50 mg every 7–14 days.

Maintenance doses
- *Without valproate and without enzyme-inducing drugs:*
  - PO (2–11 yrs): Initial target dose 1–10 mg/kg/day in 1–2 divided doses (max. 200 mg/day)
  - PO (>12 yrs): 100–200 mg daily in 1–2 divided doses.
- *Without valproate but with enzyme-inducing drugs:*
  - PO (2–11 yrs): 5–15 mg/kg daily in 1–2 divided doses (max 400 mg/day)
  - PO (>12 yrs): 200–400 mg daily in 2 divided doses, increased if necessary to 700 mg/day.
- *With valproate*:
  - PO (2–11 yrs): 1–5 mg/kg/day in 1–2 divided doses (max. 200 mg/day).
  - PO (12–17 yrs): 100–200 mg daily in 1–2 divided doses.

Preparations

Tablets (25 mg, 50 mg, 100 mg, 200 mg). Dispersible tablets (2 mg, 5 mg, 25 mg, 100 mg) may be chewed: the child should drink a glass of water, squash, or fruit juice after they have chewed the tablet.

Important interactions and unwanted effects

Rash which is occasionally serious including Stevens–Johnson syndrome. Mood disturbance. Rarely hepatic dysfunction, lymphadenopathy, leukopenia, thrombocytopenia.

Comments

- Initial desensitizing dose and slow escalation are used to reduce the otherwise high incidence of rash. Warn families to report any rash or signs and symptoms of blood disorder (such as anaemia, unexplained bruising, or infection) urgently and to discontinue treatment.
  Lamotrigine can sometimes be cautiously reintroduced despite previous rash formation if indicated, using the increments above but increasing at intervals of 2–3 months. Dose titration should be repeated if restarting after an interruption of >4 days.

- Not licensed for use as monotherapy in children under 12 yrs, or as adjunctive treatment in children under 2 yrs.
- Round dose up or down to the nearest solid dosage (e.g. half or quarter of a tablet).
- For interactions between antiseizure medicines, see this chapter ➲ p. 709.

Levetiracetam

Neurological indications

Generalized, absence, and focal seizures. Second-line treatment in convulsive status epilepticus.

Dosing

Convulsive status epilepticus (or frequent recurrent, clustering seizures)
- IV (all ages): 40 mg/kg iv bolus over 5 mins (max 3 g/dose).

Regular use: starting doses and escalation regimen
- PO (1–5 months): 7 mg/kg/day in 1–2 divided doses, incrementing by 7 mg/mg/day every 14 days.
- PO (>6 months and <50 kg): 10 mg/kg/day in 1–2 divided doses, incrementing by 10 mg/kg/day every 7 days.
- PO (12–17 yrs and >50 kg): 250 mg BD, incrementing by 500 mg BD every 7–14 days.

Maintenance doses
- PO (1–5 months): Up to 21 mg/kg BD
- PO (>6 months and <50 kg): 40 mg/kg/day occasionally up to 60 mg/kg/day in 1–2 divided doses
- PO (12–17 yrs and >50 kg): up to 1.5 g BD.

Preparations

Tablet (250 mg, 500 mg, 750 mg, 1 g) can be crushed and dispersed in water. Granules (250 mg, 500 mg, 750 mg, 1 g): prepare suspension immediately before administration. Oral solution (500 mg/5 mL). Solution for IV infusion (500 mg/5 mL).

Important interactions and unwanted effects

Drowsiness, weakness, behavioural disturbance. Rarely precipitates non-convulsive status epilepticus. Reduce dose if eGFR <80 mL/min/1.73 m².

Comments

Generally well tolerated. For discontinuation, decreased dose gradually over several weeks. For interactions between antiseizure medicines, see this chapter ➲ p. 709. IV dose same as PO maintenance.

Levodopa (L-DOPA)

Neurological indications
Treatment of DOPA-responsive conditions including DOPA-responsive dystonia and tetrahydrobiopterin synthesis disorders.

Dosing
Starting doses and escalation regimen
- PO (all ages): 1–2 mg/kg/day in 4–6 divided doses increasing by 1 mg/kg/day every 3–5 days.

Maintenance doses
Increase progressively until clinical effect, or unwanted effects (particularly vomiting) supervene. Typical doses for DOPA-responsive dystonias (DRD) are around 10–12 mg/kg/day. Lack of response after 3 months at maximum clinically tolerated dose is sufficient to exclude DRD (response can be delayed).

Preparations
1 part carbidopa: 4 parts levodopa preparation is recommended; at higher doses consider preparation containing 1:10 carbidopa: levodopa.
    Tablets may be crushed and dispersed in water immediately prior to administration.
- Sinemet® 62.5 mg scored tablet containing carbidopa 12.5 mg:levodopa 50 mg. Also available: Sinemet® 110, Sinemet® Plus, and Sinemet® 275.
- Madopar® 10/12.5: soluble tablet containing 50 mg levodopa:12.5 mg benserazide. Also available Madopar®100/25 tablets.

Contraindications
Closed angle glaucoma.

Important interactions and unwanted effects
Sudden onset of sleep, excessive sedation. Nausea and vomiting, autonomic disturbance (e.g. postural hypotension and syncope).

Comments
Amino acid precursor of dopamine which replenishes striatal dopamine. Usually administered with a DOPA decarboxylase inhibitor to reduce unwanted systemic effects. In prolonged therapy psychiatric, hepatic, haematological, renal, and cardiovascular monitoring is advisable. Prescribed doses are expressed as levodopa. Avoid abrupt withdrawal.

Lisdexamfetamine
See Dexamfetamine in this chapter p. 665.

Lorazepam

Neurological indications

Emergency treatment of status epilepticus.

Dosing

- IV (all ages):100 microgms/kg (max. 4 mg/dose) over 60 seconds via a large vein, repeated once if initial dose is ineffective after 5–10 mins. Can also be given sublingually or rectally.

Preparations

Intravenous injection (2 mg/mL, 4 mg/mL).

Contraindications

See under diazepam in this chapter ➲ p. 666.

Important interactions and unwanted effects

See under diazepam in this chapter ➲ p. 666.

Comments

Superior to parenteral diazepam as the latter tends to enter adipose tissue lowering circulating levels, and where repeated doses can accumulate before re-entering the bloodstream, causing late respiratory effects. One larger dose is typically more effective than repeated partial doses.

Dilute with equal volume of 0.9% saline or water for injection and inject slowly through a large vein. In neonates, dilute to 100 microgms/mL (i.e. 1 mL/kg total volume). Avoid injections containing benzyl alcohol in neonates.

Mannitol

Neurological indications

Emergency treatment of known or suspected cerebral oedema but inferior to hypertonic saline (see hypertonic saline in this chapter ➲ p. 676).

Dosing

- IV (>1 months): 0.25–1.5 g/kg (1.25–7.5 mL/kg of 20% solution) over 30–60 min. Repeated if necessary after 4–8 h, max. twice.

Preparations

10% and 20% solutions. Examine infusion for crystals. If crystals are present: warm to 60°C, allow to cool to body temperature, and administer via an in-line filter (15-micron filter is suitable).

Contraindications

Cardiac failure or pulmonary oedema. Pre-existing hypernatraemia or hypovolaemia. Intracranial bleeding. Anuria.

Important interactions and unwanted effects

Hypovolaemia due to obligatory diuresis. Extravasation may occur.

Comments

Increasingly replaced by hypertonic saline (see hypertonic saline in this chapter ⟳ p. 676). A transient artefactual hypertonic hyponatraemia typically occurs on initial use (the mannitol causes water shift from the intracellular to the extracellular compartment and a dilutional hyponatraemia with normal total body sodium). Prolonged or frequent use will result in hypernatraemia, limiting further use. After prolonged repeated use mannitol will eventually cross into the intracellular compartment thus having entirely the opposite effect to that desired, drawing water into cells.

Melatonin

Neurological indications

Sleep induction for EEG; treatment of sleep–wake cycle disorders particularly in children with neurodisability (most studied in children with visual impairment).

Dosing

Maintenance doses
- For sleep EEG. PO: <5 yrs, 3 mg; >5 yrs, 6 mg. Up to 12 mg for older teenagers.
- For sleep–wake cycle disorders. Under 2 yrs, 2.5–5 mg; over 2 yrs, 2.5–10 mg at night.

Preparations

Capsule (2 mg, 3 mg, 5 mg) can be opened and dispersed in drink (water, milk, or fruit juice) prior to administration. Controlled-release tablet (1 mg, 2 mg, 5 mg). Oral solution (1 mg/mL).

Comments

Standard formulation is effective for 5 h. Treatment with a combination of standard and controlled-release preparation has been described. Use in visual impairment argued based on loss of physiological light/dark sleep cues. Does not affect EEG. Safety of long-term use is not established. Doses >10 mg for sleep–wake disorders show no additional efficacy.

Methylphenidate

Neurological indications

Treatment of attention-deficit hyperactivity disorder. Symptomatic treatment of narcolepsy.

Dosing

Starting doses and escalation regimen
These doses relate to standard-release tablets. For controlled-release tablet dosing refer to relevant product literature.
- PO (4–5 yrs): 2.5 mg BD, increased at weekly intervals by 2.5 mg/day.
- PO (>6 yrs): 5 mg OD-BD increased at weekly intervals by 5–10 mg/day.

Maintenance doses
- PO (4–6 yrs): up to 1.4 mg/kg/day in 2–3 divided doses.
- PO (>6 yrs): 1–2 mg/kg/day up to 60 mg/day, typically at 8 am and 1 pm. Max 2.1 mg/kg/day or 90 mg/day. Avoid giving last dose later than 4 pm.

Preparations

Tablets and controlled-release tablets. Caution if switching between products due to difference in formulations and biphasic profiles of some.

Contraindications

See under dexamfetamine in this chapter ➲ p. 665.

Important interactions and unwanted effects

See under dexamfetamine in this chapter ➲ p. 665.

Comments

Short duration of action permits tailored use, e.g. omitting doses at weekends and during school holidays. Consider initial and subsequent blinded trials omitting doses: ideally with a semi-objective symptom severity measure (e.g. Connor questionnaire for parents and teachers). Many children with attention-deficit hyperactive disorder may have co-existing epilepsy. It has been reported that stimulants may exacerbate pre-existing seizure tendencies: in our opinion, this risk is not high and epilepsy is not a contraindication to stimulant therapy if otherwise clinically indicated.

Discontinue if no effect after 1 month. Not recommended under 4 yrs old.

NOTE Controlled drug (CD) regulations apply in the UK.

Methylprednisolone

Neurological indications

'Pulse' remission-initiating treatment of non-infectious CNS inflammation including demyelination and vasculitis.

Dosing
- IV (all ages): 30 mg/kg (max. 1 g) OD for 3 to 5 days.

Preparations

Powder for reconstitution—diluted in 0.9% saline or glucose 5% and administered over at least 30 min.

Contraindications

Active systemic infection.

Important interactions and unwanted effects

Rapid infusion may be associated with severe hypertension and cardiovascular collapse. May cause insomnia: if possible, avoid giving in the evening. See typical unwanted steroid effects under ACTH in this chapter ➲ p. 651). High-dose methylprednisolone may increase blood ciclosporin levels.

Comments

Usually followed by a maintenance course of oral prednisolone.

Midazolam

Neurological indications

Rescue for prolonged seizures; status epilepticus (in emergency room/in-patient settings); sedation for minor procedures.

Dosing

<u>Buccal</u> use as an emergency rescue treatment for prolonged seizures, single dose to be repeated once after 5–10 mins if required

- <3 months: 300 microgms/kg (max 2.5 mg)
- 3–11 months: 2.5 mg
- 1–4 yrs: 5 mg
- Child 5–9 yrs: 7.5 mg
- Child 10–17 yrs: 10 mg

Intravenous use for refractory status epilepticus in PICU settings

- All ages: IV injection 150–200 microgms/kg (maximum 10 mg) over 2–3 mins, followed by continuous infusion of 1 microgms/kg/min.
- Increase by 1 microgms/kg/min every 15 min until seizure control achieved: maximum 300 microgms/kg/h, occasionally higher when ventilated.

Sedation for procedures (See Acute sedation protocols in this Chapter ➜ p. 708)

Preparations

Injection 1 mg/mL, 2 mg/mL. Buccal liquid (prefilled syringes containing 2.5 mg, 5 mg, 7.5 mg, or 10 mg; bottles containing 10 mg/mL).

Important interactions and unwanted effects

Rapid IV injection (<2 min) may cause seizure like myoclonus in preterm neonates. Monitor closely for respiratory depression, laryngospasm, bronchospasm, respiratory arrest, hypotension, heart rate changes, cardiac arrest, anaphylaxis. Rarely involuntary movement on withdrawal, paradoxical excitement and aggression, urinary retention, and incontinence.

NOTE Controlled drug (CD) regulations apply in the UK.

Neostigmine

Neurological indications

Short-term treatment of myasthenia and disorders of neuromuscular transmission.

Dosing

IM/SC

A test dose of 0.05 mg/kg should be given then:
- Neonate: 150 microgms/kg every 6–8 h, 30 min before feeds, increasing as necessary to max 300 microgms/kg every 4 h.
- 1 mth–11 yrs: 200–500 microgms repeated every 3–4 h as required.
- Over 12 yrs: 1–2.5 mg every 3–4 h as required.

Oral

- Neonate: 1–2 mg, then 1–5 mg every 3–4 h, 30 min before feeds.
- 1 month–5 yrs: 7.5 mg repeated every 3–4 h as required, max 90 mg/day.
- 6–11 yrs: 15 mg repeated every 3–4 h as required, max 90 mg/day.
- >12 yrs: 15–30 mg repeated every 3–4 h as required, max 300 mg/day.

Preparations

Injection (2.5 mg/mL) tablets 15 mg (scored).

Contraindications

Intestinal obstruction, urinary retention.

Important interactions and unwanted effects

Has strong muscarinic action, and concomitant atropine or propantheline treatment may be required to treat abdominal cramps, excess salivation, or diarrhoea. Bronchoconstriction suggests overdose.

Nitrazepam

Neurological indications

Treatment of myoclonic seizures in infants and second-line treatment of infantile spasms.

Dosing

Starting doses and escalation regimen
- PO: 125 microgms/kg at night increasing by 125 microgms/kg/day increments divided in 3 doses every 3–4 days.

Maintenance doses
- PO: 0.3–1 mg/kg/day divided into 3 doses.

Discontinuation regimen
- 75% of the dose for 2 months; 50% of the dose for 2 months; 25% of the dose for 2 months: then stop.

Preparations

Tablets (5 mg). Oral solution (2.5 mg/5 mL).

Contraindications

See under diazepam in this chapter ⟿ p. 666.

Important interactions and unwanted effects

See under diazepam in this chapter ⟿ p. 666.

Oxcarbazepine

Neurological indications

See under carbamazepine in this chapter ➲ p. 659: particularly useful in situations of partial response to carbamazepine where higher doses are being prevented by emerging unwanted effects. Will *worsen* primary generalized epilepsies (especially JME), tonic, atonic, and absence seizures.

Dosing

Starting doses and escalation regimen
- PO (>6 yrs): 4–5 mg/kg/day (max. 300 mg/day) divided in 2 doses, increasing in 5–10 mg/kg/day (max. 300 mg/day) increments at weekly intervals.

Maintenance doses
- PO (>6 yrs): 15 mg/kg BD (max 46 mg/kg.day)

Discontinuation regimen
- 75% for 2 weeks; 50% for 2 weeks; 25% for 2 weeks; then stop.

Preparations

Tablets (150 mg, 300 mg, 600 mg); oral solution (300 mg/5 mL)

Important interactions and unwanted effects

See under carbamazepine in this chapter ➲ p. 659. Hyponatraemia due to SIADH is considerably more common than with carbamazepine. A past history of rash formation with carbamazepine is a relative, but not absolute contraindication to oxcarbazepine use, although extra caution is required.

❶ Test children of Han-Chinese or Thai origin for HLA-B*1502 allele (see Carbamazepine in this chapter ➲ p. 659).

Comments

Oxcarbazepine is a drug very closely related to carbamazepine, modified to prevent conversion to a particular metabolite responsible for many of the dose-related unwanted effects of the latter. In theory, therefore, it should be similarly efficacious and better tolerated. Can be directly substituted (without a transition period) for carbamazepine: typical starting dose of oxcarbazepine = 150% prior carbamazepine dose.

For interactions between antiseizure medicines, see this chapter ➲ p. 709.

Oxybate sodium

Neurological indications

Cataplexy, severe narcolepsy.

Dosing

Dosing taken at bedtime and again 2.5–4 h later (see Table 7.3).

Table 7.3 Oxybate sodium dosing recommendations

Weight (kg)	Initial daily dose (taken in 2 divided doses)	Dose increases (titrating to clinical effect)	Maximum daily dose
15–20	≤ 1 g/day	≤ 0.5 g/day weekly	0.2 g/kg
20–30	≤ 2 g/day	≤ 1 g/day weekly	0.2 g/kg
30–45	≤ 3 g/day	≤ 1 g/day weekly	0.2 g/kg
≥45	≤ 4.5 g/day	≤ 1.5 g/day weekly	9 g

Preparations

Oral solution (500 mg/mL) needs further dilution and preparation by family before ingesting. Dilute with 60 mL water.

Contraindications

Situations where poor adherence likely; unsuitable family and social situations (controlled drug); alcohol-dependency; sleep apnoea; succinic semialdehyde dehydrogenase deficiency.

Important interactions and unwanted effects

Nausea, salty taste, headache, enuresis, bowel habit alterations. Doses should only be taken in bed. Death reported in adults with multiple comorbidities and polypharmacy.

Comments

Has also been used in adult movement disorders e.g. myoclonus. Very expensive. If therapy has been stopped for more than 14 consecutive days, it should be re-titrated from initial starting dose.

Paraldehyde

Neurological indications

Status epilepticus.

Dosing

- PR (all ages): 0.4 mL/kg (max. 10 mL) of undiluted paraldehyde.
- Undiluted liquid should be mixed with 9 volumes of 0.9 % saline, or 1 volume of olive oil or sunflower oil (avoid peanut/arachis oil because of anaphylaxis risk).
- Pre-mixed preparations available.
- Doses above are expressed as mL *of paraldehyde* (i.e. volume of 1:1 pre-mixed liquid should be double the above dose).

Preparations

Liquid for rectal administration.

Contraindications

Gastric disorders; colitis (with rectal administration).

Important interactions and unwanted effects

Frequent rectal administration can result in proctitis. Plastic syringes can be used if the dose is administered immediately, otherwise use a glass syringe due to product degradation when in contact with plastic.

Comments

Intramuscular administration is possible but not recommended: risk of sterile abscess.

Perampanel

Neurological indications

Adjunctive treatment of focal seizures.

Table 7.4 Dosing

Age	4–11 yrs	4–11 yrs	4–11 yrs	>12 yrs
Weight	<20 kg	20–29.9 kg	≥30 kg	–
Starting dose	1 mg OD	1 mg OD	2 mg OD	2 mg OD
Titration	Increase by 0.5 mg/day weekly	Increase by 1 mg/day weekly	Increase by 2 mg/day weekly	
Usual dose	2–4 mg OD	4–6 mg OD	4–8 mg OD	4–8 mg OD
Max dose	6 mg OD	8 mg OD	12 mg OD	12 mg OD

Preparations

Tablets (2 mg, 4 mg, 6 mg, 8 mg, 10 mg, 12 mg); oral solution (0.5 mg/mL).

Important interactions and unwanted effects

Behavioural disturbances (aggression, anxiety). Suicidal ideation has been reported. Dizziness, drowsiness.

Comments

Slow dose escalation vital to minimizing likelihood of unwanted effects. For discontinuation reduce dose gradually. For interactions between antiseizure medicines, see this chapter ⵕ p. 709.

Phenobarbital (phenobarbitone)

Neurological indications

Status epilepticus; maintenance ASM.

Dosing

Starting doses and escalation regimen

- Status epilepticus. Slow IV injection (all ages): 20 mg/kg (max. 1 g): dilute solution 1 in 10 with water for injections and infuse at max. 1 mg/kg/min. Additional 2.5–5 mg/kg doses may be considered. In frequent recurrent seizures (i.e. clusters), oral loading may be adequate (dose unchanged).

Maintenance doses

- PO/IV (Neonate): 2.5–5 mg/kg once daily.
- PO (1 month–11 yrs): 5–8 mg/kg/day divided in 1–2 doses.
- PO (>12 yrs): 60–180 mg once daily.
- Due to auto-induction of metabolism, higher doses may be required (under specialist advice).

Missed dose regimen

- If one or more doses have been missed and breakthrough seizures have occurred, consider giving a single *additional* partial loading dose (e.g. 5 mg/kg once).

Preparations

Tablets (15 mg, 30 mg, 60 mg; may be crushed). Intravenous injection (30 mg/mL, 60 mg/mL, 200 mg/mL). Oral solution available (preferably avoid alcohol-containing products).

Contraindications

Porphyria. Severe impairment of renal or hepatic function.

Important interactions and unwanted effects

Drowsiness, respiratory depression. Skin reactions. Megaloblastic anaemia with prolonged use (treat with folate).

Comments

Aim for trough levels of 15–40 mg/L (60–180 micromol/L) although higher levels may be acceptable if no signs of toxicity as tolerance can occur. Injection may be given rectally (same as oral dose). Induces liver enzymes: many important interactions (see other sources). For interactions between antiseizure medicines, see this chapter p. 709.

Phenobarbital use in pregnancy has been associated with dose-dependent increased rates of congenital malformation. Its use in female patients should only be after informed discussion of risks (see Contraception and reproductive health in Chapter 4 p. 320).

Avoid alcohol-containing solutions in children.

Phenytoin

Neurological indications

Status epilepticus. Acute seizure management particularly in ICU setting (e.g. post-neurosurgery). Maintenance ASM for all seizure types except absence epilepsy and absence status (may aggravate).

Dosing

Status epilepticus and urgent initiation of maintenance ASM
See Box 7.1.
- Neonates (specialist advice only) to 18 yrs: 20 mg/kg slow IV infusion (over 30 min with cardiac monitoring; max. rate 1 mg/kg/min to max. 50 mg/min).
- In less urgent situations, oral loading (same doses) may be appropriate.

Maintenance doses
- PO/IV (<12 yrs): 5–10 mg/kg/day (max. 300 mg daily) divided in 2 doses. Dose requirements are toward the top end of this range (and sometimes higher) in neonates and infants.
- PO (12–18 yrs): 150–200 mg BD (max. 300 mg BD).
- Due to near zero-order elimination kinetics particularly at higher blood levels, dose increments should be small to prevent inadvertent overdosing (ideally <10% increases at >fortnightly intervals).

Missed dose regimen
- If one or more doses have been missed and breakthrough seizures have occurred, consider giving an *additional* partial loading dose (e.g. 5 mg/kg single dose).

Box 7.1 Levels and loading doses

Phenytoin, and to a lesser extent phenobarbital, have reputations as difficult drugs to titrate. It is common to see inexperienced prescribers struggling with over- and undershooting levels. The main reason for this is failure to appreciate how long it can take to establish the new steady-state drug level after a dose change, which is often several days and for phenytoin **can be up to 2 weeks**.

This period can be shortened by the use of *ad hoc* loading doses (or 'negative loading doses': i.e. missing a dose if trying to reduce a high level). The ultimate steady-state level is determined solely by the maintenance dose, but loading doses will expedite the attainment of that steady state.

Thus if a blood level is still low and seizures are occurring a few days after starting phenytoin, give a further partial load (e.g. 5 or 10 mg/kg) but do not increase the maintenance dose (because of the risk of a subsequent overshoot) unless further measurements clearly show the effect of this loading dose to have passed because levels are falling again.

In general, if a child is seizure free and alert on phenobarbital or phenytoin, do not adjust the dose even if the level is outside the 'reference range' (i.e. treat the child, not the drug level).

▶ Adjustments of maintenance doses in light of steady-state blood levels should be in small increments (~10% previous dose).

Preparations

As phenytoin sodium: capsules (25 mg, 50 mg, 100 mg, 300 mg); tablets (100 mg). As phenytoin: chewable Infatabs® (50 mg); suspension (30 mg/ 5 mL); injection 50 mg/mL.

Contraindications

Porphyria.

Will typically *worsen* primary generalized epilepsies (especially JME), tonic, atonic, and absence seizures. Avoid in Dravet syndrome.

Important interactions and unwanted effects

Nausea, headache, tremor, ataxia (dose-dependent). Dyskinesias after intravenous use particularly in children with underlying neurodisability (not uncommon on ICU). Rarely blood dyscrasias, rash including Stevens–Johnson syndrome. Osteomalacia (consider calcium/vitamin D supplementation if prolonged treatment is anticipated).

Hirsutism and gum hyperplasia are common fully reversible unwanted effects. Gum hyperplasia may be limited by scrupulous attention to teeth-cleaning (it is accelerated by the presence of plaque). Dental surgeons can offer cosmetic gum resection in established cases where continuing phenytoin use is required.

Comments

Aim for trough level 10–20 mg/L (6–15 mg/L in neonates). Phenytoin is highly protein bound and levels may need to be adjusted for serum albumin.

Phenytoin liquid is a *suspension* (i.e. particles floating in liquid) not a solution. Left standing, the drug will settle in the bottle resulting in under-dosing at the top of the bottle and toxicity as the bottle empties unless it is vigorously shaken (consider use of Infatabs® as an alternative).

Nasogastric feeds should be suspended for 1h before and after oral/enteral phenytoin to improve absorption.

Intravenous phenytoin infusion is strongly alkaline and must be infused slowly into a large vein to avoid phlebitis and/or tissue injury due to extravasation. Use in-line filter (0.22–0.5°μm), flush with saline before and after infusion and dilute to 10 mg/mL.

Phenytoin use in pregnancy has been associated with increased rates of congenital malformation. Its use in female patients should only be after informed discussion of risks (see Contraception and reproductive health in Chapter 4 ➲ p. 320).

For interactions between antiseizure medicines, see this chapter ➲ p. 709.

Pimozide

Neurological indications

Tourette's syndrome.

Dosing

Starting doses and escalation regime:
- PO (2–11 yrs): 1–4 mg daily.
- PO (12–18 yrs): 2–10 mg daily.
- *Discontinuation regime.* Slowly over three weeks.

Preparation

Tablets (4 mg).

Contraindications

History of arrhythmias or congenital QT prolongation. It is recommended to carry out an ECG before use looking for prolonged QT syndrome and annual ECG during treatment.

Important interactions and unwanted effects

Some sedation, serious arrhythmias; glycosuria, and rarely hyponatraemia. Antimuscarinic effects.

Piracetam

Neurological indications:

Cortical or segmental myoclonus.

Dosing

- PO: Initially 150 mg/kg/day in 2–3 divided doses to a maximum of 300 mg/kg/day in 2–3 divided doses.
- Stop escalation if wanted or unwanted effects appear.
- Reduce dose in renal impairment:
  - two-thirds of normal dose if eGFR 50–80 mL/min/1.73 m²;
  - one-third of normal dose in 2 divided doses if eGFR 30–50 mL/min/1.73 m²;
  - one-sixth normal dose as a single dose if eGFR 20–30 mL/min/1.73 m²;
  - do not use if eGFR less than 20 mL/min/1.73 m².

Preparations

Scored 800 mg tablets; oral solution 333 mg/mL (33%).

Contraindications

Cerebral haemorrhage. Hepatic or severe renal impairment.

Important interactions and unwanted effects

Weight gain, nervousness, hyperkinesia; less commonly, drowsiness, and depression.

Comments

Oral solution has a bitter taste. Should be administered undiluted followed by a glass of water or soft drink.

Pizotifen

Neurological indications

Prophylaxis of migraine.

Dosing

Starting doses and escalation regimen
- PO (2–18 yrs): 500 microgms at night.

Maintenance doses
- 2–18 yrs: max 1.5 mg/day, max. single dose 1 mg.

Preparations

Tablets (500 microgms, 1.5 mg).

Important interactions and unwanted effects

Dry mouth, constipation, increased appetite and weight gain, drowsiness.

Prednisolone

Neurological indications

Treatment of infantile spasms and epileptic encephalopathies. Treatment of non-infectious CNS inflammation (e.g. demyelination, vasculitis).

Dosing

Starting doses and escalation regimen
- Infantile spasms (usually in combination with vigabatrin). PO: 10 mg QDS for 14 days; increasing to 20 mg TDS after 7 days if no response.
- Epileptic encephalopathies. 2–4 mg/kg/day (max. 60 mg) in 2–4 divided doses.
- CNS inflammation. 2 mg/kg/day (max. 60 mg) once daily.

Maintenance doses
- Infantile spasms. If not controlled after 7 days increase to 20 mg TDS for 7 days.
- Epileptic encephalopathies. 2–4 mg/kg/day (max. 60 mg) In 2–4 divided doses; regimen of 4 mg/kg as a single *weekly* dose permits prolonged use over several months with minimization of Cushingoid effects.
- CNS inflammation. 2 mg/kg/day (max. 60 mg) once daily.

Discontinuation regimen
Generally, systemic corticosteroids may be stopped abruptly in those whose disease is unlikely to relapse and who have received treatment for 3 weeks or less.

Gradual withdrawal recommended if:
- Received more than 40 mg or 2 mg/kg prednisolone (or equivalent of other steroids) daily for 1 week or 1 mg/kg daily for 1 month;
- Been given repeated *evening* doses;
- Received more than 3 weeks' treatment;
- Recently received repeated courses (particularly if taken for longer than 3 weeks);

- Taken a short course within 1 year of stopping long-term therapy;
- Other possible causes of adrenal suppression.

Weaning schedules
- Infantile spasms. If taking 10 mg QDS for 14 days, reduce by 10 mg every 5 days then stop. If dose increased to 20 mg TDS for 7 days, reduce to 40 mg/day for 5 days, then 20 mg/day for 5 days, then 10 mg/day for 5 days, then stop.
- Epileptic encephalopathies. Typically maintained at full dose for up to 4 weeks before reducing to alternate day regimen for up to 2 weeks and then withdrawal over a further 2 weeks.
- CNS inflammation. Typically maintained at full dose for up to 4 weeks before reducing to alternate day regimen. For ADEM and acute demyelination, would then typically withdraw over 2 weeks. For CNS vasculitides and steroid-dependent conditions, long-term treatment over many months may be required.
- Discuss with endocrinology whether treatment dose/duration warrants short synacthen test (assessing potential adrenal suppression) to guide withdrawal.

Preparations
Crushable (1 mg, 5 mg, 25 mg), enteric-coated (2.5 mg, 5 mg), and soluble (5 mg) tablets.

Contraindications
Active infection.

Important interactions and unwanted effects
Steroid effects. See ACTH in this chapter ➲ p. 651.

Comments
Prolonged steroid treatment over months requires monitoring of bone mineral density and calcium/vitamin D supplementation. Provide steroid card. Take with food. Gastric protection with a proton-pump inhibitor or H_2-antagonist may be required at high doses or prolonged courses. Note that whilst for systemic use prednisolone and prednisone can be used interchangeably, only prednisolone crosses the BBB well.

Pregabalin

Neurological indications
Neuropathic pain and paraesthesiae; also adjunctive treatment of focal seizures.

Dosing
Starting doses and escalation regimen
- PO (>12 yrs): 25 mg TDS; 75 mg/day increments at weekly intervals.

Maintenance doses
- PO (>12 yrs): 100 mg TDS (adult max. 600 mg/day).

Preparations

Capsule (25 mg, 50 mg, 75 mg, 100 mg, 150 mg, 200 mg, 300 mg) may be opened and dispersed in water prior to administration.

Comments

Generally well tolerated and free of interactions. Adjust dose to renal function. For interactions between antiseizure medicines, see this chapter ➔ p. 709.

Prochlorperazine

Neurological indications

Treatment of nausea and vomiting in migraine (with separately prescribed analgesia)

Dosing

Oral
- 1–11 yrs (>10 kg): 250 microgms/kg 2–3 times a day.
- 12–17 yrs: 5–10 mg up to 3 times a day if required.

Buccal
- 12–17 yrs: 3–6 mg twice daily, tablets to be placed high between upper lip and gum and left to dissolve.

Preparations

Oral tablet (5 mg) can be dispersed in water; buccal tablet (3 mg).

Procyclidine

Neurological indications

Emergency treatment of acute dystonia and oculogyric crises.

Dosing

- Single intravenous dose: <2 yrs, 0.5–2 mg; 2–9 yrs, 2–5 mg; 10–18 yrs, 5–10 mg. Repeat after 30 min if necessary. Can also be given IM or PO. IV/IM to be given over at least 2 mins.

Preparations

Tablets (5 mg), oral solution (2.5 mg/5 mL, 5 mg/5 mL), injection (10 mg/2 mL).

Contraindications

See Trihexyphenidyl in this chapter ➔ p. 705.
Important interactions and unwanted effects; see Trihexyphenidyl in this chapter ➔ p. 705.

Comments

Onset of effect in 5–10 min: may take 30min for full effect.

Propranolol

Neurological indications

Migraine prophylaxis. Treatment of essential tremor.

Dosing

- PO (2–11 yrs): 20–40 mg/day divided in 2 doses (max 4 mg/kg/day).
- PO (>12 yrs): 80–160 mg/day divided in 2 doses (max 4 mg/kg/day).

Discontinuation regimen
- (In migraine) try withdrawal after 2–3 months' symptom freedom.

Preparations

Tablets (10 mg, 40 mg, 80 mg, 160 mg). Oral solution (5 mg/5 mL, 10 mg/5 mL, 40 mg/mL, 50 mg/5 mL).

Contraindications

Significant asthma, uncontrolled heart failure, sick-sinus syndrome, second- or third-degree heart block, metabolic acidosis, phaeochromocytoma.

Important interactions and unwanted effects

Postural hypotension at excessive doses. Bronchospasm in susceptible individuals. Depression and self-harm in vulnerable individuals. Cold peripheries. Sleep disorders. Can mask symptoms of hypoglycaemia.

Pyridostigmine

Neurological indications

Treatment of myasthenia gravis.

Dosing

Starting doses and escalation regimen
- PO (neonate to 11 yrs): 0.5–1 mg/kg/dose (give 1 h before feeds) repeated as required up to 4–6 hourly.
- PO (>12 yrs): 30–60 mg/dose repeated as required up to 4–6 times daily.
- Increase by increments of 25–50% daily until no further improvement is seen.

Maintenance doses
- PO (<12 yrs): 30–360 mg/day divided in 4–6 doses; max. 60 mg 4 hourly.
- PO (>12 yrs): 300–600 mg/day divided in 4–6 doses (but see Comment next).

Preparations

Tablets (60 mg). Oral solution (12 mg/mL).

Contraindications

Intestinal or urinary obstruction. Care in asthma, bradycardia, hypotension, epilepsy.

Important interactions and unwanted effects

Nausea, vomiting, increased salivation, abdominal cramps.

Comments

Weaker muscarinic action than neostigmine but longer acting and fewer gastrointestinal side effects. Avoid doses >450 mg/day because of risk of AChR down-regulation. Immunosuppressant therapy is usually considered if the dose is >360 mg/day.

Pyridoxal phosphate

Neurological indication

Refractory epilepsy in infants (may be superior to pyridoxine). Consider if trial of pyridoxine fails especially in infantile spasms.

Dosing

• PO: 10 mg/kg/day; increase by 10 mg/day weekly to 50 mg/kg/day.

Preparation

Tablets 15 mg (can be crushed and mixed with water).

Important interactions and unwanted effects

Anorexia, GI disturbances, sedation.

Comments

See Vitamin B6 in Chapter 4 p. 524.

Pyridoxine (vitamin B6)

Neurological indications

Treatment of refractory epilepsy in infants: See Neonatal seizures in Chapter 5 p. 551. See also Vitamin B6 in Chapter 4 p. 524.

Dosing

• Test dose 50–100 mg oral or IV ideally with EEG monitoring.
• Maintenance (if responsive) PO/IV:
  • neonates: typically 100–200 mg/day divided in 2 doses;
  • older children: 400 mg/day (max. 30 mg/kg/day or 1 g/day).

Preparation

Tablets (10 mg, 20 mg, 50 mg; can be halved crushed and dissolved in water), capsules (100 mg), injection (50 mg/2 mL), oral solution (100 mg/5 mL).

Important interactions and unwanted effects

Severe apnoea, hypotension, and bradycardia have been reported with first doses (usually when given intravenously, give as a slow IV injection over 5 min). Otherwise well tolerated. Peripheral neuropathy on long-term treatment of higher doses.

Comments

Use for a minimum of 3 weeks. Try not to make any other changes in antiepileptics during this period to aid interpretation. Measure urinary AASA to exclude pyridoxine/pyridoxal deficiency. See Vitamin B6 in Chapter 4 ➲ p. 524 for further details. The dose for optimal neurodevelopmental outcome may be greater than the dose that controls seizures.

Risperidone

Neurological indications

Treatment of severe chorea and tic disorders. Treatment of acutely disturbed behaviour (see comment).

Dosing

Starting doses and escalation regimen
- Movement disorder. PO (>12 yrs): 1 mg/day divided in 2 doses increasing at weekly intervals by 1 mg/day if required.
- Acutely disturbed behaviour. PO (>12 yrs): 2 mg/day divided in 2 doses with rapid titration according to response.

Maintenance doses
- Movement disorder. PO (>12 yrs): up to 4 mg/day divided in 2 doses.
- Acutely disturbed behaviour. PO (>12 yrs): 4–8 mg/day but doses up to 10 mg/day may be used for brief periods.

Preparations

Tablet (0.25 mg, 0.5 mg, 1 mg, 2 mg, 3 mg, 4 mg, 6 mg). Dispersible tablet (0.5 mg, 1 mg, 2 mg, 3 mg, 4 mg). Oral solution (1 mg/mL, can be diluted in water or juice for immediate use).

Contraindications

See Haloperidol in this chapter ➲ p. 675.

Important interactions and unwanted effects

See Haloperidol in this chapter ➲ p. 675. Risk of neuroleptic malignant syndrome particularly at high doses.

Comments

Use of antipsychotics to manage acutely disturbed behaviour should only be considered in extreme situations (e.g. a large adolescent with severe learning difficulties and/or autism with a risk of injury to themselves or others) and in consultation with liaison psychiatry service. Reduce dose in hepatic and renal impairment.

Rufinamide

Neurological indications

Epilepsy, particularly Lennox–Gastaut syndrome.

Dosing

- PO (1–3 yrs): 5 mg/kg twice daily, increase by 5 mg/kg twice daily at 7–14 days intervals; max. 22.5 mg/kg twice daily.
- PO (4–18 yrs; <30 kg): 100 mg twice daily increase by 100 mg twice daily at 7–14 day intervals; max. 500 mg twice daily.
- PO (4–18 yrs; >30 kg): 200 mg twice daily increasing if required by 200 mg twice daily at 7–14 day intervals.
  - Max. doses: 900 mg twice daily for body weight 30–50 kg; 1.2 g twice daily for body weight 50–70 kg; 1.6 g twice daily for body weight over 70 kg.
- Doses may be escalated more rapidly at two-day intervals under specialist supervision.
- If on valproate, maximum doses are lower: consult product literature.

Preparations

Tablet (100 mg, 200 mg, and 400 mg): may be crushed and mixed with water. Oral solution (40 mg/mL).

Contraindications

Severe liver impairment; breast feeding.

Important interactions and unwanted effects

May raise phenytoin levels; metabolism inhibited by valproate.

Comments

A serious hypersensitivity syndrome has been reported in children after initiating therapy; consider withdrawal if rash or signs or symptoms of hypersensitivity syndrome develop.

Stiripentol

Neurological indications

Anti-epileptic drug particularly for Dravet Syndrome (see Dravet syndrome in Chapter 4 ⊃ p. 278.)

Dosing

Starting doses and escalation regimen
- PO (>3 yrs): initially 10 mg/kg in 2–3 divided doses; titrate dose over minimum of 3 days to max. 50 mg/kg/day in 2–3 divided doses.

Preparations

Capsule, powder for suspension (250 mg, 500 mg). Capsules and powder for suspension are not bio-equivalent.

Important interactions and unwanted effects

Stiripentol reduces clearance of other ASMs (particularly benzodiazepines) and unwanted effects relate largely to such accumulation. Nausea may occur when used with valproate.

Comments

Most commonly used in conjunction with valproate and/or clobazam in treatment of Dravet syndrome (see Dravet syndrome in Chapter 4 ⟲ p. 278). Valproate and clobazam doses may need to be halved. Other ASMs metabolized by the cytochrome P450 system (phenobarbital, phenytoin, carbamazepine) will also accumulate. Avoid giving with milk/dairy products, carbonated drinks, or fruit juice. Avoid caffeine.

Sulthiame (sultiame)

Neurological indications

Focal epilepsies, particularly used in atypical epilepsy with centrotemporal spikes.

Dosing

- PO (all ages): Initially 3 mg/kg/day divided into 2–3 doses.
- PO (all ages): Maintenance 5–10 mg/kg/day divided into 3 doses.

Preparations

Tablets 50 mg and 200 mg. Tablets can be divided.

Contraindications

Hypersensitivity to sulphonamides; porphyria; hyperthyroidism.

Important interactions and unwanted effects

Gastric irritation in 10%. Dose-dependent adverse effects similar to ethosuximide and acetazolamide. Hypersalivation. Stevens–Johnson. Can increase phenytoin and lamotrigine levels.

Comments

Widespread use and experience in German-speaking countries but little elsewhere. Needs to be imported.

Sumatriptan

Neurological indications

Acute symptom relief in migraine episode.

Dosing

- PO (6–9 yrs): 25 mg as single dose. Repeat after 2 h if needed.
- PO (10–12 yrs): 50 mg as single dose. Repeat after 2 h if needed.
- >12 yrs: 50–100 mg PO single dose *or* 10 mg as nasal spray single dose. Repeat after 2 h if needed: no more than 2 doses in 24 h.

Preparations

Tablets (50 mg, 100 mg). Nasal spray (10 mg, 20 mg). Autoinjector (3 mg, 6 mg).

Contraindications

Vasospasm, previous cerebrovascular accident or transient ischaemic attack, peripheral vascular disease, hypertension, previous myocardial infarction. Use with caution in hemiplegic migraine.

Important interactions and unwanted effects

Taste disturbance, mild irritation, or burning sensation in the nose or throat, heat, heaviness, pressure, or tightness, flushing in any part of the body, dizziness, weakness, fatigue, drowsiness, and transient increases in blood pressure.

Comments

Other triptans are not direct equivalents: rizatriptan has a short half-life, and frovatriptan has a much longer half-life than sumatriptan. Zolmitriptan and rizatriptan available as dissolvable wafers.

Tetrabenazine

Neurological indications

Involuntary movement; choreoathetosis.

Dosing

- PO (<5 yrs): 3.125 mg BD; increasing by this dose at weekly intervals according to response; likely max. 12.5 mg BD.
- PO (5–10 yrs): 6.25 mg BD, increasing by this dose at weekly intervals according to response; likely maximum 37.5 mg BD.
- PO (10–18 yrs): 12.5 mg BD, increasing by this dose at weekly intervals according to response; likely max. 62.5 mg BD.

Preparations

Tablets (25 mg) may be crushed and mixed with water.

Contraindications

Severe hepatic or renal impairment. Parkinsonism. Phaeochromocytoma. Prolactin-dependent tumours.

Important interactions and unwanted effects

Interacts with metoclopramide: increased risk of dystonia. Drowsiness, gastrointestinal disturbances, depression, extrapyramidal dysfunction, hypotension; rarely parkinsonism; neuroleptic malignant syndrome reported. Daily doses greater than 50 mg should not be given without CYP2D6 genotyping.

Thiamine

Neurological indications

Prevention and treatment of Wernicke encephalopathy (see Wernicke encephalopathy in Chapter 4 p. 522). Treatment of biotin responsive basal ganglia disease (together with biotin, see Thiamine transporter 2 deficiency in Chapter 4 ⟩ p. 523).

Dosing

- PO (neonate): 50–100 mg daily (can be divided into 2–3 doses).
- PO (>1 months): 100 mg daily (can be divided into 2–3 doses) increased occasionally to as much as 2 g daily in biotin responsive basal ganglia disease.

Preparations

- Tablets (50 mg and 100 mg). Oral solution (100 mg/5 mL). Solutions for iv infusion given over 30 mins.

Comments

Long-term treatment usually only required in confirmed cases of transporter deficiency: addressing causes of dietary thiamine insufficiency usually sufficient in other situations.

Tizanidine

Neurological indications

Increased tone due to cortico-spinal tract pathology.

Dosing

- PO: 0.03 mg/kg/day, increasing by 0.03–0.05 mg/kg/day at three daily intervals up to 0.75 mg/kg/day (max 36 mg) in 3 divided doses.

Preparations

Tablet (2 mg and 4 mg) may be crushed and mixed with water.

Contraindications

Severe hepatic or renal impairment.

Important interactions and unwanted effects

Interacts with ciprofloxacin and phenytoin. Dry mouth, sleepiness, or light-headedness, GI haemorrhage. Can prolong QT interval.

Topiramate

Neurological indications

Broad-spectrum ASM. Migraine prophylaxis.

Dosing

Starting doses and escalation regimen

- PO (2–17 yrs): 0.5–1 mg/kg/day (max. 25 mg/dose) increasing by 1 mg/kg/day (max. 50 mg/day) divided in 2 doses every 1–2 weeks.

Maintenance doses
- Epilepsy. PO: 5–10 mg/kg/day (occasionally up to 15 mg/kg/day) in two divided doses. Adult max. 400 mg/day.
- Migraine prophylaxis. PO: 50–100 mg/day.

Preparations

Tablet (25 mg, 50 mg, 100 mg, 200 mg). Sprinkle capsule (15 mg, 25 mg, 50 mg). Oral suspension (50 mg/5 mL, 100 mg/5 mL). Tablets can be crushed and dispersed in water. A crushed-tablet suspension (e.g. 10 mg/mL) can be given rectally for short periods if oral administration is not possible (see Parenteral maintenance of antiseizure medications in Chapter 5 ➲ p. 549).

Contraindications

Narrow or closed angle glaucoma.

Important interactions and unwanted effects

Nausea, anorexia with weight loss, paraesthesiae. Somnolence and cognitive impairment. Renal stones in 5%.

Comments

Adverse effects are less common with slower introduction.

For interactions between antiseizure medicines, see this chapter ➲ p. 709.

Topiramate use in pregnancy has been associated with dose-dependent increased rates of congenital malformation. Its use in female patients should only be after informed discussion of risks (see Contraception and reproductive health in Chapter 4 ➲ p. 320).

Trihexyphenidyl

Neurological indications

Dystonia and extrapyramidal movement disorders.

Dosing

Starting doses and escalation regimen
- PO (3 months–18 yrs): 1–2 mg/day divided in 1–2 doses, increase by 1 mg/day every 3–7 days, divided in 3–4 doses according to response.

Maintenance doses
- PO (3 months to 18 yrs): 5–10 mg/day, max. 2 mg/kg/day (adult max. 20 mg/day) in 3–4 divided doses.

Preparations

Tablet (2 mg, 5 mg) disintegrates rapidly in water. Oral solution (5 mg/5 mL).

Contraindications

Intestinal obstruction, urinary retention, closed angle glaucoma, myasthenia gravis.

Important interactions and unwanted effects

Urinary retention, constipation, tachycardia, anhidrosis (and hyperpyrexia), dry mouth, blurred vision, confusion, agitation, hallucination.

Comments

Previously known as benzhexol. Gradual dose escalation allows toleration of comparatively high doses.

Ubiquinone

See co-enzyme Q10 in this chapter ➲ p. 664.

Valproate

Neurological indications

Broad-spectrum ASM. Migraine prophylaxis, mood-stabilizer (e.g. in bipolar disorder). Treatment of (particularly non-convulsive) status epilepticus.

Dosing

Starting doses and escalation regimen
- Epilepsy and migraine. PO/PR: Neonates: 20 mg/kg/day. >1months: 10 mg/kg/day. >12 yrs: 600 mg/day divided in 2 doses increasing by 10 mg/kg/day (>12 yrs 200 mg/day) every 5–7 days.
- Non-convulsive status epilepticus. 10 mg/kg IV loading dose over 30 min then 30–40 mg/kg/day continuous IV infusion for 24–48 h (max 2.5 g/day).

Maintenance doses
- PO/IV/PR: 20–40 mg/kg/day divided in 2 doses, max 60 mg/day (adult 1–2 g/day, occasionally 2.5 g/day).

Preparations

Crushable tablet (100 mg). Enteric-coated tablet (200 mg, 500 mg). Controlled-release tablet (200 mg, 300 mg, 500 mg). Oral solution (200 mg/5 mL). Intravenous injection (100 mg/mL). Modified-release granules (50 mg, 100 mg, 250 mg, 500 mg, 750 mg, 1 g). Modified-release capsules (150 mg, 300 mg).

Contraindications

Active liver disease or family history of severe liver disease. Known or suspected Alpers syndrome. Porphyria. Pregnancy.

Important interactions and unwanted effects

- Valproate is a known teratogen causing a distinct fetal valproate syndrome and/or neural tube defects, and adverse developmental outcomes in babies exposed *in utero*. **Valproate should not be prescribed to young women of reproductive age** unless absolutely necessary and only after completion of an annually renewed risk assessment (see Contraception and reproductive health in Chapter 4 ❷ p. 320). In the UK, MHRA guidance (2023) states valproate must not be started in new patients (male or female) younger than 55 years, unless two specialists independently consider and document that there is no other effective or tolerated treatment, or there are compelling reasons that the reproductive risks do not apply.

- Transient thinning of the hair; hair invariably re-grows and this is rarely a reason to stop the drug. Weight gain. Gastric irritation (usually helped by enteric-coated preparation). Thrombocytopenia (tends to be dose-related).

- Valproate-induced Fanconi syndrome (proximal renal tubular dysfunction) results in glycosuria (without hyperglycaemia), subsequent osmotic diuresis and dehydration, proteinuria, electrolyte disturbances, hypophosphatasia, and in severe cases osteomalacia and fractures.

- Impaired hepatic function leading rarely to fatal hepatic failure (some cases likely to be due to unidentified beta-oxidation or mitochondrial depletion (Alpers) syndromes: avoid use if mitochondrial disease suspected).

Comments

Routine monitoring of liver function in an asymptomatic child is not indicated. Carers should be taught to seek medical attention in case of unexplained nausea, vomiting, darkened urine, or jaundice. For interactions between antiseizure medicines, see this chapter ❷ p. 709.

Vigabatrin

Neurological indications

Treatment of infantile spasms particularly in tuberous sclerosis. Adjunctive treatment of severe epilepsies. May worsen generalized tonic–clonic, absence, and myoclonic seizures.

Dosing

Starting doses and escalation regimen
- Infantile spasms. PO: 50 mg/kg/day increasing if required every 48 h to 100 mg/kg/day and then 150 mg/kg/day divided in 2 doses.

Maintenance doses
- Infantile spasms. PO: Up to 150 mg/kg/day (max 3 g/day).

Discontinuation regimen
- Infantile spasms. Withdraw slowly e.g. by 20% per month.

Preparations

Tablet (500 mg). Soluble tablet (100 mg, 500 mg). Powder (500 mg). Powder can be dispersed in 10 mL of water and the appropriate volume used to give small doses. Tablets can be crushed and dispersed in water or squash. Sachets can be administered rectally.

Contraindications

Pre-existing or potential for visual impairment (particularly visual field impairments).

Important interactions and unwanted effects

Visual field defects: occur in 30–50% of adults on drug for more than 1–2 yrs. Often small and asymptomatic; however, they may be significant and are *irreversible*. Unable to monitor in children with developmental age <8yrs. Consequent desire to limit duration of use of vigabatrin in treatment of infantile spasms where possible.

Reversible basal ganglia changes (in 20–30%) ± reversible encephalopathy.

Zonisamide

Neurological indications

Broad-spectrum ASM.

Dosing

Starting doses and escalation regimen
- PO (>6 yrs): 1 mg/kg/day increasing by 1 mg/kg/day divided in 2 doses every 1–2 weeks.

Maintenance doses
- PO (>6 yrs): 8 mg/kg/day (very occasionally up to 30 mg/kg/day) divided in 2 doses. Adult max. 500 mg/day.

Preparations

Capsules (25 mg, 50 mg, 100 mg). Oral solution (20 mg/mL).

Important interactions and unwanted effects

Somnolence, poor concentration. More rarely nephrolithiasis, (encourage to report back/abdominal pain or urinary symptoms), Stevens–Johnson syndrome, agranulocytosis, oligohydrosis, and hyperthermia (beware in small children). Teratogenesis (risk in teenage pregnancy).

Acute sedation protocols

NICE guidelines ('Sedation in under 19s: using sedation for diagnostic and therapeutic procedures', NICE guideline CG112 December 2010) emphasize that adequate monitoring of sedation in children, by staff with appropriate training and expertise, is much more important to the procedure's success and safety than the specifics of drugs, doses, and routes.

All children should have iv access established prior to sedation.

Painless procedure lasting <60 min (e.g. MRI)

Infant <4 months
Feed and swaddle.

Child <5 yrs
Chloral hydrate 50 mg/kg (max. 1 g) po 60 min before scan + melatonin 5 mg po just prior.

Child >5 yrs
Consider decision to attempt scan under oral sedation carefully. General anaesthesia is usually more satisfactory (avoiding movement artefacts in images) and always safer. A child with a developmental age of 9 or above can usually manage an awake MRI with parental encouragement although there will be exceptions. If necessary, between 5 and 7 yrs chloral hydrate 75 mg/kg (max. 2 g) po 60 min before scan + melatonin 5 mg po just prior to procedure may be tried, though paradoxical agitation is sometimes seen.

Risks of adverse events rise rapidly with attempts to 'top up' failed sedations and *should not be attempted*: re-book a study under GA.

Anxiolysis before distressing procedures
- Midazolam 0.025–0.05 mg/kg iv 5 min before procedure; *or*
- Midazolam 0.3 mg/kg (max 10mg) buccally 15 min before procedure.

Note midazolam has no analgesic properties. Child will be amnestic but may still move!

If procedure is painful as well as anxiety-provoking (e.g. LP, NCV) consider 0.3 mg/kg buccal midazolam + morphine 0.1 mg/kg orally. Nitrous oxide can also be very effective for older, cooperative children but requires nursing staff to be trained in its administration.

Interactions of antiseizure medicines

- Enzyme-inducing drugs such as carbamazepine, oxcarbazepine, eslicarbazepine, phenobarbital, phenytoin, and topiramate may *lower* plasma concentrations of clobazam, clonazepam, lamotrigine, perampanel; active metabolites of oxcarbazepine, phenytoin, tiagabine, topiramate, and valproate; and at times ethosuximide and zonisamide.
- Protein binding is often competitive so oxcarbazepine, eslicarbazepine, etc may *raise* the plasma concentration of phenytoin.
- Lamotrigine is reported to sometimes *raise* the plasma concentration of carbamazepine and phenytoin, making unwanted effects more likely.
- Valproate *raises* the plasma concentration of the active metabolite of carbamazepine, lamotrigine, phenobarbital, and phenytoin.
- Vigabatrin *lowers* the concentration of phenytoin and at times phenobarbital.
- Cannabidiol and clobazam mutually *increase* levels of metabolites: clobazam doses are typically reduced.
- Acetazolamide *raises* levels of carbamazepine (although it would be unusual to use these together).
- Gabapentin and levetiracetam are not reported to have interactions.
- Oral contraceptives may *lower* the concentrations of enzyme-inducing drugs which may in turn lower the concentration of the oral contraceptive. Alternative contraceptive options may need to be considered: see Contraception and reproductive health in Chapter 4 ⮕ p. 320.

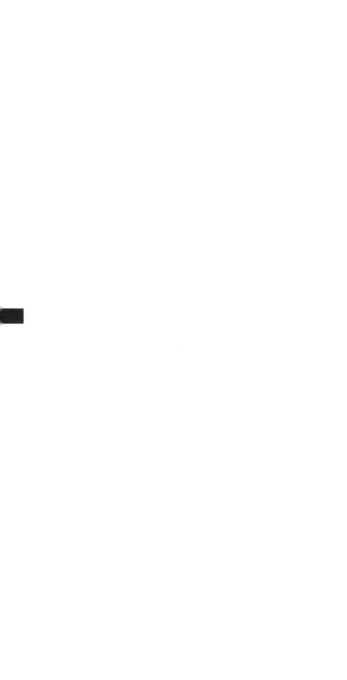

Index

For the benefit of digital users, indexed terms that span two pages (e.g., 52–53) may, on occasion, appear on only one of those pages.
Note: Tables, figures, and boxes are indicated by an italic *t*, *f*, and *b* following the page number.